Non-Obstetric Surgery During Pregnancy

Ceana H. Nezhat
Editor

Michael S. Kavic
Raymond J. Lanzafame
Michael K. Lindsay • Travis M. Polk
Associate Editors

Non-Obstetric Surgery During Pregnancy

A Comprehensive Guide

Springer

Editor
Ceana H. Nezhat
Nezhat Medical Center
Atlanta, GA
USA

Minimally Invasive Surgery and
Robotics Northside Hospital
Atlanta, GA
USA

Department of Gynecology and Obstetrics
Emory University
Atlanta, GA
USA

Associate Editors
Michael S. Kavic
Department of Surgery
Northeast Ohio Medical University
Youngstown, OH
USA

Raymond J. Lanzafame
School of Dental Medicine
State University of New York at Buffalo
Buffalo, NY
USA

Society of Laparoendoscopic Surgeons
Rochester, NY
USA

Michael K. Lindsay
Department of Gynecology and
Obstetrics
Emory University
Atlanta, GA
USA

Travis M. Polk
Division of Trauma and Surgical Critical
Care
LAC+USC Medical Center
Keck School of Medicine
University of Southern California
Los Angeles, CA
USA

ISBN 978-3-030-08090-7 ISBN 978-3-319-90752-9 (eBook)
https://doi.org/10.1007/978-3-319-90752-9

Printed on acid-free paper

This Springer imprint is published by the registered company Springer Nature Switzerland AG
The registered company address is: Gewerbestrasse 11, 6330 Cham, Switzerland

To the mother and twins whose story planted the first seed of this project years ago and to all mothers and infants worldwide, past, present, and future.

Foreword I

"She's Pregnant"

No two words create more doubt, angst, and heartburn for a surgical consultant.
Every surgeon has been there. After hearing about a case from an ER doctor or a trainee and formulating a mental model and plan, the conversation closes with "by the way, she's pregnant."

Suddenly a twinge, perhaps a jolt, or maybe even a cold sweat ensues. The consultant surgeon's mind kicks into overdrive churn. The clinical problem and solution, previously obvious, is now in question! There is an agonizing reappraisal. Do the fundamental principles of care for a general surgical or specialty surgical problem remain valid, or do they "go out the window"? Now every intervention holds the possibility of a 200% morbidity or 200% mortality.

While concurrent surgical disease arises infrequently during pregnancy, pregnancy is common. Thus, this is a nontrivial problem, usually arising at the worst possible time.

"What to Do?"

Enter Nezhat's volume *Non-obstetric Surgery During Pregnancy: A Comprehensive Guide*. More than just a "how to do cookbook" this book provides a rational framework of thinking about the health of both the fetus and the pregnant mother. Dr. Nezhat brings three decades of deep experience and expertise in obstetrics and gynecology to us all in this superb book. Ceana is recognized as a leading authority and he does not disappoint.

In crisp clean sequence, the fundamental groundwork is laid; preferred imaging strategies, anesthesia considerations, and OR setup are wonderfully outlined. Subsequent sections target general surgical and specialty surgical conditions often arising during pregnancy. Each, in turn, is methodically covered. Treatment options, risks, and benefits are all carefully and thoroughly described. Finally, gynecological conditions, obstetric complications, and in utero operative approaches to spinal bifida round out this exceptional book.

Forearmed with the knowledge gained from this book, the general surgeon or the specialty surgeon will no longer quake when they hear the words, "She's pregnant!"

Thomas M. Krummel
Stanford Byers Center for Biodesign
Stanford University
Stanford, CA
USA

Foreword II

I congratulate Dr. Ceana H. Nezhat and his associate editors Drs. Michael S.Kavic, Raymond J. Lanzafame, Michael K. Lindsay, and Travis M. Polk on highlighting the much ignored topic of non-obstetrical surgery during pregnancy. In addition to the surgical procedures themselves, it is imperative the surgeon is knowledgeable about the pathophysiology of pregnancy and its impact on both the mother and fetus. Hypertension and diabetes during pregnancy can result in increased morbidity and mortality when compared to women who are not pregnant. A 50% increase in blood volume, as well as changes in renal function, can impact the procedures being performed. This book provides the reader with an in-depth knowledge of surgical procedures and anesthesia challenges in the gravid patient. Procedures reviewed range from establishing a pneumoperitoneum in pregnancy to exploratory laparotomy.

Abdominal surgery is presently the most common surgical procedure for the pregnant patient. Unfortunately, even if done by the most experienced surgeon, the procedure can result in a miscarriage and loss of pregnancy. The authors recommend surgical procedures be delayed when possible and elective procedures avoided until completion of the pregnancy. However, there are many conditions that require emergent surgery, such as appendicitis. The authors have provided their readers with a road map to perform these procedures. The ultimate goal is to protect both the mother and the unborn fetus.

This book provides an evaluative review of the surgical management of urgent and emergent procedures during pregnancy as well as a thorough analysis of gynecologic surgery and the surgical management of obstetrical complications. This comprehensive guide is a must-read not only for obstetrician gynecologists but also for any clinician involved in the management of a pregnant patient.

Dr. Nezhat has brought together both national and international experts to contribute their years of experience for this book. It is through knowledge we will be able to decrease the unacceptable morbidity and mortality of the pregnant and postpartum patient observed throughout the world today.

Ira R. Horowitz
Department of Gynecology and Obstetrics
Emory University School of Medicine
Atlanta, GA
USA

Emory Clinic, Atlanta, GA
USA

Emory Healthcare, Atlanta, GA
USA

Emory University School of Medicine
Atlanta, GA
USA

Preface

Non-obstetrics Surgery During Pregnancy: A Comprehensive Guide was conceptualized from an identified gap in education and fills a major void as one of a few texts which provides a comprehensive evidence-based approach to the management of major non-obstetric surgical procedures. Surgery for non-obstetric causes during pregnancy is not uncommon and a timely topic. The book is written in "cookbook style" and geared towards most specialties. It is my intention that this book provides a compendium that will assist clinicians by guiding their management of pregnant patients and hopefully improving outcomes for both mother and baby.

The text flows logically with introductory chapters, such as history of laparoscopy, instrumentation, room setup, and patient positioning, laying the groundwork for performing non-obstetric surgery in a pregnant patient. Moreover, there will be individual chapters covering various specialties and detailing surgical complications that may arise specific to each field. The book concludes with an overview of various obstetrics-related complications that require surgical management. I trust the readers will find this to be a useful, well-rounded, and educative resource.

Ideally, every child is "well-born," physically, mentally, and emotionally which is fundamental to human dignity. The contributors to this book represent the vanguard in their respective specialties. They highlight critical factors for consideration while caring for the pregnant woman and her unborn child, aspiring to build human dignity one birth at a time. I greatly appreciate the editorial assistance/review provided by my associate editors whose extensive experience in varying disciplines brought expert-level evaluation to the review process. Special thanks to Ms. Sarah Kyle McClellan, MPH, who contributed greatly to the review process and preparation of the book. We are very proud of the depth of information we are providing to our readers owing to the knowledge and experience of our contributors.

Atlanta, GA, USA — Ceana H. Nezhat
Youngstown, OH, USA — Michael S. Kavic
Rochester, NY, USA — Raymond J. Lanzafame
Atlanta, GA, USA — Michael K. Lindsay
Los Angeles, CA, USA — Travis M. Polk

Contents

Contributors

Farshad Adib, MD Department of Orthopaedics, University of Maryland Medical Center, Baltimore, MD, USA

Ali Akdemir, MD Department of Obstetrics and Gynecology, Ege University Hospital, Bornova, İzmir, Turkey

Wayne L. Ambroze Jr, MD Department of Surgery, Northside Hospital, Atlanta, GA, USA

Ali Amiri, BS in Biomedical Engineering Marketing Research and Product Development, KARL STORZ Endoscopy-America, Inc., El Segundo, CA, USA

Sabahattin Anıl Arı, MD Department of Obstetrics and Gynecology, Ege University Hospital, Bornova, İzmir, Turkey

Shahrokh C. Bagheri, DMD, MD, FACS, FICD Department of Surgery, Northside Hospital, Georgia Oral and Facial Surgery, Atlanta, GA, USA

Sudheer Balakrishnan, BS, MS, MD Department of Radiology, University of Southern California, LAC-USC, Los Angeles, CA, USA

James M. Bardes, MD Department of Trauma and Acute Care Surgery, LAC+USC Medical Center, Los Angeles, CA, USA

Vicki Barnett, RN, MSN, CNOR Surgical Services, Northside Hospital, Atlanta, GA, USA

Ashley N. Bartalot, MD Department of Obstetrics and Gynecology, New York Presbyterian Brooklyn Methodist Hospital, Brooklyn, NY, USA

Benedict B. Benigno, MD Ovarian Cancer Institute, Northside Hospital, Atlanta, GA, USA

Gynecologic-Oncology, Northside Hospital, Atlanta, GA, USA

Behnam Bohluli, DMD, OMFS Deaprtment of Oral and Maxillofacial Surgery, University of Toronto, Toronto, ON, Canada

Jason H. Boulter, MD Department of Neurosurgery, Walter Reed National Military Medical Center-Bethesda, Bethesda, MD, USA

Megan Kennedy Burns, MD, MA Stanford Medical Center, Palo Alto, CA, USA

Frank Van Calenbergh, MD, PhD Department of Neurosurgery, University Hospitals Leuven, Campus Gasthuisberg, Leuven, Belgium

Laura Cancelliere, BHsc, MD Faculty of Medicine, Department of Obstetrics and Gynecology, University of Toronto, Toronto, ON, Canada

Luc De Catte, MD, PhD Department of Obstetrics and Gynaecology, University Hospitals Leuven, Campus Gasthuisberg, Leuven, Belgium

Bradley Paul Champagne, MD Department of Surgery, Our Lady of Lourdes Regional Medical Center, Lafayette, LA, USA

Ramen H. Chmait, MD The USFetus Research Consortium, Miami, FL, USA

Department of Obstetrics and Gynecology, Keck School of Medicine, University of Southern California, Los Angeles, CA, USA

Jan Deprest, MD, PhD, FRCOG Department of Obstetrics and Gynaecology, University Hospitals Leuven, Campus Gasthuisberg, Leuven, Belgium

Roland Devlieger, MD, PhD Department of Obstetrics and Gynaecology, University Hospitals Leuven, Campus Gasthuisberg, Leuven, Belgium

Sarah Devroe, MD Department of Anesthesiology, University Hospitals Leuven, Campus Gasthuisberg, Leuven, Belgium

Tracey DeYoung, MD Department of Women's Health, Naval Medical Center Portsmouth, Norfolk, VA, USA

Amelia Donlan, BS Athens, GA, USA

Angela L. Du, MD Department of Obstetrics, Gynecology and Reproductive Sciences, Magee-Womens Hospital of UPMC, Pittsburgh, PA, USA

Pooyan Sadr-Eshkevari, DDS Department of Oral and Maxillofacial Surgery, University of Louisville, Louisville, KY, USA

Laura Fluke, DO Department of General Surgery, Naval Medical Center Portsmouth, Portsmouth, VA, USA

Sandro Gerli, MD, PhD Clinic for Gynecology and Obstetrics, Clinical Centre of Serbia, Belgrade, Serbia

Laura E. Gilbertson, MD Division of Pediatric Anesthesiology, Emory University, Atlanta, GA, USA

Jonathan E. Gilhooly, MD Department of Neurosurgery, Walter Reed National Military Medical Center-Bethesda, Bethesda, MD, USA

Harcharan Gill, MD Department of Urology, Stanford University School of Medicine, Stanford, CA, USA

Daniel Grabo, MD Department of Surgery, West Virginia University, Morgantown, WV, USA

Joy A. Greer, MD, CDR, MC, USN Department of Women's Health, Naval Medical Center Portsmouth, Norfolk, VA, USA

Shabnam Gupta, MD Department of Gynecology and Obstetrics, Emory University Hospital Midtown, Atlanta, GA, USA

Tracy Nicole Hadnott, MD Division of Reproductive Endocrinology and Infertility, Department of Reproductive Medicine, University of California, San Diego, La Jolla, CA, USA

Ivy N. Haskins, MD Department of Digestive Disease and Surgical Institute, Cleveland Clinic Foundation, Cleveland, OH, USA

Michael S. Jacobson, MD Georgia Retina, Tucker, GA, USA

Northside Hospital, Atlanta, GA, USA

Georgia Retina Surgery Center, LLC, Atlanta, GA, USA

Dekalb Medical Center, Decatur, GA, USA

Luc Joyeux, MD, MSc Department of Development and Regeneration, Cluster Woman and Child, Katholieke Universiteit Leuven, Leuven, Belgium

Sasa Kadija, MD, PhD Clinic for Gynecology and Obstetrics, Clinical Centre of Serbia, Belgrade, Serbia

Christine M. Kariya, MD Department of Surgery, University of Maryland Medical Center, Baltimore, MD, USA

Stephen M. Kavic, MD Department of Surgery, University of Maryland School of Medicine, Baltimore, MD, USA

Natalie Kessler, BSc Sandy Springs, GA, USA

Eftichia V. Kontopoulos, MD, PhD The Fetal Institute, Miami, FL, USA
The USFetus Research Consortium, Miami, FL, USA

Iris Krishna, MD, MPH Division of Maternal-Fetal Medicine, Department of Gynecology and Obstetrics, Emory University Hospital Midtown, Atlanta, GA, USA

Raymond J. Lanzafame, MD, MBA, FACS School of Dental Medicine, State University of New York at Buffalo, Buffalo, NY, USA

Society of Laparoendoscopic Surgeons, Miami, FL, USA

Nucelio L. B. M. Lemos, MD, PhD Department of Obstetrics and Gynecology, Pelvic Functional Surgery and Neuropelveology Clinic, Mount Sinai Hospital and Women's College Hospital, Toronto, ON, Canada

Pelvic Neurodysfunctions Division, Department of Gynecology, Federal University of São Paulo, São Paulo, SP, Brazil

Liesbeth Lewi, MD, PhD Department of Obstetrics and Gynaecology, University Hospitals Leuven, Campus Gasthuisberg, Leuven, Belgium

Adrienne L. K. Li, MD, FRCSC Department of Obstetrics and Gynecology, Mount Sinai Hospital, Toronto, ON, Canada

Grant C. Lynde, MD, MBA Department of Anesthesiology, Practice and Process Improvement, Emory University, Atlanta, GA, USA

Antonio Malvasi Laboratory of Human Physiology, Phystech BioMed School, Faculty of Biological and Medical Physics, Moscow Institute of Physics and Technology (State University), Moscow Region, Russia

Department of Obstetrics and Gynecology, Santa Maria Hospital GVM Care and Research, Bari, Italy

Roger A. Meyer, DDS, MD, MS, FACS Northside Hospital, Atlanta, GA, USA

Baharak Moshiree, MD, MS-CI Department of Gastroenterology, Carolinas Healthcare System, Charlotte, NC, USA

Ospan A. Mynbaev, MD, MSc, MedPharm, PhD, ScD Laboratory of Human Physiology, Phystech BioMed School, Faculty of Biological and Medical Physics, Moscow Institute of Physics and Technology (State University), Moscow Region, Russia

Division of Molecular Technologies, Research Institute of Translational Medicine, N.I. Pirogov Russian National Research Medical University, Moscow, Russia

Institute of Numerical Mathematics, RAS, Moscow, Russia

Chris J. Neal, MD Department of Neurosurgery, Walter Reed National Military Medical Center-Bethesda, Bethesda, MD, USA

Uniformed Services University of the Health Sciences, Bethesda, MD, USA

Michael Franklin Neblett II, MD Department of Gynecology and Obstetrics, Emory University Hospital Midtown, Atlanta, GA, USA

Camran Nezhat, MD Stanford Medical Center, Palo Alto, CA, USA

University of California, San Francisco, San Francisco, CA, USA

Ceana H. Nezhat, MD Nezhat Medical Center, Atlanta, GA, USA

Minimally Invasive Surgery and Robotics, Northside Hospital, Atlanta, GA, USA

Department of Gynecology and Obstetrics, Emory University, Atlanta, GA, USA

Farr Nezhat, MD, FACOG, FACS Department of Obstetrics and Gynecology, Weill Cornell Medical College of Cornell University, New York, NY, USA

Hakan Orbay, MD, PhD Department of Surgery, University of Maryland Medical Center, Baltimore, MD, USA

Douglas E. Ott, MD, MBA Biomedical Engineering, Mercer University, Macon, GA, USA

William Parker, MD Department of Ob Gyn and Reproductive Sciences, UC San Diego, La Jolla, CA, USA

Travis M. Polk, MD, FACS Division of Trauma and Surgical Critical Care, LAC+USC Medical Center, Keck School of Medicine, University of Southern California, Los Angeles, CA, USA

Rubén A. Quintero, MD The Fetal Institute, Miami, FL, USA

The USFetus Research Consortium, Miami, FL, USA

Atoosa Rabiee, MD Washington DC VA Medical Center, Washington, MD, USA

Meredith Redden, MD Northside Hospital, Atlanta, GA, USA

Michael J. Rosen, MD Department of Digestive Disease and Surgical Institute, Cleveland Clinic Foundation, Cleveland, OH, USA

Joseph S. Sanfilippo, MD, MBA Department of Obstetrics, Gynecology and Reproductive Sciences, Magee-Womens Hospital of UPMC, Pittsburgh, PA, USA

Morgan Schellenberg, MD, MPH Division of Trauma and Surgical Critical Care, LAC+USC Medical Center, University of Southern California, Los Angeles, CA, USA

Marion Schertzer, MD Department of Colon and Rectal Surgery, Northside Hospital, Atlanta, GA, USA

Fatih Sendag, MD Department of Obstetrics and Gynecology, Ege University Hospital, Bornova, İzmir, Turkey

Corey Sermer, BMSc, MSc Department of Obstetrics and Gynecology, Mount Sinai Hospital, Toronto, ON, Canada

Milad Sharifpour, MD, MS Department of Anesthesiology and Critical Care, Emory University Hospital, Atlanta, GA, USA

Michal Rosen Shaubi, MD Department of Obstetrics and Gynecology, Mount Sinai Hospital, Toronto, ON, Canada

Radmila Sparic, MD Clinic for Gynecology and Obstetrics, Clinical Centre of Serbia, Belgrade, Serbia

Medical Faculty, University of Belgrade, Belgrade, Serbia

Michael Stark, MD New European Surgical Academy, Berlin, Germany

Nicholas S. Szuflita, MD, MPH Department of Neurosurgery, Walter Reed National Military Medical Center-Bethesda, Bethesda, MD, USA

Meaghan E. Tenney, MD University Gynecologic Oncology, Northside Hospital, Atlanta, GA, USA

Andrea Tinelli Department of Obstetrics and Gynecology, Division of Experimental Endoscopic Surgery, Imaging, Technology and Minimally Invasive Therapy, Vito Fazzi Hospital, Lecce, Italy

Laboratory of Human Physiology, Phystech BioMed School, Faculty of Biological and Medical Physics, Moscow Institute of Physics and Technology (State University), Moscow Region, Russia

Mehmet Cihat Unlu, MD Department of Obstetrics and Gynecology, Bakirkoy Hospital, Acibadem University, Istanbul, Turkey

Hannes Van der Merwe, MD Department of Development and Regeneration, Cluster Woman and Child, Katholieke Universiteit Leuven, Leuven, Belgium

Nancy N. Wang, MD, MPH Department of Urology, Stanford University School of Medicine, Stanford, CA, USA

Pengfei Wang, MD, PhD Department of Obstetrics and Gynecology, NYU-Winthrop Hospital, Mineola, NY, USA

Annie Weber, MD Department of Orthopaedics, University of Maryland Medical Center, Baltimore, MD, USA

Julie Yetso, MPAS, PA-C Department of Orthopaedics, University of Maryland Medical Center, Baltimore, MD, USA

Gazi Yildirim, MD Department of Obstetrics and Gynecology, Yeditepe University Hospital, Istanbul, Turkey

Stacy Young, MD Stanford Medical Center, Palo Alto, CA, USA

Cici Zhang, MD Department of Colon and Rectal Surgery, Northside Hospital, Atlanta, GA, USA

Introduction

As I reflect upon the days when I delivered babies, I recall hearing the much-awaited cry of the newborn filling the room with joy and a sense of relief. It was one of the most rewarding moments of my career. Months of caring for both mother and her unborn child had finally come to fruition. During my last call as a chief resident in obstetrics, I was called on a code for an antepartum mother in cardiac arrest around 30 weeks twin gestation in preterm labor on tocolysis. When I arrived, Emergency Medical Services (EMS) announced unsuccessful resuscitation attempts on the mother. I proceeded with emergency bedside cesarean delivery of the twins in seconds. Following delivery, the mother responded to resuscitation and all survived. What I did not know at the time was this event would stay with me throughout my career and one day blossom into the idea for a comprehensive guide on maternal obstetric and non-obstetric complications for all physicians caring for a pregnant mother.

Obstetrics is a multifaceted specialty relating closely to other branches in medicine. Since pregnant and nonpregnant women are subject to the same diseases, physicians must be well versed with surrounding various ailments. Extensive knowledge of pregnancy physiology and pathophysiology of obstetric disorders must then be applied, improving perinatal outcome.

Fetal and infant safety and survival have taken priority over maternal health and well-being during pregnancy. Neonatal wards today are staffed by highly trained specialists who are ready for the worst in regard to infants, while mothers are tended to by nurses and doctors who expect the best and are unprepared when complications arise. Research has shown that pregnant women who undergo non-obstetric surgery have a higher risk of postoperative septicemia, pneumonia, and urinary tract infections (UTIs). They are also at an approximate fourfold higher risk of in-hospital mortality following non-obstetric surgery compared with nonpregnant patients [1]. The lack of education provided to doctors, nurses, and other health care professionals regarding maternal health in pregnancy demonstrates the absence of risk the modern world associates with childbearing.

Historically, pregnancy has been a time of joy and apprehension. During the Renaissance, women would write out their wills as soon as they became pregnant [2]. History is, in fact, full of maternal death. Thomas Jefferson lost his wife after childbirth in 1782. Princess Charlotte of Wales, granddaughter of King George III and cousin to Queen Victoria, died after giving birth to a stillborn in 1817. Charlotte Bronte died of hyperemesis gravidarum in 1855.

In the seventeenth century, childbirth predominantly took place in the home in the presence of a midwife and a group of *female* friends, neighbors, and family members [3]. However, in France, the "man-midwife" was becoming more accepted [4], and in Britain, the Chamberlen family had developed obstetrical forceps, which would be kept a secret for more than 100 years [3, 5].

Early on, successful cesarean sections typically occurred in remote rural areas without access to adequate medical care or hospitals. The first record of a successful cesarean section was performed by a "sow gelder" in Switzerland in 1500. Not only did both mother and baby survive, but fertility was preserved and the woman went on to conceive and deliver five more children naturally [3, 4]. Cesarean section can be traced back to ancient times in both Western and non-Western cultures. The initial purpose of cesarean section was to retrieve the infant from a dead or dying mother, either in an attempt to save the baby or for religious purposes. Regardless, it was a measure of last resort and the mother was not expected to survive.

There are several possible explanations as to why operations in remote rural areas yielded more successful outcomes; first, with the absence of professional care, cesarean sections were executed without delay in earlier stages of labor in stronger women and less distressed fetuses, resulting in greater chances of success; and second, hospitals were riddled with infections spreading between patients by the unclean hands of the medical staff. In rural areas, cesarean sections were performed in people's homes, which were less contaminated with sickness and disease. However, it was urbanization and the growth of hospitals when cesarean sections became largely accepted and regularly performed [3].

Today, the average global rate of cesarean section is 18.6%. Latin America and the Caribbean report the highest rate of births by cesarean section (40.5%), followed by North America (32.3%), Oceania (31.1%), Europe (25.0%), Asia (19.2%), and Africa (7.3%) [6]. In 2015, the World Health Organization (WHO) released a statement on cesarean section rates. They concluded that cesarean sections are effective in saving maternal and infant lives, but only when medically necessary, as they can cause significant and sometimes permanent complications. WHO further reported, at population level, that cesarean section rates higher than 10% have no association with further reductions in maternal or newborn mortality rates [7].

Advancing knowledge and development of anesthesia opened doors for obstetrics. Opium and its derivatives, including laudanum, morphine, and heroin, are the oldest method of pain relief and have been used in childbirth for thousands of years. In the nineteenth century, chloroform was popular owing to the support of several prominent women: Frances Longfellow, wife of the American poet Henry Wadsworth Longfellow; Emma Darwin, wife of Charles Darwin; and Queen Victoria, who was given chloroform by Dr. John Snow during the births of her eighth and ninth children [2, 8–10]. Today, anesthesiologists know the physiological effects anesthesia have on developing fetuses and should be consulted before any surgery is performed on a pregnant patient.

Maternal mortality ratio (MMR) is defined as pregnancy-related deaths per 100,000 live births. In 2015, the estimated global MMR was 216 (80%

uncertainty interval (UI) 207–249) showing roughly a 44% drop over the past 25 years; the MMR in 1991 was 385 (80% UI 359–427) [11]. Trends for maternal mortality mirror those for many other health statistics; developing regions accounted for approximately 99% of the global maternal deaths in 2015. WHO Sustainable Development Goals (SDGs) explain, "Drivers of success in reducing maternal mortality range from making improvements at the provider and health system level to implementing interventions aimed at reducing social and structural barriers" [11]. According to data collected by WHO and its partners, the United States is one of only 11 countries worldwide and the only developed country to have experienced a negative (−16.7%) change in MMR between 1990 and 2015 [11]. A study published in *Lancet* (2016) systematically compiled and processed all available data sources from 186 of 195 countries and territories. Researchers reported a 56% rise in MMR in the United States between 1990 (MMR = 16.9 [95% UI 16.2–17.8]) and 2015 (MMR = 26.4 [95% UI 24.6–28.4]) [12]. The reason behind this unexpected increase in maternal mortality in the United States is unclear. Possible explanations include the implementation or improvement of surveillance systems, such as the addition of pregnancy questions to state death certificates starting in 2003 [13]. MacDorman et al. estimate that 79.9% of the increase in MMR was a result of improved surveillance. Other possible explanations for the observed increase in maternal mortality could be advanced maternal age and/or the increasing number of pregnant women in the United States with a chronic disease [14]. The Centers for Disease Control and Prevention (CDC) launched its nationwide surveillance system for pregnancy-related deaths in 1986. Data released in 2017 revealed 26.5% of maternal mortality is associated with cardiovascular disease including cardiomyopathy [15]. The obesity epidemic in the United States may play a role due to increased risk for cardiovascular disease. The 2013 ACOG Committee opinion on obesity in pregnancy reported that "more than one third of women are obese, more than one half of pregnant women are overweight or obese, and 8% of reproductive-aged women are extremely obese, putting them at a greater risk of pregnancy complications" [16]. Rates of severe maternal morbidity or mortality increased from 143.2/10,000 births among women with normal body mass index (BMI) to 167.9, 178.3, and 202.9/10,000 in women with Class I, II, and III obesity, respectively [17]. Other medical noncardiovascular disease was attributed to 14.5% of maternal deaths, followed by infection and sepsis (12.7%) and hemorrhage (11.4%) [15]. One factor that could play a role, regardless, is the lack of associated risk afforded to pregnancy and childbirth in a "healthy" mother in the modern world.

Throughout a pregnancy, attention must be paid to both mother and fetus. However, this is not always the case. Poor communication between health care providers, hospital staff, and departments is a structural barrier within the health care system that can result in life-threatening situations for both mother and baby. For example, neonatal intensive care units (NICUs) and labor and delivery staff operate independently of each other. NICU nurses may come in to check on an infant and not notice the mother's elevated blood pressure. The same dynamic occurs between other departments. There is a need for physicians of all specialties to know how to handle a pregnant patient; odds are they will be confronted with such complications. If a pregnant woman comes through the emergency department with a head injury that requires immediate surgery, there is not always time to consult an obstetrician regarding the appropriate anesthesia or anesthetic to use, proper patient positioning, or appropriate postoperative instructions and warning signs.

Physicians need to stay up to date with organizational recommendations regarding antibiotic use in pregnant patients. UTI occurs in about 8% of women, most commonly during the first trimester. Some UTIs are "asymptomatic bacteriuria," which has been associated with premature birth, low birth weight, and death in newborns and developing fetuses. If a UTI goes untreated, it can spread and cause permanent maternal kidney damage. Since 2011, the American College of Obstetricians and Gynecologists (ACOG) has recommended against the use of two types of antibiotics, sulfonamides and nitrofurantoin, during the first trimester of pregnancy. In 2017, ACOG revisited its stance to add that nitrofurantoin and sulfonamides may be used in the first trimester when "no other suitable alternative antibiotics are available." Sulfonamides and nitrofurantoin have both been associated with birth defects, including brain malformations, heart defects, and cleft lips and palates [18]. However, according to a report published in January 2018 by the CDC, doctors do not seem to be following recommendations or do not know they exist [19]. In 2014, about 35% of privately insured first-trimester moms filled prescriptions for nitrofurantoin and 8% filled prescriptions for the sulfonamide antibiotic, trimethoprim-sulfamethoxazole. Since UTIs occur most commonly during the first trimester, some patients do not yet know they are pregnant. It is important for doctors to always ask patients complaining of UTI symptoms if they are sexually active and possibly pregnant before prescribing any antibiotics.

Changing trends in maternal age at first birth are of particular interest and importance to obstetricians due to the varying risks of complications and maternal outcomes in pregnancy. The CDC published a report in January 2016 [20] stating that mean age of first-time mothers increased 5.3% from 24.9 in 2000 to 26.3 in 2014. First births in women aged 30–34 rose the most (28%) from 16.5% to 21.1% followed by women aged 35+ from 7.4% to 9.1% (23%). Women aged 35+ have been found to be at greater odds of preterm delivery, hypertension, severe preeclampsia, and superimposed preeclampsia. Furthermore, analysis showed women aged ≥40 years at time of delivery were associated with increased odds of mild preeclampsia, poor fetal growth, and fetal distress [21]. The number of first births for women under 20 decreased 42% from 2000 (23.1%) to 2014 (13.4%). Women aged ≤19 years, compared to 25–29-year-old women, have elevated odds of preterm delivery, chorioamnionitis, endometritis, and mild preeclampsia. Within the same age group, women 15–19 years of age also have significantly elevated odds for severe preeclampsia, eclampsia, postpartum hemorrhage, fetal distress, and poor fetal growth [21].

Looking past external, structural, and maternal risk factors such as medical advancements, communication issues, and maternal age, undergoing non-obstetric surgery while pregnant incurs risks of its own. In a recent study by Balinskaite et al., researchers identified pregnancies where non-obstetric surgery occurred via maternity admissions using hospital administrative data. Of all recorded pregnancies, less than 1% (47,628/6,484,280) had undergone non-obstetric surgery. Abdominal surgery (any kind) (26.2%) was the most common surgical group and patients who underwent abdominal surgery were found to have a high risk of miscarriage associated with hospital admission aRR = 1.90 (95% CI 1.81–1.99) and preterm delivery aRR = 1.62 (95% CI 1.54–1.70) compared to women who did not undergo surgery while pregnant. Abdominal surgery was followed by dental (11.3%), nail-skin (10.0%), orthopedic (9.6%), ENT (6.4%), perianal (6.3%), and breast (4.0%). Further analysis found fewer than 6% of operations occurred within 1 week of the end of pregnancy. Researchers estimated that every 287 surgical operations were associated with one additional stillbirth, every 31 operations were associated with one additional preterm delivery, every 39 operations were associated with an extra-low-birth-weight baby, every 25 operations were associated with an additional cesarean section, and every 50 operations were associated with one additional long inpatient stay [22].

Trauma, appendicitis, cholecystitis, pancreatitis, and bowel obstruction are some of the major non-obstetric abdominal indications for surgical intervention during pregnancy. Approximately 7% of pregnant women will experience physical trauma during pregnancy. Trauma is the leading cause of maternal death, accounting for approximately 50% of deaths during pregnancy. Roughly 1 in 500 pregnant women require surgery and the most common non-obstetric surgical condition during pregnancy is acute appendicitis. Acute cholecystitis is the second most frequently reported non-obstetric emergency in pregnancy, with approximately 40% of acute cases requiring surgery. The incidence of acute pancreatitis in pregnancy ranges from 1 in 1066 live births to 1 in 3000 pregnancies. It appears to be more prevalent with advancing gestational age and occurs more commonly in the third trimester or during the postpartum period. Bowel obstruction, or more specifically, adhesive small bowel disease and volvulus, is the third highest cause of surgical admissions in the pregnant patient.

Elective surgery is generally avoided during pregnancy if observational and medical management are possible. Ideally, it is best to perform surgeries during the second trimester as risks from teratogenicity and preterm labor are lower. However, carefully planned non-obstetric surgeries may be performed during any trimester, if required, while still ensuring the safety of two patients, mother and fetus. Any physician contemplating surgery on a gravid patient should obtain an obstetric consultation prior to surgery, if possible, as obstetricians are uniquely qualified and familiar with the physiological changes in pregnancy and the pathophysiology of obstetric disorders [23]. A multidisciplinary team should also be present during all non-obstetric surgeries. Pathologies may present differently or inconsistently due to changes in pregnancy requiring good physician understanding of altered pelvic neuroanatomy and neurophysiologic pathways of pain to accurately diagnose and effectively manage conditions. The configuration of a safe and effective operating room, active monitoring of patient positioning throughout surgery, and adherence to appropriate protocols for prophylactic measures for peripheral neuropathy are vital components when performing non-obstetric surgery.

The aim of this book is to provide health care professionals and students with a comprehensive resource for non-obstetric surgery to better prepare for appropriate intervention and surgery, be it of a routine or emergent nature that may arise in a pregnant patient.

Ceana H. Nezhat, MD
Nezhat Medical Center, Atlanta, GA, USA

Minimally Invasive Surgery and Robotics, Northside Hospital, Atlanta, GA, USA

Department of Gynecology and Obstetrics, Emory University, Atlanta, GA, USA

References

1. Huang SY, Lo PH, Liu WM, Cherng YG, Yeh CC, Chen TL, et al. Outcomes after nonobstetric surgery in pregnancy patients: a nationwide study. Mayo Clin Proc. 2016;91(9):1166–72. doi: 10.1016/j.mayocp.2016.06.021.
2. Victoria and Albert Museum. Renaissance childbirth. 2016. [cited 2017 Nov 2]. Available from http://www.vam.ac.uk/content/articles/r/renaissance-childbirth/.
3. Sewell JE. Cesarean section—a brief history. NIH U.S. National Library of Medicine [Internet]. 1993 April 30 [cited 2017 Aug 15]. Available from https://www.nlm.nih.gov/exhibition/cesarean/index.html.
4. Drife J. The start of life: a history of obstetrics. Postgrad Med J 2002;78:311–5.
5. Dunn PM. The Chamberlen family (1560–1728) and obstetric forceps. Arch Dis Child Fetal Neonatal Ed. 1999;81:F232–5.
6. Betrán AP, Ye J, Moller A-B, Zhang J, Gülmezoglu AM, Torloni MR. The Increasing Trend in Caesarean Section Rates: Global, Regional and National Estimates: 1990–2014. PLoS ONE 2016;11(2):e0148343. doi:10.1371/journal.pone.0148343.
7. World Health Organization. WHO Statement on Caesarean section rates. Geneva: World Health Organization; 2015 (WHO/RHR/15.02).
8. Skowronski GA. Pain relief in childbirth: changing historical and feminist perspectives. Anaesth Intensive Care. 2015;43 Suppl:25–8.
9. Walzer Leavitt J. Joseph B. DeLee and the practice of preventive obstetrics. Am J Public Health. 1988;78(10):1353–1361.
10. Feldhusen AE. The history of midwifery and childbirth in America: a time line. Midwifery Today 2000.
11. World Health Organization (WHO). Trends in maternal mortality: 1990 to 2015: estimates by WHO, UNICEF, UNFPA, World Bank Group and the United Nations Population Division; 2015.
12. Kassebaum N, et al. Global, regional, and national levels of maternal mortality, 1990–2015: a systematic analysis for the Global Burden of Disease Study 2015. Lancet. 2016;388:1775-812.
13. MacDorman MF, Declercq E, Cabral H, Morton C. Recent increases in the U.S. maternal mortality rate: disentangling trends from measurement issues. Obstet Gynecol. 2016; 128(3):447-455.
14. Campbell KH, Savtiz D, Werner EF, Pettker CM, Goffman D, Chazotte C, et al. Maternal morbidity and risk of death at delivery hospitalization. Obstet Gynecol. 2013; 122(3):627–33. doi: 10.1097/AOG.0b013e3182a06f4e.
15. Creanga AA, Syverson C, Seed K, Callaghan WM. Pregnancy-related mortality in the United States, 2011–2013. Obstet and Gynecol. 2017;130(2):366–73.
16. Obesity and pregnancy. Committee Opinion No. 549. American College of Obstetricians and Gynecologists. Obstet Gynecol. 2013;121(1):213–7.

17. Lockwood CJ. A call to arms against maternal mortality. Contemporary OB/GYN. 2018;63(1):6–7.
18. Sulfonamides, nitrofurantoin, and risk of birth defects. Committee Opinion No. 717. American College of Obstetricians and Gynecologists. Obstet Gynecol. 2017;130:e150–2.
19. Ailes EC, Summers AD, Tran EL, Gilboa SM, Arnold KE, Meaney-Delman D, et al. Antibiotics dispensed to privately insured pregnant women with urinary tract infections—United States, 2014. Centers for Disease Control and Prevention (CDC) Morbidity Mortality Weekly Rep. 2018;67(1):18–21.
20. Mathews TJ, Hamilton BE. Mean age of mothers in on the rise: United States, 2000–2014. Centers for Disease Control and Prevention. 2016 Jan; NCHS Data Brief No. 232. Available from https://www.cdc.gov/nchs/data/databriefs/db232.pdf.
21. Cavazos-Rehg PA, Krauss MJ, Spitznagel EL, Bommarito K, Madden T, Olsen MA, et al. Maternal age and risk of labor and delivery complications. Matern Child Health J. 2015; 19(6):1202–1211. doi:10.1007/s10995-014-1624-7.
22. Balinskaite V, Bottle A, Sodhi V, Rivers A, Bennett PR, Brett SJ, et al. The risk of adverse pregnancy outcomes following nonobstetric surgery during pregnancy: estimates from a retrospective Cohort study of 6.5 million pregnancies. Ann Surg. 2017;266(2):260–266. doi: 10.1097/SLA.0000000000001976.
23. Gabbe SG, Niebyl JR, Simpson JL, editors. Obstetrics normal & problem pregnancies. 2nd ed. New York: Churchill Livingstone; 1991.

Part I

Laying the Groundwork

The History of Non-obstetric Endoscopic Surgery During Pregnancy

1

Megan Kennedy Burns, Stacy Young, and Camran Nezhat

History of Surgery in Pregnancy

Approximately 1 in 500 women will require non-obstetric surgery during pregnancy, but it was not until the 1970s and 1980s that researchers began looking critically at the effects of non-obstetric surgery on the pregnant mother and developing fetus [1, 2]. Surgical intervention in pregnancy, regardless of the operative approach or trimester of pregnancy, can increase the incidence of adverse pregnancy outcome, with the most serious of these complications being pregnancy loss and preterm labor [3]. Earlier studies in the 1960s demonstrated that intra-abdominal procedures were associated with a greater risk of preterm labor than extra-abdominal procedures and intra-operative cervical manipulation increased the risk even further [4, 5].

In 1989 Mazze and Kallen published a study of adverse fetal outcomes after non-obstetric surgery in pregnancy, examining the Swedish Birth Registry between 1973 and 1981 and finding no increased risk of congenital malformation or stillbirth [6]. This study showed that patients who underwent non-obstetric surgery during pregnancy had an increased risk for low birth weight (<2500 g) and very low birth weight (<1500 g) infants, due to growth restriction as well as preterm delivery. Another finding from this study was the increased rate of neonatal death within the first 7 days of life [6]. The study did not, however, differentiate between complications due to the surgical procedure and complications due to underlying pathology that necessitated surgical intervention.

Cohen-Kerem et al., in 2005, published a review of the surgical literature critically evaluating maternal and fetal outcomes following non-obstetric surgery [7]. This study revealed a miscarriage rate of 5.8% of all patients who underwent surgical intervention in pregnancy and 10.5% of patients who underwent surgical intervention in their first trimester. The rate of preterm delivery induced by the surgical procedure or the underlying pathology was 3.5% and was most prevalent in patients undergoing appendectomy, while the overall preterm delivery rate was 8.2%. A total of 2.5% of patients experienced fetal loss, and 2.0% of pregnancies were complicated by a major birth defect. Importantly, this study demonstrated that surgical intervention and general anesthesia are not major risk factors for miscarriage and do not increase the risk of major birth defects, concluding that surgical interventions

M. K. Burns · S. Young (✉)
Stanford Medical Center, Palo Alto, CA, USA
e-mail: megan.burns@camrannezhatinstitute.com; stacy.young@camrannezhatinstitute.com

C. Nezhat
Stanford Medical Center, Palo Alto, CA, USA

University of California, San Francisco, San Francisco, CA, USA
e-mail: camran.nezhat@camrannezhatinstitute.com

C. H. Nezhat (ed.), *Non-Obstetric Surgery During Pregnancy*,
https://doi.org/10.1007/978-3-319-90752-9_1

should be performed when indicated in pregnancy [7].

A later study published by Balinskaite et al. in 2017 confirmed these findings, looking at a retrospective cohort of 6.5 million pregnancies in the United Kingdom [8]. This study measured adverse outcome in attributable risk, with an AR of 0.4% for stillbirth and 2.6% for low birth weight in patients who underwent surgery compared to patients who did not, but there was no difference between patients who underwent laparoscopy and open abdominal surgery. This study also demonstrated that risks increased with increasing gestational age. Again, investigators were unable to differentiate the risk of the underlying pathology from the risk of the surgery itself, but the overall risk of adverse birth outcome in women who underwent non-obstetric surgery in pregnancy was generally low compared to women who did not, providing reassurance to both expectant mothers and the practitioners caring for them [8].

History of Laparoscopy

It was not long before the time when researchers were beginning to more critically look at the effects of non-obstetric surgery during pregnancy that Camran Nezhat was revolutionizing the world of surgery with the invention of video-assisted laparoscopy (Table 1.1) [9–11]. Prior to this development, surgeons directly visualized intra-abdominal pathology through the eyepiece of the laparoscope, requiring them to bend over the operating table [12–14] and limiting them to relatively simple procedures such as cyst drainage, lysis of adhesions, biopsies, cautery of lesions, and tubal ligations [15–18]. The invention and pioneering of video-assisted laparoscopy allowed them to stand upright and operate "off the monitor," allowing the entire operative team to visualize the surgical procedure from a television screen in the operating room. In 1985, Camran Nezhat finally reported the use of videolaparoscopy for the treatment of severe endometriosis with ureteral resection at the annual meeting of the American Society of Fertility after years of skepticism and intense criticism [19–22].

Camran Nezhat invented and pioneered the use of video-assisted endoscopy and its use for the most extensive pathology for the first time in 1979 [9–11, 19, 22]. By doing so, he revolutionized surgery and opened the vista for endoscopic surgeons all over the world to help their patients. He has advocated and proven that a majority of procedures previously performed by laparotomy can be converted into minimally invasive procedures, providing countless benefits to patients, opening the door for other surgeons to further advance the field and improve outcomes for patients around the world. Early in this field's development, he declared that, "wherever in the body a cavity exists or can be created, minimally invasive surgery is possible and probably preferable. The limiting factors are only the skill and experience of the surgeon and availability of proper instrumentation" [19, 23].

The development of videolaparoscopy was by no means smooth. Dr. Kurt Semm of Germany performed the first laparoscopic appendectomy in 1983 and was greeted with derision and condemned by the German Board of Surgery [24]. The first laparoscopic cholecystectomy was similarly received when presented at the Congress of the German Surgical Society by Erich Muhe in 1986 [25]. A year later, Philippe Mouret performed the first laparoscopic cholecystectomy with video assistance, followed by Francois Dubois in 1988 [26]. In October 1989, video-assisted laparoscopic cholecystectomy was presented at the American College of Surgeons' annual meeting, sparking a rapid expansion of the horizons of minimally invasive surgery. Leonard Schulz and John Corbitt developed several approaches to laparoscopic herniorrhaphy [27–30], and Petelin, Reddick, and Olsen reported on laparoscopic common bile duct exploration [10]. Camran Nezhat published the first video-assisted laparoscopic partial colectomy in 1991 [31], followed by Redwine, Fowler, and Jacobs performing minimally invasive segmental colon resections [32–34]. That year, Katkhouda, Dallemagne, Zucker, and Bailey developed a minimally invasive vagotomy tech-

Table 1.1 Procedures performed by Camran Nezhat and collaborators for the first time in surgical history [23, 31, 40, 42, 64, 222–250]

1985	**Videolaparoscopy for the treatment of severe endometriosis involving the bowel, bladder, and ureter** Nezhat C, Nezhat F. Videolaseroscopy for the treatment of endometriosis, American Fertility Society (ASRM) 1985, Canada. American College of Obstetricians and Gynecologists Annual Meeting, Las Vegas, Nevada, 1987
1988	**Videolaparoscopy for the treatment of bowel endometriosis** Nezhat C, Nezhat F. Evaluation of safety of videolaseroscopic treatment of bowel endometriosis, Scientific Paper, 44th Annual Meeting of the American Fertility Society, Atlanta Hilton and Towers, Atlanta, Georgia, October 8–13, 1988
1989	**Safe laser excision and vaporization of endometriosis with laparoscopic repair of the bowel after disk excision** Nezhat CR, Nezhat FR. Fertil Steril, 1989; P 52(1): 149–151 (reported repair of the bowel after disk excision of endometriosis)
	Laparoscopic removal of dermoid cysts Nezhat C, Winer WK, Nezhat F. Laparoscopic removal of dermoid cysts. Obstet Gynecol, February 1989;73(2): 278–281
1990	**Laparoscopic management of interstitial pregnancy** Nezhat, C. & Nezhat, F. Conservative Management of Ectopic Gestation. Fertil Steril 53, 382–383 (1990)
1991	**Laparoscopically assisted anterior rectal wall resection and reanastomosis for deeply infiltrating endometriosis** Nezhat C, Pennington E, Nezhat F, Silfen SL. Laparoscopically assisted anterior rectal wall resection and reanastomosis for deeply infiltrating endometriosis. Surg Laparosc Endosc, June 1991;1(2): 106–108
	Laparoscopic ovarian cystectomy during advanced pregnancy Nezhat F, Nezhat C, Silfen SL, Fehnel SH. Laparoscopic ovarian cystectomy during pregnancy. J Laparoendosc Surg, June 1991;1(3): 161–164
	Laparoscopic radical hysterectomy with para-aortic and pelvic lymph node dissection Nezhat, C.R., Burrell, M.O., Nezhat, F.R., Benigno, B.B. & Welander, C.E. Laparoscopic Radical Hysterectomy with Para-aortic and Pelvic Node Dissection. Am J Obstet Gynecol 166, 864–865 (1992) Nezhat C, Nezhat F. Silfen SL. Videolaseroscopy: the CO_2 laser for advanced operative laparoscopy. Obstet Gynecol Clin North Am. 1991; 18:585–604 Nezhat CR, Nezhat FR, Ramirez CE, et al. Laparoscopic radical hysterectomy and laparoscopic assisted vaginal radical hysterectomy with pelvic and para-aortic node dissection, *J Gynecol Surg*. 1993;9:105–120
1992	**Laparoscopic ureteroureterostomy** Nezhat C, Nezhat F. Laparoscopic repair of ureter resected during operative laparoscopy. Obstet Gynecol, September 1992; 80(3 Pt 2): 543–544
	Laparoscopic segmental bowel resection/proctectomy for infiltrating endometriosis of the rectum Nezhat F, Nezhat C, Pennington E. Laparoscopic proctectomy for infiltrating endometriosis of the rectum. Fertil Steril, May 1992;57(5): 1129–1132
	Laparoscopic segmental bowel resection of the rectosigmoid colon Nezhat F, Nezhat C, Pennington E, Ambroze W Jr. Laparoscopic segmental resection for infiltrating endometriosis of the recto sigmoid colon: a preliminary report. *Surg Laparosc Endosc*. 1992;2:212–216
	Laparoscopic treatment of ovarian remnant syndrome Nezhat F, Nezhat C. Operative laparoscopy for the treatment of ovarian remnant syndrome. Fertil Steril, May 1992;57(5): 1003–1007
	Laparoscopic ureteral resection and ureteroureterostomy for ureteral obstruction Nezhat C, Nezhat F, Green B. Laparoscopic treatment of obstructed ureter due to endometriosis by resection and ureteroureterostomy: a case report. J Urol, September 1992;148(3): 865–868
	New theory regarding pathogenesis and clinical and histologic classification of endometriomas Nezhat F, Nezhat C, Allan CJ, Metzger DA, Sears DL. Clinical and histologic classification of endometriomas: implications for a mechanism of pathogenesis. Journal of Reproductive Medicine, September 1992;Vol. 37, No. 9, Pp: 771–776
	Laparoscopic vaginal vault suspension for vaginal vault prolapse Nezhat C, Nezhat F, Nezhat CH. Operative Laparoscopy Minimally Invasive Surgery: State of the Art, 1992. Obstetrics and Gynecology Journal, 1994
	Laparoscopic treatment of diaphragmatic endometriosis Nezhat F, Nezhat C, Levy JS. Laparoscopic treatment of symptomatic diaphragmatic endometriosis: a case report. Fertil Steril 1992;58(3): 614–616 Nezhat C, King LP, Paka C, Odegaard J, Beygui R. Bilateral thoracic endometriosis affecting the lung and diaphragm. JSLS. 2012 Jan-Mar; 16(1): 140–142

(continued)

Table 1.1 (continued)

1993	**Laparoscopic segmental bladder resection for endometriosis** Nezhat C, Nezhat F. Laparoscopic segmental bladder resection for endometriosis: A report of two cases. Obstet Gynecol, Vol. 81, No. 5, Pp: 882–884, 1993
	Laparoscopic repair of small bowel and colon Nezhat C., Nezhat F. Ambroze W. & Pennington E. Laparoscopic repair of small bowel and colon: A report of 26 cases. Surg Endosc. P 7(2): 88–8 9. (1993)
1994	**Laparoscopic repair of vesicovaginal fistula** Nezhat CH, Nezhat F, Nezhat C, Rottenberg H. Laparoscopic repair of a vesicovaginal fistula: A case report. Obstet. Gynecol, Vol. 83, No. 5, Pp: 899–901, 1994
	Laparoscopic-assisted myomectomy Nezhat C, Nezhat F, Bess O, Nezhat CH, Mashiach R. Laparoscopically assisted myomectomy: a report of a new technique in 57 cases. Int J Fertil Menopausal Stud. P 39(1): 39–44. (1994)
	Laparoscopic disk excision and primary repair of the anterior rectal wall Nezhat C, Nezhat F, Pennington E, et al. Laparoscopic disk excision and primary repair of the anterior rectal wall for the treatment of full thickness bowel endometriosis. *Surg Endosc.* 1994;8:682–685
	In collaboration with robotic pioneers, Drs. Ajit Shah and Phil Green, Nezhat was involved with the development of the da Vinci Robot
1996	**First case of vaginal vault evisceration after total laparoscopic hysterectomy** Nezhat CH, Nezhat F, Seidman DS, Nezhat C. Vaginal vault evisceration after total laparoscopic hysterectomy. Obstet Gynecol 1996;87: 868–870
	Laparoscopic management of advanced ovarian cancer Amara DP, Nezhat C, Teng NN, Nezhat F, Nezhat C, Rosati M. Operative laparoscopy in the management of ovarian cancer. Surgical Laparoscopy 1996 Endoscopy & Percutaneous Techniques. P 6(1): 38–45. (1996)
1997	**Laparoscopic repair of major retroperitoneal vascular injury** Nezhat C, Childers J, Nezhat F, Nezhat CH, Seidman D. Major Retroperitoneal Vascular Injury During Laparoscopic Surgery. Human Reprod 1997; P 12, 480–483
1999	**Laparoscopic ureteroneocystostomy with vesicopsoas hitch for ureteral endometriosis** Nezhat C, Nezhat F, Nezhat CH, Frieha F. Laparoscopic Vesicopsoas Hitch for Infiltrative Ureteral Endometriosis. Fert Stert 1999 Vol 71, No. 2, P 376–379
2002	**Laparoscopic control of a leaking inferior mesenteric vessel secondary to trocar injury** Jacobson M, Oesterling S, Milki A, Nezhat CR. Laparoscopic control of a leaking inferior mesenteric vessel secondary to trocar injury. JSLS. 2002; 6:389–391
2003	**Laparoscopic repair of uteroperitoneal fistula (niche, isthmocele, cesarean section scar defect, diverticulum)** Nezhat C, Jacobson MT, Osias J, Velasco A, Charles R. Laparoscopic Repair of Uteroperitoneal Fistula. JSLS 2003; 7:367–369
2005	**Laparoscopic treatment of liver endometriosis** Nezhat, C. et al. Laparoscopic management of hepatic endometriosis: report of two cases and review of the literature. Journal of Minimally Invasive Gynecology. P 12, 196–200. (2005)

nique for treatment of peptic ulcer disease, and Philippe Mouret repaired a perforated peptic ulcer laparoscopically [25, 35, 36]. In urology, Flowers and Tierney popularized laparoscopic pelvic lymphadenectomy [37, 38], while Ralph Clayman performed a minimally invasive nephrectomy [39]. In 1992, video-assisted laparoscopic radical hysterectomy with pelvic and para-aortic lymphadenectomy was developed by Camran and Farr Nezhat [40–42]. Also in that year, Hashizume, Phillips, Petelin, and Flowers performed a minimally invasive splenectomy [43, 44]; Petelin and Gagner performed a minimally invasive adrenalectomy [45]. By 1997, video-assisted laparoscopic aortofemoral bypass had been pioneered by Dion and Gracia [46].

Benefits of Laparoscopy

Today, video-assisted laparoscopy is the gold standard in many fields of surgery [36, 43, 45, 47–53]. Camran Nezhat has long been one of the greatest pioneers and proponents of minimally invasive surgery, declaring, "wherever a cavity exists in the body, or can be created, endoscopic surgery is indicated, and most probably, preferable" [23]. Avoiding the large incisions involved with laparotomy means that patients undergoing minimally invasive surgery are able to avoid many of the complications of these operations, including the prolonged inflammatory response caused by extensive tissue injury [42, 54, 55]. The increased blood loss associated with laparotomy is also avoided, and the subsequent increased need for transfusion [56, 57]. Patients undergoing video-assisted laparoscopic surgery have less postoperative pain and fatigue, require less narcotic pain medication, and have a shorter duration of recovery [58]. These patients also experience a more rapid resumption of peristalsis and initiation of oral intake [59, 60]. Further advantages of video-assisted laparoscopy include better exposure and visualization of the pertinent anatomy, improved cosmesis, and decreased chronic wound complications [61–63].

Surgical Considerations in Pregnancy

Until 1990, laparoscopy was considered to be contraindicated in pregnancy, but in 1991, Nezhat et al. showed the safety of laparoscopic surgery during advanced pregnancy by reporting the first laparoscopic ovarian cystectomy in pregnancy [64]. Laparoscopy has numerous advantages over laparotomy, similar to those found in nonpregnant patients. These include improved visualization and magnification, less postoperative pain and opioid requirements resulting in less fetal depression, faster recovery time, and earlier ambulation resulting in a lower risk of atelectasis and thromboembolism [65].

Prior to 1991, concerns over laparoscopy during pregnancy included unknown effects of anesthesia on the fetus, difficulty with laparoscopic entry due to an enlarged uterus, and uterine injury during initial trocar placement. Physiologic changes in pregnancy to the respiratory, cardiovascular, renal, gastrointestinal, and hematologic systems decrease patients' ability to tolerate surgical stressors. Although there is a theoretical concern over fetal exposure to carbon monoxide from electrocautery and laser [66, 67], a study by Nezhat et al. in 1996 did not demonstrate increased levels of carboxyhemoglobin in women undergoing prolonged laparoscopic procedures [68].

There are numerous unique effects of pneumoperitoneum in the pregnant patient, such as reduced blood flow to the uterus due to decreased venous return and increased peripheral vascular resistance, difficulty with ventilation due to increased intra-abdominal pressure and decreased functional residual lung capacity, fetal hypercarbia, and acidosis due CO_2 insufflation [69–73]. A study in pregnant sheep performed in 1995 demonstrated fetal acidosis after exposure to 90 to 120 min of CO_2 pneumoperitoneum. However, there were no changes in fetal hemodynamics or signs of fetal stress for intra-abdominal pressures less than 20 mmHg. Furthermore, average fetal pH did not fall below 7.2 and recovered after release of pneumoperitoneum [71]. Likewise, a study by Candiani in 1992 showed no change in uteroplacental perfusion with pneumoperitoneum during adnexal surgery during pregnancy based on measurements of mean uterine resistance and umbilical artery pulsatility indices [74].

Due to obvious limitations, no randomized controlled studies have been conducted to evaluate the safety of laparoscopy in pregnancy. However, all literature published on surgery during pregnancy to date have been reassuring. Since the 1970s, there have been only two case reports of CO_2 embolism due to intrauterine insufflation [75, 76]. Laparoscopy has been shown to be safe in multiple studies and has been performed in patients up to 31 weeks gestation [6, 7, 77–86].

Surgery should be performed in the second trimester, if possible, after fetal organogenesis is complete. After 10 weeks, the placenta takes over progesterone production and no longer relies on the corpus luteum to sustain the pregnancy. Thus, adnexal surgery may damage the corpus luteum in the first trimester and could result in adverse pregnancy outcomes, requiring progesterone supplementation. Surgery in the third trimester is associated with a high risk of preterm labor and preterm delivery [87, 88], in addition to technical difficulties associated with an enlarged uterus [89]. However, surgery, when indicated, can be performed in any trimester. Although anesthetic agents are not known to be teratogenic, the effects are not known with certainty. Anesthetic agents do cross the placenta, and exposure to anesthetics should be limited as much as possible. The patient should be placed in the left lateral tilt position to reduce compression of the IVC by the gravid uterus, which can reduce preload and cause hypotension. Due to the hypercoagulable state in pregnancy, sequential compression devices (SCDs) should be placed prior to induction of anesthesia and remain in place until the patient is fully ambulatory. Initial trocar placement should be at Palmer's point or 4–5 cm above the gravid uterus to prevent inadvertent uterine injury and perforation. According to the Society of American Gastrointestinal and Endoscopic Surgeons (SAGES) guidelines for laparoscopic surgery during pregnancy (Table 1.2), either Veress needle or open Hasson entry techniques may be used [86]. $ETCO_2$ should be monitored to measure maternal hypercapnia [90] and, indirectly, fetal acidosis, which results from peritoneal absorption of CO_2 and decreased lung ventilation in pregnant patients. Surgery time and anesthesia exposure should be kept to a minimum and pneumoperitoneum maintained at or below 15 mmHg [91–94].

Isobaric (gasless) laparoscopy was proposed as an alternative in 1995 to avoid the complications of pneumoperitoneum. Performed by manually lifting the abdominal wall, isobaric laparoscopy avoids the need for CO_2 insufflation, thus preventing complications such as maternal and fetal hypercarbia. This technique has been used in pregnant patients undergoing adnexal surgery, cholecystectomy, and myomectomy [95–97]. Romer reported a case of a torsed hematosalpinx that was managed using gasless laparoscopy at 13 weeks gestation in 2002. There were no surgical complications, and the patient proceeded to have a normal pregnancy [96]. In 2005, Melgrati performed an isobaric laparoscopic myomectomy during pregnancy at 24 weeks gestation under spinal anesthesia with conscious sedation. The remainder of the pregnancy was uneventful. Although they reported that uterine closure was performed as safely and quickly as laparotomy [97], a randomized study by Goldberg et al. in 1997 demonstrated gasless laparoscopy to be inferior in terms of visualization, longer operating times, and increased risk of complications [98].

Uterine manipulation should be minimized to prevent uterine contractions and irritability. Postoperative pain control is important, as pain can also cause uterine irritability. Opioids can be used postoperatively for pain control, although it should be limited due to its fetal depressive effects and risk of neonatal abstinence syndrome with prolonged use near delivery. NSAIDs should be avoided greater than 32 weeks gestation due to the risk of premature closure of the ductus arteriosus. Prophylactic tocolysis is not recommended as there is no difference in rate of preterm delivery between patients who received tocolysis and those who did not [99]. SAGES recommends preoperative and postoperative fetal heart tone auscultation only, as intraoperative fetal monitoring may not be an accurate measure of fetal distress, due to fetal heart rate changes as a result of fetal depressive effects of anesthesia [100] and technical difficulties of ultrasound monitoring. ACOG recommends an individualized approach to intraoperative fetal monitoring depending on gestational age, type of surgery, and available facilities [89].

In 1997, Gurbuz et al. proposed that laparoscopy is safe in pregnancy for treatment of non-obstetric abdominal pain without additional risk to the fetus, regardless of gestational age, in patients who require urgent surgical intervention [101]. That same year, Reedy et al. published the results of their review of the Swedish Health Registry, showing no significant differences in fetal morbidity, malformations, or fetal loss between patients who had undergone surgical intervention pregnancy and patients who had not [80]. Years later, in 2010, Corneille et al. published a review of pregnant women presenting with non-obstetric acute abdomen, declaring that morbidity and mortality for laparoscopy and laparotomy are similar and that perinatal complications are due primarily to disease severity and not

Table 1.2 2017 SAGES guidelines for the use of laparoscopy during pregnancy [251]

Summary of recommendations				
			Quality of evidence	Strength of recommendation
Diagnosis and workup				
Guideline 1	*Ultrasound*	Ultrasound imaging during pregnancy is safe and effective in identifying the etiology of acute abdominal pain in many patients and should be the initial imaging test of choice	+++	*Strong*
Guideline 2	*Risk of ionizing radiation*	Ionizing radiation exposure to the fetus increases the risk of teratogenesis and childhood leukemia. Cumulative radiation dosage should be limited to 50–100 mGy during pregnancy	+++	*Strong*
Guideline 3	*Computed tomography*	Abdominal CT scan may be used in emergency situations during pregnancy. CT scan should not be the initial imaging test of choice	++	*Weak*
Guideline 4	*Magnetic resonance imaging*	MR imaging without the use of intravenous gadolinium can be performed at any stage of pregnancy. MRI is preferred over CT scan for diagnosis of non-obstetric abdominal pain in the gravid patient	++	*Strong*
Guideline 5	*Nuclear medicine*	Administration of radionucleotides for diagnostic studies is safe for mother and fetus	++	*Weak*
Guideline 6	*Cholangiography*	Intraoperative and endoscopic cholangiography exposes the mother and fetus to minimal radiation and may be used selectively during pregnancy. The lower abdomen should be shielded when performing cholangiography during pregnancy to decrease the radiation exposure to the fetus	++	*Weak*
Guideline 7	*Diagnostic laparoscopy*	In the absence of access to imaging modalities, laparoscopy may be used selectively in the workup and treatment of acute abdominal processes in pregnancy	++	*Weak*
Patient selection				
Guideline 8	*Preoperative decision-making*	Laparoscopic treatment of acute abdominal disease offers similar benefits to pregnant and nonpregnant patients compared to laparotomy	+++	*Strong*

(continued)

Table 1.2 (continued)

Summary of recommendations				
			Quality of evidence	Strength of recommendation
Guideline 9	*Laparoscopy and trimester of pregnancy*	Laparoscopy can be safely performed during any trimester of pregnancy when operation is indicated	+++	*Strong*
Treatment				
Guideline 10	*Patient positioning*	Gravid patients beyond the first trimester should be placed in the left lateral decubitus position or partial left lateral decubitus position to minimize compression of the vena cava	++	*Strong*
Guideline 11	*Initial port placement*	Initial abdominal access can be safely accomplished with an open (Hasson), Veress needle, or optical trocar technique, by surgeons experienced with these techniques, if the location is adjusted according to fundal height	++	*Weak*
Guideline 12	*Insufflation pressure*	CO_2 insufflation of 10–15 mmHg can be safely used for laparoscopy in the pregnant patient. The level of insufflation pressure should be adjusted to the patient's physiology	++	*Weak*
Guideline 13	*Intraoperative CO_2 monitoring*	Intraoperative CO_2 monitoring by capnography should be used during laparoscopy in the pregnant patient	+++	*Strong*
Guideline 14	*Venous thromboembolism (VTE) prophylaxis*	Intraoperative and postoperative pneumatic compression devices and early postoperative ambulation are recommended prophylaxis for deep venous thrombosis in the gravid patient	++	*Weak*
Guideline 15	*Gallbladder disease*	Laparoscopic cholecystectomy is the treatment of choice in the pregnant patient with symptomatic gallbladder disease, regardless of trimester	++	*Weak*
Guideline 16	*Choledocolithiasis*	Choledocholithiasis during pregnancy can be managed safely with preoperative endoscopic retrograde cholangiopancreatography (ERCP) with sphincterotomy followed by laparoscopic cholecystectomy, laparoscopic common bile duct exploration at the time of cholecystectomy, or postoperative ERCP. Comparative studies are lacking	++	*Weak*

Table 1.2 (continued)

Summary of recommendations				
			Quality of evidence	Strength of recommendation
Guideline 17	*Laparoscopic appendectomy*	Laparoscopic appendectomy is the treatment of choice for pregnant patients with acute appendicitis	+++	*Strong*
Guideline 18	*Solid organ resection*	Laparoscopic adrenalectomy, nephrectomy, and splenectomy are safe procedures in appropriately selected pregnant patients	+	*Weak*
Guideline 19	*Adnexal mass*	Laparoscopy is a safe and effective treatment in gravid patients with symptomatic ovarian cystic masses. Observation is acceptable for all other cystic lesions, provided ultrasound is not concerning for malignancy and tumor markers are normal. Initial observation is warranted for most cystic lesions <6 cm in size	++	*Weak*
Guideline 20	*Adnexal torsion*	Laparoscopy is recommended for both diagnosis and treatment of adnexal torsion	++	*Strong*
Perioperative care				
Guideline 21	*Fetal heart monitoring*	Fetal heart monitoring of a fetus considered viable should occur preoperatively and postoperatively in the setting of urgent abdominal surgery during pregnancy	++	*Weak*
Guideline 22	*Tocolytics*	Tocolytics should not be used prophylactically in pregnant women undergoing surgery but should be considered perioperatively when signs of preterm labor are present	+++	*Strong*

to operative technique [102]. Now, many abdominal pathologies requiring surgical management are treated laparoscopically in pregnancy, as addressed below.

Abdominal Diseases and Disorders

Appendicitis

Appendicitis [94, 103–105] is the most common cause of non-obstetric surgery in pregnant patients, [106] and accounts for 25% of non-obstetric surgery. It is estimated to have an incidence of 1/500–1/2000 of all pregnancies [106] and is most commonly diagnosed during the second trimester, comprising 40% of cases [107, 108]. Pregnancy does not appear to affect the incidence of appendicitis, although pregnancy is associated with a higher rate of perforation [109], most likely due to a delay in diagnosis. The perforation rate when surgery is delayed more than 24 h is 66%, while it is practically nonexistent when patients are operated on within 24 h [108].

Appendicitis is a difficult diagnosis to make during pregnancy [110, 111], due to physiologic changes in pregnancy that imitate appendicitis: nausea, vomiting, and abdominal discomfort due to round ligament pain. Leukocytosis is normal in pregnancy, although a left shift may indicate an infectious etiology of leukocytosis. Stretching of the abdominal wall leads to diminished perception of peritoneal irritation and precise localization of pain. Right lower quadrant pain and tenderness is the most common sign [107, 112, 113], but rebound and guarding may not be present due to the position of the uterus between the appendix and abdominal wall. Hesitation to perform imaging and surgery during pregnancy results in further delays in diagnosis. Appendicitis may have an atypical presentation in advanced pregnancies, due to the upward displacement of the appendix by the gravid uterus after 12 weeks gestation, reaching the iliac crest by 6 months, and returning to its normal location by postpartum day 10. A retrocecal appendix can present with flank or back pain and be confused with pyelonephritis [108].

Prompt diagnosis and treatment is important to prevent sepsis and rupture, which significantly increases maternal and fetal morbidity and even mortality [114]. Fetal morbidity is 1.5% in cases of unruptured appendicitis but up to 20–35% with ruptured appendicitis [1, 108, 112, 115–119]. Peritonitis and infection can also cause preterm contractions, especially in the third trimester. Thus, appendicitis should be promptly treated surgically as soon as it is diagnosed. There is no role for conservative treatment in appendicitis. Laparoscopic appendectomy has been shown to be safe and associated with fewer complications compared with open appendectomy in numerous studies [7, 84, 94, 99, 102, 116, 117, 119–134]. In 1990 Schreiber et al. reported six cases of laparoscopic appendectomies during pregnancy, from 8 to 25 weeks of gestation, with no complications [103].

Graded compression ultrasound is the initial imaging of choice, as it is considered safe in pregnancy. However, it has a low sensitivity for detection of appendicitis, especially after 32 weeks due to limited view from the enlarged uterus and in cases of ruptured appendicitis [135]. Abdominal MRI [136–139] has high sensitivity (91%) and specificity (85%) [140] for the diagnosis of appendicitis and has not been shown to have adverse fetal effects [141–145]. Although gadolinium has not been shown to have adverse effects on the fetus [142, 143], it is classified as Category C, and therefore use should be avoided when possible. Although CT provides a higher sensitivity and specificity compared with MRI (93%) [146], it is avoided when possible due fetal radiation exposure. The most susceptible period to the harmful effects of radiation is during organogenesis (2–8 weeks gestation), whereas fetal demise is the highest in the first 2 weeks of gestation. After 8 weeks, the major risk is mental retardation. After 20 weeks, the risk of radiation is associated with a small increase in childhood leukemia [147]. Cumulative doses less than 5 rads are considered safe during pregnancy. A single CT delivers approximately 2.5 rads and so may be considered only after diagnostic testing with ultrasound or MRI is equivocal.

Biliary Disease: Cholecystitis, Cholelithiasis, and Choledocolithiasis

Acute cholecystitis is the second most common non-obstetric condition requiring surgery during pregnancy and occurs in 1/2000 to 1/2500 of pregnancies. The incidence of gallstones in pregnant women is 1–3%, and symptomatic biliary disease is 0.05–8%. There is an increased incidence of gallstones found during pregnancy, due to estrogenic and progestational effects. Estrogen increases cholesterol levels, and progesterone causes smooth muscle relaxation, decreasing bile acid secretion and inhibiting gallbladder emptying. Cholelithiasis is the most common cause of cholecystitis, causing over 90% of cases [1].

Ultrasound is the imaging method of choice for diagnosis of cholecystitis, with a sensitivity of 80–90% and specificity of 88–100% [108, 109, 148]. Findings on ultrasound suggestive of cholecystitis include sonographic Murphy's sign, gallbladder thickening, and pericholecystic fluid. Elevated transaminases and particularly direct hyperbilirubinemia may indicate cholecystitis; elevated alkaline phosphatase is less reliable as it is normally elevated in pregnancy.

There is emerging evidence that surgical treatment during pregnancy may be beneficial even in cases of symptomatic cholelithiasis. In 2008, Jelin et al. reported an increased risk of fetal death and preterm labor with conservative management of symptomatic biliary disease, as well as increased risk of recurrent symptoms, cholecystitis, and biliary pancreatitis [108, 149–151]. Silvestri et al. later reported in 2011 on the safety of laparoscopic cholecystectomy in pregnancy after comparing 32,479 nonpregnant and 436 pregnant women, with decreased rates of complications in the pregnant women compared to the nonpregnant population [152]. In a systematic review of 590 patients in 2016 by Nasioudis et al., laparoscopic cholecystectomy was shown to be safe and associated with fewer complications compared to laparotomy [153].

Choledocolithiasis is uncommon and estimated to occur in 1 in 1200 pregnant women [108]. Ultrasound may demonstrate a dilated common bile duct. ERCP with sphincterotomy during pregnancy is safe and recommended for treatment of choledocolithiasis. It is important to counsel patients on the risk of pancreatitis, preterm labor, or post-sphincterotomy bleeding [154].

Acute Pancreatitis

The incidence of pancreatitis in pregnancy is 1 in 1000 to 1 in 5000 [155, 156] and occurs more frequently in the third trimester and postpartum. The most common causes of pancreatitis are gallstones, which account for the majority of cases, followed by alcohol, medications, infections, and hyperlipidemia [157, 158]. Extremely elevated lipase levels are the most reliable laboratory finding in these cases. Ultrasound or MRI should be performed to evaluate the severity of disease, which dictates treatment. Gallstone pancreatitis is usually managed conservatively during pregnancy, with hydration, bowel rest, and antibiotics, followed by cholecystectomy or ERCP with sphincterotomy for gallstone pancreatitis once the acute inflammation has subsided to prevent future recurrence, which can be up to 70% [159, 160]. Morphine for analgesia should be avoided as it can cause sphincter of Oddi spasm. Severe hemorrhagic or necrotizing pancreatitis, ruptured pseudocysts, or pancreatitis nonresponsive to initial conservative management requires surgery, as it can be associated with a high fetal mortality rate of 10–20% [159].

Acute Intestinal Obstruction

Acute intestinal obstruction is the third most common cause of acute abdomen in pregnancy and complicates 1 in 1500 to 1 in 3000 pregnancies [161]. The risk is greatest during periods of rapid uterine size changes, between 16 to 20 weeks and 32 to 36 weeks, and in the postpartum period [162]. Abdominal X-ray may demonstrate dilated small bowel loops and air-fluid levels and may be used for either diagnosis or to monitor response to treatment. A single abdominal X-ray provides 0.325 rad of radiation exposure. A CT may be performed if abdominal X-ray is inconclusive and there is a high clinical suspicion. Obstruction may occur as a result of adhesions from prior abdominal surgeries or pelvic infections, which account for 60–70% of cases [163, 164]. Volvulus is the second most common cause of intestinal obstruction in pregnancy, accounting for 25% of cases. Of these, cecal volvulus is the most common as the enlarging uterus displaces the colon, but the cecum remains fixed [163, 165]. Other less common causes include intussusception (5%), hernia, cancer, and diverticulitis/diverticulosis [165].

Obstruction should be initially managed conservatively, with hydration, electrolyte replacement, bowel rest, and decompression, with surgical management reserved for those who fail conservative therapy. Colonoscopy can be both diagnostic and therapeutic in cases of sigmoid volvulus but is less effective for cecal volvulus. In 1984, Orchard reported a case series of three large bowel obstructions caused by volvulus that were managed by colonoscopy [166]. Due to the high risk (>50%) of recurrent volvulus, surgery postpartum is indicated [166]. Any signs of ischemia or strangulation require immediate laparotomy and resection of gangrenous bowel. Maternal mortality is high, estimated to be 6–20%, fetal mortality is 20–26%, and bowel strangulation requiring resection is 23%, with the incidence of maternal and fetal mortality increasing with advancing gestations [162, 164].

Gastric Cancer

In 2016 Kim et al. reported a case of a 36-year-old patient at 18 weeks gestation who underwent laparoscopic gastrectomy at 23 weeks gestation and then received four cycles of chemotherapy. The patient delivered a healthy infant at 36 weeks and remained in remission 1 year after surgery [167]. The same year, Alshahrani and Yoo published a case of laparoscopic distal gastrectomy in a woman at 17 weeks gestation, followed by a spontaneous vaginal delivery at 39 weeks, and the mother remained in remission at follow-up 4 months after delivery [168].

Renal Cancer

In 2005 Basten reported a case of laparoscopic nephrectomy performed for a 30-year-old patient at 16 weeks gestation with renal cell carcinoma, demonstrating both maternal and fetal safety of the procedure [169].

Pelvic Diseases and Disorders [65]

Adnexal Masses [64, 65, 170–175]

In 1991, Nezhat et al. reported the first case of adnexal surgery in pregnancy. The patient presented with a history of endometriosis and persistent bilateral adnexal masses who underwent laparoscopic ovarian cystectomy at 16 weeks. There were no complications, and the patient went on to have an uneventful pregnancy and delivery [64]. Later that year, Shalev reported two cases of laparoscopic detorsion of ovaries during early pregnancy. Both patients had uneventful pregnancies [176]. In 2003, Mathevet et al. published a case series of 47 expectant mothers who underwent laparoscopic management of ovarian cysts, torsion, or pelvic masses. In this study, 17 women presented in the first trimester, 27 in the second trimester, and 4 in the third trimester. One pregnancy loss occurred following an uncomplicated ovarian cystectomy at 17 weeks gestation. The authors concluded that laparoscopic adnexal surgery is safe and effective when performed by a skilled surgical team [83]. Three years later, Purnichescu et al. reported a case series of 21 women, with no adverse events documented, including eight procedures performed in the first trimester [177]. A later retrospective review by Ko et al. in 2009 analyzed 11 patients who underwent emergent laparoscopic adnexal surgery in the first trimester of pregnancy, with no maternal or fetal complications [178]. In 2016, Myounghwan Kim published a case report of a patient at 10 weeks gestation with a torsed pedunculated ovarian leiomyoma which was managed with salpingo-oophorectomy. There were no maternal or fetal complications [179].

Adnexal masses are estimated to complicate 2% of pregnancies [180–182]. The most common adnexal masses in pregnancy are mature cystic teratomas (24–40%) or persistent corpus luteum cysts (30%). Although many adnexal masses regress during pregnancy [183, 184], persistent masses greater than 5–6 cm [183, 185–188] should be removed in the second trimester to prevent ovarian torsion, rupture, obstruction of labor, and to rule out malignancy [186, 188–191]. Only 1–8% of adnexal masses are found to be malignant [188, 191–194]. Emergent surgery is associated with higher maternal morbidity and fetal mortality compared to elective surgery [186, 195, 196]. The risk of significant morbidity as a result of torsion, rupture, infection, or hemorrhage is estimated to be 10–42% [186, 197]. Laparoscopic surgery for adnexal masses has been performed safely during pregnancy in numerous studies [64, 83, 88, 173, 177, 178, 198–202]. Other indications for adnexal surgery include adnexal torsion [203–208], heterotopic pregnancy [77, 209], and solid ovarian tumors.

Leiomyomas [210, 211]

Myomectomy during pregnancy has been reported in symptomatic patients, often due to the increase in leiomyoma size during pregnancy causing increased pain. In 2000, an observational study was published by Dubuisson et al. of 100 patients who underwent laparoscopic myomectomy. Of these, 72 patients had a trial of labor, and 58 delivered vaginally. There were three cases of uterine rupture, although only one case ruptured at the site of the uterine scar, none ruptured during a trial of labor [212]. A retrospective analysis published in 2002 reviewed 18 patients who underwent isobaric myomectomy between 6 and 24 weeks gestation and demonstrated no adverse outcomes [82, 213]. In 2005, Melgrati et al. published a case report of isobaric myomectomy in a patient at 24 weeks gestation, followed by a full-term normal spontaneous vaginal delivery [97]. Concerns regarding myomectomy during pregnancy include the risk of preterm labor, preterm rupture of membranes, fetal injury, technical difficulty, and uterine rupture during pregnancy and labor. The risk of uterine rupture after laparoscopic myomectomy has been estimated to be less than 1% [97, 214].

Cervical Cancer

Cervical cancer is the most common malignancy diagnosed during pregnancy, estimated to affect 1 in 1000 to 1 in 10,000 pregnant women [215–218]. The optimal treatment for cervical cancer during pregnancy has not been well established and depends on maternal desires, clinical stage of disease, and gestational age at time of diagnosis. Historically, the standard treatment for cervical cancer diagnosed prior to 20 weeks' gestation was pregnancy termination in order to not delay treatment of the malignancy. Options now include preservation of pregnancy if desired, with scheduled delay of treatment until fetal viability, neoadjuvant chemotherapy followed by cesarean hysterectomy at fetal viability, and radical trachelectomy in pregnancy [219]. Patients with stage IB1 cervical cancer or less may choose conservative surgical management with radical vaginal trachelectomy and laparoscopic pelvic lymphadenectomy [219–221]. Delay of treatment is associated with a 5% risk of recurrence, similar to the risk of recurrence in nonpregnant patients.

In order to help guide management decisions, and whether conservative management is an option, Hertel et al. performed laparoscopic lymph node staging of cervical cancer on a 39-year-old G1P0 woman at 19 weeks' gestation in 2001. The patient was diagnosed with stage IB1, grade 2 adenosquamous cervical cancer with positive margins on cone biopsy and lymphovascular space invasion. Eighteen parametric and pelvic lymph nodes were removed. One positive lymph node was detected, and therefore the patient underwent an open radical hysterectomy with para-aortic lymphadenectomy [216].

In 2010, Favero et al. proposed that laparoscopic pelvic lymphadenectomy is both feasible and safe in pregnancy prior to a planned treatment delay in 18 patients at gestational ages ranging from 6 to 23 weeks. In this study, no surgical complications nor maternal or fetal complications were noted, and 14 patients with negative lymph nodes successfully carried to fetal maturity and showed no evidence of disease at 38 months postpartum [218]. In 2012 Bravo et al. published the first case of radical vaginal trachelectomy with laparoscopic pelvic lymphadenectomy in a patient with stage IB1 cervical adenocarcinoma at 11 weeks' gestational age, followed by cesarean hysterectomy at 36 weeks' gestational age with remission noted at 40 months postpartum [219].

Conclusion

The development of non-obstetric endoscopic surgery in pregnancy is relatively recent, starting with the 1991 publication of laparoscopic ovarian cystectomy in advanced pregnancy by Camran Nezhat. Other laparoscopic surgical procedures were rapidly applied to the pregnant population, with demonstrated safety in all trimesters of pregnancy. Now, surgery is recommended in the pregnant population when indicated, regardless of gestational age, and laparoscopic approaches should be strongly considered when appropriate.

References

1. Kammerer WS. Nonobstetric surgery during pregnancy. Med Clin North Am. 1979;63(6):1157–64.
2. Kort B, Katz VL, Watson WJ. The effect of nonobstetric operation during pregnancy. Surg Gynecol Obstet. 1993;177(4):371–6.
3. Schwarzman P, Baumfeld Y, Bar-Niv Z, Baron J, Mastrolia SA, Sheiner E, et al. The effect of non-obstetric invasive procedures during pregnancy on perinatal outcomes. Arch Gynecol Obstet. 2015;292(3):603–8.
4. Levine W, Diamond B. Surgical procedures during pregnancy. Am J Obstet Gynecol. 1961;81:1046–52.
5. Smith BE. Fetal prognosis after anesthesia during gestation. Anesth Analg. 1963;42:521–6.
6. Mazze RI, Kallen B. Reproductive outcome after anesthesia and operation during pregnancy: a registry study of 5405 cases. Am J Obstet Gynecol. 1989;161(5):1178–85.
7. Cohen-Kerem R, Railton C, Oren D, Lishner M, Koren G. Pregnancy outcome following non-obstetric surgical intervention. Am J Surg. 2005;190(3):467–73.
8. Balinskaite V, Bottle A, Sodhi V, Rivers A, Bennett PR, Brett SJ, et al. The risk of adverse pregnancy outcomes following nonobstetric surgery during pregnancy: estimates from a retrospective cohort study of 6.5 million pregnancies. Ann Surg. 2017;266(2):260–6.
9. Carter JE. Biography of Camran Nezhat, MD, FACOG, FACS. JSLS. 2006;10(2):275–80.
10. Kelley WE Jr. The evolution of laparoscopy and the revolution in surgery in the decade of the 1990s. JSLS. 2008;12(4):351–7.
11. Podratz K. Degrees of Freedom: Advances in Gynecological and Obstetrical Surgery. Remembering Milestones and Achievements in Surgery: Inspiring Quality for a Hundred Years 1913-2012. Tampa: Faircount Media Group; 2013. American College of Surgeons; 2012.
12. Nance ML, Nance FC. It is time we told the Emperor about his clothes. J Trauma. 1996;40(2):185–6.
13. Clinical Outcomes of Surgical Therapy Study Group. A comparison of laparoscopically assisted and open colectomy for colon cancer. N Engl J Med. 2004;350:2050–9.
14. Pappas TN, Jacobs DO. Laparoscopic resection for colon cancer—the end of the beginning? N Engl J Med. 2004;350(20):2091–2.
15. Frangeheim H. Endoscopy and gynecology. In: Phillips JM, editor. The range and limits of operating laparoscopy in the diagnosis of sterility. Downey, CA: AAGL; 1978.
16. Hulka JF. Textbook of laparoscopy. Orlando, FL: Grune and Stratton, Inc.; 1985.
17. Martin DC. AAGL manual of endoscopy. Downey, CA: AAGL; 1988.
18. Wheeless CR. Atlas of pelvic surgery. Philadelphia, PA: Lippincott Williams & Wilkins; 1988.
19. Nezhat C, Crowgey SR, Garrison CP. Surgical treatment of endometriosis via laser laparoscopy. Fertil Steril. 1986;45(6):778–83.
20. Nezhat C, Hood J, Winer W, Nexhat F, Crowgey SR, Garrison CP. Videolaseroscopy and laser laparoscopy in gynaecology. Br J Hosp Med. 1987;38(3):219–24.
21. Nezhat C, Crowgey S, Nezhat F. Videolaseroscopy for the treatment of endometriosis associated with infertility. Fertil Steril. 1989;51(2):237–40.
22. Nezhat C, Nezhat F. Evaluation of safety of videolaseroscopic treatment of bowel endometriosis. Scientific Paper, 44th Annual Meeting of the American Fertility Society; Atlanta Hilton and Towers, Atlanta, GA, October 8–13, 1988.
23. Nezhat C, Nezhat F, Nezhat C. Operative laparoscopy (minimally invasive surgery): state of the art. J Gynecol Surg. 1992;8(3):111–41.
24. Semm K. Endoscopic appendectomy. Endoscopy. 1983;15(2):59–64.
25. Perissat J, Collet D, Monguillon N. Advances in laparoscopic surgery. Digestion. 1998;59(5):606–18.
26. Dubois F, Icard P, Berthelot G, Levard H. Coelioscopic cholecystectomy. Preliminary report of 36 cases. Ann Surg. 1990;211(1):60–2.
27. Corbitt JD Jr. Laparoscopic herniorrhaphy. Surg Laparosc Endosc. 1991;1(1):23–5.
28. Corbitt JD Jr. Laparoscopic herniorrhaphy. A preperitoneal tension-free approach. Surg Endosc. 1993;7(6):550–5.
29. Corbitt JD Jr. Transabdominal preperitoneal herniorrhaphy. Surg Laparosc Endosc. 1993;3(4):328–32.
30. MacFadyen BV Jr, Arregui ME, Corbitt JD Jr, Filipi CJ, Fitzgibbons RJ Jr, Franklin ME, et al. Complications of laparoscopic herniorrhaphy. Surg Endosc. 1993;7(3):155–8.
31. Nezhat C, Pennington E, Nezhat F, Silfen SL. Laparoscopically assisted anterior rectal wall resection and reanastomosis for deeply infiltrating endometriosis. Surg Laparosc Endosc. 1991;1(2):106–8.
32. Fowler DL, White SA. Laparoscopy-assisted sigmoid resection. Surg Laparosc Endosc. 1991;1(3):183–8.
33. Jacobs M, Verdeja JC, Goldstein HS. Minimally invasive colon resection (laparoscopic colectomy). Surg Laparosc Endosc. 1991;1(3):144–50.
34. Redwine DB, Sharpe DR. Laparoscopic segmental resection of the sigmoid colon for endometriosis. J Laparoendosc Surg. 1991;1(4):217–20.
35. Bailey RW, Flowers JL, Graham SM, Zucker KA. Combined laparoscopic cholecystectomy and selective vagotomy. Surg Laparosc Endosc. 1991;1(1):45–9.
36. Katkhouda N, Mouiel J. A new technique of surgical treatment of chronic duodenal ulcer without laparotomy by videocoelioscopy. Am J Surg. 1991;161(3):361–4.

37. Flowers JL, Feldman J, Jacobs SC. Laparoscopic pelvic lymphadenectomy. Surg Laparosc Endosc. 1991;1(2):62–70.
38. Tierney JP, Kusminsky RE, Boland JP, Oliver RS Jr. Laparoscopic pelvic lymph node dissection. W V Med J. 1991;87(4):151–2.
39. Clayman RV, Kavoussi LR, Soper NJ, Dierks SM, Merety KS, Darcy MD, et al. Laparoscopic nephrectomy. N Engl J Med. 1991;324(19):1370–1.
40. Nezhat CR, Burrell MO, Nezhat FR, Benigno BB, Welander CE. Laparoscopic radical hysterectomy with paraaortic and pelvic node dissection. Am J Obstet Gynecol. 1992;166(3):864–5.
41. Nezhat F, Nezhat C, Gordon S, Wilkins E. Laparoscopic versus abdominal hysterectomy. J Reprod Med. 1992;37(3):247–50.
42. Nezhat CR, Nezhat FR, Burrell MO, Ramirez CE, Welander C, Carrodeguas J, et al. Laparoscopic radical hysterectomy and laparoscopically assisted vaginal radical hysterectomy with pelvic and paraaortic node dissection. J Gynecol Surg. 1993;9(2):105–20.
43. Carroll BJ, Phillips EH, Semel CJ, Fallas M, Morgenstern L. Laparoscopic splenectomy. Surg Endosc. 1992;6(4):183–5.
44. Hashizume M, Sugimachi K, Ueno K. Laparoscopic splenectomy with an ultrasonic dissector. N Engl J Med. 1992;327(6):438.
45. Gagner M, Lacroix A, Bolte E. Laparoscopic adrenalectomy in Cushing's syndrome and pheochromocytoma. N Engl J Med. 1992;327(14):1033.
46. Dion YM, Gracia CR. A new technique for laparoscopic aortobifemoral grafting in occlusive aortoiliac disease. J Vasc Surg. 1997;26(4):685–92.
47. Sgambati SA, Ballantyne GH. Minimally invasive surgery in the diseases of the colon and rectum: the legacy of an ancient tradition. In: Jager RM, Wexner S, editors. Laparoscopic colectomy. New York: Churchill Livingstone; 1995. p. 13–23.
48. Schuessler WW, Schulam PG, Clayman RV, Kavoussi LR. Laparoscopic radical prostatectomy: initial short-term experience. Urology. 1997;50(6):854–7.
49. Kelley WE, Bailey R, Bertelsen C, et al. Stereotactic automated surgical biopsy using the ABBI biopsy device: a multicenter study. Breast J. 1998;4:302–6.
50. Jobe BA, Duncan W, Swanstrom LL. Totally laparoscopic abdominal aortic aneurysm repair. Surg Endosc. 1999;13(1):77–9.
51. McMahon AJ, Fischbacher CM, Frame SH, MacLeod MC. Impact of laparoscopic cholecystectomy: a population-based study. Lancet. 2000;356(9242):1632–7.
52. Matsumoto M, Hata T, Tsushima Y, Hamanaka S, Yoshitaka H, Shinoura S, et al. Minimally invasive vascular surgery for repair of infrarenal abdominal aortic aneurysm with iliac involvement. J Vasc Surg. 2002;35(4):654–60.
53. Katz MR, Van Praet F, de Canniere D, Murphy D, Siwek L, Seshadri-Kreaden U, et al. Integrated coronary revascularization: percutaneous coronary intervention plus robotic totally endoscopic coronary artery bypass. Circulation. 2006;114(1 Suppl):I473–6.
54. Haynes AB, Weiser TG, Berry WR, Lipsitz SR, Breizat AH, Dellinger EP, et al. A surgical safety checklist to reduce morbidity and mortality in a global population. N Engl J Med. 2009;360(5):491–9.
55. Medeiros LR, Rosa DD, Bozzetti MC, Fachel JM, Furness S, Garry R, et al. Laparoscopy versus laparotomy for benign ovarian tumour. Cochrane Database Syst Rev. 2009;2:CD004751.
56. Lee M, Kim SW, Paek J, Lee SH, Yim GW, Kim JH, et al. Comparisons of surgical outcomes, complications, and costs between laparotomy and laparoscopy in early-stage ovarian cancer. Int J Gynecol Cancer. 2011;21(2):251–6.
57. Galaal K, Bryant A, Fisher AD, Al-Khaduri M, Kew F, Lopes AD. Laparoscopy versus laparotomy for the management of early stage endometrial cancer. Cochrane Database Syst Rev. 2012;9:CD006655.
58. Schwenk W, Bohm B, Muller JM. Postoperative pain and fatigue after laparoscopic or conventional colorectal resections. A prospective randomized trial. Surg Endosc. 1998;12(9):1131–6.
59. Lacy AM, Garcia-Valdecasas JC, Delgado S, Grande L, Fuster J, Tabet J, et al. Postoperative complications of laparoscopic-assisted colectomy. Surg Endosc. 1997;11(2):119–22.
60. Lacy AM, Garcia-Valdecasas JC, Delgado S, Castells A, Taura P, Pique JM, et al. Laparoscopy-assisted colectomy versus open colectomy for treatment of non-metastatic colon cancer: a randomised trial. Lancet. 2002;359(9325):2224–9.
61. Cruse PJ, Foord R. The epidemiology of wound infection. A 10-year prospective study of 62,939 wounds. Surg Clin North Am. 1980;60(1):27–40.
62. Bucknall TE, Cox PJ, Ellis H. Burst abdomen and incisional hernia: a prospective study of 1129 major laparotomies. Br Med J (Clin Res Ed). 1982;284(6320):931–3.
63. Nezhat C. Operative endoscopy will replace almost all open procedures. JSLS. 2004;8(2):101–2.
64. Nezhat F, Nezhat C, Silfen SL, Fehnel SH. Laparoscopic ovarian cystectomy during pregnancy. J Laparoendosc Surg. 1991;1(3):161–4.
65. Tazuke SI, Nezhat FR, Nezhat CH, Seidman DS, Phillips DR, Nezhat CR. Laparoscopic management of pelvic pathology during pregnancy. J Am Assoc Gynecol Laparosc. 1997;4(5):605–8.
66. Beebe DS, Swica H, Carlson N, Palahniuk RJ, Goodale RL. High levels of carbon monoxide are produced by electro-cautery of tissue during laparoscopic cholecystectomy. Anesth Analg. 1993;77(2):338–41.
67. Ott D. Smoke production and smoke reduction in endoscopic surgery: preliminary report. Endosc Surg Allied Technol. 1993;1(4):230–2.
68. Nezhat C, Seidman DS, Vreman HJ, Stevenson DK, Nezhat F, Nezhat C. The risk of carbon monoxide

poisoning after prolonged laparoscopic surgery. Obstet Gynecol. 1996;88(5):771–4.
69. Callery MP, Soper NJ. Physiology of the pneumoperitoneum. Baillieres Clin Gastroenterol. 1993;7(4):757–77.
70. Barnard JM, Chaffin D, Droste S, Tierney A, Phernetton T. Fetal response to carbon dioxide pneumoperitoneum in the pregnant ewe. Obstet Gynecol. 1995;85(5 Pt 1):669–74.
71. Hunter JG, Swanstrom L, Thornburg K. Carbon dioxide pneumoperitoneum induces fetal acidosis in a pregnant ewe model. Surg Endosc. 1995;9(3):272–7. discussion 7-9
72. Curet MJ, Vogt DA, Schob O, Qualls C, Izquierdo LA, Zucker KA. Effects of CO2 pneumoperitoneum in pregnant ewes. J Surg Res. 1996;63(1):339–44.
73. Uemura K, McClaine RJ, de la Fuente SG, Manson RJ, Campbell KA, McClaine DJ, et al. Maternal insufflation during the second trimester equivalent produces hypercapnia, acidosis, and prolonged hypoxia in fetal sheep. Anesthesiology. 2004;101(6):1332–8.
74. Candiani M, Maddalena S, Barbieri M, Izzo S, Alberico D, Ronzoni S. Adnexal masses in pregnancy: fetomaternal blood flow indices during laparoscopic surgery. J Minim Invasive Gynecol. 2012;19(4):443–7.
75. Barnett MB, Liu DT. Complication of laparoscopy during early pregnancy. Br Med J. 1974;1:328.
76. Reedy M, Galan H, Richards W, et al. Laparoscopy during pregnancy: a survey of the Society of Laparoendoscopic Surgeons. Am J Obstet Gynecol. 1995;172:289.
77. Remorgida V, Carrer C, Ferraiolo A, Natucci M, Anserini P. Laparoscopic surgery in pregnancy. A case report with a brief review of the topic. Surg Endosc. 1995;9(2):195–6.
78. Parker WH, Childers JM, Canis M, Phillips DR, Topel H. Laparoscopic management of benign cystic teratomas during pregnancy. Am J Obstet Gynecol. 1996;174(5):1499–501.
79. Reedy MB, Galan HL, Richards WE, Preece CK, Wetter PA, Kuehl TJ. Laparoscopy during pregnancy. A survey of laparoendoscopic surgeons. J Reprod Med. 1997;42(1):33–8.
80. Reedy MB, Kallen B, Kuehl TJ. Laparoscopy during pregnancy: a study of five fetal outcome parameters with use of the Swedish Health Registry. Am J Obstet Gynecol. 1997;177(3):673–9.
81. Andreoli M, Servakov M, Meyers P, Mann WJ Jr. Laparoscopic surgery during pregnancy. J Am Assoc Gynecol Laparosc. 1999;6(2):229–33.
82. Al-Fozan H, Tulandi T. Safety and risks of laparoscopy in pregnancy. Curr Opin Obstet Gynecol. 2002;14(4):375–9.
83. Mathevet P, Nessah K, Dargent D, Mellier G. Laparoscopic management of adnexal masses in pregnancy: a case series. Eur J Obstet Gynecol Reprod Biol. 2003;108(2):217–22.
84. Oelsner G, Stockheim D, Soriano D, Goldenberg M, Seidman DS, Cohen SB, et al. Pregnancy outcome after laparoscopy or laparotomy in pregnancy. J Am Assoc Gynecol Laparosc. 2003;10(2):200–4.
85. Melnick DM, Wahl WL, Dalton VK. Management of general surgical problems in the pregnant patient. Am J Surg. 2004;187(2):170–80.
86. Guidelines Committee of the Society of American G, Endoscopic S, Yumi H. Guidelines for diagnosis, treatment, and use of laparoscopy for surgical problems during pregnancy: this statement was reviewed and approved by the Board of Governors of the Society of American Gastrointestinal and Endoscopic Surgeons (SAGES), September 2007. It was prepared by the SAGES Guidelines Committee. Surg Endosc. 2008;22(4):849–61.
87. Buttery BW, Beischer NA, Fortune DW, Macafee CA. Ovarian tumours in pregnancy. Med J Aust. 1973;1(7):345–9.
88. Soriano D, Yefet Y, Seidman DS, Goldenberg M, Mashiach S, Oelsner G. Laparoscopy versus laparotomy in the management of adnexal masses during pregnancy. Fertil Steril. 1999;71(5):955–60.
89. Practice ACoO. ACOG Committee Opinion No. 474: nonobstetric surgery during pregnancy. Obstet Gynecol. 2011;117(2 Pt 1):420–1.
90. Bhavani-Shankar K, Steinbrook RA, Brooks DC, Datta S. Arterial to end-tidal carbon dioxide pressure difference during laparoscopic surgery in pregnancy. Anesthesiology. 2000;93(2):370–3.
91. Curet MJ, Allen D, Josloff RK, Pitcher DE, Curet LB, Miscall BG, et al. Laparoscopy during pregnancy. Arch Surg. 1996;131(5):546–50. discussion 50-1
92. Guidelines for laparoscopic surgery during pregnancy. Surg Endosc. 1998;12(2):189–90.
93. Reynolds JD, Booth JV, de la Fuente S, Punnahitananda S, McMahon RL, Hopkins MB, et al. A review of laparoscopy for non-obstetric-related surgery during pregnancy. Curr Surg. 2003;60(2):164–73.
94. Moreno-Sanz C, Pascual-Pedreno A, Picazo-Yeste JS, Seoane-Gonzalez JB. Laparoscopic appendectomy during pregnancy: between personal experiences and scientific evidence. J Am Coll Surg. 2007;205(1):37–42.
95. Iafrati MD, Yarnell R, Schwaitzberg SD. Gasless laparoscopic cholecystectomy in pregnancy. J Laparoendosc Surg. 1995;5(2):127–30.
96. Romer T, Bojahr B, Schwesinger G. Treatment of a torqued hematosalpinx in the thirteenth week of pregnancy using gasless laparoscopy. J Am Assoc Gynecol Laparosc. 2002;9(1):89–92.
97. Melgrati L, Damiani A, Franzoni G, Marziali M, Sesti F. Isobaric (gasless) laparoscopic myomectomy during pregnancy. J Minim Invasive Gynecol. 2005;12(4):379–81.
98. Goldberg JM, Maurer WG. A randomized comparison of gasless laparoscopy and CO2 pneumoperitoneum. Obstet Gynecol. 1997;90(3):416–20.
99. Walsh CA, Tang T, Walsh SR. Laparoscopic versus open appendicectomy in pregnancy: a systematic review. Int J Surg. 2008;6(4):339–44.

100. Reitman E, Flood P. Anaesthetic considerations for non-obstetric surgery during pregnancy. Br J Anaesth. 2011;107(Suppl 1):i72–8.
101. Gurbuz AT, Peetz ME. The acute abdomen in the pregnant patient: is there a role for laparoscopy? Surg Endosc. 1997;11(2):98–102.
102. Corneille MG, Gallup TM, Bening T, Wolf SE, Brougher C, Myers JG, et al. The use of laparoscopic surgery in pregnancy: evaluation of safety and efficacy. Am J Surg. 2010;200(3):363–7.
103. Schreiber JH. Laparoscopic appendectomy in pregnancy. Surg Endosc. 1990;4(2):100–2.
104. Mazze RI, Kallen B. Appendectomy during pregnancy: a Swedish registry study of 778 cases. Obstet Gynecol. 1991;77(6):835–40.
105. Cristalli B, Nos C, Heid M, Levardon M. Laparoscopy, appendicitis and pregnancy. J Gynecol Obstet Biol Reprod (Paris). 1992;21(4):449.
106. Andersen B, Nielsen TF. Appendicitis in pregnancy: diagnosis, management and complications. Acta Obstet Gynecol Scand. 1999;78(9):758–62.
107. Cunningham FG, McCubbin JH. Appendicitis complicating pregnancy. Obstet Gynecol. 1975;45:415–20.
108. Augustin G, Majerovic M. Non-obstetrical acute abdomen during pregnancy. Eur J Obstet Gynecol Reprod Biol. 2007;131(1):4–12.
109. Diegelmann L. Nonobstetric abdominal pain and surgical emergencies in pregnancy. Emerg Med Clin North Am. 2012;30(4):885–901.
110. Guttman R, Goldman RD, Koren G. Appendicitis during pregnancy. Can Fam Physician. 2004;50:355–7.
111. Humes DJ, Simpson J. Acute appendicitis. BMJ. 2006;333(7567):530–4.
112. Babaknia A, Parsa H, Woodruff JD. Appendicitis during pregnancy. Obstet Gynecol. 1977;50(1):40–4.
113. Gomez A, Wood M. Acute appendicitis during pregnancy. Am J Surg. 1979;137(2):180–3.
114. Ghazanfar A, Nasir SM, Choudary ZA, Ahmad W. Acute appendicitis complicating pregnancy; experience with the management of 50 patients. J Ayub Med Coll Abbottabad. 2002;14(3):19–21.
115. Fallon WF Jr, Newman JS, Fallon GL, Malangoni MA. The surgical management of intra-abdominal inflammatory conditions during pregnancy. Surg Clin North Am. 1995;75(1):15–31.
116. Rollins MD, Chan KJ, Price RR. Laparoscopy for appendicitis and cholelithiasis during pregnancy: a new standard of care. Surg Endosc. 2004;18(2):237–41.
117. Halkic N, Tempia-Caliera AA, Ksontini R, Suter M, Delaloye JF, Vuilleumier H. Laparoscopic management of appendicitis and symptomatic cholelithiasis during pregnancy. Langenbecks Arch Surg. 2006;391(5):467–71.
118. McGory ML, Zingmond DS, Tillou A, Hiatt JR, Ko CY, Cryer HM. Negative appendectomy in pregnant women is associated with a substantial risk of fetal loss. J Am Coll Surg. 2007;205(4):534–40.
119. Lemieux P, Rheaume P, Levesque I, Bujold E, Brochu G. Laparoscopic appendectomy in pregnant patients: a review of 45 cases. Surg Endosc. 2009;23(8):1701–5.
120. Affleck DG, Handrahan DL, Egger MJ, Price RR. The laparoscopic management of appendicitis and cholelithiasis during pregnancy. Am J Surg. 1999;178(6):523–9.
121. de Perrot M, Jenny A, Morales M, Kohlik M, Morel P. Laparoscopic appendectomy during pregnancy. Surg Laparosc Endosc Percutan Tech. 2000;10(6):368–71.
122. Wu JM, Chen KH, Lin HF, Tseng LM, Tseng SH, Huang SH. Laparoscopic appendectomy in pregnancy. J Laparoendosc Adv Surg Tech A. 2005;15(5):447–50.
123. Palanivelu C, Rangarajan M, Parthasarathi R. Laparoscopic appendectomy in pregnancy: a case series of seven patients. JSLS. 2006;10(3):321–5.
124. Page AJ, Pollock JD, Perez S, Davis SS, Lin E, Sweeney JF. Laparoscopic versus open appendectomy: an analysis of outcomes in 17,199 patients using ACS/NSQIP. J Gastrointest Surg. 2010;14(12):1955–62.
125. Sadot E, Telem DA, Arora M, Butala P, Nguyen SQ, Divino CM. Laparoscopy: a safe approach to appendicitis during pregnancy. Surg Endosc. 2010;24(2):383–9.
126. Wei B, Qi CL, Chen TF, Zheng ZH, Huang JL, Hu BG, et al. Laparoscopic versus open appendectomy for acute appendicitis: a metaanalysis. Surg Endosc. 2011;25(4):1199–208.
127. Eom JM, Hong JH, Jeon SW, Choi JS, Lee JH, Kim HO, et al. Safety and clinical efficacy of laparoscopic appendectomy for pregnant women with acute appendicitis. Ann Acad Med Singapore. 2012;41(2):82–6.
128. Mohamed AA, Mahran KM. Laparoscopic appendectomy in complicated appendicitis: is it safe? J Minim Access Surg. 2013;9(2):55–8.
129. Peled Y, Hiersch L, Khalpari O, Wiznitzer A, Yogev Y, Pardo J. Appendectomy during pregnancy--is pregnancy outcome depending by operation technique? J Matern Fetal Neonatal Med. 2014;27(4):365–7.
130. Cheng HT, Wang YC, Lo HC, Su LT, Soh KS, Tzeng CW, et al. Laparoscopic appendectomy versus open appendectomy in pregnancy: a population-based analysis of maternal outcome. Surg Endosc. 2015;29(6):1394–9.
131. Thomson JE, Kruger D, Jann-Kruger C, Kiss A, Omoshoro-Jones JA, Luvhengo T, et al. Laparoscopic versus open surgery for complicated appendicitis: a randomized controlled trial to prove safety. Surg Endosc. 2015;29(7):2027–32.
132. Cox TC, Huntington CR, Blair LJ, Prasad T, Lincourt AE, Augenstein VA, et al. Laparoscopic appendectomy and cholecystectomy versus open: a study in 1999 pregnant patients. Surg Endosc. 2016;30(2):593–602.

133. Laustsen JF, Bjerring OS, Johannessen O, Qvist N. Laparoscopic appendectomy during pregnancy is safe for both the mother and the fetus. Dan Med J. 2016;63(8):A5259.
134. Segev L, Segev Y, Rayman S, Shapiro R, Nissan A, Sadot E. Appendectomy in pregnancy: appraisal of the minimally invasive approach. J Laparoendosc Adv Surg Tech A. 2016;26(11):893–7.
135. Puylaert JB, Rutgers PH, Lalisang RI, de Vries BC, van der Werf SD, Dorr JP, et al. A prospective study of ultrasonography in the diagnosis of appendicitis. N Engl J Med. 1987;317(11):666–9.
136. Greenhalgh R, Punwani S, Taylor SA. Is MRI routinely indicated in pregnant patients with suspected appendicitis after equivocal ultrasound examination? Abdom Imaging. 2008;33:21–5.
137. Spalluto LB, Grand DJ. MRI of acute appendicitis in the pregnant patient. Med Health R I. 2012;95(2):39–40.
138. Yan J, Sabbagh R, Adu A, Gilet A. MRI of early appendicitis during pregnancy. BMJ Case Rep. 2012;2012:bcr2012006878.
139. Burke LM, Bashir MR, Miller FH, Siegelman ES, Brown M, Alobaidy M, et al. Magnetic resonance imaging of acute appendicitis in pregnancy: a 5-year multi-institutional study. Am J Obstet Gynecol. 2015;213(5):693.e1–6.
140. Baron KT, Arleo EK, Robinson C, Sanelli PC. Comparing the diagnostic performance of MRI versus CT in the evaluation of acute nontraumatic abdominal pain during pregnancy. Emerg Radiol. 2012;19(6):519–25.
141. Leyendecker JR, Gorengaut V, Brown JJ. MR imaging of maternal diseases of the abdomen and pelvis during pregnancy and the immediate postpartum period. Radiographics. 2004;24(5):1301–16.
142. Patel SJ, Reede DL, Katz DS, Subramaniam R, Amorosa JK. Imaging the pregnant patient for nonobstetric conditions: algorithms and radiation dose considerations. Radiographics. 2007;27(6):1705–22.
143. Katz DS, Klein MA, Ganson G, Hines JJ. Imaging of abdominal pain in pregnancy. Radiol Clin North Am. 2012;50(1):149–71.
144. Karul M, Berliner C, Keller S, Tsui TY, Yamamura J. Imaging of appendicitis in adults. Rofo. 2014;186(6):551–8.
145. Masselli G, Brunelli R, Monti R, Guida M, Laghi F, Casciani E, et al. Imaging for acute pelvic pain in pregnancy. Insights Imaging. 2014;5(2):165–81.
146. Timins JK. Radiation during pregnancy. N J Med. 2001;98(6):29–33.
147. Hurwitz LM, Yoshizumi T, Reiman RE, Goodman PC, Paulson EK, Frush DP, et al. Radiation dose to the fetus from body MDCT during early gestation. AJR Am J Roentgenol. 2006;186(3):871–6.
148. Tseng JY, Yang MJ, Yang CC, Chao KC, Li HY. Acute cholecystitis during pregnancy: what is the best approach? Taiwan J Obstet Gynecol. 2009;48(3):305–7.
149. Lu EJ, Curet MJ, El-Sayed YY, Kirkwood KS. Medical versus surgical management of biliary tract disease in pregnancy. Am J Surg. 2004;188(6):755–9.
150. Jelin EB, Smink DS, Vernon AH, Brooks DC. Management of biliary tract disease during pregnancy: a decision analysis. Surg Endosc. 2008;22(1):54–60.
151. Othman MO, Stone E, Hashimi M, Parasher G. Conservative management of cholelithiasis and its complications in pregnancy is associated with recurrent symptoms and more emergency department visits. Gastrointest Endosc. 2012;76(3):564–9.
152. Silvestri MT, Pettker CM, Brousseau EC, Dick MA, Ciarleglio MM, Erekson EA. Morbidity of appendectomy and cholecystectomy in pregnant and nonpregnant women. Obstet Gynecol. 2011;118(6):1261–70.
153. Nasioudis D, Tsilimigras D, Economopoulos KP. Laparoscopic cholecystectomy during pregnancy: a systematic review of 590 patients. Int J Surg. 2016;27:165–75.
154. Chong VH, Jalihal A. Endoscopic management of biliary disorders during pregnancy. Hepatobiliary Pancreat Dis Int. 2010;9(2):180–5.
155. Jouppila P, Mokka R, Larmi TK. Acute pancreatitis in pregnancy. Surg Gynecol Obstet. 1974;139(6):879–82.
156. Woodhouse CR. Acute pancreatitis associated with pregnancy. Br J Clin Pract. 1977;31(6):79–84.
157. Nathan L, Huddleston JF. Acute abdominal pain in pregnancy. Obstet Gynecol Clin North Am. 1995;22(1):55–68.
158. Ramin KD, Ramin SM, Richey SD, Cunningham FG. Acute pancreatitis in pregnancy. Am J Obstet Gynecol. 1995;173(1):187–91.
159. Scott LD. Gallstone disease and pancreatitis in pregnancy. Gastroenterol Clin North Am. 1992;21(4):803–15.
160. Swisher SG, Schmit PJ, Hunt KK, Hiyama DT, Bennion RS, Swisher EM, et al. Biliary disease during pregnancy. Am J Surg. 1994;168(6):576–9. discussion 80-1
161. Beck WW Jr. Intestinal obstruction in pregnancy. Obstet Gynecol. 1974;43(3):374–8.
162. Connolly MM, Unti JA, Nora PF. Bowel obstruction in pregnancy. Surg Clin North Am. 1995;75(1):101–13.
163. Hill LM, Symmonds RE. Small bowel obstruction in pregnancy. A review and report of four cases. Obstet Gynecol. 1977;49(2):170–3.
164. Perdue PW, Johnson HW Jr, Stafford PW. Intestinal obstruction complicating pregnancy. Am J Surg. 1992;164(4):384–8.
165. Pratt AT, Donaldson RC, Evertson LR, Yon JL Jr. Cecal volvulus in pregnancy. Obstet Gynecol. 1981;57(6 Suppl):37S–40S.
166. Orchard JL, Mehta R, Khan AH. The use of colonoscopy in the treatment of colonic volvulus: three cases and review of the literature. Am J Gastroenterol. 1984;79(11):864–7.

167. Kim EY, Jun KH, Jung JH, Jo YS, Chin HM. Laparoscopic gastrectomy followed by chemotherapy for advanced gastric cancer diagnosed during pregnancy: a case report. Anticancer Res. 2016;36(9):4813–6.
168. Alshahrani AS, Yoo MW. Gastric cancer in pregnancy: is laparoscopic gastrectomy with lymph node dissection feasible and safe? Ann Surg Treat Res. 2017;92(1):51–3.
169. van Basten JP, Knipscheer B, de Kruif J. Case report: retroperitoneoscopic tumor nephrectomy during pregnancy. J Endourol. 2006;20(3):186–7.
170. Parker WH, Levine RL, Howard FM, Sansone B, Berek JS. A multicenter study of laparoscopic management of selected cystic adnexal masses in postmenopausal women. J Am Coll Surg. 1994;179(6):733–7.
171. Tazuke S, Nezhat CR, Phillips DR, Roemisch M. Removal of adnexal masses by operative laparoscopy during pregnancy. J Am Assoc Gynecol Laparosc. 1996;3(4 Suppl):S50.
172. Yuen PM, Chang AM. Laparoscopic management of adnexal mass during pregnancy. Acta Obstet Gynecol Scand. 1997;76(2):173–6.
173. Stepp KJ, Tulikangas PK, Goldberg JM, Attaran M, Falcone T. Laparoscopy for adnexal masses in the second trimester of pregnancy. J Am Assoc Gynecol Laparosc. 2003;10(1):55–9.
174. Balthazar U, Steiner AZ, Boggess JF, Gehrig PA. Management of a persistent adnexal mass in pregnancy: what is the ideal surgical approach? J Minim Invasive Gynecol. 2011;18(6):720–5.
175. Koo YJ, Kim HJ, Lim KT, Lee IH, Lee KH, Shim JU, et al. Laparotomy versus laparoscopy for the treatment of adnexal masses during pregnancy. Aust N Z J Obstet Gynaecol. 2012;52(1):34–8.
176. Shalev E, Bustan M, Yarom I, Peleg D. Recovery of ovarian function after laparoscopic detorsion. Hum Reprod. 1995;10(11):2965–6.
177. Purnichescu V, Cheret-Benoist A, Von Theobald P, Mayaud A, Herlicoviez M, Dreyfus M. Laparoscopic management of pelvic mass in pregnancy. J Gynecol Obstet Biol Reprod (Paris). 2006;35(4):388–95.
178. Ko ML, Lai TH, Chen SC. Laparoscopic management of complicated adnexal masses in the first trimester of pregnancy. Fertil Steril. 2009;92(1):283–7.
179. Kim M. Laparoscopic management of a twisted ovarian leiomyoma in a woman with 10 weeks' gestation. Medicine (Baltimore). 2016;95(44):e5319.
180. Lavery JP, Koontz WL, Layman L, Shaw L, Gumpel U. Sonographic evaluation of the adnexa during early pregnancy. Surg Gynecol Obstet. 1986;163(4):319–23.
181. Giuntoli RL 2nd, Vang RS, Bristow RE. Evaluation and management of adnexal masses during pregnancy. Clin Obstet Gynecol. 2006;49(3):492–505.
182. Leiserowitz GS. Managing ovarian masses during pregnancy. Obstet Gynecol Surv. 2006;61(7):463–70.
183. Struyk AP, Treffers PE. Ovarian tumors in pregnancy. Acta Obstet Gynecol Scand. 1984;63(5):421–4.
184. Bernhard LM, Klebba PK, Gray DL, Mutch DG. Predictors of persistence of adnexal masses in pregnancy. Obstet Gynecol. 1999;93(4):585–9.
185. Tawa K. Ovarian tumors in pregnancy. Am J Obstet Gynecol. 1964;90:511–6.
186. Hess LW, Peaceman A, O'Brien WF, Winkel CA, Cruikshank DP, Morrison JC. Adnexal mass occurring with intrauterine pregnancy: report of fifty-four patients requiring laparotomy for definitive management. Am J Obstet Gynecol. 1988;158(5):1029–34.
187. Grendys EC Jr, Barnes WA. Ovarian cancer in pregnancy. Surg Clin North Am. 1995;75(1):1–14.
188. Whitecar MP, Turner S, Higby MK. Adnexal masses in pregnancy: a review of 130 cases undergoing surgical management. Am J Obstet Gynecol. 1999;181(1):19–24.
189. Kumari I, Kaur S, Mohan H, Huria A. Adnexal masses in pregnancy: a 5-year review. Aust N Z J Obstet Gynaecol. 2006;46(1):52–4.
190. Leiserowitz GS, Xing G, Cress R, Brahmbhatt B, Dalrymple JL, Smith LH. Adnexal masses in pregnancy: how often are they malignant? Gynecol Oncol. 2006;101(2):315–21.
191. Yen CF, Lin SL, Murk W, Wang CJ, Lee CL, Soong YK, et al. Risk analysis of torsion and malignancy for adnexal masses during pregnancy. Fertil Steril. 2009;91(5):1895–902.
192. Roberts JA. Management of gynecologic tumors during pregnancy. Clin Perinatol. 1983;10(2):369–82.
193. Nezhat FR, Tazuke S, Nezhat CH, Seidman DS, Phillips DR, Nezhat CR. Laparoscopy during pregnancy: a literature review. JSLS. 1997;1(1):17–27.
194. Sayar H, Lhomme C, Verschraegen CF. Malignant adnexal masses in pregnancy. Obstet Gynecol Clin North Am. 2005;32(4):569–93.
195. Logsdon-Pokorny VK. Gynecologic surgery during pregnancy. Clin Obstet Gynecol. 1994;37(2):294–305.
196. Wang PH, Chao HT, Yuan CC, Lee WL, Chao KC, Ng HT. Ovarian tumors complicating pregnancy. Emergency and elective surgery. J Reprod Med. 1999;44(3):279–87.
197. Hill LM, Johnson CE, Lee RA. Ovarian surgery in pregnancy. Am J Obstet Gynecol. 1975;122(5):565–9.
198. Moore RD, Smith WG. Laparoscopic management of adnexal masses in pregnant women. J Reprod Med. 1999;44(2):97–100.
199. Fatum M, Rojansky N. Laparoscopic surgery during pregnancy. Obstet Gynecol Surv. 2001;56(1):50–9.
200. Lin YH, Hwang JL, Huang LW, Seow KM. Successful laparoscopic management of a huge ovarian tumor in the 27th week of pregnancy. A case report. J Reprod Med. 2003;48(10):834–6.
201. Yuen PM, Ng PS, Leung PL, Rogers MS. Outcome in laparoscopic management of persistent adnexal mass during the second trimester of pregnancy. Surg Endosc. 2004;18(9):1354–7.
202. Ribic-Pucelj M, Kobal B, Peternelj-Marinsek S. Surgical treatment of adnexal masses in preg-

nancy: indications, surgical approach and pregnancy outcome. J Reprod Med. 2007;52(4):273–9.
203. Mage G, Canis M, Manhes H, Pouly JL, Bruhat MA. Laparoscopic management of adnexal torsion. A review of 35 cases. J Reprod Med. 1989;34(8):520–4.
204. Shalev E, Rahav D, Romano S. Laparoscopic relief of adnexal torsion in early pregnancy. Case reports. Br J Obstet Gynaecol. 1990;97(9):853–4.
205. Ozcan U, Vicdan K, Oguz S, Taner MZ, Caglar AT. Torsion of the normal adnexa in early pregnancy and laparoscopic detorsion. J Pak Med Assoc. 1992;42(5):127–8.
206. Morice P, Louis-Sylvestre C, Chapron C, Dubuisson JB. Laparoscopy for adnexal torsion in pregnant women. J Reprod Med. 1997;42(7):435–9.
207. Pezzuto A, Steinkasserer M, Tricolore C, Ferrari B, Nardelli GB, Minelli L. Successful laparoscopic management of adnexal torsion during week 15 of a single pregnancy. J Minim Invasive Gynecol. 2010;17(6):686.
208. Weiner E, Mizrachi Y, Keidar R, Kerner R, Golan A, Sagiv R. Laparoscopic surgery performed in advanced pregnancy compared to early pregnancy. Arch Gynecol Obstet. 2015;292(5):1063–8.
209. Louis-Sylvestre C, Morice P, Chapron C, Dubuisson JB. The role of laparoscopy in the diagnosis and management of heterotopic pregnancies. Hum Reprod. 1997;12(5):1100–2.
210. Currie A, Bradley E, McEwen M, Al-Shabibi N, Willson PD. Laparoscopic approach to fibroid torsion presenting as an acute abdomen in pregnancy. JSLS. 2013;17(4):665–7.
211. Sesti F, Pietropolli A, Sesti FF, Piccione E. Gasless laparoscopic surgery during pregnancy: evaluation of its role and usefulness. Eur J Obstet Gynecol Reprod Biol. 2013;170(1):8–12.
212. Dubuisson JB, Fauconnier A, Deffarges JV, Norgaard C, Kreiker G, Chapron C. Pregnancy outcome and deliveries following laparoscopic myomectomy. Hum Reprod. 2000;15(4):869–73.
213. De Carolis S, Fatigante G, Ferrazzani S, Trivellini C, De Santis L, Mancuso S, et al. Uterine myomectomy in pregnant women. Fetal Diagn Ther. 2001;16(2):116–9.
214. Hurst BS, Matthews ML, Marshburn PB. Laparoscopic myomectomy for symptomatic uterine myomas. Fertil Steril. 2005;83(1):1–23.
215. Duggan B, Muderspach LI, Roman LD, Curtin JP, d'Ablaing G 3rd, Morrow CP. Cervical cancer in pregnancy: reporting on planned delay in therapy. Obstet Gynecol. 1993;82(4 Pt 1):598–602.
216. Hertel H, Possover M, Kuhne-Heid R, Schneider A. Laparoscopic lymph node staging of cervical cancer in the 19th week of pregnancy. A case report. Surg Endosc. 2001;15(3):324.
217. Marnitz S, Schmittel A, Bolbrinker J, Schmidt FP, Fons G, Kalache K, et al. The therapeutic management of a twin pregnancy complicated by the presence of cervical cancer, following laparoscopic staging and chemotherapy, with an emphasis on cisplatin concentrations in the fetomaternal compartments amnion fluid, umbilical cord, and maternal serum. Fertil Steril. 2009;92(5):1748 e1–4.
218. Favero G, Chiantera V, Oleszczuk A, Gallotta V, Hertel H, Herrmann J, et al. Invasive cervical cancer during pregnancy: laparoscopic nodal evaluation before oncologic treatment delay. Gynecol Oncol. 2010;118(2):123–7.
219. Bravo E, Parry S, Alonso C, Rojas S. Radical vaginal trachelectomy and laparoscopic pelvic lymphadenectomy in IB1 cervical cancer during pregnancy. Gynecol Oncol Case Rep. 2012;2(3):78–9.
220. Shepherd JH, Crawford RA, Oram DH. Radical trachelectomy: a way to preserve fertility in the treatment of early cervical cancer. Br J Obstet Gynaecol. 1998;105(8):912–6.
221. Dargent D, Martin X, Sacchetoni A, Mathevet P. Laparoscopic vaginal radical trachelectomy: a treatment to preserve the fertility of cervical carcinoma patients. Cancer. 2000;88(8):1877–82.
222. Nezhat C, Nezhat F, editors. Videolaseroscopy for the treatment of endometriosis. Monteral, QC: American Fertility Society (ASRM); 1985.
223. Nezhat C, Nezhat F, editor Videolaseroscopy for the treatment of endometriosis. American College of Obstetricians and Gynecologists Annual Meeting; Las Vegas, NV. 1987.
224. Nezhat C, Nezhat F. Evaluation of safety of videolaseroscopic treatment of bowel endometriosis. 1988.
225. Nezhat C, Winer WK, Nezhat F. Laparoscopic removal of dermoid cysts. Obstet Gynecol. 1989;73(2):278–81.
226. Nezhat C, Nezhat F. Conservative management of ectopic gestation. Fertil Steril. 1990;53(2):382–3.
227. Nezhat CR, Nezhat FR, Silfen SL. Videolaseroscopy. The CO2 laser for advanced operative laparoscopy. Obstet Gynecol Clin North Am. 1991;18(3):585–604.
228. Nezhat C, Nezhat F. Laparoscopic repair of ureter resected during operative laparoscopy. Obstet Gynecol. 1992;80(3 Pt 2):543–4.
229. Nezhat C, Nezhat F, Green B. Laparoscopic treatment of obstructed ureter due to endometriosis by resection and ureteroureterostomy: a case report. J Urol. 1992;148(3:865–8.
230. Nezhat F, Nezhat C. Operative laparoscopy for the treatment of ovarian remnant syndrome. Fertil Steril. 1992;57(5):1003–7.
231. Nezhat F, Nezhat C, Allan CJ, Metzger DA, Sears DL. Clinical and histologic classification of endometriomas. Implications for a mechanism of pathogenesis. J Reprod Med. 1992;37(9):771–6.
232. Nezhat F, Nezhat C, Levy JS. Laparoscopic treatment of symptomatic diaphragmatic endometriosis: a case report. Fertil Steril. 1992;58(3):614–6.
233. Nezhat F, Nezhat C, Pennington E. Laparoscopic proctectomy for infiltrating endometriosis of the rectum. Fertil Steril. 1992;57(5):1129–32.
234. Nezhat F, Nezhat C, Pennington E, Ambroze W Jr. Laparoscopic segmental resection for infil-

trating endometriosis of the rectosigmoid colon: a preliminary report. Surg Laparosc Endosc. 1992;2(3):212–6.
235. Nezhat CR, Nezhat FR. Laparoscopic segmental bladder resection for endometriosis: a report of two cases. Obstet Gynecol. 1993;81(5 (Pt 2)):882–4.
236. Nezhat C, Nezhat F, Ambroze W, Pennington E. Laparoscopic repair of small bowel and colon. A report of 26 cases. Surg Endosc. 1993;7(2):88–9.
237. Nezhat CH, Nezhat F, Nezhat C. Laparoscopic sacral colpopexy for vaginal vault prolapse. Obstet Gynecol. 1994;84(5):885–8.
238. Nezhat CH, Nezhat F, Nezhat C, Rottenberg H. Laparoscopic repair of a vesicovaginal fistula: a case report. Obstet Gynecol. 1994;83(5 Pt 2):899–901.
239. Nezhat C, Nezhat F, Bess O, Nezhat CH, Mashiach R. Laparoscopically assisted myomectomy: a report of a new technique in 57 cases. Int J Fertil Menopausal Stud. 1994;39(1):39–44.
240. Nezhat C, Nezhat F, Pennington E, Nezhat CH, Ambroze W. Laparoscopic disk excision and primary repair of the anterior rectal wall for the treatment of full-thickness bowel endometriosis. Surg Endosc. 1994;8(6):682–5.
241. Amara DP, Nezhat C, Teng NN, Nezhat F, Nezhat C, Rosati M. Operative laparoscopy in the management of ovarian cancer. Surg Laparosc Endosc. 1996;6(1):38–45.
242. Nezhat CH, Nezhat F, Seidman DS, Nezhat C. Vaginal vault evisceration after total laparoscopic hysterectomy. Obstet Gynecol. 1996;87(5 Pt 2):868–70.
243. Nezhat C, Childers J, Nezhat F, Nezhat CH, Seidman DS. Major retroperitoneal vascular injury during laparoscopic surgery. Hum Reprod. 1997;12(3):480–3.
244. Nezhat CH, Nezhat FR, Freiha F, Nezhat CR. Laparoscopic vesicopsoas hitch for infiltrative ureteral endometriosis. Fertil Steril. 1999;71(2):376–9.
245. Jacobson MT, Oesterling S, Milki A, Nezhat C. Laparoscopic control of a leaking inferior mesenteric vessel secondary to trocar injury. JSLS. 2002;6(4):389–91.
246. Jacobson MT, Osias J, Velasco A, Charles R, Nezhat C. Laparoscopic repair of a uteroperitoneal fistula. JSLS. 2003;7(4):367–9.
247. Nezhat CH, Malik S, Nezhat F, Nezhat C. Laparoscopic ureteroneocystostomy and vesicopsoas hitch for infiltrative endometriosis. JSLS. 2004;8(1):3–7.
248. Nezhat C, Kazerooni T, Berker B, Lashay N, Fernandez S, Marziali M. Laparoscopic management of hepatic endometriosis: report of two cases and review of the literature. J Minim Invasive Gynecol. 2005;12(3):196–200.
249. Nezhat C, King LP, Paka C, Odegaard J, Beygui R. Bilateral thoracic endometriosis affecting the lung and diaphragm. JSLS. 2012;16(1):140–2.
250. Nezhat C, Main J, Paka C, Nezhat A, Beygui RE. Multidisciplinary treatment for thoracic and abdominopelvic endometriosis. JSLS. 2014;18(3):e2014.00312.
251. Pearl JP, Price RR, Tonkin AE, Richardson WS, Stefanidis D. SAGES guidelines for the use of laparoscopy during pregnancy. Surg Endosc. 2017;31(10):3767–82.

Neurological Pathway of Non-obstetric Pain During Pregnancy

2

Michal Rosen Shaubi, Laura Cancelliere, Corey Sermer, Adrienne L. K. Li, and Nucelio L. B. M. Lemos

Introduction

Although physiologic to pregnancy, adaptations in the bony pelvis and pelvic floor muscles, vasculature, and viscera themselves may cause pain. In addition, any coincidental conditions known to cause or worsen pain may also occur during pregnancy; however, in the altered physiological environment of pregnancy, such known pathologies may present differently or inconsistently. This dynamic interplay between modified physiology and pathology poses a challenge to accurate diagnosis and effective management of these conditions.

Extensive knowledge of the pelvic neuroanatomy and pain pathways is essential to navigate through these often blurred clinical pictures, allowing for a better understanding of the topographical origin of the pain. In this chapter, we will review pelvic neuroanatomy and explore the neurophysiologic pathways of pain during pregnancy in order to provide the reader with this necessary tool for diagnosis and treatment. We will then highlight common nerve entrapments and related neuropathies caused and/or exacerbated by pregnancy.

Topographical Innervation of the Lower Body

The foundation of accurately mapping the topographical origin of pain begins with understanding the innervation and related dermatomes of somatic and autonomic nerves, which are displayed in Fig. 2.1. In this chapter, we will focus on the intrapelvic and intra-abdominal pathways, which encompass virtually all of the bundles of the lumbosacral plexus.

Innervation of the Abdominal Wall

The thoracoabdominal nerves are branches of the ventral primary rami of spinal nerves T7–T11. They travel anteroinferiorly between the internal oblique and transverse abdominal muscles and supply motor and sensory fibers along the abdominal wall, mostly above the umbilicus and the umbilical level.

M. R. Shaubi · C. Sermer · A. L. K. Li
Department of Obstetrics and Gynecology, Mount Sinai Hospital, Toronto, ON, Canada

L. Cancelliere
Faculty of Medicine, Department of Obstetrics and Gynecology, University of Toronto, Toronto, ON, Canada
e-mail: laura.cancelliere@mail.utoronto.ca

Nucelio L. B. M. Lemos (✉)
Department of Obstetrics and Gynecology, Pelvic Functional Surgery and Neuropelveology Clinic, Mount Sinai Hospital and Women's College Hospital, Toronto, ON, Canada

Pelvic Neurodysfunctions Division, Department of Gynecology, Federal University of São Paulo, São Paulo, SP, Brazil
e-mail: nucelio.lemos@utoronto.ca

C. H. Nezhat (ed.), *Non-Obstetric Surgery During Pregnancy*,
https://doi.org/10.1007/978-3-319-90752-9_2

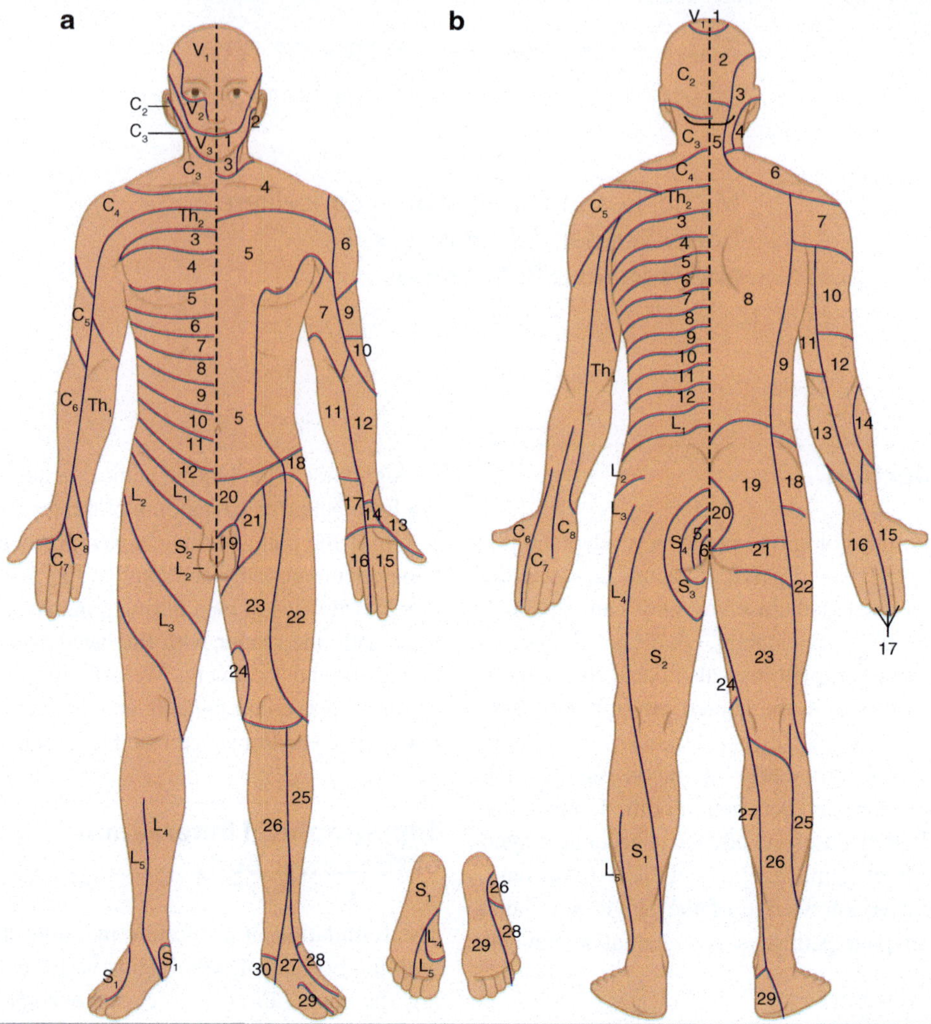

1. N. trigeminus
2. N. auricularis magnus
3. N. transversus colli
4. Nn. supraclaviculares
5. Rr. cutanei anteriores nn.inter-costalium
6. N. cutaneus brachii lateralis superior (N. axillaris)
7. N. cutaneus brachii medialis
8. Rr. mammarii laterales nn. inter-costalium
9. N. cutaneus brachii posterior (N.radialis)
10. N. cutaneus antebrachii posterior
11. N. cutaneus antebrachii medialis
12. N. cutaneus antebrachii lateralis
13. R. superficialis n. radialis
14. R. palmaris n. mediani
15. N. medianus
16. Nn. digitales palmares communes
17. R. palmaris n. ulnaris
18. N. iliohypogastricus (R. cut. lat.)
19. N. ilioinguinalis (Nn. scrotales anteriores)
20. N. iliohypogastricus (R. cutaneus anterior)
21. N. genitofemoralis (R. femoralis)
22. N. cutaneus femoris lateralis
23. N. femoralis (Rr. cutanei anteriores)
24. N. obturatorius (R. cut.)
25. N. cutaneus surae lateralis
26. N. saphenus
27. N. peronaeus superficialis
28. N. suralis
29. N. peronaeus profundus
30. N. tibialis (Rr. calcanei)

1. N. frontalls(V1)
2. N. occipitalis major
3. N. occipitalis minor
4. N. auricularis magnus
5. Rr. dorsales nn. cervicales
6. Nn. supraclaviculares
7. N. cutaneus brachii lateralis superior (N. axillaris)
8. Rr. dors. nn. spin. cervic., thorac., lumb.
9. Rr. cutanei laterales nn. inter-costalium
10. N. cutaneus brachii posterior
11. N. cutaneus brachii medialis
12. N. Cutaneus antebrachi posterior
13. N. cutaneus antebrachii medialis
14. N. cutaneus antebrachii lateralis
15. R. superficialis n. radialis
16. R. dorsalis n. ulnaris
17. N. medianus
18. N. iliohypogastricus (R. cut. lat.)
19. Nn. clunium superiores
20. Nn. clunium medil
21. Nn. clunium inferiores
22. N. cutaneus femoris lateralis
23. N. cutaneus femoris posterior
24. N. obturatorius (R. cut.)
25. N. cutaneus surae lateralis
26. N. suralis
27. N. saphenus
28. N. plantaris lateralis
29. N. plantaris medialis

Fig. 2.1 Dermatomes of the cranial and spinal nerves

The lower abdominal wall, inferior to the umbilicus, has few origins for motor and sensory innervations.

The subcostal nerves (T12) also travel antero-inferiorly between the internal oblique and transverse abdominal muscles.

The iliohypogastric and ilioinguinal nerves (T12–L1) enter the retroperitoneal space emerging on the lateral border of the psoas muscle. They then course anteriorly and distally to pierce the internal abdominal oblique muscle close to the anterosuperior iliac spine. The genitofemoral (T12–L2) nerve emerges from the anterior border of the psoas muscle, and its two branches leave the abdomen through the femoral (femoral branch) and inguinal (genital branch) canals (Fig. 2.2). Their fibrotic entrapment is related to post-herniorrhaphy inguinodynia.

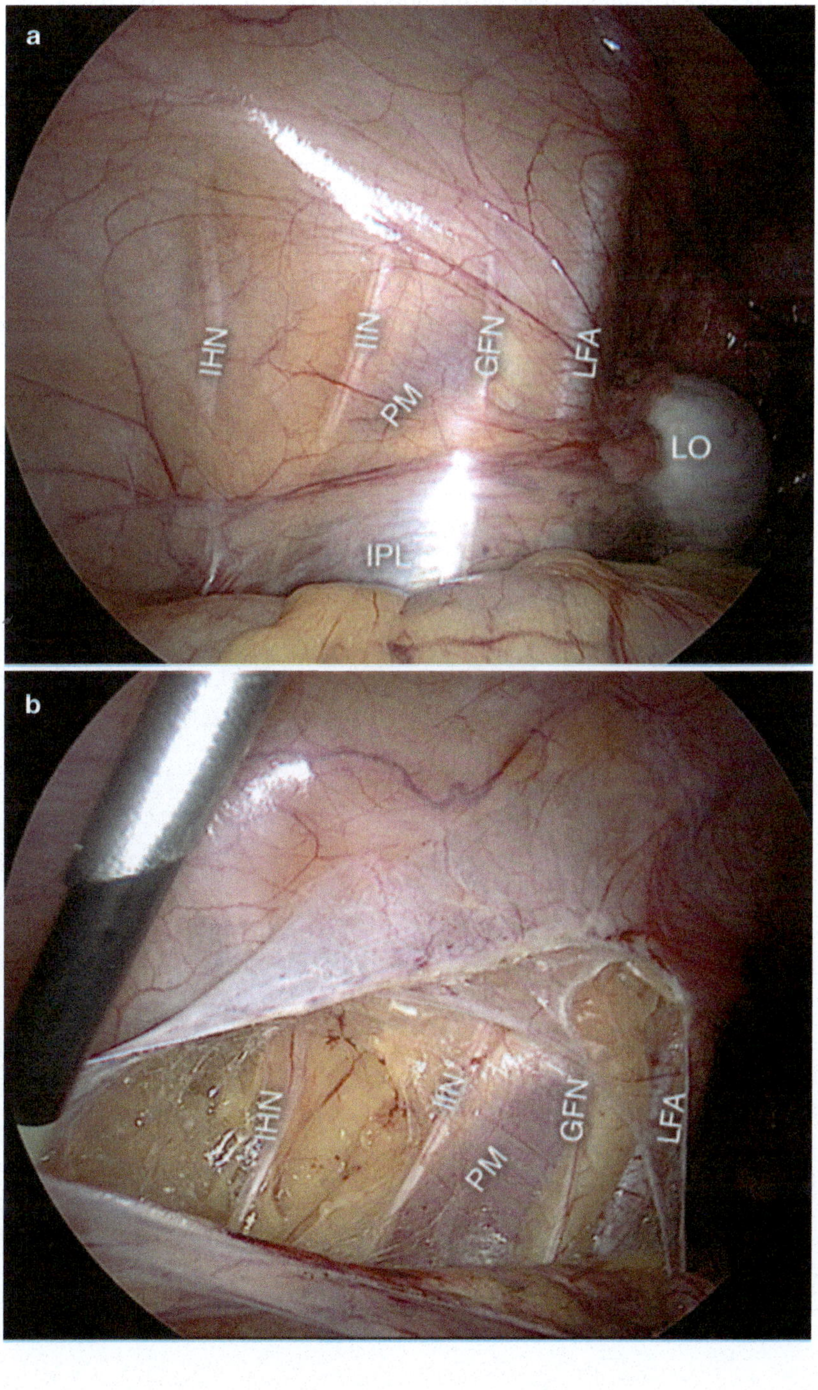

Fig. 2.2 Iliohypogastric (IHN), ilioinguinal (IIN), and genitofemoral (GFN) nerves, with the overlying peritoneum intact (**a**) and reflected (**b**) *PM* psoas muscle, *LO* left ovary, *IPL* infundibulopelvic ligament, *LFA* left femoral artery

Innervation of the Lower Back

The innervation of the back arises from the meningeal branches and dorsal rami of the spinal nerves. Each spinal nerve gives off a recurrent meningeal branch (or sinuvertebral nerve), which then reenters the vertebral canal and supplies vasomotor and sensory fibers to the dura, ligaments, periosteum, and blood vessels.

The dorsal primary rami of the spinal nerves contain motor, sensory, and sympathetic fibers. They supply the muscles, bones, joints, and skin of the back. Most dorsal rami divide into medial and lateral branches. Through most of the trunk, the sensory distribution of dorsal primary rami appears in regular bands. However, in the skin overlying the buttocks, the lumbar and sacral dorsal primary rami overlap as a series of cluneal nerves.

Innervation of the Pelvic Viscera

The superior hypogastric plexus, which is formed by fibers from the para-aortic sympathetic trunk, gives rise to the hypogastric nerves. The hypogastric nerves run over the hypogastric fascia in an anterior and distal direction. After crossing about two thirds of the distance between the sacrum and the uterine cervix or the prostate, its fibers spread to join the pelvic splanchnic nerves, thereby forming the inferior hypogastric plexus (Fig. 2.3). The hypogastric nerves carry the sympathetic signals to the internal urethral and anal sphincters, rectum, and bladder. These signals cause detrusor relaxation and bladder contraction, thus promoting urinary continence. The hypogastric nerves also carry proprioceptive and nociceptive afferent signals from the pelvic viscera.

The sacral nerve roots can be found juxtalaterally to the hypogastric fascia, which is formed by the medial fibers of the endopelvic fascia. They leave the sacral foramina and course anteriorly and distally, lying over the piriformis muscle and crossing the internal iliac vessels, laterally, to merge and form the nerves of the sacral plexus. Before crossing the internal iliac vessels, sacral nerve roots give off thin parasympathetic branches known as the pelvic splanchnic nerves (Fig. 2.4). The pelvic splanchnic nerves promote detrusor contraction and provide extrinsic parasympathetic innervation to the descending colon, sigmoid colon, and rectum. They also carry nociceptive afferent signals from the pelvic viscera. Finally, the pelvic splanchnic nerves join the hypogastric nerves to form the inferior hypogastric plexus in the pararectal fossa.

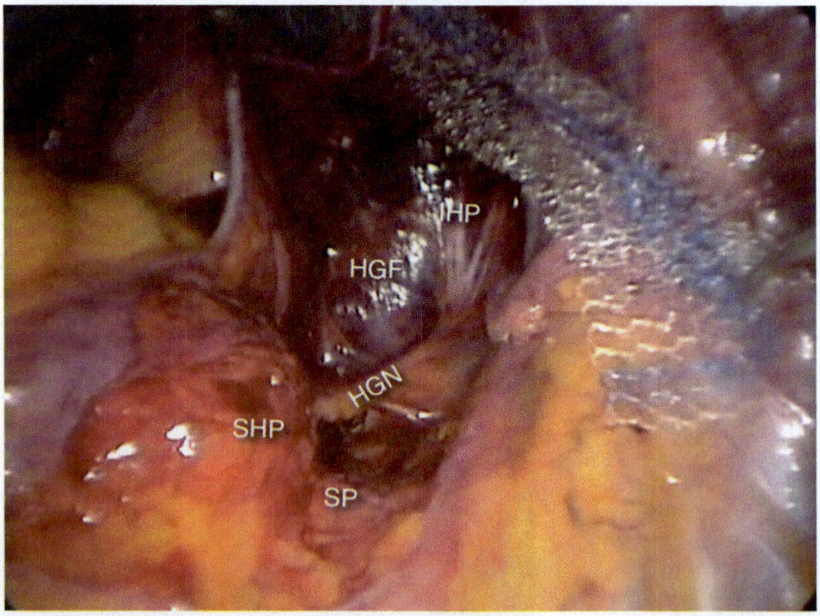

Fig. 2.3 The hypogastric nerve (HN) emerges from the superior hypogastric plexus (SHP) at the level of the sacral promontory (SP) and runs anteriorly and distally, juxtalaterally to the hypogastric fascia (HF), to merge with the pelvic splanchnic nerves to form the inferior hypogastric plexus (IHP)

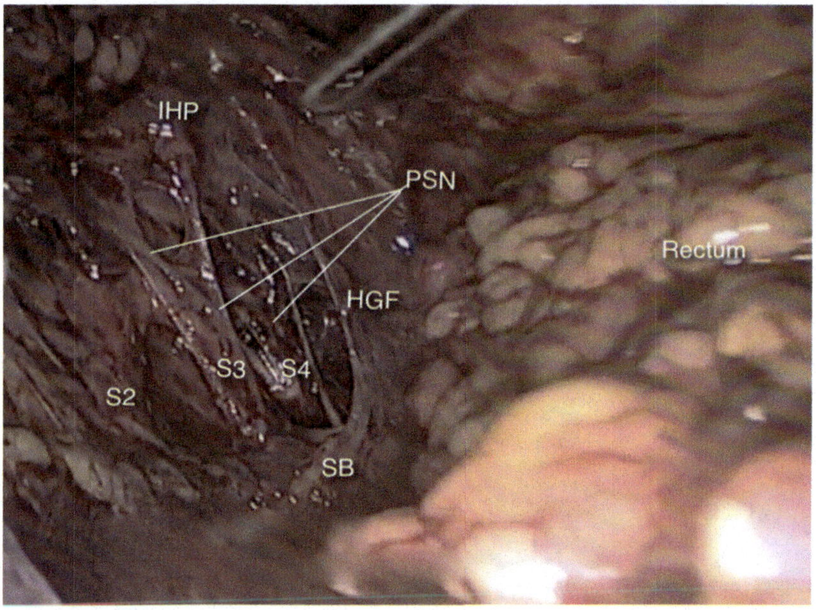

Fig. 2.4 The sacral nerve roots (S2–S4), found juxta-laterally to the hypogastric fascia (HGF), give origin to the pelvic splanchnic nerves (PSN), which run anteriorly and distally to merge the hypogastric nerve and form the inferior hypogastric plexus (IHP)

Innervation of the Pelvic Floor and Perineum

The pudendal nerve is formed by fibers of S2, S3, and S4 nerve roots and leaves the pelvis through the pudendal (Alcock's) canal (Fig. 2.5). It gives sensory branches to the lower gluteal region and the perineal skin. It also sends motor branches to the perineal muscles and the anterior fibers of the levator ani. Finally, there are direct motor and sensory nerves from the S3 and S4 nerve roots to the posterior fibers of the levator ani [1, 2].

Innervation of the Lower Limbs

The femoral nerve is the largest motor and sensory nerve of the lumbar plexus. It enters the abdomen by the posterolateral aspect of the psoas muscle and leaves through the femoral canal to innervate the quadriceps muscle and the skin overlying the anterior thigh (Fig. 2.6).

The obturator nerve enters the obturator space at the level of the pelvic brim and exits through the obturator canal. It provides motor branches to the hip adductors and sensory branches to the skin of the medial thigh (Fig. 2.7a).

The lumbosacral trunk and distal portions of the S1, S2, S3, and S4 nerve roots merge into the obturator space and form the sciatic and pudendal nerves (Fig. 2.7b).

The sciatic nerve is formed by the L4 and L5 fibers of the lumbosacral trunk and fibers from the S1, S2, and S3 nerve roots. It leaves the pelvis through the sciatic notch, giving off sensory branches to the upper gluteal region, posterolateral thigh, leg, ankle, and foot. It also controls the hip extensors, abductors and rotators, knee flexors, and all the muscles of the ankle and foot.

Central Nerve Pathways

The Spinal Cord and Brain Stem

Ascending Tracts in the Spinal Cord

There are two main pathways that carry nociceptive signals to higher centers in the brain: the spinothalamic tract and the spinoreticular tract.

The cell bodies of the secondary afferent neurons of the spinothalamic tract are located at the dorsal horn of the spinal gray matter. From there, they decussate within a few segments of the level of entry into the spinal cord and ascend in the contralateral spinothalamic tract to nuclei

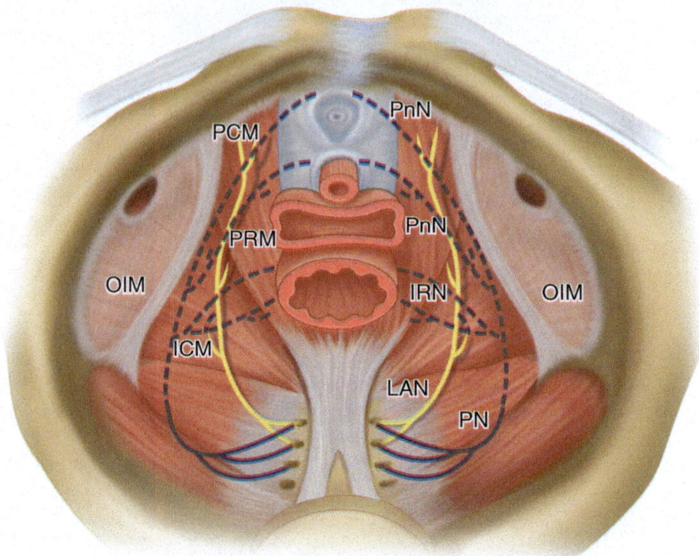

Fig. 2.5 Schematic diagram illustrating the most common pattern of innervation of the levator ani muscles (LAM)—superior view. The nerves traveling on the superior surface of LAM are shown as a continuous line, and the nerves coursing inferior to LAM are illustrated by a dashed line. *IRN* inferior rectal nerve, *PN* pudendal nerve. The PN branches into the dorsal nerve of the clitoris (DNC), perineal nerve (PnN), and the inferior rectal nerve (IRN). The perineal nerve and the IRN send branches that enter the inferior surface of the iliococcygeus (ICM), pubococcygeus (PCM), and puborectalis (PRM) muscles. The PN innervates the visceral bundles of the PCM, the PRM, and the external urethral sphincter

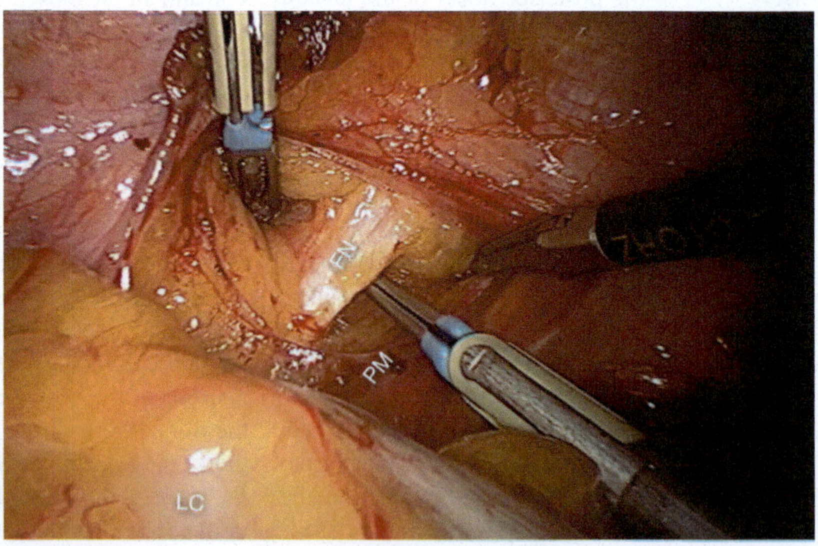

Fig. 2.6 The left femoral nerve (FN) enters the retroperitoneal space on the posterolateral aspect of the psoas muscle (PM). *LC* left colon

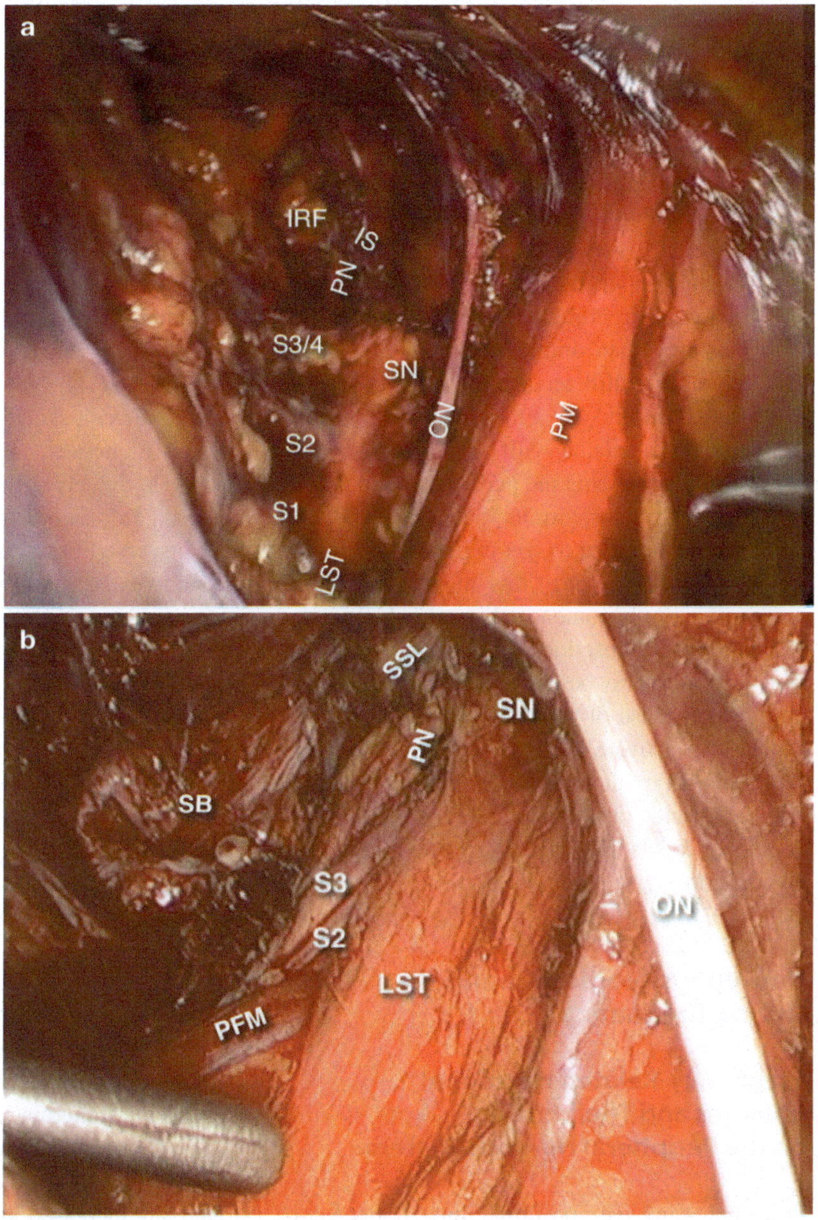

Fig. 2.7 Nerves of the obturator space (right side). (**a**) The final step of a laparoscopic approach to Alcock's canal syndrome, where the sacrospinous ligament has been transected to expose the pudendal nerve (PN). (**b**) The sacrospinous ligament (SSL) is intact. In both pictures, the internal and external iliac vessels are retracted medially. *ON* obturator nerve, *PM* psoas muscle, *SN* sciatic nerve, *LST* lumbosacral trunk, *PN* pudendal nerve, *IRF* ischiorectal fossa, *IS* ischial spine, *SB* sacral bone, *PFM* piriformis muscle

within the thalamus. Third-order neurons then ascend to terminate in the somatosensory cortex. There are also projections to the periaqueductal gray (PAG) matter. The spinothalamic tract transmits signals that are important for pain localization.

The spinoreticular tract fibers also decussate and ascend in the contralateral cord to reach the brain stem reticular formation, before projecting to the thalamus and hypothalamus and many further projections to the cortex. This pathway is involved in the emotional aspects of pain.

Cortical Representation and Brain Processing

Pain stimuli received from the spinal cord are interpreted in different forebrain areas, known as the *central pain matrix*. In previous studies, it has been shown that different pain stimuli cause different neural activity within this matrix [3, 4]. The processing of pain stimuli involves three parts of the central nervous system: the first part localizes the pain and depicts it; the second part allows the understanding of the pain; and the third part is responsible for the emotional aspect of the pain. Visceral pain usually initiates stronger emotional responses, when compared to somatic pain. The emotional structures of the brain—the hypothalamus, amygdala, and anterior cingulated cortex—therefore fulfill an important role in pain perception. The activity of these regions is related to emotions associated with past events, consequently individualizing the perception of pain. In addition, this creates correlations with events and sensations not related to, yet experienced during, the pain period; in turn, this may precipitate a cross-memory phenomenon through which experience of such sensations causes the associated pain experience to be perceived, even after the physiologic cause of pain is removed. Mild pain stimuli that activate the amygdala may be interpreted in a more intense way and may cause anxiety, fear, and obsession. Therefore, previous emotional events may have a key function in pain nociception.

Neurophysiological Changes During Pregnancy

Pregnancy-Related Hormonal Changes and Their Effects on the Peripheral Nervous System

Pregnancy can have a profound impact on the normal physiology of several components of the peripheral nervous system. Most notably, electrophysiological studies show that median nerve latency is prolonged in the pregnant population (2.1 ms compared to 1.8 ms in nonpregnant population), often leading to symptoms of carpal tunnel syndrome [5]. Furthermore, gustatory thresholds of both the chorda tympani and the glossopharyngeal nerve are increased during the first trimester of pregnancy [6]. By the third trimester, the gustatory thresholds have returned to nonpregnant levels [6]. Animal studies have also suggested changes in peripheral nerve physiology during pregnancy. For example, pregnant rats require a greater stimulus (higher right atrial pressure) to initiate discharge of their afferent cardiac receptors [7]. The pregnant rats also lack the high-frequency discharge seen in nonpregnant rats, further suggesting physiological changes [7].

Unfortunately, the mechanisms responsible for these changes are poorly understood; however, several theories have been postulated. Soft tissue edema due to fluid overload and/or hormonally-induced musculoskeletal changes can cause compression of nerves, thereby compromising their function [8]. Specifically, relaxin, which is increased in pregnancy, can cause tightening of the transverse flexor retinaculum leading to compression of the median nerve and altered nerve function. Moreover, other hormones of pregnancy including progesterone and estrogen, have been linked to increased nociceptive threshold [9] and increased pain latency [10] all of which could play a role in the physiological changes in the peripheral nervous system during pregnancy.

Neurophysiological Changes of the Central Nervous System

Different systems have different alterations as a modification for pregnancy. These modifications may have different effects on pain perception.

An increased pain threshold during pregnancy has been illustrated in rat models [11, 12]. Studies suggest that this is due to activation of an endogenous spinal opioid system. Iwasaki et al. demonstrated an increased threshold for somatic and visceral pain on day 21 of pregnancy, as compared to thresholds on day 7 and in nonpregnant rats.

Moreover, in response to stress, animals (including humans) increase their plasma levels of β-endorphin released by the pituitary. Pregnancy imposes a significant stress on the body; hence, β-endorphin levels are high [13]. The placenta is also an endorphin-releasing site for the mother and the fetus [14].

Sex steroids - including the major hormones of pregnancy estrogen and progesterone - play an important role in pain perception within both the peripheral and central nervous sytems. During the menstrual cycle there are fluctuations of pain sensitivity, thereby suggesting that the associated hormonal fluctuations in sex steroid levels affects sensitivity to pain stimuli. High levels of estrogen during pregnancy may lower pain tolerance by increasing the sensitivity of afferent nociceptors and dorsal horn neurons in the spinal cord.

Intrapelvic Nerve Entrapments in Pregnancy

A significant portion of the lumbosacral plexus crosses the pelvic brim and is subject to entrapments by endometriosis, fibrosis, nerve sheath tumors, varicose veins, and abnormal bundles of the piriformis. The latter two etiologies are of particular interest during pregnancy, because of the mechanical and vascular changes that could directly affect their behavior [15].

During pregnancy, the uterus grows from ~70 g prior to conception to ~1100 grams at full term, when it fills most of the abdominal cavity [16]. As early as the second trimester, the uterus of a pregnant woman in the supine position can compress the aorta and the inferior vena cava, diverting the venous return from the legs and pelvis to the vertebral venous system. Nerve entrapment, or compression neuropathy, can occur in pregnancy because of mechanical compression of the uterus on adjacent structures, or directly on nerves or nerve roots. This produces symptoms including pain, tingling, numbness, and muscle weakness along the affected nerve's dermatome and/or myotome [17]. Autonomic nerve entrapment or distention will produce visceral and vegetative symptoms, such as urinary frequency or urgency, dysuria, rectal pain, suprapubic, and/or abdominal cramps and chills.

Lumbosacral pain affects more than 50% of women at some time during pregnancy [18]. Although it is also common in women who are not pregnant, pain may be more severe and disabling in the pregnant population [19]. The discomfort can be pregnancy-related pelvic girdle pain, which is often near the sacroiliac joints and can radiate to the pubic symphysis and/or the posterior thighs [19]. Other women have lumbar spine pain, which is sometimes accompanied by pelvic girdle pain. Lumbar pelvic pain usually resolves after delivery but may persist for many months postpartum. Additionally, the pain can begin in the postpartum period [20]. There are several factors that contribute to back pain during pregnancy, including increased lumbar lordosis, direct pressure from the gravid uterus, postural stress, and ligamentous laxity due to the hormone relaxin. Severe lumbar disk displacement with objective clinical signs of radiculopathy occurs in 1 in 10,000 pregnancies [21]. In these cases, the L5 or S1 root is commonly affected by lateral compression. Women can develop low back pain, sciatica, and other typical findings of lumbar or lumbosacral radiculopathy [22]. Surgical emergencies, such as cauda equina syndrome leading to bilateral leg or sphincter dysfunction can occur with large central disk herniations. Less than 2% of disk herniations result in cauda equina syndrome or severe neurologic deficit [23].

The musculoskeletal and hematologic adaptations of pregnancy may aggravate or unmask intrapelvic causes of lumbosacral radiculopathy. To accommodate for a growing uterus and changing center of gravity, the lordosis of the lumbar spine and anterior tilt of the pelvis significantly increase. This subsequently increases forces on joints in the pelvis and lower limbs, strains the paraspinal and hip extensor and abductor muscles, and changes the spatial relationships between the pelvic sidewalls and floor, intrapelvic nerves, and vasculature [24]. An increase in blood volume and uterine blood flow, coupled with a decrease in systemic vascular resistance and venous return, creates intrapelvic vascular distention. This can exacerbate or trigger pain due to pelvic congestion in previously symptomatic or asymptomatic patients, respectively. Pelvic congestion syndrome is a well-described, multifactorial cause of cyclic pelvic pain. Dilated ovarian veins and subsequent pelvic varicosities have been identified as the underlying structural etiology in symptomatic patients. Pain is therefore worse during times of increased vascular distention, which occurs during prolonged walking and standing, and during the premenstrual period and pregnancy [25–28].

Varicosities or aberrant vessels may also cause pelvic pain by entrapping the lumbosacral nerves [29]. The sacral plexus covers the pelvic sidewalls and is covered itself by branches of the internal iliac vessels. Therefore, dilated or variant branches of iliac vessels may entrap the lumbosacral plexus against structures of the pelvic sidewalls and floor. Specifically, variant superior gluteal veins compressing the lumbosacral nerve roots have been identified in patients with sciatica with no identifiable spinal or musculoskeletal cause. This anatomical variation in symptomatic patients—referred to as superior gluteal vein syndrome—has been identified as a novel intrapelvic cause of sciatica (Fig. 2.8) [29]. A significant improvement in pain with a 92.3% success rate after nerve decompression by laparoscopic vessel ligation strongly suggests a potential causative role of this neurovascular conflict in the pathophysiology of atypical sciatica [29]. Associated symptoms of perineal or gluteal pain, anorectal dysfunction, rectal pain, and/or lower urinary tract symptoms in the absence of pelvic organ prolapse or other identifiable causes suggest an intrapelvic source of nerve entrapment [26, 28, 29].

Women with varicosities or aberrant iliac vessels overlying lumbosacral nerve roots may experience sciatica with the aforementioned urinary, perineal, gluteal, and anorectal symptoms when such vessels become further dilated in pregnancy. While some patients present with exacerbation of preexisting pain, many patients experience the onset of symptoms in pregnancy. A recent cadaver study identified variant superior gluteal veins in 35.6% (CI 21.6–49.5%) of dissected female cadavers [30]. Given that the prevalence of sciatica in the general population is much lower at an estimated 3–5%, not all individuals with variant pelvic vessels develop symptoms of lumbosacral nerve entrapment [31]. However, these vascular variants leave otherwise asymptomatic women vulnerable to neurovascular compression should fluctuations in the intrapelvic environment occur. Specifically, veins overlying nerve roots may become dilated, and/or postural changes affecting the relationship between the bony pelvis and sacral plexus may trigger symptomatic neurovascular conflict in pregnancy. Therefore, pregnancy may function as a stress test to identify women at risk of developing vascular entrapments of the sacral plexus in the future.

Piriformis syndrome is a common entity described as buttock pain that is exacerbated by hip flexion when combined with internal or external rotation of the affected leg. However, these symptoms may also present secondary to entrapment by the hamstring, gluteal, and obturator internus-gemellus complex muscles and/or

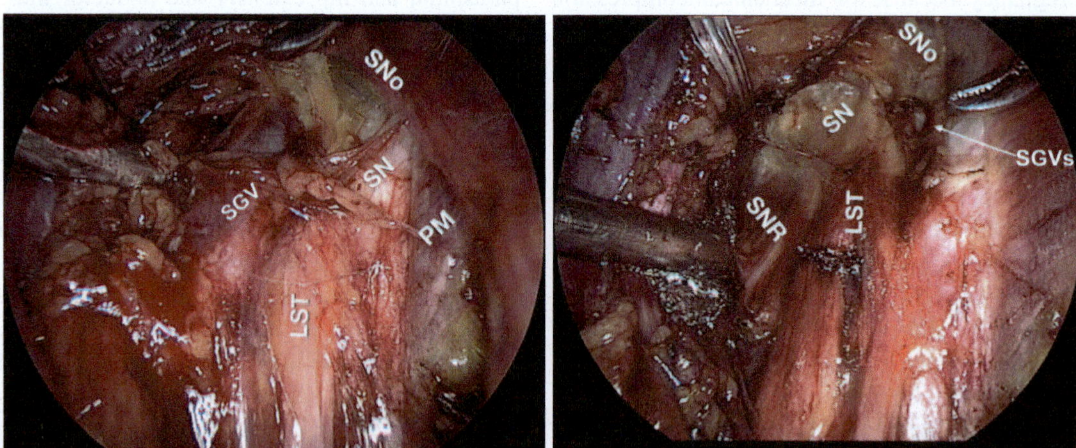

Fig. 2.8 Anatomical variation of the superior gluteal vein causing entrapment of the sciatic nerve. Top: variant of the superior gluteal vein (SGV) compressing the lumbosacral trunk (LST)

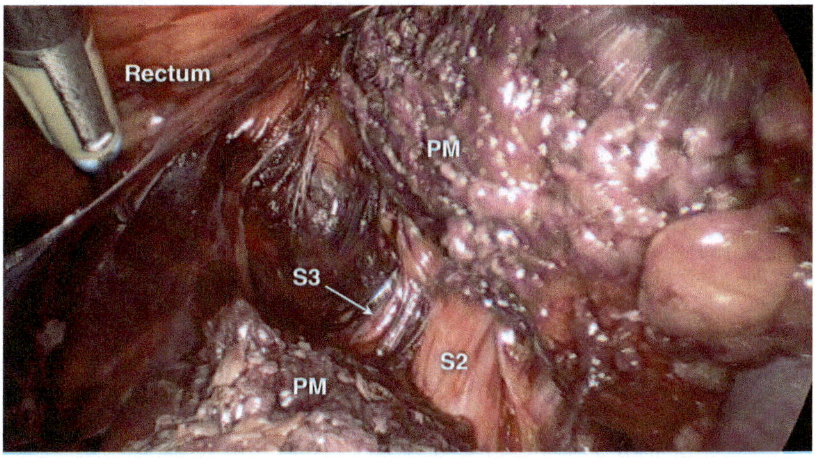

Fig. 2.9 Laparoscopic view of a transected abnormal bundle of the piriformis muscle which was causing the entrapment of nerve roots S3 and S4. *PM* piriformis muscle

fibrous bands and aberrant vessels [29, 32, 33]. In pregnancy, this group of deep gluteal muscles must compensate for the increase in lumbar lordosis and the anterior tilt of the pelvis. Intrapelvic entrapment of sacral nerve roots by abnormal bundles of the piriformis have also been identified in patients presenting with symptoms of piriformis syndrome (Fig. 2.9). We have recently performed a cadaver study (data not yet published) and found a 37.5% (CI 20.7–54.3%) prevalence of variant piriformis bundles in a general population of female cadavers. The postural changes in pregnancy may therefore also aggravate or trigger symptoms of piriformis syndrome in women with this variant. This may also serve as a prognostic marker for women at risk of developing the piriformis syndrome in the future. Therefore, when symptoms resolve after delivery, these women should be counseled not to perform exercises that cause hypertrophy of the piriformis and to routinely stretch the muscle.

Other Pelvic Entrapment Neuropathies Directly Related to Pregnancy

Meralgia Paresthetica

Meralgia paresthetica is a common syndrome in pregnancy. It is strictly a sensory neuropathy caused by compression of the lateral femoral cutaneous nerve under or within the inguinal ligament. In approximately 80% of cases, symptoms are unilateral and consist of tingling, numbness, and pain in the lateral thigh [34]. Increased abdominal girth and lumbar lordosis are risk factors for developing this neuropathy during pregnancy [35]. The lateral femoral cutaneous nerve may also be injured during thigh flexion during the second stage of labor. In women who undergo caesarean delivery, the lateral femoral cutaneous nerve may be injured by the incision or pressure from a retractor. Treatment during pregnancy consists of supportive care, as spontaneous recovery after delivery typically occurs. The sensory branches of the femoral nerve form the anterior femoral cutaneous and saphenous nerves. Femoral neuropathy is rare during pregnancy [36]. The femoral nerve may be compressed at the inguinal ligament during delivery by thigh flexion, external rotation, and abduction [35]. This mononeuropathy usually presents as painless weakness when the patient attempts to walk after delivery.

Obturator Neuropathy

The obturator nerve is derived from the anterior divisions of the ventral rami of the L2–L4 nerve roots. The nerve travels along the lateral pelvic wall, enters the obturator foramen, and innervates the thigh adductor muscles. Obturator nerve lesions are uncommon because the nerve is protected deep within the pelvis and the medial thigh [37]. Unilateral or bilateral lesions can be associated with delivery. Contributing factors include compression by the fetal head against the pelvic wall, use of forceps, and the lithotomy position. Obturator neuropathy can cause pain along the medial thigh as well as weakness. Prognosis is similar to that of femoral neuropathy.

Conclusion

Pregnancy is a unique physiologic condition of stress where the adaptive changes of virtually all systems contribute to the multifactorial perception of pain. Non-obstetric pain can be an extremely bothersome situation to many pregnant women. The dynamic interplay between modified physiology and pathology often causes altered and/or inconsistent presentations in pregnancy, thereby posing a challenge to accurate diagnosis. A deep understanding of the normal neuroanatomy and physiology of pain, paired with appreciation for the mechanical, hormonal, and vascular changes of pregnancy prove essential to the topographic and etiological diagnosis of pain, which is the basis for effective treatment.

References

1. Wallner C, Maas CP, Dabhoiwala NF, Lamers WH, DeRuiter MC. Innervation of the pelvic floor muscles: a reappraisal for the levator ani nerve. Obstet Gynecol. 2006;108(3 Pt 3):529–34.
2. Grigorescu BA, Lazarou G, Olson TR, Downie SA, Powers K, Greston WM, Mikhail MS. Innervation of the levator ani muscles: description of the nerve branches to the pubococcygeus, iliococcygeus, and puborectalis muscles. Int Urogynecol J Pelvic Floor Dysfunction. 2008;19(1):107–16.
3. Ingvar M. Pain and functional imaging. Philos Trans R Soc Lond Ser B Biol Sci. 1999;354(1387):1347–58.
4. May A. Neuroimaging: visualising the brain in pain. Neurol Sci. 2007;28(Suppl 2):S101–7.
5. Eogan M, O'Brien C, Carolan D, Fynes M, O'Herlihy C. Median and ulnar nerve conduction in pregnancy. Int J Gynaecol Obstet. 2004;87(3):233–6.
6. Kuga M, Ikeda M, Suzuki K, Takeuchi S. Changes in gustatory sense during pregnancy. Acta Otolaryngol Suppl. 2002;546:146–53.
7. Hines T, Hodgson TM. Pregnancy alters cardiac receptor afferent discharge in rats. Am J Physiol Regul Integr Comp Physiol. 2000;278(1):R149–56.
8. Turgut F, Cetinsahinahin M, Turgut M, Bolukbasi O. The management of carpal tunnel syndrome in pregnancy. J Clin Neurosci. 2001;8(4):332–4.
9. Liu NJ, Gintzler AR. Prolonged ovarian sex steroid treatment of male rats produces antinociception: identification of sex-based divergent analgesic mechanisms. Pain. 2000;85(1–2):273–81.
10. Gordon FT, Soliman MR. The effects of estradiol and progesterone on pain sensitivity and brain opioid receptors in ovariectomized rats. Horm Behav. 1996;30(3):244–50.
11. Sander HW, Portoghere PS, Gintzler AR. Spinal ×-opiate receptor involvement in the analgesia of pregnancy: effect of intrathecal nor-binaltorphimine, a ×-selective antagonist. Brain Res. 1988;474(2):343–7.
12. Iwasaki H, Collins JG, Saito Y. Pregnancy induced naloxone reversible analgesia in rats. Anesth Analog (Abstract). 1989;68:S131.
13. Carr DB, Murphy MT. Operation, anesthesia and the endorphin system. Int Anesthesiol Clin. 1989;26:199–205.
14. Sirinathsinghji DJS, Heavens RP. Stress-related peptide hormones in the placenta: their possible physiological significance. J Endocrinol. 1989;122:435–7.
15. Lemos NLBM, et al. Intrapelvic nerve entrapment as a cause of pelvic floor dysfunction and refractory pudendal pain: a review of 50 cases. ICS 2017.
16. Cunningham F, Leveno KJ, Bloom SL. Williams obstetrics. 22nd ed. New York: McGraw-Hill Companies; 2005.
17. Bouche P. Compression and entrapment neuropathies. Handb Clin Neurol. 2013;115:311–66. https://doi.org/10.1016/B978-0-444-52902-2.00019-9.
18. Fast A, Shapiro D, Ducommun EJ, Friedmann LW, Bouklas T, Floman Y. Low-back pain in pregnancy. Spine. 1987;12:368–71.
19. Gutke A, Ostgaard HC, Oberg B. Pelvic girdle pain and lumbar pain in pregnancy: a cohort study of the consequences in terms of health and functioning. Spine. 2006;31:E149–55.
20. Russell R, Dundas R, Reynolds F. Long term backache after childbirth: prospective search for causative factors. BMJ. 1996;312:1384–8.
21. LaBan MM, Perrin JCS, Latimer FR. Pregnancy and the herniated lumbar disc. Arch Phys Med Rehabil. 1983;64:319–21.
22. Garmel SH, Guzelian GA, D'Alton JG, D'Alton ME. Lumbar disk disease in pregnancy. Obstet Gynecol. 1997;89:821–2.
23. Brown MD, Levi ADO. Surgery for lumbar disc herniation during pregnancy. Spine. 2001;26:440–3.
24. Foti T, Davids JR, Bagley A. A biomechanical analysis of gait during pregnancy. J Bone Joint Surg Am. 2000;82(5):625.
25. Ganeshan A, Upponi S, Hon LQ, et al. Chronic pelvic pain due to pelvic congestion syndrome: the role of diagnostic and interventional radiology. Cardiovasc Intervent Radiol. 2007;30(6):1105–11.
26. Possover M, Schneider T, Henle KP. Laparoscopic therapy for endometriosis and vascular entrapment of sacral plexus. Fertil Steril. 2011;95(2):756–8.

27. D'Archambeau O, Maes M, De Schepper AM. The pelvic congestion syndrome: role of the "nutcracker phenomenon" and results of endovascular treatment. JBR–BTR. 2004;87:1–8.
28. Lemos N, Possover M. Laparoscopic approach to intrapelvic nerve entrapments. J Hip Preserv Surg. 2015;2(2):92–8.
29. Cancelliere L, Li ALK, Moretti Marques R, Fernandes GL, Sermer C, Kumar K, Sebastiao Afonso J, Girão MJBC, Lemos N. Superior gluteal vein syndrome: an intrapelvic cause of sciatica. NAU [submitted for review 2018].
30. Cancelliere L, Lemos N, Li ALK, et al. Superior gluteal vein variation in laparoscopic cadaver dissection, data collected June 2017. [unpublished].
31. Tarulli AW, Raynor EM. Lumbosacral radiculopathy. Neurol Clin. 2007;25(2):387.
32. Martin HD, Shears SA, Johnson JC, Smathers AM, Palmer IJ. The endoscopic treatment of sciatic nerve entrapment/deep gluteal syndrome. Arthroscopy. 2011;27(2):172–81.
33. McCrory P, Bell S. Nerve entrapment syndromes as a cause of pain in the hip, groin and buttock. Sports Med. 1999;27(4):261–74.
34. Tsen LC. Neurologic complications of labor analgesia and anesthesia. Int Anesthesiol Clin. 2002;40:67–88.
35. Wong CA, Scavone BM, Dugan S, Smith JC, Prather H, Ganchiff JN, et al. Incidence of postpartum lumbosacral spine and lower extremity nerve injuries. Obstet Gynecol. 2003;101:279–82.
36. Kofler M, Kronenberg MF. Bilateral femoral neuropathy during pregnancy. Muscle Nerve. 1998;21:1106–10.
37. Nogajski JH, Shnier RC, Zagami AS. Postpartum obturator neuropathy. Neurology. 2004;63:2450–1.

Non-obstetric Imaging in Pregnant Women

3

Sudheer Balakrishnan

Introduction

The patient's pregnancy status should be determined when considering non-sonographic imaging for a woman of childbearing age that will include the abdomen and pelvis. The exception to this standard is the scenario of life-threatening trauma, in which case the patient may be imaged without delay. Once a pregnancy is confirmed, the main predicament healthcare providers face when deciding whether to order diagnostic imaging is the associated risk to the developing fetus. Choosing an imaging modality and deciding on the necessity of a contrast agent involve a careful balance between maximizing diagnostic yield and minimizing harmful exposure to the fetus. It is vital for healthcare providers to educate themselves on these topics so they can engage in thoughtful risk-benefit discussions with patients and make confident decisions without delaying patient care. Knowledge on this subject matter will also be instrumental in creating a multidisciplinary institutional policy when it comes to imaging pregnant patients.

S. Balakrishnan
Department of Radiology, University of Southern California, LAC-USC, Los Angeles, CA, USA
e-mail: sbalakrishnan@dhs.lacounty.gov

Pregnancy Screening

Current ACR (American College of Radiology) guidelines for pregnancy screening before imaging studies using ionizing radiation are based on whether the evaluation will involve a high fetal absorbed radiation dose (typically studies that include the abdominopelvic region) [1]. For these studies, a urine pregnancy test is recommended. If the study is not likely to expose the fetus to a high radiation dose (e.g., extremity radiograph), a verbal/written confirmation should be obtained from the patient confirming that she is not pregnant. If the patient expresses any uncertainty during this questioning, a urine pregnancy test should be obtained. It is recommended that pregnancy screening also be performed before MRI evaluations [2].

Informed Consent

Informed consent should be obtained from patients before any imaging evaluation that involves ionizing radiation or before an MRI evaluation. The exception to this standard is the pregnant patient with life-threatening traumatic injuries, for which imaging should proceed without delay. Consent includes a discussion of potential risks to the pregnant patient and fetus, as well as the benefits of obtaining potentially valuable clinical information using imaging.

C. H. Nezhat (ed.), *Non-Obstetric Surgery During Pregnancy*,
https://doi.org/10.1007/978-3-319-90752-9_3

Ionizing Radiation: Radiography, Fluoroscopy, Computed Tomography (CT), and Nuclear Medicine

While the fetal effects of both ultrasound and magnetic resonance imaging (MRI) have been studied, it is the effect of ionizing radiation on the developing fetus that has produced the most research as well as anxiety from healthcare providers. These potential effects include death of the embryo, organ malformations, intrauterine growth restriction, microcephaly, mental retardation, decreased intelligence quotient, and increased incidence of childhood cancers [3, 4]. Most of the data we have on this topic are based on results of animal model research, epidemiologic studies of atomic bomb survivors in Japan, and studies of patients exposed to treatment-related radiation. Ionizing radiation includes particles and photon radiation (e.g., gamma rays used in nuclear medicine, X-rays used in radiography/mammography/fluoroscopy/CT). Fetal radiation-induced effects are the product of either mutagenesis (changes in nuclear DNA) or cell death and can be subdivided into those that are teratogenic and those that are carcinogenic.

Teratogenesis is a process by which congenital malformations are induced in an embryo or fetus. Fetal susceptibility to teratogens depends on the gestational age and the estimated exposure dose incurred by the fetus (Table 3.1) [3, 4]. Teratogenesis falls under the category of deterministic effects, which are those effects that do not occur below a certain threshold. Once this threshold is exceeded, however, the severity of the effect increases with increasing dose. Fetal radiation doses of less than 50 mGy are not associated with a higher risk of teratogenesis or fetal loss [1, 5], and most diagnostic imaging employing ionizing radiation falls well below this threshold (Table 3.2). It is important to note, however, that this threshold refers to the cumulative dose incurred by the fetus throughout the duration of the pregnancy, not just the dose incurred during a single examination. Thus, a patient who is imaged several times throughout her pregnancy or an injured pregnant patient undergoing several consecutive imaging evaluations may possibly exceed this threshold, particularly during lifesaving interventional procedures and fluoroscopy. During the first 2 weeks of gestation, a fetal radiation dose of greater than 50 mGy will result in death of the embryo or will have no effect. This is referred to as the "all or none" phenomenon.

Table 3.1 Estimated threshold dose and effects of ionizing radiation

Gestational period (weeks after conception)	Effects	Estimated threshold dose [3–7]
Before implantation (0–2 weeks)	Embryo death or no effect ("all or none")	50–100 mGy
Organogenesis (2–8 weeks)	Congenital anomalies (skeletal, ocular, genital)	200 mGy
	Growth retardation	200–250 mGy
Fetal period (8–15 weeks)	Severe mental retardation (high risk)	60–310 mGy
	Intellectual deficit	25 IQ point loss per gray
	Microcephaly	200 mGy
Fetal period (16–25 weeks)	Severe mental retardation (low risk)	250–280 mGy

Table 3.2 Estimated mean fetal absorbed dose (mGy) [3, 8, 9]

Cervical spine radiograph (AP, lateral)	<0.001
Extremity radiograph	<0.001
Chest radiograph (PA, lateral)	0.002
Lumbar spine radiograph (AP, lateral)	1
Abdominal radiograph (AP)	1–3
CT head	0
CTPA	0.03 in early pregnancy, 0.2 in late pregnancy
CT chest	0.2
CT abdomen/pelvis	25
CTA aorta	34
V/Q scan	*Perfusion*: 0.6 early pregnancy, 0.8 late pregnancy *Ventilation*: 0.3

The risk of congenital malformations from radiation-induced teratogenesis is greatest during gestational weeks 2–8, the period of fetal organogenesis. The risk of adverse central nervous system effects is greatest during gestational weeks 8–15 [6].

Carcinogenesis is the transformation of normal cells to cancerous cells. Cancer induction as a consequence of radiation exposure falls under the category of stochastic effects. Stochastic effects do not have a threshold, and while the risk increases with increasing radiation dose, the severity does not (i.e., the patient will either develop cancer or they will not). There is some debate as to whether the risk of radiation-induced fetal carcinogenesis is increased during any particular period of the pregnancy, with some primate studies indicating an increased risk during the first trimester [10]. Although there is significant evidence to support the claim of increased risk of childhood cancers as a result of fetal irradiation, the previously estimated excess cases per gray of exposure have fallen under increased scrutiny due to less than the expected number of cases found among atomic bomb survivors [3]. The estimated relative risk of a fatal childhood cancer after fetal exposure to 50 mGy is 2, which signifies an increased baseline risk from 1 in 2000 to 1 in 1000 [11]. While there is an increased risk of all childhood cancers, the risk of leukemia is the highest postradiation exposure [3]. A fetal radiation dose of 50 mGy will also increase the overall lifetime risk for cancer by 2% [3, 12, 13].

The estimated fetal radiation exposure is less than 50 mGy (the threshold for radiation-induced teratogenesis) during most imaging studies that employ ionizing radiation (Table 3.2). To put things in perspective, the natural background radiation dose incurred by the fetus during pregnancy is 1 mGy. According to the 1977 Report 54 of the National Council on Radiation Protection and Measurements, "the risk of abnormality is considered to be negligible at 5mGy or less when compared to other risks of pregnancy, and the risk of malformation is significantly increased above control levels only at doses above 150 mGy" [14]. The other risks of pregnancy referenced in this statement include spontaneous abortion (15%), prematurity/growth retardation (4%), spontaneous birth defects (3%), and mental retardation (1%). The ACR issued the following policy statement concerning therapeutic abortion following radiation exposure during pregnancy: "The interruption of pregnancy is rarely justified because of radiation risk to the embryo or fetus from a radiologic examination" [15]. The American College of Obstetricians and Gynecologists agrees that "exposure to less than 5 rad (50 mGy) has not been associated with an increase in fetal anomalies or pregnancy loss" [5].

MRI

MRI uses a magnetic field and radiofrequency (RF) pulses to generate images of the body. Most notably it does not employ ionizing radiation. There is currently no evidence that MR imaging during pregnant at 1.5 tesla (T) or lower magnetic field strengths causes detrimental effects to the fetus [16]. Two aspects of this modality that have caused some concern are fetal exposure to acoustic noise from generation of the magnetic gradient and heating effects associated with energy absorption from RF pulses. Thus far, studies have not shown any evidence of cochlear injury or significant increased risk of neonatal hearing loss associated with fetal exposure to 1.5 T MRI in utero [17, 18]. Due to the highly conductive nature of amniotic fluid and its limited capacity to dissipate heat, absorption of RF energy with subsequent heating of fetal tissues has raised some concern. The specific absorption rate (SAR) is a measure of RF energy deposition in tissues and indicates the potential for tissue heating. SAR is dependent on both scanner (strength of the magnetic field, type of pulse used, etc.) and patient (body size, anatomic region being exposed, etc.) characteristics. The FDA has set acoustic noise limits as well as SAR limits for the whole body, head, torso, and extremities. One study which evaluated RF energy deposition in an anatomic model of a pregnant patient found that the temperature rise in fetal model tissues was not significant when recommended SAR limits were followed [19]. The ACR's 2007 white paper on safe MR practices states that MRI may be used in pregnant patients during any trimester if deemed necessary by referring clinicians and radiologists [2]. MRI may be considered "necessary" if the desired clinical information cannot be obtained with ultrasound and could possibly affect clinical management of the patient or fetus during the pregnancy. Due to the lack of data and experience with use of magnetic fields strengths greater than 2.5 T in evaluating pregnant patients, these should be avoided.

Ultrasound

Ultrasound uses high-frequency sound waves to generate images of the body. It also does not employ ionizing radiation. There is currently no evidence that diagnostic ultrasound evaluations during pregnancy cause detrimental effects to the human fetus. However, as with any modality, a lack of evidence does not definitively confirm absent risk. The thermal effect of ultrasound refers to heating within tissues after absorption of ultrasound beam energy. This effect is dependent on the thermal characteristics of the imaged tissues, the intensity of the ultrasound beam, and the length of the evaluation [20]. The thermal index (TI) is an on-screen guide that indicates potential for tissue heating. In addition, there are nonthermal effects of ultrasound, principally cavitation and acoustic streaming. Cavitation arises when negative pressure in an ultrasonic pulse draws gas bubbles out of solution into tissues, where their interaction may affect cell membrane transport or cause direct tissue damage. Acoustic streaming refers to energy absorption within liquids in the sonographic field, which may lead to velocity gradients and associated shear stress. The mechanical index (MI) is an on-screen guide that indicates potential for nonthermal effects. Most animal research on these effects have employed ultrasound exposures that are more typical of therapeutic application rather than diagnostic. There are no documented cases of these effects occurring during diagnostic ultrasound evaluation on a human [21]. With the introduction of newer ultrasound techniques requiring higher acoustic output levels, it is imperative that we continue to follow cautionary measures. In general, the sonographer should regularly check both the TI and MI and keep them as low as possible while still maintaining the diagnostic integrity of the exam. Exam times should be kept as short as possible. Doppler imaging (color, spectral, power) has a higher potential to produce a biologically significant rise in temperature, so this modality should be used sparingly, especially in the first trimester, with the lowest possible power output that still produces diagnostic images [21].

Intravenous Iodinated Contrast

It is well documented that iodinated contrast crosses the placenta [22]; thus fetal exposure to these agents warrants discussion. The FDA classifies iodinated contrast as a category B drug, indicating that while animal studies have not revealed a fetal risk, there have been no controlled studies in pregnant women [23]. These agents should be administered only after evaluating the associated risk-benefit ratio. Because current iodinated contrast mediums are water soluble, they are quickly cleared through fetal and maternal circulation; thus deleterious effects on fetal thyroid function are highly unlikely [24]. Evaluation of neonatal thyroid function during the first week of life is already standard practice, regardless of the mother's history of iodinated contrast exposure during pregnancy. Because there have been no controlled studies in pregnant women, iodinated contrast should only be used when it will provide valuable information for patient management that a non-contrast evaluation would not [25]. One such clinical scenario is the evaluation of a traumatized pregnant patient, in which case intravenous iodinated contrast should always be administered to exclude life-threatening vascular and visceral injuries.

Intravenous Paramagnetic Contrast

The FDA classifies paramagnetic contrast as a category C drug. This designation is a result of animal studies revealing toxic fetal side effects (i.e., growth retardation, congenital malformations) after the administration of intravenous gadolinium at a two to seven times higher dose than that which is routinely administered to humans [26]. Gadolinium-based agents also pass through the placenta into fetal circulation and are subsequently excreted into the amniotic fluid via the fetal kidneys [2]. Chelated gadolinium may reside in the amniotic fluid for an indeterminate time before being resorbed and eliminated. The main concern is the dissociation of the potentially toxic gadolinium ion from its chelate while residing in the amniotic fluid. In a retrospective review of the Canadian birth database, exposure to gadolinium-based contrast agents at any time during pregnancy was associated with an increased risk of stillbirth or neonatal death, as well as rheumatologic and inflammatory skin conditions [27]. It should be noted that the control group in this study was pregnant patients who did not undergo MRI, rather than patients who underwent MRI without gadolinium-based contrast agents. There are no known cases of nephrogenic systemic fibrosis, which is a syndrome involving connective tissue and visceral fibrosis after gadolinium exposure, associated with use of gadolinium-based contrast agents in pregnant patients [25]. Because the fetal effects of intravenous gadolinium-based contrast agents have not been completely elucidated, its use is restricted to only those situations in which contrast is absolutely critical to gain valuable clinical information for patient management [25].

Intravenous Contrast Administration During Lactation

Neonatal blood levels of both iodinated contrast and gadolinium-based contrast agents after breastfeeding are very low [25]. Thus there is no need for breastfeeding cessation after these agents are administered to a lactating mother [25].

Oral and Rectal Contrast

Oral and rectal contrast agents (i.e., barium sulfate, Gastrografin) are not absorbed by the body and may be administered without affecting the fetus. Oral contrast may be considered in patients with a history of bowel surgery or to assist with bowel evaluation in patients with low BMI or decreased intra-abdominopelvic fat. Rectal contrast may be considered to evaluate for bowel trauma in the setting of penetrating injury to the pelvis.

Contrast Reaction

Aside from cases of life-threatening trauma, patients should always be questioned about prior contrast reactions and allergies. Management of contrast reactions in pregnant patients is the same as that for nonpregnant adults [28]. For pregnant patients with hypotension, appropriate treatment may include placing the patient in a left lateral decubitus position to alleviate inferior vena cava (IVC) compression by the gravid uterus. If cardiac compressions are required, the patient should be placed back into the supine position.

Specific Clinical Scenarios

Acute Appendicitis

Acute appendicitis is the most common non-obstetric emergency warranting surgical intervention in pregnant patients [29]. Associated risks during pregnancy include a higher rate of appendiceal perforation due to delayed diagnosis, premature labor, and increased fetal morbidity and mortality [29, 30]. Imaging is essential not only to avoid these complications but also to decrease the number of negative laparotomies which one study described as high as 14–43% without preoperative imaging [31]. See Fig. 3.1.

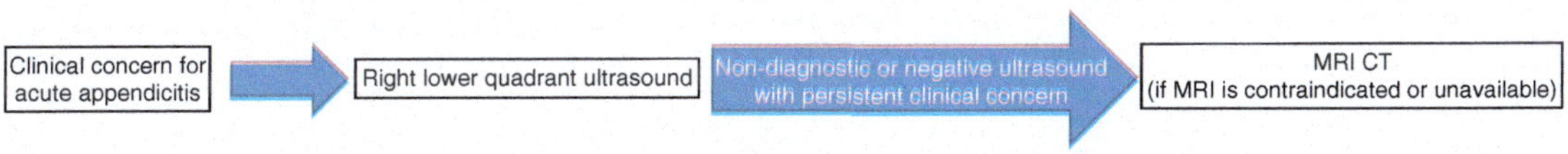

Fig. 3.1 Imaging algorithm for evaluation of appendicitis

Ultrasound

Ultrasound is recommended as the initial imaging study for acute appendicitis during pregnancy as it does not involve fetal radiation exposure and can simultaneously evaluate the pelvis for alternative sources of pain. Studies evaluating ultrasound diagnosis of acute appendicitis in pregnant patients have shown consistently high specificity (95–96%) and varying sensitivity (66–100%) [32]. The appendix is more easily evaluated during the first and second trimester due to superior migration and rotation of the appendix that may occur in the third trimester. Placing the patient in the left lateral decubitus position may aid evaluation during the third trimester [32]. Limitations of ultrasound evaluation include poor visualization due to increased abdominal girth, overlying bowel gas, or operator proficiency. In the setting of clinically suspected acute appendicitis with a negative or inconclusive ultrasound, further imaging is warranted.

CT

A recent study demonstrated CT to be 92% sensitive and 99% specific for the diagnosis of acute appendicitis during pregnancy [33]. The main drawback of this modality is fetal radiation exposure which makes it a tertiary option after ultrasound and MRI. The estimated fetal radiation dose from a CT abdomen/pelvis is 25 mGy, and while this still falls below the threshold of 50 mGy for induction of fetal teratogenesis, there is still a theoretical risk of carcinogenesis that is estimated to be approximately 1 cancer per 500 fetuses exposed to 30 mGy [34]. Consultation with a diagnostic radiologist is recommended to make protocol adjustments that will reduce fetal radiation dose. CT may also be considered after a nondiagnostic ultrasound if MRI is contraindicated or not available. Administering both intravenous and oral contrast will improve visualization of the appendix.

MRI

Studies have shown MRI to have a high sensitivity and specificity for detection of appendicitis as well as other lower abdominal and pelvic pathologies causing acute right lower quadrant abdominal pain [35]. MRI should be used as a second-line imaging study after an inconclusive ultrasound [36, 37]. Intravenous paramagnetic contrast is not required for this study.

Biliary Disease

Complications of biliary calculi and cholecystitis are associated with high maternal and fetal mortality and may require ERCP or surgical intervention [38]. The estimated fetal radiation dose during ERCP is reported to be within safe limits [39, 40]. See Fig. 3.2.

Ultrasound

Ultrasound is the initial study of choice for evaluating biliary disease. Depending on the patient's clinical condition and surgical preference, sonographic findings of cholecystitis may be managed medically, evaluated further with MRI or MR cholangiopancreatography (MRCP), or may warrant endoscopic retrograde cholangiopancreatography (ERCP) and/or surgical intervention.

MRI

MRCP has a high sensitivity (98%) and specificity (84%) for biliary disease [41] and does not require the use of intravenous paramagnetic contrast. MRCP avoids the known complications of ERCP which include pancreatitis, hemorrhage, infection, and bowel perforation. One study concluded that MRCP is comparable to ERCP for diagnosis of choledocholithiasis in pregnant patients and ERCP should be reserved for those patients requiring an intervention [42]. Additionally, abdominal MRI with MRCP may

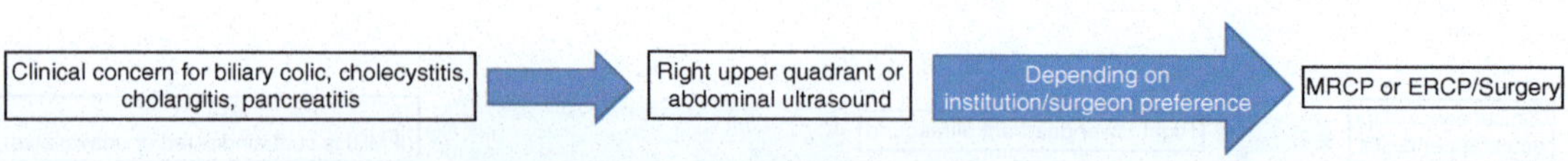

Fig. 3.2 Imaging algorithm for evaluation of biliary colic, cholecystitis, cholangitis, pancreatitis

detect alternative causes of elevated liver enzymes.

Pulmonary Embolism (PE)

Pulmonary venous thromboembolism occurs more frequently during pregnancy and is associated with a higher mortality in pregnant patients [43, 44]. The clinical manifestations of PE are nonspecific, and the utility of the D-dimer test is limited as this value may be elevated in normal pregnancy. Thus the diagnosis of PE during pregnancy is almost wholly reliant on imaging. See Fig. 3.3.

Ultrasound

Compression ultrasound of the lower extremities to evaluate for deep venous thrombosis (DVT) is the recommended initial imaging study. Because the treatment for DVT and pulmonary embolus (PE) is the same in both pregnant and nonpregnant patients, a positive lower-extremity ultrasound can preclude any further imaging. A negative lower-extremity ultrasound however does not exclude systemic venous thromboembolism. One study showed that 10% of nonpregnant patients with a high clinical suspicion of PE and a negative lower-extremity ultrasound had angiographically proven PE [45]. Patients with a high clinical suspicion of PE and a negative lower-extremity ultrasound warrant further imaging with either CT pulmonary angiography (CTPA) or ventilation/perfusion (V/Q) scan. Limitations of lower-extremity ultrasound include a low sensitivity for detection of iliac vein thrombosis which occurs more frequently during pregnancy [44].

CT Pulmonary Angiography (CTPA) vs. Ventilation/Perfusion (V/Q) Scan

CTPA has a higher sensitivity (81–91%) and specificity (93–97%) than V/Q scanning for main, lobar, and segmental pulmonary arterial emboli [43]. The sensitivity of a high-probability V/Q scan for these types of emboli is 41% [43]. While the average estimated fetal radiation dose from CTPA is lower than that from V/Q scanning, the radiation dose administered to the maternal breasts from CTPA is higher [45]. The consulting diagnostic radiologist can assist with protocol adjustments to decrease breast radiation exposure during CTPA. An additional advantage of CTPA is that it can evaluate for an alternative etiology of the patient's symptoms (pneumonia, pulmonary edema, pleural effusion, etc.).

Magnetic Resonance Angiography (MRA)

Most MRA protocols for detection of pulmonary embolism employ gadolinium-based contrast agents which are not routinely recommended for use in pregnant patients. Studies evaluating non-contrast MRA for detection of pulmonary emboli have shown a per vessel sensitivity of 69% as compared to CTPA, with the missed emboli occurring in segmental and subsegmental pulmonary arteries [46].

Trauma

Traumatic injury is the most common cause of non-obstetric maternal mortality, with the highest percentage of these cases involving motor vehicle collisions [47–49]. The primary goal in caring for a pregnant trauma patient is to stabilize the mother. Imaging is vital in evaluation of maternal traumatic injuries as non-obstetric laparotomy is associated with a 26% incidence of preterm labor in the second trimester and an 82% incidence in the third trimester [50, 51]. The reported fetal mortality rate after blunt trauma ranges from 3 to 38%, most commonly due to placental abruption, maternal death, or

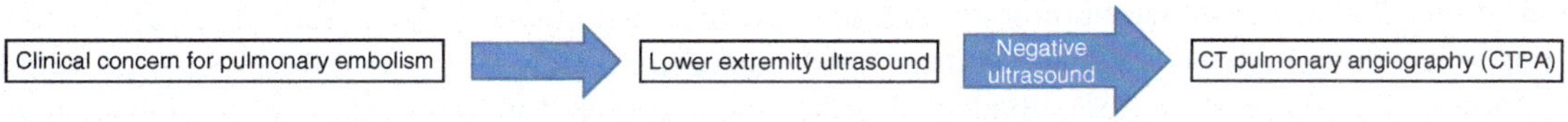

Fig. 3.3 Imaging algorithm for evaluation of pulmonary embolism

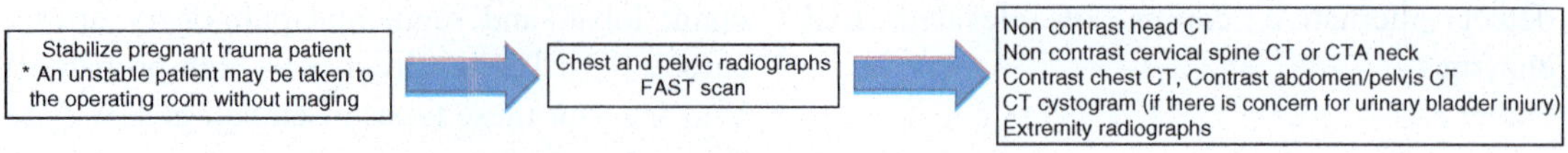

Fig. 3.4 Imaging algorithm for evaluation of traumatic injuries

shock [48]. While fetal loss occurs at a much higher rate with life-threatening trauma (i.e., 40–50%) than minor trauma (i.e., 1–5%), minor trauma is much more common [52]. Thus the majority of fetal losses are secondary to minor trauma [52]. For imaging evaluations that would require the patient to lie supine for extended periods of time, consideration may be given to having the patient lie in a 30° left lateral decubitus position to avoid exacerbation of hypotension from IVC compression by the gravid uterus. After the mother has been stabilized, a fetal ultrasound may be performed to assess gestational age and confirm a fetal heart rate. If the gestational age is less than 24–26 weeks, intermittent fetal monitoring may be used as a fetus this age would not survive outside of the uterus. If the gestational age is greater than 24–26 weeks, the fetus is considered viable, and continuous external fetal monitoring should be used [53]. See Fig. 3.4.

Ultrasound

Initial imaging of the mother may begin with a focused assessment with sonography in trauma (FAST) to evaluate for intraperitoneal or pericardial fluid. It should be noted that the reported sensitivity of this exam exhibits significant variation, and it is limited in detection of small (<400 mL) amounts of intraperitoneal fluid [54–56] as well as detection of retroperitoneal injuries. Confounding this is the actual relevance of small amounts of intraperitoneal fluid in pregnant patients, which may be a normal, expected finding. In pregnant patients, ultrasound demonstrates a 61–83% sensitivity and 94–100% specificity in detection of traumatic intra-abdominal injuries [57–59]. Ultrasound is not a substitute for CT in evaluation of traumatic injuries as its ability to detect solid and hollow organ injuries is substantially less than CT [54, 60–62].

Radiographs

The estimated fetal radiation dose from radiographs obtained to evaluate traumatic injury in a pregnant patient falls well below the threshold of 50 mGy for induction of fetal loss/fetal anomalies. Clinicians should not hesitate in obtaining chest and extremity radiographs in pregnant trauma patients. If there is concern for an unstable pelvic injury, an AP pelvic radiograph can be obtained with the chest radiograph during the initial evaluation. Abdominal and lumbar spine radiographs are associated with relatively higher fetal radiation dose that is typically 1–3 mGy and should not be obtained in trauma evaluations as injuries in these regions can be identified on a CT of the abdomen/pelvis.

CT

CT is the workhorse imaging modality in the evaluation of the traumatized pregnant patient and is more sensitive than ultrasound in detection of small-volume free peritoneal fluid, retroperitoneal hemorrhage, and visceral organ injury [54, 60–62]. When imaging body segments that do not include the fetus in the field of view, the estimated fetal radiation dose is well below that of background radiation during pregnancy (0.5–1.0 mGy). Imaging which includes the fetus within the field of view will incur a higher estimated fetal radiation dose; however even the dose associated with a CT abdomen/pelvis (25 mGy) is still below the threshold of 50 mGy for induction of fetal loss/congenital anomalies. One scenario in which a single imaging study of a traumatized pregnant patient could exceed 50 mGy would be a prolonged fluoroscopic abdominopelvic evaluation/intervention for life-threatening hemorrhage [8]. Another scenario in which cumulative fetal radiation dose may exceed 50 mGy throughout the pregnancy would be multiple follow-up CT and/or fluoroscopic imaging evaluations for a patient with extensive traumatic injuries. Intravenous iodinated contrast administration is absolutely vital in the assessment of both visceral and vascular traumatic injuries and should not be withheld due to concerns about fetal exposure. While gastrointestinal contrast is not routinely administered during CT evaluations of the traumatized patient, rectal contrast may be considered in the setting of penetrating pelvic trauma to evaluate for possible bowel injury. The healthcare provider will determine which regions of the body require evaluation with CT. If there is concern for traumatic injury to the head and neck, a non-contrast head and non-contrast cervical spine CT should be obtained. Alternatively, if there is concern for cervical vascular injury, a CT angiography (CTA) of the neck may be substituted for the non-contrast cervical spine CT. Neck CTA will not only exclude major cervical vascular injury but will also evaluate for cervical spine injury. If there is concern for thoracic injury, a contrast-enhanced chest CT should be obtained. If there is concern for abdominopelvic injury, a contrast-enhanced abdomen/pelvis CT should be obtained. At our institution, a typical CT evaluation for traumatic injury dubbed as "pan-scan" includes non-contrast head CT, non-contrast cervical spine CT or CTA neck, contrast-enhanced CT of the chest and upper abdomen in the arterial phase, and a contrast-enhanced CT of the abdomen/pelvis in the portal venous phase. The initial images from the abdomen/pelvis are previewed by the radiologist at the scanner to assess whether delayed imaging is required. Delayed imaging that is obtained at 3–5 min after the initial scan may be helpful in differentiating pseudoaneurysm vs. active arterial contrast extravasation as well as detecting urinary collecting system/urinary bladder injuries. If there is concern for urinary bladder injury, a CT cystogram should be obtained, as delayed imaging itself does not effectively exclude traumatic urinary bladder injury [63].

MRI

Although MRI offers diagnostic evaluation without the use of ionizing radiation, there are several disadvantages with the use of MRI rather than CT as the initial modality to exclude acute traumatic injury. These include long examination times which make MR imaging more susceptible to motion artifact, increased difficulty with patient monitoring and resuscitation efforts, and the controversial use of intravenous paramagnetic contrast, given the known teratogenic effects of these agents in animal models.

Urolithiasis

Urolithiasis is one of the most common non-obstetric indications for hospitalization of pregnant patients [64, 65]. To further complicate the issue, hormone-related physiologic dilatation of the collecting system and compression of distal ureters by the enlarged uterus may mimic obstructive hydronephrosis. It is reported that 70–80% of ureteral calculi will pass spontaneously in pregnant patients [65]. However, if obstructive urolithiasis is not appropriately addressed, it may lead to pyelonephritis or premature labor induced by renal colic [65]. See Fig. 3.5.

Ultrasound

Ultrasound is the initial imaging modality of choice in evaluation of urolithiasis in pregnant patients. Sensitivity for detection of renal/ureteral calculi with ultrasound ranges from 34 to 95% [65, 66]. Use of Doppler ultrasound with calculation of resistive indices (RI) has been advocated to differentiate obstructive hydronephrosis from physiologic dilatation of the collecting systems. Typically, pregnancy should not affect intrarenal RI; thus an abnormally elevated RI >0.70 should be considered pathologic [67]. It should be noted that RI elevation usually

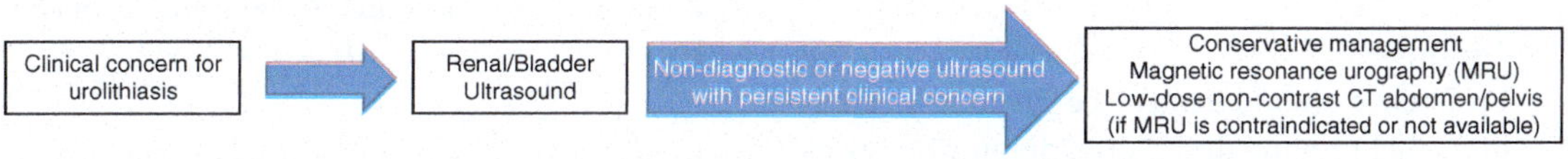

Fig. 3.5 Imaging algorithm for evaluation of urolithiasis

occurs within 6 h after acute obstruction. An absent ureteral jet on the symptomatic side has a reported sensitivity of 100% and specificity of 91% [68]. However approximately 15% of asymptomatic pregnant patients have absent unilateral ureteral jets; thus the patient should be imaged in the contralateral decubitus position to decrease the false positive rate [68, 69]. Transvaginal US may be considered to evaluate for distal ureteral calculi if the transabdominal US is normal or nondiagnostic [70].

CT

Low-dose non-contrast CT has gained favor as a possible second-line imaging test for urolithiasis in pregnant patients if MRI is contraindicated or not available. One article reports an estimated fetal radiation dose of 4–7.2 mGy at 0 months gestation and 8.5–11.7 mGy at 3 months gestation using a protocol that employs low-tube current (i.e., 160 mA, 140 kVp) and a 16-row multidetector CT [71]. The reported sensitivity and specificity for these exams are >95% and >98%, respectively.

MRI

Non-contrast MR urography is also considered to be a second-line imaging test when ultrasound is non-diagnostic in a patient with persistent symptoms despite conservative management. These studies have a high reported sensitivity for identifying urinary tract dilatation and locating the site of obstruction [72]. Limitations include a lack of institutional availability, high cost, and poor visualization of small calculi.

Therapeutic Intervention

While conservative treatment is recommended as the initial management for patients with renal colic, if therapeutic intervention is required, a ureteral stent may be placed with ultrasound guidance or under direct visualization using a ureteroscope [64]. Percutaneous nephrostomies may also be placed via ultrasound [64].

Conclusion

Preference should always be given to evaluations that provide the desired diagnostic information without the use of ionizing radiation when imaging non-traumatized pregnant patients. The healthcare provider should discuss risks and benefits of the examination with the patient when ordering an imaging study that employs ionizing radiation or an MRI for a pregnant patient and should obtain consent in cases that do not involve life-threatening trauma. While there are no documented adverse human fetal effects from diagnostic ultrasound, judicious use is advocated to keep fetal exposure as low as possible. The estimated fetal radiation dose should be kept as low as possible (i.e., below the cumulative threshold of 50 mGy) if an imaging evaluation that employs ionizing radiation must be used. Consideration should also be given to the number and type of imaging evaluations employing ionizing radiation a pregnant patient has already had during her current pregnancy, as these studies will contribute to the cumulative fetal radiation dose. Intravenous iodinated contrast administration is typically very useful for CT evaluations, especially for evaluation of traumatic injuries. Administration of intravenous paramagnetic contrast agents for MRI evaluations during pregnancy should only be considered when it is absolutely vital for patient management. Consultation with a diagnostic radiologist is helpful not only with choosing the appropriate imaging evaluation but also with tailoring study parameters to decrease radiation exposure while still maintaining the diagnostic integrity of the exam.

References

1. ACR–SPR practice parameter for imaging pregnant or potentially pregnant adolescents and women with ionizing radiation. Resolution 39. [Internet]. American College of Radiology. 2014 [cited 23 October 2017]. http://www.acr.org/~/media/9e2ed55531fc4b4fa53ef3b6d3b25df8.pdf.
2. Kanal E, Barkovich A, Bell C, Borgstede J, Bradley W, Froelich J, et al. ACR guidance document on MR safe practices: 2013. J Magn Reson Imaging. 2013;37(3):501–30.
3. International Commission on Radiologic Protection. Biological effects after prenatal irradiation (embryo

and fetus). IRCP publication no. 90. New York, NY: Pergamon; 2003. p. 153–82.
4. De Santis M, Di Gianantonio E, Straface G, Cavaliere A, Caruso A, Schiavon F, et al. Ionizing radiations in pregnancy and teratogenesis: a review of literature. Reprod Toxicol. 2005;20(3):323–9.
5. ACOG Committee opinion #299: guidelines for diagnostic imaging during pregnancy. Obstet Gynecol. 2004;104(3):647.
6. Wagner L, Lester R, Saldana L. Exposure of the pregnant patient to diagnostic radiations. Medical Physics Pub: Madison, WI; 1997.
7. Parry RA, Glaze SA, Archer BR. Typical patient radiation doses in diagnostic radiology. Radiographics. 1999;19:1289–302.
8. McCollough C, Schueler B, Atwell T, Braun N, Regner D, Brown D. Radiation exposure and pregnancy: when should we be concerned? Radiographics. 2007;27(4):909–17.
9. Osei E, Faulkner K. Fetal doses from radiological examinations. Br J Radiol. 1999;72(860):773–80.
10. Rice J. Prenatal susceptibility to carcinogenesis by xenobiotic substances including vinyl chloride. Environ Health Perspect. 1981;41:179–88.
11. Raptis C, Mellnick V, Raptis D, Kitchin D, Fowler K, Lubner M, et al. Imaging of trauma in the pregnant patient. Radiographics. 2014;34(3):748–63.
12. Chen M, Coakley F, Kaimal A, Laros R. Guidelines for computed tomography and magnetic resonance imaging use during pregnancy and lactation. Obstet Gynecol. 2008;112(2, Part 1):333–40.
13. Nguyen C, Goodman L. Fetal risk in diagnostic radiology. Semin Ultrasound CT MRI. 2012;33(1):4–10.
14. NCRP. Medical radiation exposure of pregnant and potentially pregnant women. Bethesda: NCRP Report No 54; 1977.
15. American College of Radiology. ACoR 04-05 bylaws. Reston, VA: American College of Radiology; 2005.
16. Shellock F, Crues J. MR procedures: biologic effects, safety, and patient care. Radiology. 2004;232(3):635–52.
17. Reeves M, Brandreth M, Whitby E, Hart A, Paley M, Griffiths P, et al. Neonatal cochlear function: measurement after exposure to acoustic noise during in utero MR imaging. Radiology. 2010;257(3):802–9.
18. Strizek B, Jani J, Mucyo E, De Keyzer F, Pauwels I, Ziane S. Safety of MR imaging at 1.5 T in fetuses: a retrospective case-control study of birth weights and the effects of acoustic noise. Radiology. 2015;275(2):530–7.
19. Hand J, Li Y, Hajnal J. Numerical study of RF exposure and the resulting temperature rise in the foetus during a magnetic resonance procedure. Phys Med Biol. 2010;55(4):913–30.
20. Abramowicz J, Barnett S, Duck F, Edmonds P, Hynynen K, Ziskin M. Fetal thermal effects of diagnostic ultrasound. J Ultrasound Med. 2008;27(4):541–59.
21. Abramowicz J, Kossoff G, Marsal K, Ter Haar G. Safety statement, 2000 (reconfirmed 2003). Ultrasound Obstet Gynecol. 2003;21(1):100.
22. Dean P. Fetal uptake of an intravascular radiologic contrast medium. Rofo. 1977;127(09):267–70.
23. Ultravist package insert. Montville, NJ: Berlex; 2004.
24. Bourjeily G, Chalhoub M, Phornphutkul C, Alleyne T, Woodfield C, Chen K. Neonatal thyroid function: effect of a single exposure to iodinated contrast medium in utero. Radiology. 2010;256(3):744–50.
25. ACR Manual on Contrast Media v10.3 [Internet]. 2017 [cited 24 October 2017]. http://www.acr.org/Quality-Safety/Resources/Contrast-Manual.
26. Omniscan package insert. Princceton, NJ: GE Healthcare; 2005.
27. Ray J, Vermeulen M, Bharatha A, Montanera W, Park A. Association between MRI exposure during pregnancy and fetal and childhood outcomes. JAMA. 2016;316(9):952.
28. Sikka A, Bisla J, Rajan P, Chalifoux L, Goodhartz L, Miller F. How to manage allergic reactions to contrast agent in pregnant patients. Am J Roentgenol. 2016;206(2):247–52.
29. Tamir I, Bongard F, Klein S. Acute appendicitis in the pregnant patient. Am J Surg. 1990;160(6):571–6.
30. Tracey M, Fletcher HS. Appendicitis in pregnancy. Am Surg. 2000;66:555–9.
31. Weiss C, Macura K. Diagnosis of ruptured appendicitis during pregnancy: role of magnetic resonance imaging. J Women Imaging. 2003;5(4):192–8.
32. Lim H, Bae S, Seo G. Diagnosis of acute appendicitis in pregnant women: value of sonography. Am J Roentgenol. 1992;159(3):539–42.
33. Lazarus E, Mayo-Smith W, Mainiero M, Spencer P. CT in the evaluation of nontraumatic abdominal pain in pregnant women. Radiology. 2007;244(3):784–90.
34. Wagner L, Huda W. When a pregnant woman with suspected appendicitis is referred for a CT scan, what should a radiologist do to minimize potential radiation risks? Pediatr Radiol. 2004;34(7):589–90.
35. Birchard K, Brown M, Hyslop W, Firat Z, Semelka R. MRI of acute abdominal and pelvic pain in pregnant patients. Am J Roentgenol. 2005;184(2):452–8.
36. Pedrosa I, Zeikus E, Levine D, Rofsky N. MR imaging of acute right lower quadrant pain in pregnant and nonpregnant patients. Radiographics. 2007;27(3):721–43.
37. Pedrosa I, Levine D, Eyvazzadeh A, Siewert B, Ngo L, Rofsky N. MR imaging evaluation of acute appendicitis in pregnancy. Radiology. 2006;238(3):891–9.
38. Lu E, Curet M, El-Sayed Y, Kirkwood K. Medical versus surgical management of biliary tract disease in pregnancy. Am J Surg. 2004;188(6):755–9.
39. Kahaleh M, Hartwell G, Arseneau K, Pajewski T, Mullick T, Isin G, et al. Safety and efficacy of ERCP in pregnancy. Gastrointest Endosc. 2004;60(2):287–92.
40. Gupta R, Tandan M, Lakhtakia S, Santosh D, Rao GV, Reddy DN. Safety of therapeutic ERCP in pregnancy: an Indian experience. Indian J Gastroenterol. 2005;24:161–3.
41. Shanmugam V, Beattie G, Yule S, Reid W, Loudon M. Is magnetic resonance cholangiopancreatography

the new gold standard in biliary imaging? Br J Radiol. 2005;78(934):888–93.
42. Moon J, Cho Y, Cha S, Cheon Y, Ahn H, Kim Y. The detection of bile duct stones in suspected biliary pancreatitis: comparison of MRCP, ERCP, and intraductal US. Am J Gastroenterol. 2005;100(5):1051–7.
43. Winer-Muram H, Boone J, Brown H, Jennings S, Mabie W, Lombardo G. Pulmonary embolism in pregnant patients: fetal radiation dose with helical CT. Radiology. 2002;224(2):487–92.
44. Nijkeuter M, Ginsberg J, Huisman M. Diagnosis of deep vein thrombosis and pulmonary embolism in pregnancy: a systematic review. J Thromb Haemost. 2006;4(3):496–500.
45. Scarsbrook A, Evans A, Owen A, Gleeson F. Diagnosis of suspected venous thromboembolic disease in pregnancy. Clin Radiol. 2006;61(1):1–12.
46. Mudge C, Healey T, Atalay M, Pezzullo J. Feasibility of detecting pulmonary embolism using noncontrast MRI. ISRN Radiol. 2013;2013:1–5.
47. Baerga-Varela Y, Zietlow S, Bannon M, Harmsen W, Ilstrup DM. Trauma in pregnancy. J Trauma Injury Infect Crit Care. 1999;46(1):208.
48. Grossman NB. Blunt trauma in pregnancy. Am Fam Physician. 2004;70:1303–10.
49. Esposito T, Gens DR, Smith LG, Scorpio R, Buchman T. Trauma during pregnancy. Arch Surg. 1991;126(9):1073.
50. Visser B, Glasgow R, Mulvihill K, Mulvihill S. Safety and timing of nonobstetric abdominal surgery in pregnancy. Dig Surg. 2001;18(5):409–17.
51. Puri A, Khadem P, Ahmed S, Yadav P, Al-Dulaimy K. Imaging of trauma in a pregnant patient. Semin Ultrasound CT MRI. 2012;33(1):37–45.
52. Mattox K, Goetzl L. Trauma in pregnancy. Crit Care Med. 2005;33(Supplement):S385–9.
53. Sadro C, Bittle M, O'Connell K. Imaging the pregnant trauma patient. Ultrasound Clin. 2011;6(1):97–103.
54. Rose JS. Ultrasound in abdominal trauma. Emerg Med Clin North Am. 2004;22(3):581–99. vii
55. Branney SW, Wolfe RE, Moore EE, Albert NP, Heinig M, Mestek M, et al. Quantitative sensitivity of ultrasound in detecting free intraperitoneal fluid. J Trauma. 1995;39(2):375–80.
56. Shackford SR, Rogers FB, Osler TM, Trabulsy ME, Clauss DW, Vane DW. Focused abdominal sonogram for trauma: the learning curve of nonradiologist clinicians in detecting hemoperitoneum. J Trauma. 1999;46(4):553–62. discussion 562-564
57. Richards JR, Ormsby EL, Romo MV, Gillen MA, McGahan JP. Blunt abdominal injury in the pregnant patient: detection with US. Radiology. 2004;233(2):463–70.
58. Goodwin H, Holmes JF, Wisner DH. Abdominal ultrasound examination in pregnant blunt trauma patients. J Trauma. 2001;50(4):689–693; discussion 694. discussion 694
59. Brown MA, Sirlin CB, Farahmand N, Hoyt DB, Casola G. Screening sonography in pregnant patients with blunt abdominal trauma. J Ultrasound Med. 2005;24(2):175–81. quiz 183-184
60. Richards JR, McGahan JP, Jones CD, Zhan S, Gerscovich EO. Ultrasound detection of blunt splenic injury. Injury. 2001;32(2):95–103.
61. Richards JR, McGahan JP, Pali MJ, Bohnen PA. Sonographic detection of blunt hepatic trauma: hemoperitoneum and parenchymal patterns of injury. J Trauma. 1999;47(6):1092–7.
62. Brown MA, Casola G, Sirlin CB, Hoyt DB. Importance of evaluating organ parenchyma during screening abdominal ultrasonography after blunt trauma. J Ultrasound Med. 2001;20(6):577–83. quiz 585
63. Mee SL, McAnnich JW, Federle MP. Computerized tomography in bladder rupture: diagnostic limitations. J Urol. 1987;137:207–9.
64. McAleer S, Loughlin K. Nephrolithiasis and pregnancy. Curr Opin Urol. 2004;14(2):123–7.
65. Parulkar B, Hopkins T, Wollin M, Howard P, Lal A. Renal colic during pregnancy: a case for conservative treatment. J Urol. 1998;159(2):365–8.
66. Stothers L, Lee L. Renal colic in pregnancy. J Urol. 1992;148(5):1383–7.
67. Hertzberg B, Carroll B, Bowie J, Paine S, Kliewer M, Paulson E, et al. Doppler US assessment of maternal kidneys: analysis of intrarenal resistivity indexes in normal pregnancy and physiologic pelvicaliectasis. Radiology. 1993;186(3):689–92.
68. Deyoe L, Cronan J, Breslaw B, Ridlen M. New techniques of ultrasound and color Doppler in the prospective evaluation of acute renal obstruction. Do they replace the intravenous urogram? Abdom Imaging. 1995;20(1):58–63.
69. Wachsberg R. Unilateral absence of ureteral jets in the third trimester of pregnancy: pitfall in color Doppler US diagnosis of urinary obstruction. Radiology. 1998;209(1):279–81.
70. Laing F, Benson C, DiSalvo D, Brown D, Frates M, Loughlin K. Distal ureteral calculi: detection with vaginal US. Radiology. 1994;192(2):545–8.
71. Hurwitz L, Yoshizumi T, Reiman R, Goodman P, Paulson E, Frush D. Radiation dose to the fetus from body MDCT during early gestation. Am J Roentgenol. 2006;186(3):871–6.
72. Roy C, Saussine C, Le Bras Y, Delepaul B, Jahn C, Steichen G. Assessment of painful ureterohydronephrosis during pregnancy by MR urography. Eur Radiol. 1996;6(3):334–8.

4 Instrumentation for Non-obstetric Surgery During Pregnancy

Ali Amiri, Ashley N. Bartalot, and Ceana H. Nezhat

Laparotomy in Pregnancy

In the hands of a skilled surgeon, many non-obstetric procedures performed during pregnancy can be completed via a minimally invasive approach. However, in the third trimester, as the uterus continues to enlarge and encompass the upper abdomen, adequate pneumoperitoneum and visualization may be difficult to achieve.

In addition to conventional laparotomy instruments (Fig. 4.1), a cesarean section tray should be readily available in case there are any signs of fetal distress and the mother does not respond to resuscitative measures.

A. Amiri (✉)
Marketing Research and Product Development, KARL STORZ Endoscopy-America, Inc., El Segundo, CA, USA
e-mail: ali.amiri@karlstorz.com

A. N. Bartalot
Department of Obstetrics and Gynecology, New York Presbyterian Brooklyn Methodist Hospital, Brooklyn, NY, USA

C. H. Nezhat
Nezhat Medical Center, Atlanta, GA, USA

Minimally Invasive Surgery and Robotics, Northside Hospital, Atlanta, GA, USA

Department of Gynecology and Obstetrics, Emory University, Atlanta, GA, USA
e-mail: ceana@nezhat.com

The Laparoscope

A high-performance laparoscope is a vital component of any laparoscopic procedure.

Besides size and configuration, laparoscopes are based on rod lens or CCD/CMOS sensor design and are used with 2D or 3D cameras. The laparoscope diameter ranges from 2 to 12 mm and may incorporate a working channel, an essential feature for laser or electrosurgery. It should be noted that the resolution of 4K cameras is outpacing the resolution of laparoscopes. For that reason, larger laparoscopes may be preferred to maximize the resolution.

The angle of view ranges from 0° to 120° in laparoscopes with a rod lens design. EndoCAMeleon® is a special variable-view

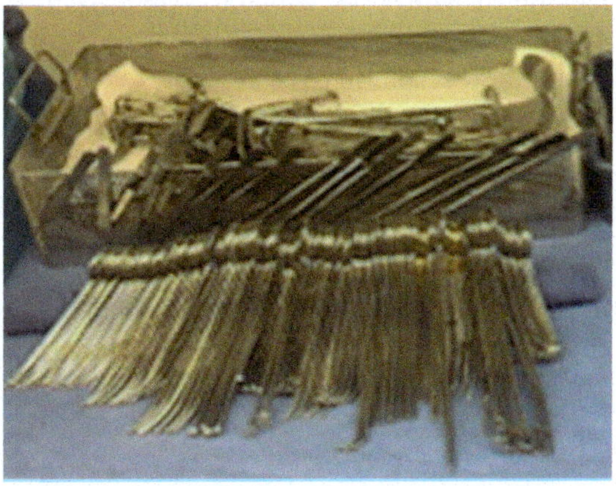

Fig. 4.1 General laparotomy tray

C. H. Nezhat (ed.), *Non-Obstetric Surgery During Pregnancy*,
https://doi.org/10.1007/978-3-319-90752-9_4

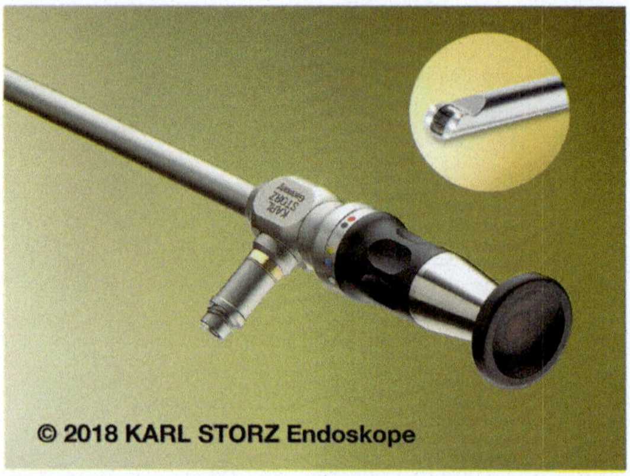

Fig. 4.2 EndoCAMeleon® variable-view laparoscope. ©2018 Photo Courtesy of KARL STORZ Endoscopy-America, Inc.

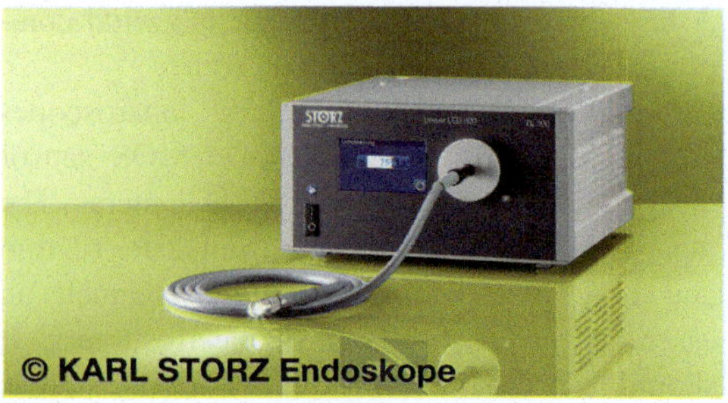

Fig. 4.3 Power LED 300 light source. ©2018 Photo Courtesy of KARL STORZ Endoscopy-America, Inc.

laparoscope manufactured by KARL STORZ and allows the angle of view to be changed intraoperatively between 0° and 120° (Fig. 4.2). Combined with a 4K camera system, such as IMAGE1 S™, it provides a look-around capability in 4K resolution.

Light Source

In recent years, there have been two noteworthy developments in light source technology. The first includes the LED-based light sources that provide brightness similar to xenon light sources but do not require a cooling fan and have a lower maintenance cost (Fig. 4.3). The second involves fluorescence imaging. Several manufacturers are also providing light sources that output a segment within or outside of the visible spectrum. Special cameras and scopes are required to visualize anatomy under near-infrared light after injection of indocyanine green (ICG) fluorescing dye. Assessment of the biliary duct system, organ perfusion, and lymph nodes are indications for use of this technology today.

The Camera

Endoscopic surgery requires the use of a camera acquiring an image. In some video imaging systems for endoscopic surgery, the camera is a separate device that attaches to an endoscope and is called a "camera head." In other video imaging systems for endoscopic surgery, the camera sensor is integrated into the endoscope, in which case the endoscope is called a video endoscope.

All camera heads and video endoscopes must be connected to a camera control unit (CCU) that houses the electronics and software. The CCU then receives the image data from the camera, processes, and distributes it for viewing on a display or documents it on a recording device.

KARL STORZ currently markets a camera system that is based on a modular design and incorporates multiple modalities.

The modular CCU, consists of one CONNECT module (top box in Fig. 4.4) and multiple video technology LINK modules (lower boxes in Fig. 4.4), which can be purchased independently. At a minimum, a CONNECT and one LINK module are required for a functioning CCU. Four LINK modules are available today, of which three can be connected with the CONNECT module at the same time:

- H3-LINK: for 4U camera heads and NIR/ICG high-definition (HD) camera head (Fig. 4.5)
- X-LINK: for single-chip camera heads and video endoscopes
- D3-LINK: for 3D HD video endoscopes (TIPCAM®)
- 4U-LINK: for 4K camera head

IMAGE1 S™ enhances the visualization of HD and ultra-high-definition (UHD/4K) images in the following ways:

- CLARA identifies and further brightens dark areas in an otherwise bright image dynamically and in real time without overexposing the bright part of the image.
- CHROMA enhances the visibility of vascularity by increasing red color contrast.
- For some surgical procedures, selecting CLARA *plus* CHROMA combines both enhancements to optimize viewing for those specific applications. NIR (near-infrared) imaging, used in conjunction with indocyanine green (ICG) fluorescing dye, enhances the visibility of blood vessels (perfusion) and biliary ducts.

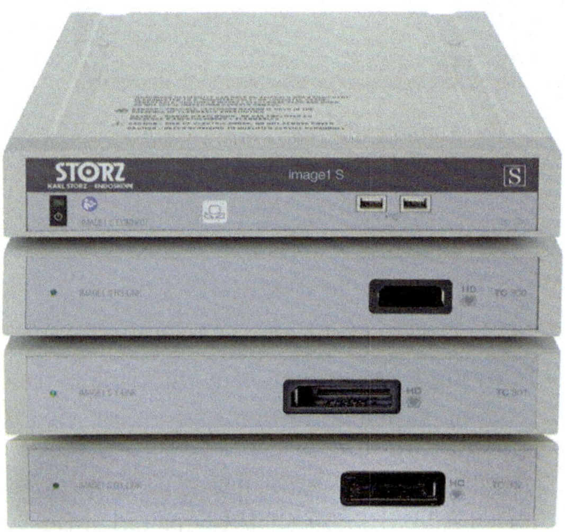

Fig. 4.4 IMAGE1 S™ Camera Control Unit with CONNECT module and three LINK modules. ©2018 Photo Courtesy of KARL STORZ Endoscopy-America, Inc.

The Monitor and Digital Capture Device

Display technology has also seen continued progress, allowing visualization of HD and 4K images. The size of surgical screens has also increased progressively with 32" becoming the norm in modern ORs. The surgical care of a pregnant woman requires close collaboration from multiple care teams, including specialty surgeons, anesthesiologists, and neonatologists. A new technology offered by KARL STORZ that assists a collaborative "care team" is called a "collaboration display" (Fig. 4.6). This large wall-mounted interactive display is available in sizes 55" up to 98" allowing the "care team" to visualize ALL relevant information, including preoperative imaging, intraoperative imaging, sonogram, and patient/fetus vitals. This technology allows for improved communication and coordination among the care team members. Remote surgical collaboration is also possible, making it possible to tap into the expertise of extended care team members who may not even be present in the OR.

Several modalities are available to digitally capture surgical footage. They range from built-in capture in CCUs to dedicated digital capture devices, such as the AIDA™ BELLA from KARL STORZ, as well as a streaming technology, e.g., StreamConnect®, that allows for cloud-based storage as part of the electronic health record of each patient (Fig. 4.7).

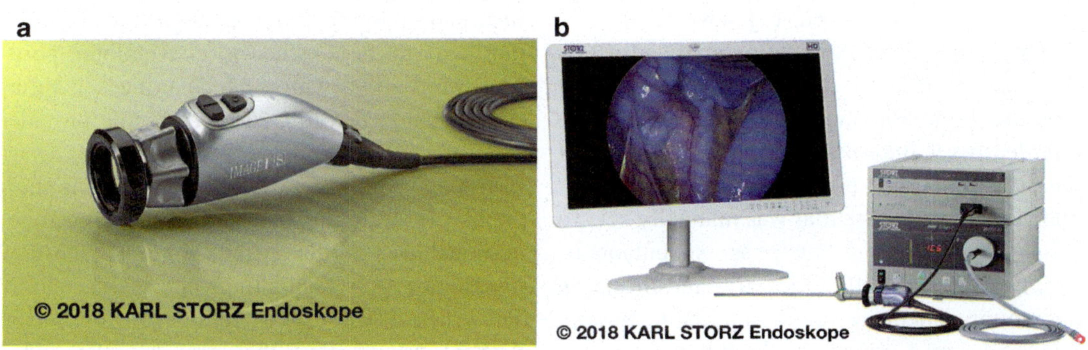

Fig. 4.5 4U camera head (**a**) and ICG system (**b**). ©2018 Photo Courtesy of KARL STORZ Endoscopy-America, Inc.

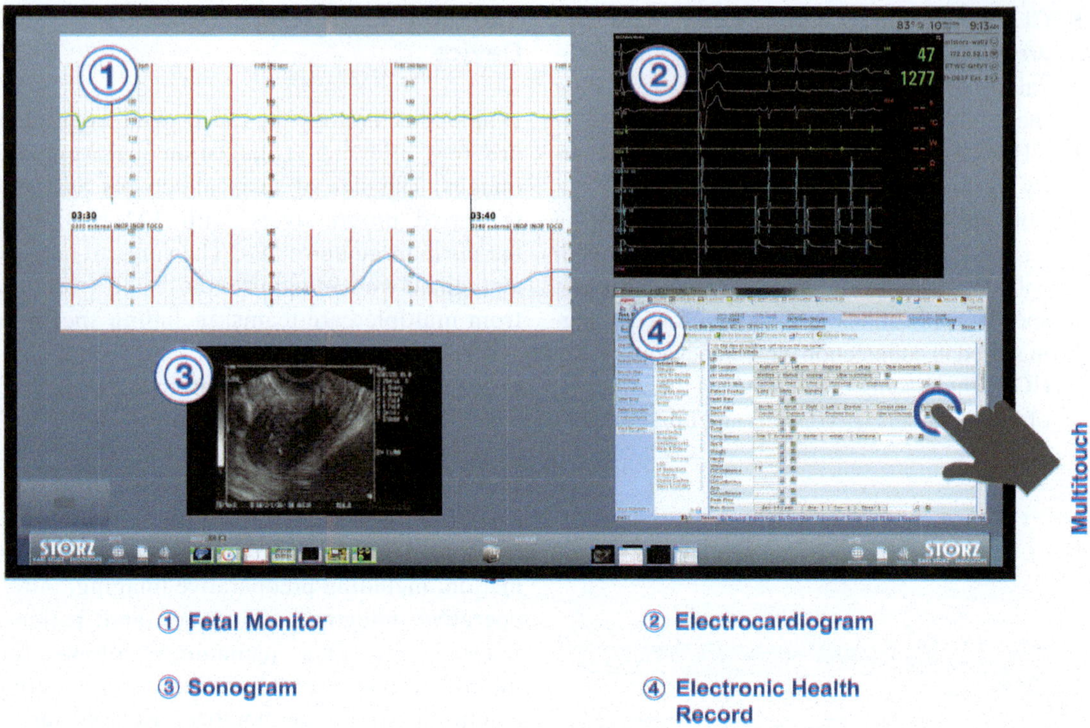

Fig. 4.6 Collaboration screen. ©2018 Photo Courtesy of KARL STORZ Endoscopy-America, Inc.

Insufflator

To adequately observe the contents of the abdominal and pelvic cavity, the abdomen is distended with CO_2 using an electronically controlled insufflator. The system has manually adjustable settings for the desired maximum intra-abdominal pressure in mmHg and the maximum CO_2 flow rate in liters per minute (L/min). There is also a digital display for the current intra-abdominal pressure, the CO_2 flow rate in L/min, and the volume of CO_2 gas consumed (Fig. 4.8).

The system is able to automatically adjust its flow rate based on the recorded intra-abdominal pressure throughout the procedure. There is also a protective feature that will sound an alarm if the intra-abdominal pressure exceeds the maximum desired pressure that was manually set. To avoid complications such as subcutaneous emphysema and difficulties for anesthesia in maintaining adequate ventilation, the maximum intra-abdominal pressure should not exceed 15 mmHg. Many commercial insufflators have a built-in heating function that heats the CO_2 to 37 °C/99 °F to help prevent the patient from becoming hypothermic and to decrease laparoscope fogging.

High-flow insufflators such as ENDOFLATOR® 50 can be paired with an S-Pilot® smoke evacuation device to maintain a clear visual field and distention.

Airseal iFS (ConMed, Utica, NY; Fig. 4.9) is a commercial insufflator that has a "3-in-1" insufflation management system that is capable of operating in three distinct modes. The Standard Insufflation Mode provides high-flow insufflation and can be attached to conventional ports. The Smoke Evacuation Mode utilizes a bifurcated, dual-lumen filtered tube set that provides high-flow insufflation and facilitates smoke evacuation and filtration. The AirSeal Mode is most popular for its ability to maintain stable pneumoperitoneum while providing high-flow insufflation and facilitating smoke evacuation. The AirSeal Mode does require the use of an AirSeal Access Port that also has the added advantage of being valve-free with unimpeded access to the abdominal cavity [1].

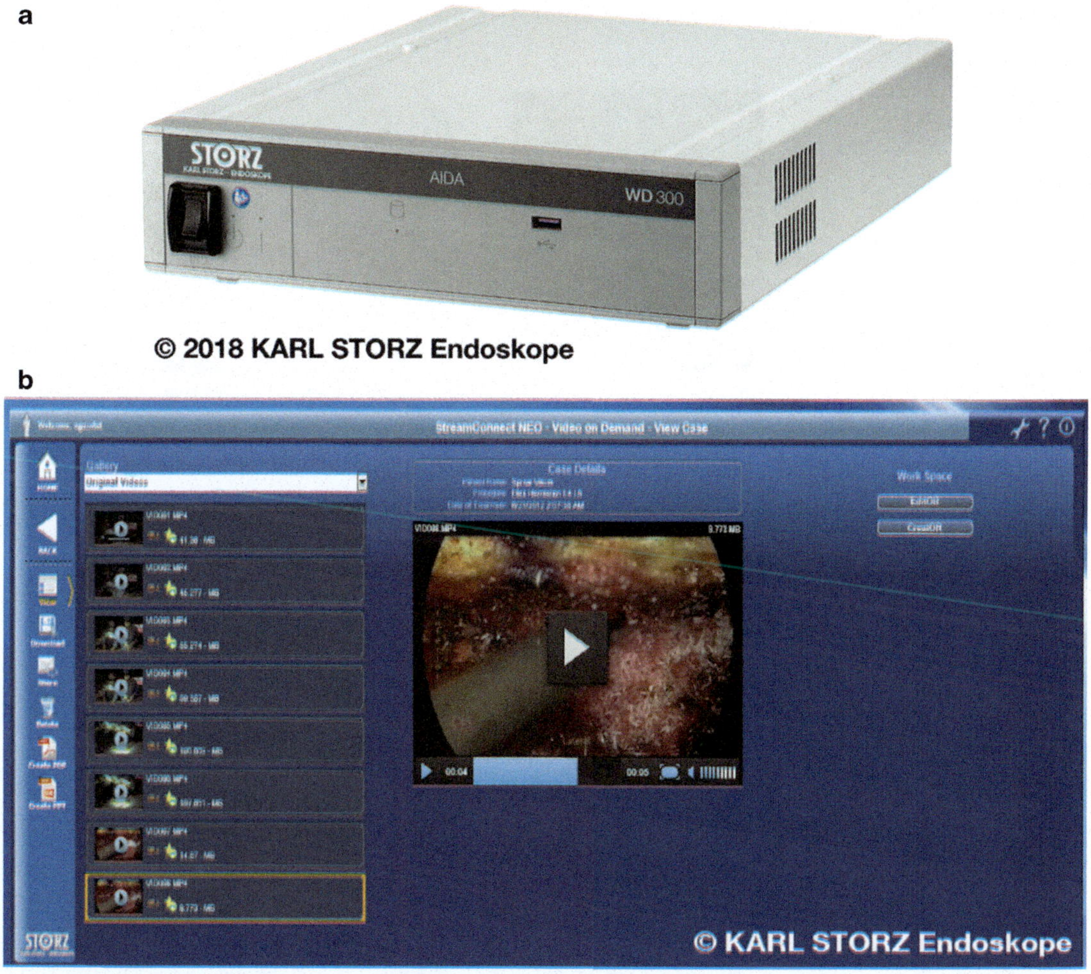

Fig. 4.7 (**a**) AIDA™ BELLA 4K Digital capture. (**b**) StreamConnect®. ©2018 Photo Courtesy of KARL STORZ Endoscopy-America, Inc.

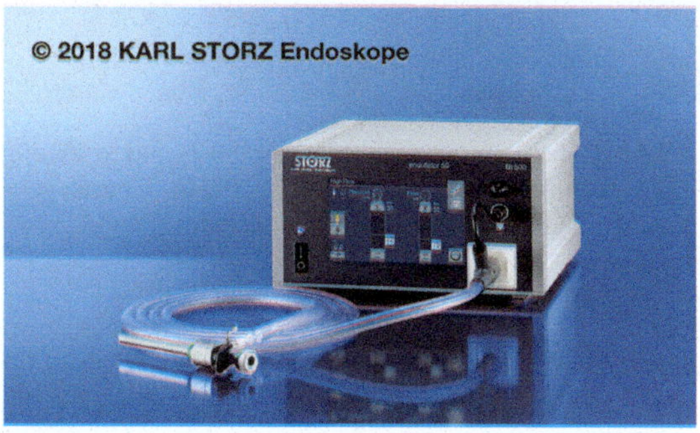

Fig. 4.8 ENDOFLATOR® 50 showing the digital display for intra-abdominal pressure, flow rate, and volume consumed. ©2018 Photo Courtesy of KARL STORZ Endoscopy-America, Inc (intra-abdominal pressure, etc…).

Integrated Operating Rooms

Like most examples of contemporary medical care, operating rooms have moved toward more complex environments. The modern OR embodies numerous critically interrelated surgical systems, technology platforms, and information systems. Each component has been developed to facilitate and enhance the flow, both into and out of the OR, of patients, personnel, and medical, as well as billing data and more (Fig. 4.10). The hurdle facing hospitals and device manufacturers is to create solutions for organizing and managing this movement.

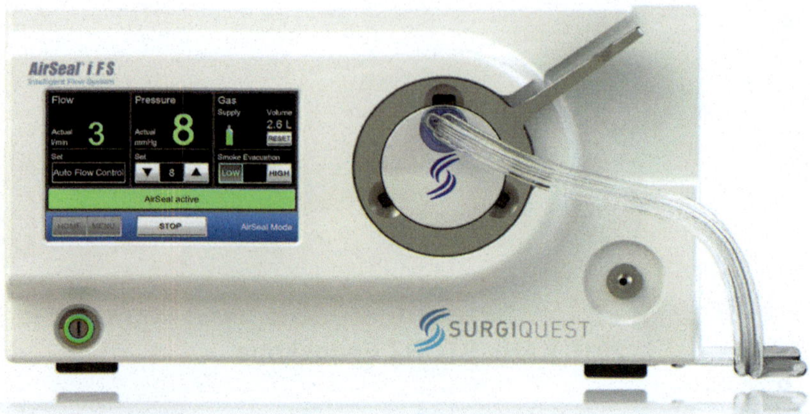

Fig. 4.9 AirSeal iFS showing the three modes available. Image courtesy of Surgiquest, ConMed, Utica, NY

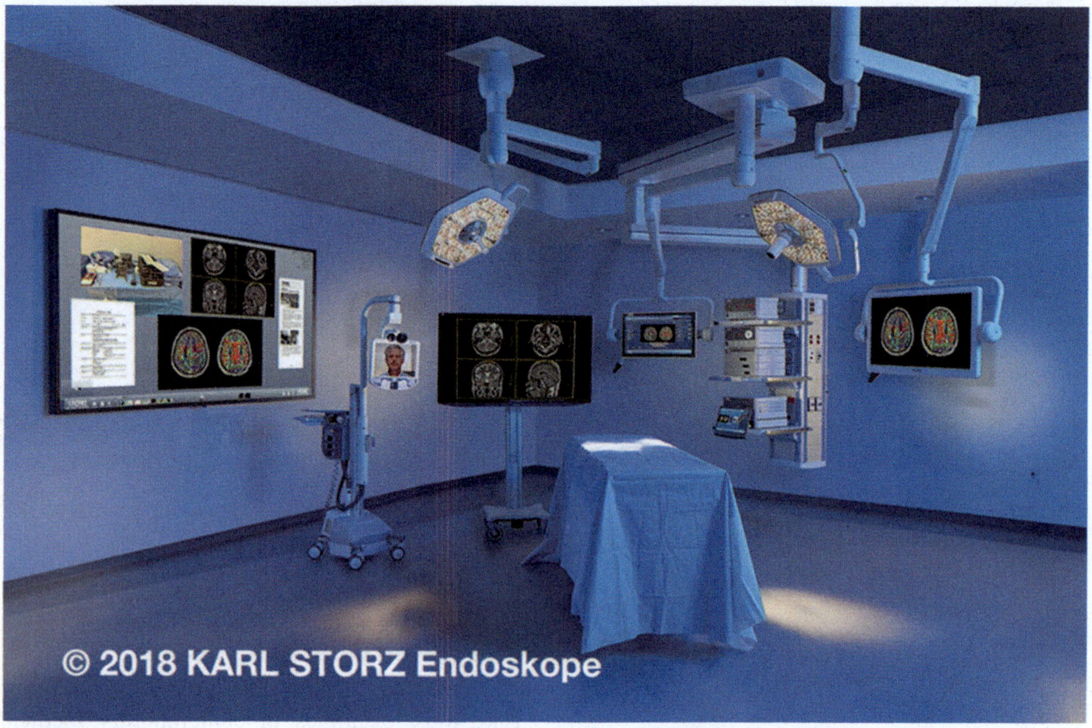

Fig. 4.10 Operating rooms today, such as the OR1® integrated suite above, must encompass a broad range of systems for data and image management, device control, and more. Each piece of equipment and its functional component must be integrated for interoperability and to streamline functional dynamics. ©2018 Photo Courtesy of KARL STORZ Endoscopy-America, Inc.

The movement of individuals, equipment, data, and more through the OR environment can be viewed in terms of workflow dynamics. The role of new generations of medical equipment within such a system can thus be envisioned as streamlining both incoming and outgoing flows while, ideally, increasing efficiency and effectiveness in terms of patient outcomes and safety.

Like most facets of medical care, the flow of people, equipment, and data into and out of the

OR has only increased in magnitude and complexity between the surgical settings of yesterday's Industrial Age and the currently evolving Information Age.

Instruments for Fetoscopy

Embryoscopy and fetoscopy were developed in the 1970s, but were displaced by high-resolution ultrasound before they were reintroduced as a surgical fetoscopy intervention. Over the past three decades, various procedures have been developed to treat the fetus for several congenital diseases, affording those patients significantly improved odds for survival and better outcomes after birth. While some of the equipment necessary to perform a fetoscopy procedure, such as light sources and cameras, are similar to those used in laparoscopic or hysteroscopic surgery, these latest interventions are enabled by new developments in endoscopes and instrumentation. KARL STORZ has been a pioneer in developing the instrumentation required for fetoscopy procedures and has supported the development of several procedures and multicenter studies in both Europe and the USA. Today, a number of surgical interventions on fetuses are performed outside of the USA. Restrictions by the regulatory body in the USA have limited the diversity of the procedures performed in the USA. Humanitarian Device Exemption (HDE) is a regulatory process within the US Food and Drug Administration (FDA) that follows the orphan drug model. Using this process, companies with an interest in marketing a device that is critical to the care of a very limited number of patients and has no predicate device to qualify for a 510(k) process can apply for a Humanitarian Use Device (HUD) designation to establish the device is used to treat diseases affecting a limited number of patients. This would be followed by the submission of an HDE application demonstrating that the probable benefit outweighs the risk. The clinical data and other relevant information are very comprehensive but less burdensome than a Premarket Approval Application that would be required with procedures with a higher prevalence. KARL STORZ is the only company in the USA that has made the required investment in resources that generate the data required to secure an HDE designation for its instrumentation used for the treatment of twin-to-twin transfusion syndrome (TTTS), which is discussed further in Chap. 33. These instruments are currently in use across more than 20 institutions in the USA, with ongoing efforts to expand the available scope and instrument designs, procedures, and sites. The current HDE-approved set (Fig. 4.11) includes fetoscopes in 1.0 to 2.0 mm in diameter and

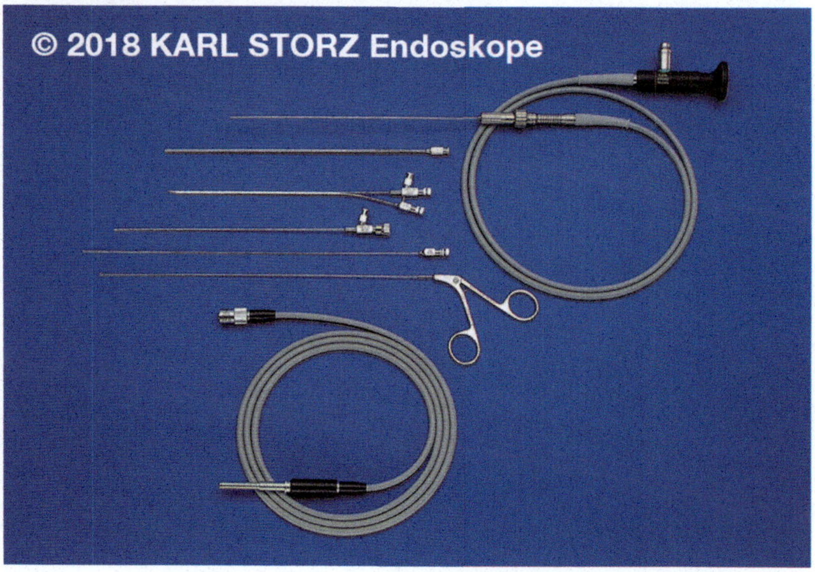

Fig. 4.11 Fetoscopy instrumentation. ©2018 Photo Courtesy of KARL STORZ Endoscopy-America, Inc.

20–30 cm in working length with accompanying instrumentation. A scope with a specially designed remote eyepiece (Fig. 4.12) reduces the weight and enables the surgeon to navigate the scope with fine movements and an ergonomic fashion. The new "Picture in Picture" feature (Fig. 4.13) of the IMAGE1 S™ camera allows a simultaneous side-by-side display of endoscopic and ultrasound images.

The Veress needle is the most common method used to insufflate the abdomen. There are disposable and reusable Veress needles available that consist of a blunt-tipped, spring-loaded inner stylet and a sharp outer needle (Fig. 4.14). The other end of the Veress needle has a valve with an adjustable occluder to allow for an injectable syringe or CO_2 tubing to be attached for insufflation. The stylet has a lateral hole that allows CO_2 to pass through.

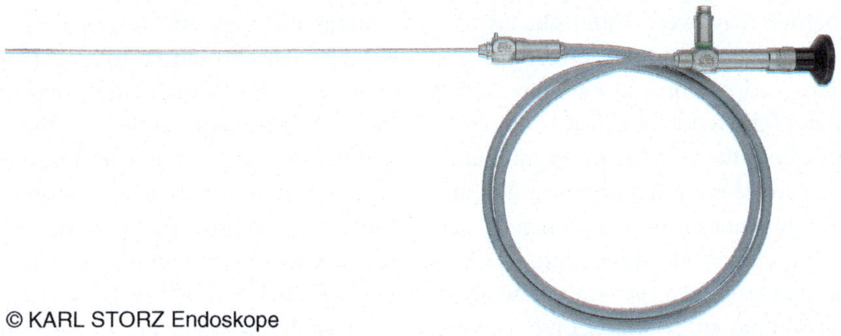

Fig. 4.12 The fetoscope used for TTTS. ©2018 Photo Courtesy of KARL STORZ Endoscopy-America, Inc.

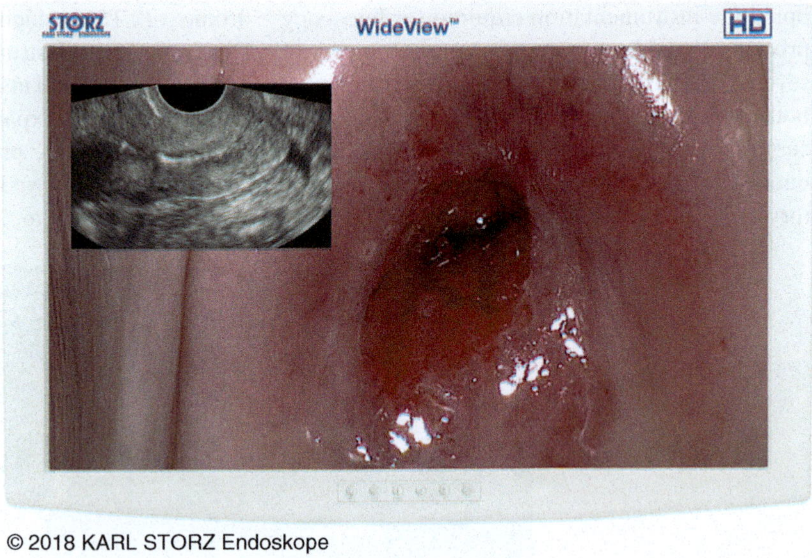

Fig. 4.13 Example of picture-in-picture display of clinical image. ©2018 Photo Courtesy of KARL STORZ Endoscopy-America, Inc.

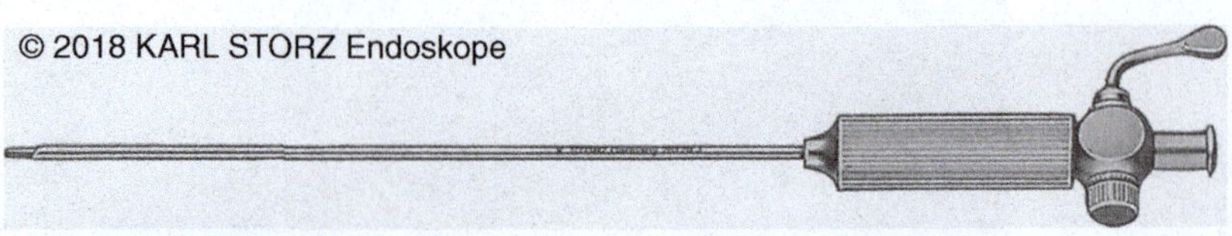

Fig. 4.14 Veress pneumoperitoneum needle with spring-loaded blunt inner cannula. ©2018 Photo Courtesy of KARL STORZ Endoscopy-America, Inc.

Access Devices

Reusable and disposable ports, which come in numerous compositions, are available for use. Trocars used with ports may be blunt, sharp, radially expanding (Fig. 4.15), shielded, and/or clear for visualization during insertion. The ports may be made of plastic, metal, or a combination of both. Commonly used port diameters range in size from 3 to 13 mm. The choice of port composition is generally up to the preference of the surgeon. If a port containing metal is selected, however, caution should be taken when using monopolar cautery as there is an increased risk for thermal injury from capacitive coupling [2]. Techniques for trocar insertion will be discussed in a later chapter.

A Gelpoint device (Applied Medical, Rancho Santa Margarita, CA) can be used during single-site video-assisted laparoscopic procedures to allow for multiple trocar insertions through a single abdominal incision.

Suction-Irrigator Probe and Hydrodissection Pump

The suction-irrigator probe has many functions during a video-assisted procedure. Its obvious functions include evacuating blood, fluid, and smoke from the operative field with the suction mode and lavage with the irrigation mode. The suction-irrigator tip can also be used as an extension of the surgeon's fingers to aid in blunt dissection, division of tissue planes and spaces, and, uniquely, hydrodissection, which dissects planes while protecting proximal structures, i.e., the ureter, pelvic vessels, bladder, and bowel, in cases of adhesion. Since the probe is sandblasted, it can also be used as a backstop for the CO_2 laser. In general, a properly designed suction-irrigation system has the following characteristics:

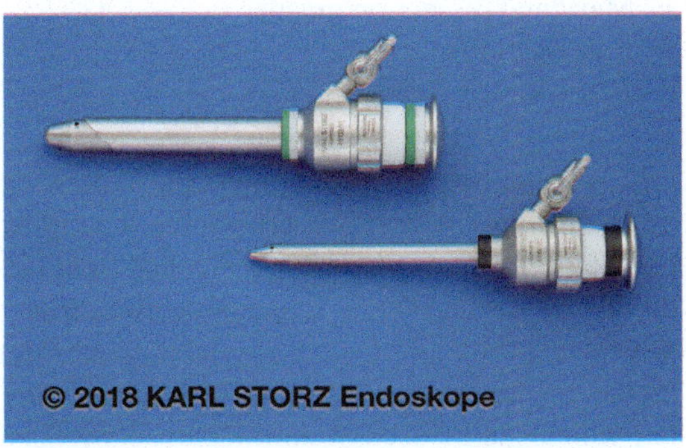

Fig. 4.15 Trocars used for access. ©2018 Photo Courtesy of KARL STORZ Endoscopy-America, Inc.

- The trumpet valve is designed ergonomically so that the valve is easy to use and provides constant control of fluid or suction, including valve regulation, rather than an on/off mechanism.
- The internal valve diameters are large enough to allow the blood and tissue to pass easily through the canister and provide sufficient irrigation flow.
- Probe tips are smooth, strong, and nonreflective, so that they can be used for blunt dissection and serve as a backstop for the CO_2 laser.
- The irrigation pump provides precise and variable irrigation pressures.

The trumpet valve can also have a metered adjustment feature incorporated into its design to allow for continuous smoke evacuation without having to manually compress the suction piston. Additional suction capability can be accessed by manually depressing the suction piston. The probe tip is available in various lengths and diameters. Care should be taken when using the probe for blunt dissection as bowel injuries have been reported during this process [3]. High pump pressures are used in hydrodissecting areas near the bowel, bladder, major blood vessels, and ureters. It is also recommended to use warmed irrigation fluid (39 °C) to help reduce risks of a drop in core temperature, which has commonly been observed with the use of large quantities of irrigation fluid during laparoscopy [4].

A higher electrically powered pump with adjustable "high" and "low" settings has been developed (Davol X-Stream Irrigation System; Davol Inc., a subsidiary of C. R. Bard, Inc.). On the low setting, the flow rate ranges from 2500 to 3800 mL/min. On the high setting, the

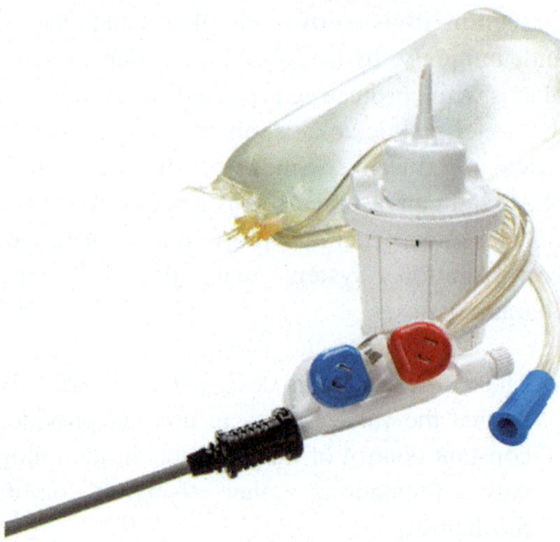

Fig. 4.16 StrykeFlow2 suction irrigator courtesy of Stryker, Inc.

flow rate ranges from 3400 to 5000 mL/min. It incorporates the effectiveness and convenience of bag irrigation with the precision and effective delivery of pressurized pump irrigation (Fig. 4.16a). The Hydro-Surg Plus system (Fig. 4.16b) is another battery-powered, high-performance system with an on/off switch for pump activation and a smoke evacuation feature that directly attaches to an I.V. pole for convenience and added security.

Electrosurgical Generator with Bipolar Forceps and Monopolar Scissors

The primary instrument used for hemostasis during operative laparoscopy is the bipolar electrocoagulator. The use of bipolar energy allows for a more controlled thermal spread over the tissue when compared to monopolar energy. Several types of bipolar forceps are available, including reusable and disposable forms. This instrument should be prepared routinely and tested prior to starting the procedure to ensure its proper function. Fine tips are used for coagulating small blood vessels during delicate operations involving the fallopian tubes, bowel, and ureters. Flatter jaws are used on larger blood vessels or pedicles, including the uterine artery and infundibulopelvic ligaments.

Monopolar scissors with and without attachment to an energy source is another instrument that should be routinely available. This instrument also comes in reusable and disposable forms. This instrument can be used for both blunt and sharp dissection of adhesions, dissecting the pelvic sidewall, resecting the diseased tissue (i.e., endometriosis), or sampling tissue for biopsy. The shaft can easily be rotated along its longitudinal axis by adjusting the dial on the handle. Care must be taken to avoid arcing when using the scissors while attached to an energy source, as this could lead to injury of the proximal tissue and blood vessels.

Grasping Instruments

As seen in Fig. 4.17, laparoscopic instrument trays with the necessary grasping instruments can be designed at the hospital or facility to be readily available and specialized for the planned procedures. A variety of graspers designed to firmly hold tissue without exerting excessive pressure that could result in injury to the tissue can be included in these trays. The following list of graspers should be included:

- At least 2–3 wavy graspers: with and without teeth
- Bowel grasper
- Maryland dissection grasper
- Babcock grasper
- Blunt-tipped probe

These graspers should include a locking mechanism and a knob on the handle that allow for the instrument to be rotated along its longitudinal axis for additional maneuverability. Many of these instruments are also available in 3.5-mm diameters, instead of the standard 5-mm diameter, which can be used in mini-laparoscopy. As a

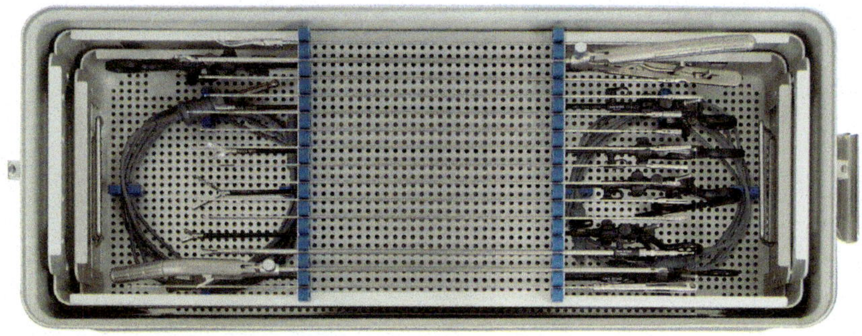

Fig. 4.17 Routine laparoscopic gynecology tray. ©2018 Photo Courtesy of KARL STORZ Endoscopy-America, Inc.

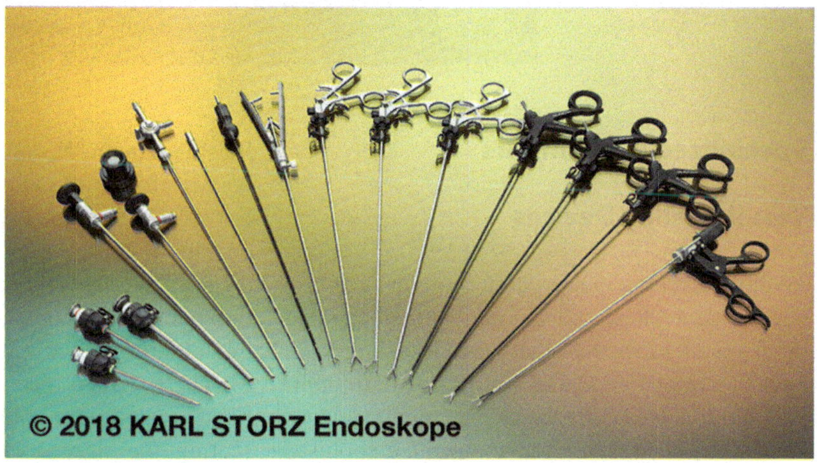

Fig. 4.18 Mini-laparoscopy instruments. ©2018 Photo Courtesy of KARL STORZ Endoscopy-America, Inc.

broad range of miniature-size instruments (Fig. 4.18) have been made available, their use has increased in recent years. This is attributed to improved cosmetics, reduced postoperative pain, faster recovery, and reduced risk of hernias, adhesions, and infections.

Da Vinci Si and Xi Basic Instruments

Although rarely necessary, computer-enhanced video-assisted laparoscopy (robotic) may be used during pregnancy. Similarly to the trays described above, specialized gynecology robotic trays can be assembled for both the Da Vinci Si and Xi compatible systems. These trays should include the following 8-mm instruments (Fig. 4.19):

- Fenestrated Bipolar Forceps[1]
- Maryland Bipolar Forceps[1]
- ProGrasp™ Forceps
- Tenaculum Forceps
- Monopolar Curved Scissors[1]
- Large or Mega Needle Driver
- Large or Mega SutureCut™ Needle Driver
- Large SutureCut™ Needle Driver
- Permanent Cautery Spatula (Xi system)[1]

Some of the specialized instruments available with the Da Vinci robotic system that might be useful are the Vessel Sealer and the Harmonic Ace® Curved Shears (Ethicon, Inc., Cincinnati, OH).

[1]Also available in 5-mm diameter for single-site applications

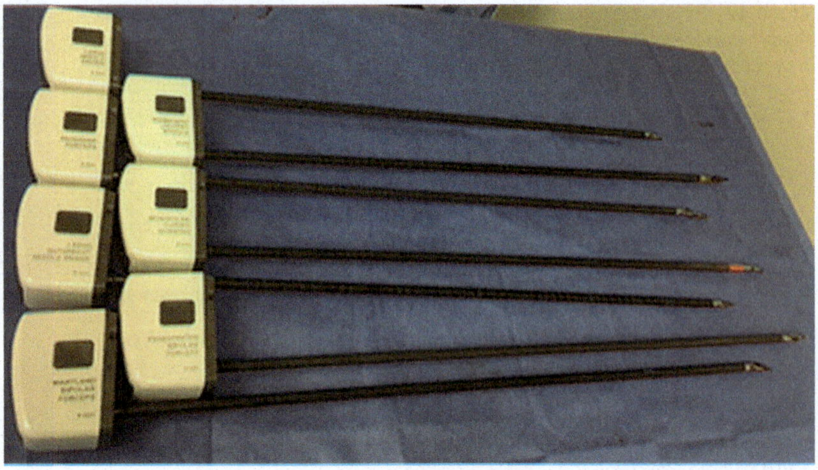

Fig. 4.19 Da Vinci Xi gynecology instruments

Specialized Instruments

Vessel-Sealing Devices

Traditional monopolar and bipolar cautery devices generate significant heat and smoke and often result in inconsistent vessel sealing with larger thermal spread and charring [5]. To compensate for these inadequacies, many devices have since been developed that utilize sophisticated energy systems for dissection and hemostasis. These advances in electrosurgical technology continue to transform the field of operative laparoscopy and have allowed for the ongoing development of devices that result in effective vessel sealing with minimal collateral damage. The most commonly utilized devices include modern feedback-controlled bipolar devices as well as ultrasonic shears.

Most commonly used modern feedback-controlled bipolar devices include the LigaSure™ sealing device (Covidien, Boulder, CO) (Fig. 4.20a, b), the Gyrus Plasma Kinetics sealer (Gyrus ACMI, Southborough, MA), and the ENSEAL® (Ethicon, Inc., Cincinnati, OH) (Fig. 4.21a, b). All of these devices use radiofrequency bipolar energy and have an impedance-based feedback loop that modifies the bipolar energy delivered. Bipolar energy differs in that the LigaSure device provides a continuous bipolar waveform, whereas the Gyrus Plasma Kinetic™ sealer delivers a pulsed bipolar waveform, allowing for a cooling-off period for cooling the blades [6]. The ENSEAL® delivers high uniform compression through the device jaws, and its dynamic thermal modulation maintains a constant temperature of approximately 100 °C, minimizing tissue charring [7, 8]. The I-shaped blade advances as the tissue is being sealed, simultaneously sealing and transecting the tissue. These devices are recommended for sealing vessels up to 7 mm in diameter.

Harmonic Scalpel

The ultrasonically activated vibrating blade of the Harmonic Ace® scalpel or shears (Ethicon, Inc., Cincinnati, OH) moves longitudinally at 55,000 vibrations per second, cutting tissue while simultaneously providing hemostasis. The vibration of the ultrasonic scalpel is thought to generate low heat at the incision site. The combination of vibration and heat causes the protein to denature. The Harmonic Ace® scalpel may limit the number of steps required for desiccation and transection of vascular pedicles. Another advantage of the harmonic scalpel is that the active blade can be used as a surgical knife. It was also found to cause less thermal spread in tissue when compared to bipolar vessel-sealing devices [5, 9].

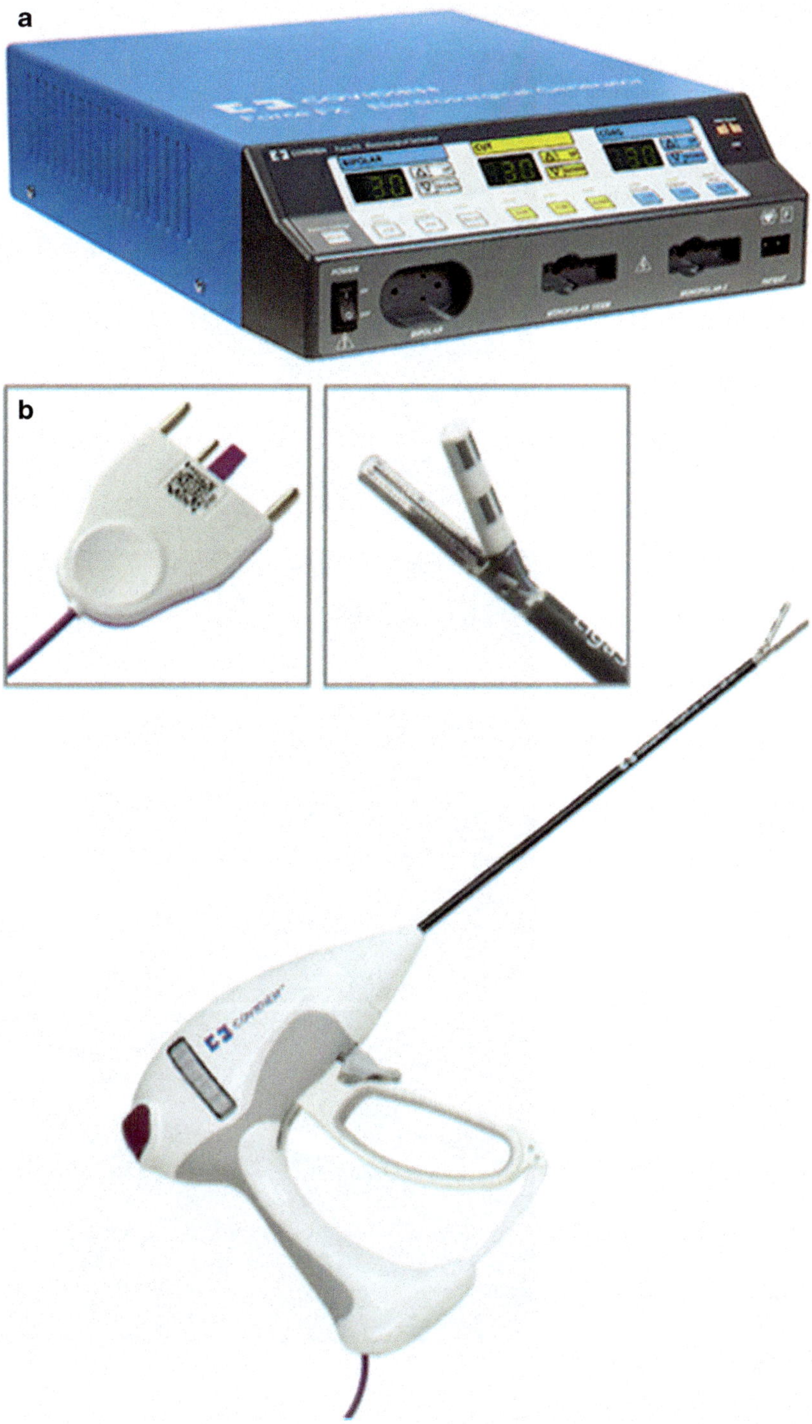

Fig. 4.20 (**a**) Covidien Electrosurgical Generator. (**b**) LigaSure 5-mm laparoscopic instrument. Photos courtesy of Covidien, Boulder, CO

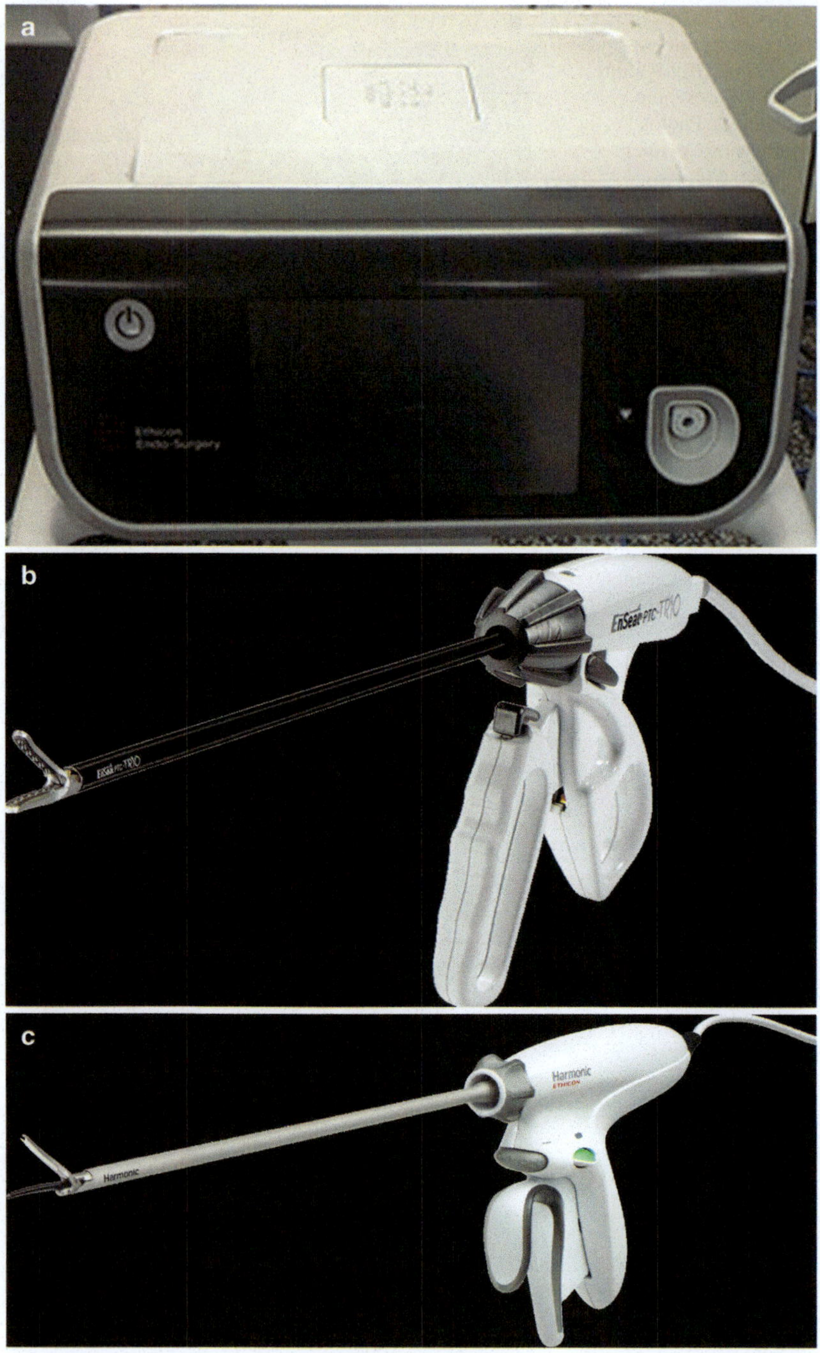

Fig. 4.21 (**a**) Ethicon electrosurgical generator. (**b**) Ethicon ENSEAL® tissue sealing device. (**c**) Ethicon Harmonic HD 1000i Shears. ©Ethicon, Inc. 2018. Reproduced with permission

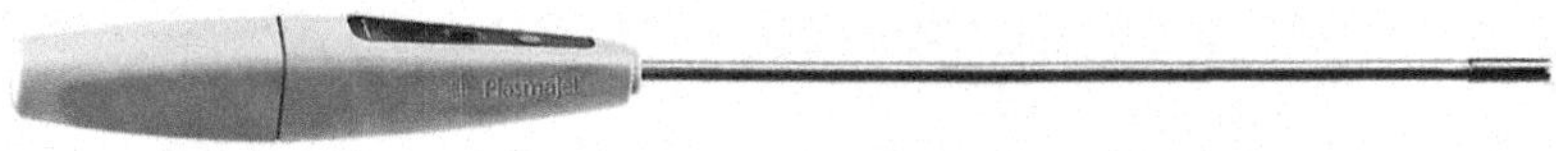

Fig. 4.22 PlasmaJet® 5-mm handpiece. Image courtesy of Plasma Surgical, Inc., Roswell, GA

In response to a few studies that showed the Harmonic Ace® scalpel to be inferior at sealing vessels greater than 4 mm when compared to bipolar vessel-sealing devices, the Harmonic Ace® + 7 Shears (Ethicon, Inc., Cincinnati, OH) was developed with the advanced hemostasis mode with improved burst pressures (1419 mmHg for 5–7-mm diameter vessels) so that the Harmonic scalpel could be utilized for sealing larger vessels up to 7 mm [5]. The HARMONIC® HD 1000i Shears (Ethicon, Inc., Cincinnati, OH; see Fig. 4.22b) was most recently developed and is now completely disposable with the energy cord already attached. This version of the harmonic scalpel is supposed to combine the advantages of the Max and Min functions into one button. There is still the advanced hemostasis mode button on the side for sealing up to 7-mm vessels. A study was published in 2016 to assess the clinical experience during a total laparoscopic hysterectomy with the use of the advanced hemostasis mode. The study included 40 patients and reported that 94.4% of transections, including the uterine artery or pedicle and the ovarian pedicles (when indicated), achieved adequate hemostasis with the Advanced Hemostasis mode alone. Five patients required the use of conventional bipolar or monopoly energy [10].

PlasmaJet

Plasma Surgical, Inc. (Roswell, GA) developed the PlasmaJet® system (Fig. 4.22), which is unique in employing a pure and electrically neutral plasma, a stream of excited argon ions and electrons at very high enthalpy, to cut, vaporize, and coagulate tissue. Because the PlasmaJet® does not use high voltage, it can be utilized in several fields of surgery, including cardiac, safe laparoscopy, neurosurgery, and spine surgery, where the use of a high-voltage device would not be appropriate. There is also no external electrical current generated by the PlasmaJet® system because it uses argon gas at 0.4 L/min, so it does not stimulate nerves and evoke action potentials or muscle twitch during surgery. The other distinct and major advantage of plasma surgery technology is that the depth of tissue damage is significantly less than that observed in electrosurgery, allowing for controlled use on delicate tissue, such as the ovary, fallopian tube, adhesions, bowel, and diaphragm and the ability at a higher-power setting to cut and coagulate denser structures.

The laparoscopic handpieces are 5 mm in diameter and 28 cm in length. The device can be controlled by the handpiece or foot pedal with both modes containing cut and coagulation function. The tissue effect is determined by the distance of the handpiece from the targeted tissue. With near-direct contact, a cutting effect may be achieved, while a greater distance from the tissue results in a coagulative effect. The PlasmaJet® produces very little plume smoke and will not overpressure the pneumoperitoneum.

Endoscopic Lasers

Three different lasers are available in the operating room: a CO_2 laser (with coupler), an argon or potassium titanyl phosphate (KTP) laser, and a neodymium-doped: yttrium-aluminum-garnet (Nd:YAG) laser. They are used through the operative channel of the laparoscope or a separate port. The CO_2 laser is on the patient's side, opposite the surgeon. The articulating arm is extended appropriately so that it does not weigh too heavily on the surgeon's hand and it can be used as free beam or fiber. YAG and argon lasers are used less frequently and are located behind the assistant standing between the patient's legs. This

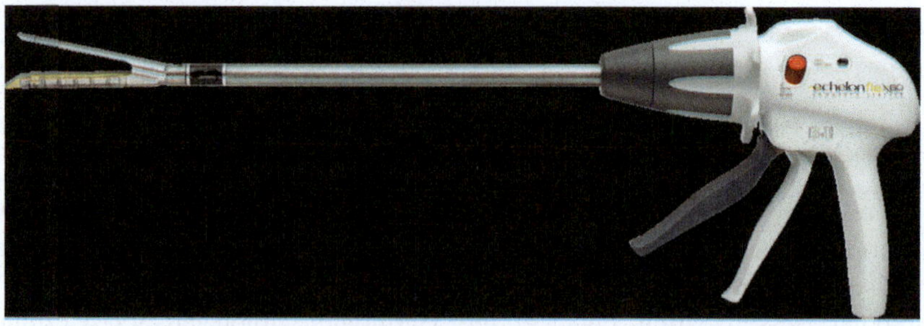

Fig. 4.23 Linear stapler designed for gynecologic use. ©Ethicon, Inc. 2018. Reproduced with permission

allows laser fibers to be passed from the back table through the second puncture site. Appropriate electrical outlets and special water connections are necessary when using fiber lasers. Typically, an outlet supplying a 220 V 30A circuit is required. The YAG laser may be either three-phase or single-phase and air or water cooled, depending on the peak wattage required for a particular procedure. Individually wrapped sterile fibers are kept with the fiber lasers, each with its own cleaver for sharpening fiber tips. Because fibers can break easily, they are handled carefully and checked repeatedly. Safety precautions are followed strictly when one is using lasers. In the CO_2 laser, the free beam is transmitted through and reflected by mirrors contained in the articulating arm. When fiber lasers are used, both the patient and the staff must wear protective tinted eyewear. CO_2 lasers have the benefit of high water absorption, with more than 95% of energy absorbed by water in 1 mm of tissue. By comparison, water transmits more than 95% of argon laser energy in 1 mm of tissue. This limits the effect of the CO_2 laser to only the most superficial layers of tissue with minimal thermal spread (approximately 0.1 mm, compared to 4 mm in the Nd: YAG laser), allowing very precise cutting and coagulation [11].

Endoscopic Stapler

Several designs of endoscopic staplers are currently available. They are very useful for rapid cutting while maintaining excellent hemostasis. In bowel surgery and appendectomy, the overlapping rows of staples prevent spillage of bowel contents within the abdomen [12]. The linear stapler designed for gynecologic use is similar to the one used for bowel operations and can be introduced through a 12-mm trocar sleeve (Fig. 4.23). Ethicon and Covidien produce endoscopic surgical staplers with different designs, but their functions overall are essentially the same. The available staplers are disposable and can be reloaded with cartridges designed for gynecologic, generally, and thoracic surgery. Each cartridge contains titanium staples that are arranged in two sets of triple-staggered rows. The instrument also contains a push-bar knife assembly, which cuts between the two sets of triple rows, ligating both ends of the incised tissue. The cut line was designed to be shorter than the staple line to prevent bleeding or spillage of bowel contents.

The endoscopic circular stapler is used most commonly in gastrointestinal and colorectal surgery, as well as gynecologic oncology for bowel resection and anastomosis, but may also be used in bowel resection or disk resection for deep infiltrating endometriosis [13, 14].

Laparoscopic Specimen Retrieval Bag

In many cases, specimens are too large to be removed directly from a standard 5-mm or even 11-mm trocar. If there is concern regarding possible malignancy or chemical peritonitis, the specimen should be contained within a specimen retrieval bag before proceeding to allow for piecemeal removal from the pelvic and abdominal

Fig. 4.24 Disposable retrieval bags. ©Ethicon, Inc. 2018. Reproduced with permission

cavities. Over the years, multiple disposable retrieval bags have been developed (Fig. 4.24). Although they have slightly different designs, the overall mechanism of action is similar. The most commonly utilized bag sizes are 5, 10, and 15 mm and are composed of a flexible plastic or polyurethane bag, introduction sleeve, and cap. The cap should be removed prior to inserting the device. Once the device is inserted within the cavity, the bag is released and opened using a plunger-like mechanism. The bag remains patent due to its attachment to a metal hoop. The specimen can then be placed within the bag and closed by pulling on the drawstring which will also separate the bag from the metal hoop. The metal hoop is simultaneously pulled back into the introduction sleeve during this process. Care should be taken prior to closing the bag to ensure that no additional tissue is within the bag's opening, i.e., bowel. If the bag and its contents are too large to be directly removed through the canula, then the bag should be pulled into the sleeve until resistance is felt. The port can then be removed and the bag brought through the incision site. The bag can then be opened, allowing the specimen contents to be aspirated and tissue extracted using forceps and/or a scalpel. The incision may need to be extended for larger specimen extraction. Care should be taken to not puncture the bag during specimen aspiration and extraction.

Aspiration-Injection Needle

A 16- or 22-gauge aspiration-injection needle can be used to aspirate and inject fluids. When attached to a 28-cm laparoscopic probe tip without fenestrations, close-chambered ovarian cyst aspiration can be performed. The needle is usually 2 cm in length and has been etched with 0.5-cm markings in order to accurately gauge tissue penetration. Once the needle is inserted to its desired depth, the cyst contents can be aspirated without leakage by attaching it to a suction device or a 60 mL syringe for manual aspiration. The aspirated cyst contents are then able to be sent for cytologic examination. The Topel (Cook Medical, Bloomington, IN) is one of the disposable laparoscopic needles available that consists of a needle with a surrounding sleeve that directly attaches to a suction-irrigator device. The suction device is first activated, allowing for the desired tissue to be pulled against the sleeve. The needle is then used to puncture the cyst while avoiding spillage of its contents.

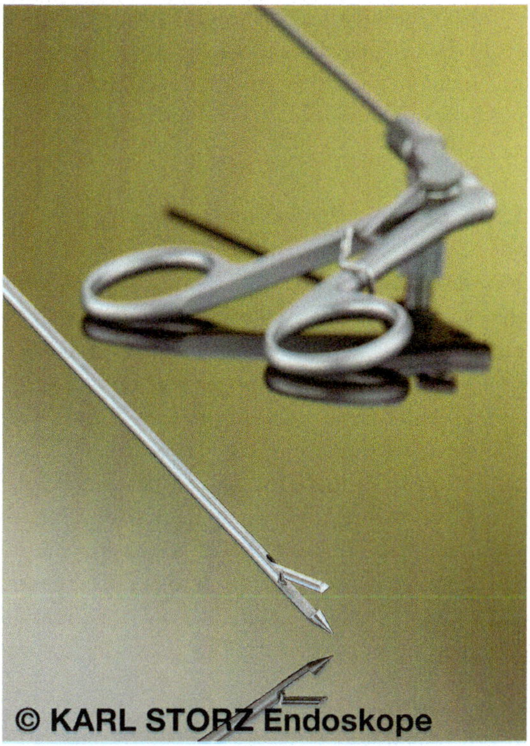

Fig. 4.25 Berci fascial closure. ©2018 Photo Courtesy of KARL STORZ Endoscopy-America, Inc.

The needle can also be used to inject dilute vasopressin into the base of fibroids before a myomectomy or into the mesosalpinx or tube before a salpingostomy for a tubal pregnancy.

Laparoscopic Port Closure Devices

It is generally accepted that the fascia from ports that are smaller than 10 mm do not need to be closed as they are not at increased risk for herniation. However, there have been reports of herniation even through ports as small as 5 mm with excessive manipulation that has led to an unintentional extension of the fascial incision [15]. If excessive manipulation has occurred throughout the procedure, then closure of the fascia should be considered. There are numerous reusable and disposable devices available on the market designed to close the fascia of port sites to prevent herniation.

The BERCI Fascial Closure Instrument by KARL STORZ (Fig. 4.25) is a simple, reusable, and cost-effective solution that is available in a 2.8-mm size with a 17-cm working length. The BERCI Fascial Closure Instrument facilitates full-thickness abdominal wall closure. It is designed for subcutaneous ligature of trocar incisions for closure of trocar incision wounds. At the completion of the procedure, the surgeon grasps the suture at mid-length with the forceps. Under direct laparoscopic vision, with adequate pneumoperitoneum, the surgeon places the BERCI Fascial Closure Instrument with suture into subcutaneous tissue directly adjacent to the trocar cannula. The instrument will pass through the tissue layers as entry is made into the peritoneal cavity. The BERCI Fascial Closure Instrument is then reinserted on the opposing lateral side of the trocar, where the suture is then grasped and pulled outside. The surgeon then ties the suture extracorporeally in a routine fashion.

The Carter-Thomason CloseSure System® has been reported as the best-reviewed and fastest-to-use device available [16]. There was also a study by Elashry that showed the Carter-Thomason device had few complications and maintained the pneumoperitoneum once the suture was tied, when compared to other closure devices [17]. Once the trocar has been removed, the appropriately sized pilot guide is inserted into the peritoneal cavity passing through the skin, muscle, fascia, and peritoneum. Next, the suture passer is placed through the hole in the pilot into the peritoneal cavity, making sure that it passes through adequate fascial tissue. The suture is grasped, preferably with a Maryland dissector grasper. The suture passer is removed and reinserted through the opposite hole in the pilot, again making sure to pass through adequate fascial tissue.

The suture passer firmly grabs the suture from the Maryland grasper and pulls it back through the pilot. The pilot is removed and the suture is finally tied extracorporeally.

References

1. ConMed. AirSeal IFS. http://www.conmed.com/en/medical-specialties/laparoscopic-robotic-and-open-surgery/general-and-bariatric-surgery/access/airseal-system/airseal-products/airseal-ifs-intelligent-flow-system. Accessed 28 May 2017.
2. Lipscomb GH, Givens VM. Preventing electrosurgical energy-related injuries. Obstet Gynecol Clin N Am. 2010;37(3):369–77.
3. Wang CW, Lee CL, Soong YK. Bowel injury by the suction-irrigator during operative laparoscopy. J Am Assoc Gynecol Laparosc. 1995;2(3):353–4.
4. Moore SS, Green CR, Wang FL, Pandit SK, Hurd WW. The role of irrigation in the development of hypothermia during laparoscopic surgery. Am J Obstet Gynecol. 1997;176(3):598–602.
5. Landman J, Kerbl K, Rehman J, Andreoni C, Humphrey PA, Collyer W, et al. Evaluation of a vessel sealing system, bipolar electrosurgery, harmonic scalpel, titanium clips, endoscopic gastrointestinal anastomosis vascular staples and sutures for arterial and venous ligation in a porcine model. J Urol. 2003;169(2):697–700.
6. Carbonell AM, Joels CS, Kercher KW, Matthews BD, Sing RF, Heniford BT. A comparison of laparoscopic bipolar vessel sealing devices in the hemostasis of small-, medium-, and large-sized arteries. J Laparoendosc Adv Surg Tech A. 2003;13(6):377–80.
7. Ethicon Endo-surgery. http://www.ees.com/Clinician/Product/energy#enseal-technology. Accessed 30 Nov 2011.
8. Person B, Vivas DA, Ruiz D, Talcott M, Coad JE, Wexner SD. Comparison of four energy-based vascular sealing and cutting instruments: a porcine model. Surg Endosc. 2008;22(2):534–8.

9. Harold KL, Pollinger H, Matthews BD, Kercher KW, Sing RF, Heniford BT. Comparison of ultrasonic energy, bipolar thermal energy, and vascular clips for hemostasis of small-, medium-, and large-sized arteries. Surg Endosc. 2003;17(8):1228–30.
10. Nieboer TE, Hinoul P, Maxson AJ, Maxson AJ, Schwiers ML, Miller CE, et al. Clinical utility of a novel ultrasonic vessel sealing device in transecting and sealing large vessels during laparoscopic hysterectomy using advanced hemostasis mode. Eur J Obstet Gynecol Reprod Biol. 2016;6(201):135–9.
11. Hunter JG, Dixon JA. Lasers in cardiovascular surgery-current status. West J Med. 1985;142(4):506–10.
12. Danielle JF, Gurley LD, Kurtz BR, Chambers JF. The use of an automatic stapling device for laparoscopic appendectomy. Obstet Gynecol. 1991;78(4):721–3.
13. Possover M, Diebolder H, Plaul K, Schneider A. Laparoscopically assisted vaginal resection of rectovaginal endometriosis. Obstet Gynecol. 2000;96(2):304–7.
14. Landi S, Pontrelli G, Surico D, Ruffo G, Benini M, Soriano D, et al. Laparoscopic disk resection for bowel endometriosis using a circular stapler and a new endoscopic method to control postoperative bleeding from the stapler line. J Am Coll Surg. 2008;207(2):205–9.
15. Nezhat C, Nezhat F, Seidman DS. Incisional hernias after operative laparoscopy. J Laparoendosc Adv Surg Tech A. 1997;7(2):111–5.
16. Shaher Z. Port closure techniques. Surg Endosc. 2007;21(8):1264–77.
17. Elashry OM, Naked SY, Wolf JS Jr, Figenshau RS, McDougall EM, Clayman RV. Comparative clinical study of port-closure techniques following laparoscopic surgery. J Am Coll Surg. 1996;183(4):335–44.

Operating Room Setup and Patient Positioning for Non-obstetric Surgery During Pregnancy

5

Vicki Barnett, Ashley N. Bartalot, and Ceana H. Nezhat

Introduction

Elective surgery is generally avoided during pregnancy if observation and medical management are possible. However, carefully planned non-obstetric surgeries may be performed if required while still ensuring the safety of both the mother and the fetus. The incidence of women requiring non-obstetric surgery during their pregnancy is similar to the frequency of nonpregnant women of child-bearing age requiring surgery. Representing about 2% of the female population in the United States, these patients require a variety of procedures and numerous surgical specialties [1]. Therefore, the perioperative surgical team requires a comprehensive knowledge of safe patient positioning for non-obstetric surgical procedures. These concepts are described in detail in this chapter based on their application in conventional operating rooms although they may be successfully adapted to various procedural settings.

Laparotomy or laparoscopy may be necessary for appendicitis, acute cholelithiasis, ovarian masses, trauma, or intestinal obstruction. Appendicitis is the most common non-obstetric surgical condition that complicates pregnancy and occurs in approximately 2 in every 1000 pregnancies [1]. This chapter provides guidance for safe and effective operating room configuration, setup, and positioning in the most common non-obstetric surgical procedures performed for pregnant surgical patients.

Team Collaboration and Safety Plan

Proper positioning is essential to the safe performance of non-obstetric surgical procedures for pregnant patients. Coordination with each member of the surgical team helps prevent patient harm, lowers the risk of health-care provider injury, and assures that the patient is safely managed. As soon as the surgery is posted to the operating room schedule, the perioperative team begins the care planning process and makes adjustments based on frequent reassessments of the patient's status. Prevention of positioning injuries requires the team to anticipate positioning

V. Barnett
Surgical Services, Northside Hospital, Atlanta, GA, USA

A. N. Bartalot
Department of Obstetrics and Gynecology, New York Presbyterian Brooklyn Methodist Hospital, Brooklyn, NY, USA

C. H. Nezhat (✉)
Nezhat Medical Center, Atlanta, GA, USA

Minimally Invasive Surgery and Robotics, Northside Hospital, Atlanta, GA, USA

Department of Gynecology and Obstetrics, Emory University, Atlanta, GA, USA
e-mail: ceana@nezhat.com

C. H. Nezhat (ed.), *Non-Obstetric Surgery During Pregnancy*,
https://doi.org/10.1007/978-3-319-90752-9_5

equipment and supplies that will be needed based on an initial comprehensive patient assessment. The evaluation is generated by a patient interview, a full history and physical examination, and a detailed review of the medical records in order to plan for transportation, transfer, and hand-off during each phase of perioperative care. Preoperatively identifying hazards that may be encountered during transport and transfer activities can prevent potential problems by assuring the required equipment, and an adequate number of appropriately skilled personnel are available to ensure the safety of both the patient and the perioperative team [2].

The assessment includes the plan for anesthesia, which may involve anesthetic procedures for the care of the patient preoperatively, intraoperatively, and postoperatively. The orientation and setup of the operating room will be determined based on which configuration will provide the most suitable access for the type of anesthetic to be delivered, the planned procedure, and the desired surgical position. Additional safety planning and precautions will need to be considered for procedure-specific positioning.

Operating Room Setup

Prior to the patient entering the operating room (OR), the table should be checked if it is functioning properly and that it is able to perform all the positions necessary for the procedure. The goal of positioning the operative equipment is to maximize the operating room space while creating a safe and comfortable environment for the entire team. The table should be centered and parallel to the longest wall positioned in the room to minimize the need for relocation. The table should be in level position, with the height lowered to allow for safe patient transfer and relaxed arm positioning for all operators (Fig. 5.1).

Patient Positioning

The pregnant patient should be attended during transport and transfer by appropriate personnel maintaining a left lateral recumbent position using a positioning wedge and avoiding a flat supine position. Active participation in safely positioning the patient initially and positioning assessment during the procedure are expected from the entire surgical team including the perioperative registered nurse and surgical technologist under the direction of and in collaboration with the surgeon and anesthesia provider [2]. Additional staff members should be available to help safely move and position the patient to protect staff members from injury. Transfer the patient to the surgical table with the stretcher, and the table should be positioned side by side and securely locked. Sliding or pulling the patient can result in shearing forces or friction on the patient's skin and should be avoided by using a sufficient number of staff. An inflatable transfer pad can also be used to aid in transferring the patient to and from the surgical table [3]. The patient should be attended at all times while on the surgical table, and the team should actively coordinate all positioning changes or table movement. A lack of clear communication about who will attend to the patient during the brief time the safety straps are removed or before the patient is transferred is a contributing factor for when the patient falls in the operating room [2].

Specifically designed equipment should be used to decrease the risk for positioning injuries (Fig. 5.2). Assemble all necessary positioning aids, such as padding, pillows, and bed accessories before induction in order to position the patient promptly after induction or regional anesthetic. Ensure all positioning aids are clean and working properly and that there is moving help to lift or turn the patient.

The number of pads and warming blankets beneath the patient has been implicated as a risk factor for pressure ulcer development [3]. Pillows, blankets, and molded-foam devices may produce only a minimum amount of pressure redistribution and are therefore less effective during long procedures (Fig. 5.3). Towels and sheet rolls do not reduce pressure and may contribute to friction injuries. Convoluted foam mattress overlays (egg crate mattresses) may be more effective in redistributing pressure and resist compression best if they are made of thick, dense foam. Several anti-skid methods may be used to

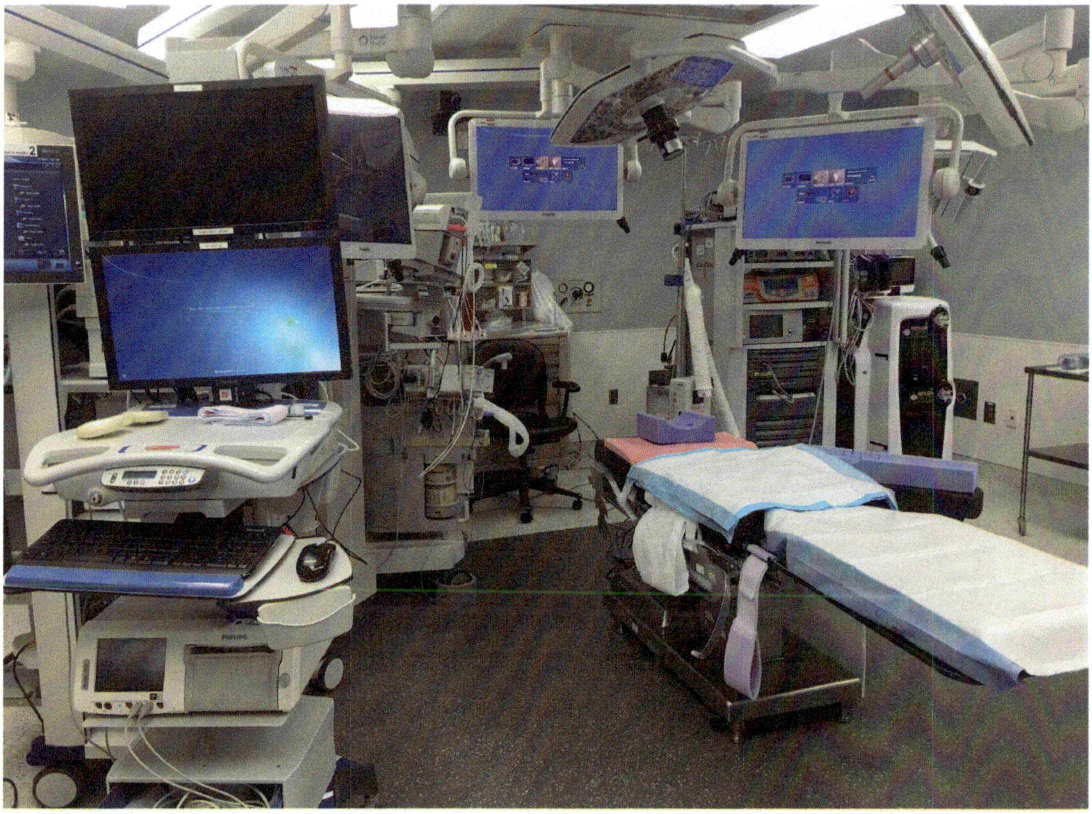

Fig. 5.1 Final OR setup

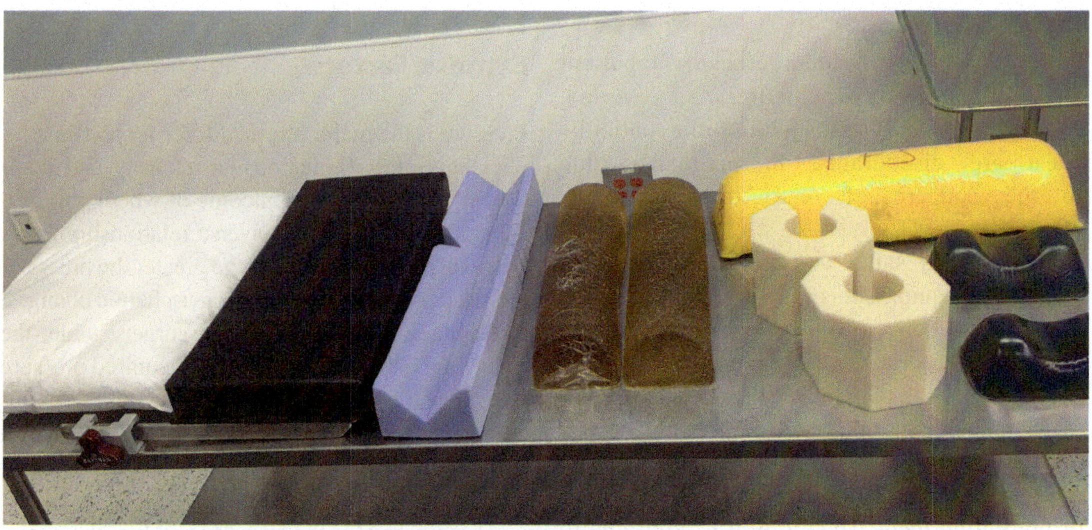

Fig. 5.2 Positioning aids assembled prior to patient induction

prevent the patient from sliding, including gel pads, egg crate, or foam mattress pads placed directly beneath the patient [3].

When using a uterine displacing wedge or chest rolls to reduce pressure from the pregnant uterus on the vena cava, the placement

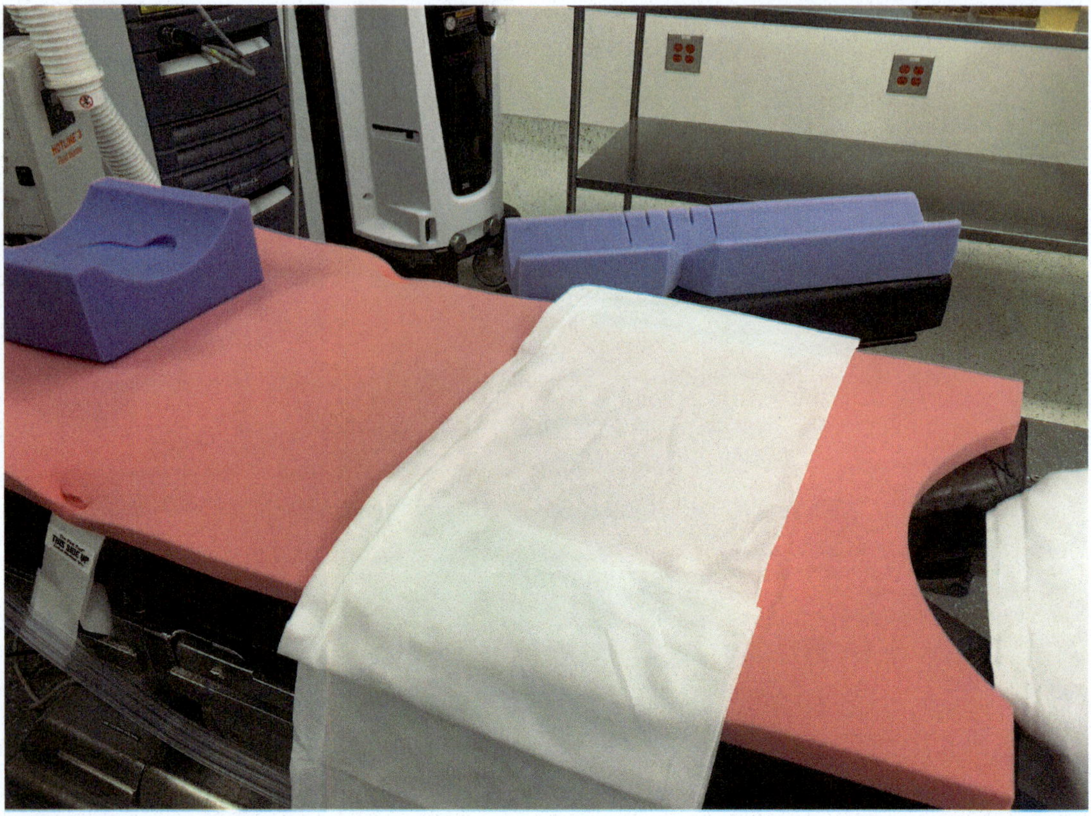

Fig. 5.3 Convoluted foam mattress effective in redistributing pressure. The Pink Pad: Pigazzi Positioning System (Xodus Medical, Inc. New Kensington, PA)

device should be placed underneath the patient and not beneath the mattress or overlay. Additional safety straps across the patient's chest are discouraged in pregnancy due to the concern of restricting respiratory effectiveness [1].

The primary safety consideration for patient positioning equipment is to redistribute pressure, especially at bony prominences on the patient's body. The need to assess the skin thoroughly before surgery is imperative. Proper skin assessment includes noting the temperature, color, moisture, turgor, and integrity. The costs of treating pressure injuries are far more than the costs of preventing them. Therefore, it is advisable to focus on preventative strategies that take into account the extrinsic and intrinsic factors that interact to contribute to the overall risk of developing pressure injuries [4].

Extrinsic Factors

Pressure is the major physical force responsible for decubitus ulcer formation. Its intensity and duration affect the ultimate outcome of whether the tissue suffers damage. An inverse relationship exists between pressure and time: the greater the pressure, the shorter time it takes to cause ischemic changes. The longer a patient is on the surgery table, the higher the risk of operating room-acquired pressure ulcer development when combined with the multiple variables of the intraoperative experience. Duration is considered more of a causative factor than is the intensity of pressure [4].

Hypothermia is the frequent result of the cooler operating room environment, exposure of external and internal body surfaces, and infusion and irrigation with unwarmed solutions. This creates peripheral vessel constriction to conserve core temperature and increases the patient's heat metabolism, which enhances the tissues need for oxygen, nutrients, and metabolic waste product removal. Ways to offset hypothermia in the OR and to reduce its detrimental effects include using forced-air warming therapy over the patient. Avoid placing a warming blanket under the patient in the areas where the pressure is greatest [4].

Intrinsic Factors

Intrinsic factors lower a patient's tissue tolerance to pressure and decrease the time and pressure required for tissue breakdown. Certain preexisting conditions are regarded as intrinsic risk factors for operating room-induced pressure injury. These risk factors [4] can be categorized into patient-specific and surgical-specific (Table 5.1).

Plan for Fetal Monitoring

The facility's ability to deliver appropriate intraoperative and postoperative care to the mother and her fetus is an important consideration. The team must carefully consider the resources available to them to manage both obstetric and neonatal emergencies, should preterm delivery occur (Fig. 5.4).

Table 5.1 Risk factors for developing peripheral neuropathy

Patient-specific	Surgical
Diabetes mellitus	Improper positioning
PVD	Prolonged operative times
Congenital cervical rib	Use of candy cane stirrups
Extreme BMI	
History of smoking	
History of alcohol intake	

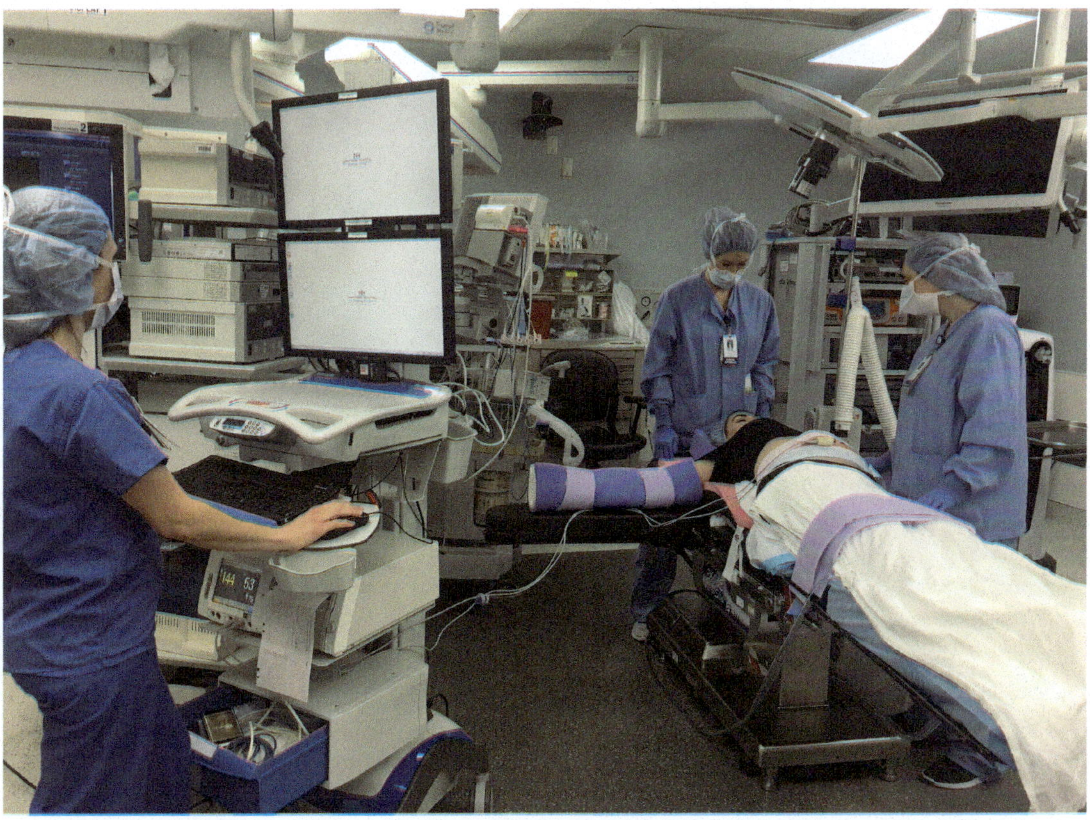

Fig. 5.4 Surgical team including labor and delivery nurse confirming patient positioning prior to induction

According to the American Academy of Pediatrics, fetal viability is determined by the age, weight, and gender of a preterm neonate before 26 weeks. For patients whose neonate is older than 26 weeks gestation, intraoperative electronic fetal monitoring may be advisable if all of the following apply [5]:

- The fetus is viable.
- It is physically possible to perform intraoperative electronic fetal monitoring.
- A health-care provider with obstetric privileges is available to intervene if needed for fetal indications.
- The surgeon obtained informed consent to perform an emergency cesarean delivery.
- The type of surgery will allow for safe interruption of the surgical procedure for physicians to perform an emergency delivery if warranted.

When the fetus is not viable, a person qualified in fetal heart rate monitoring should perform simultaneous electronic fetal heart rate and contraction monitoring before and after the surgical procedure (Fig. 5.5) [5]. The necessity for perioperative monitoring of the fetus and uterine activity remains a matter of discussion and ongoing controversy. In spite of recent improvements in surgical techniques and anesthesia, little has been written about fetal and uterine response during non-obstetric surgery. Currently, few studies exist that support the necessity and feasibility of fetal heart rate (FHR) monitoring during non-obstetric surgical procedures [6]. Although with fetal heart rate monitoring, should early compromise or contractions be detected, prompt treatment may allow rapid improvement of fetal status or uterine activity [7].

Perinatal nurses are ideally positioned to collaborate in providing comprehensive nursing care to both the fetus and mother. Because of their

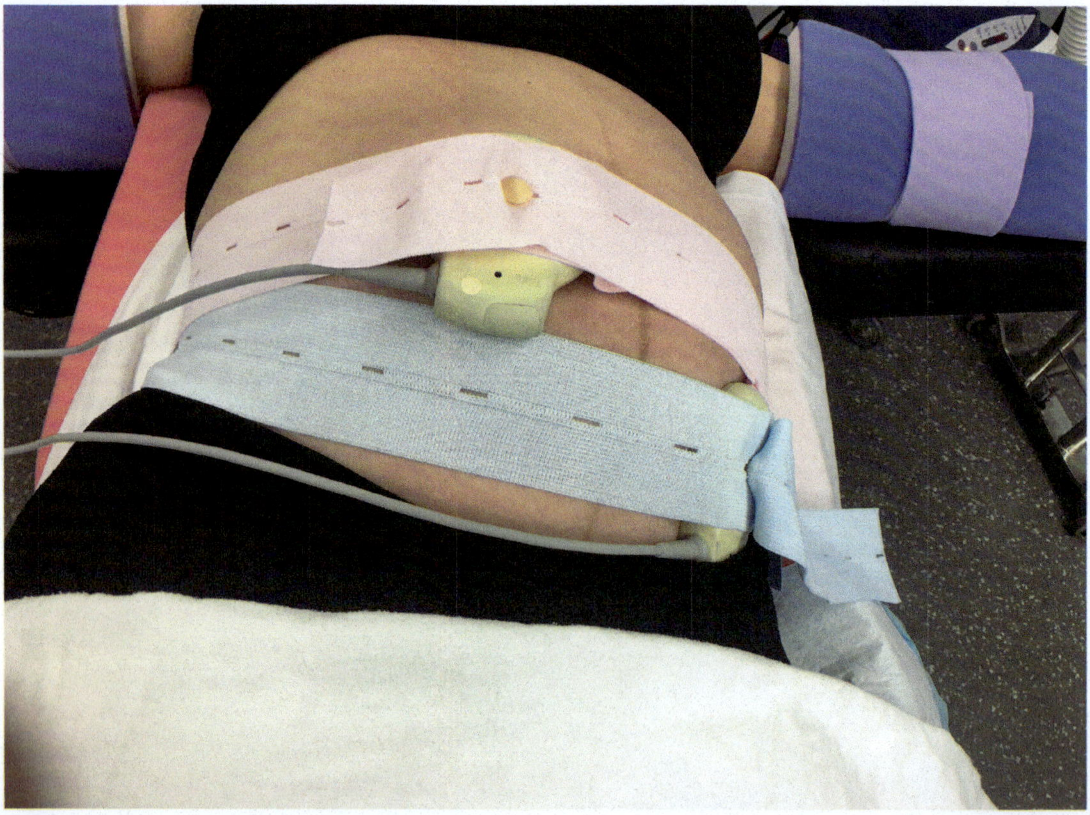

Fig. 5.5 Uterine displacing wedge and fetal monitoring in place

knowledge, experience, and education in this area, perinatal nurses have an important intraoperative role to play in the care of these patients. They are ideally suited to join the surgical team in order to provide information to the surgical team about the fetus and the mother's response to surgery.

A comprehensive and thorough surgical plan will also include the plan for potential emergency procedures. The setup necessary for any emergency procedures, including cesarean section delivery and neonatal resuscitation, is available and open or as determined necessary by the plan of care. If unrelieved fetal distress occurs, one intervention to be considered is emergency cesarean delivery. When the decision is made that an emergency cesarean delivery will be performed, the circulating nurse and surgical assistant should open the required instruments and count them before beginning the procedure.

The perinatal circulating nurse should bring the infant warming device and infant resuscitation equipment into the OR to prepare for receiving the infant. In this situation, an additional nurse is required to care for the infant, because the operating room circulating nurse is only able to care for one patient, the mother. This additional nurse should be in the OR for the entire procedure, enabling the fastest response to a potential emergency situation. The nurse or respiratory therapy practitioner who joins the team for this circumstance must be competent at resuscitating an infant should there be a need to do so. The surgeon or obstetrician also may request that a pediatrician be available in the operating room or be available on call for the emergency cesarean birth. If the pediatrician is to remain on call, ensure that the physician's correct contact information is immediately available [8].

Video- and Robot-Assisted Laparoscopic Surgery

Video-assisted and robot-assisted laparoscopic surgeries are safe for pregnant patients. Placing a video monitor directly facing each surgeon over the patient's contralateral knee at eye level helps decrease eyestrain (Fig. 5.6) [4].

If possible an additional video monitor for the assistant can also be set up toward the patient's shoulder. The video monitors can be fixed and mounted to the ceiling, placed on a portable stand, or attached to a mobile stand with an articulating arm. The video monitor provides the surgeons view of the operative field and should be set for maximal clarity and true color transmission. The laparoscopic tower should be designed to hold the

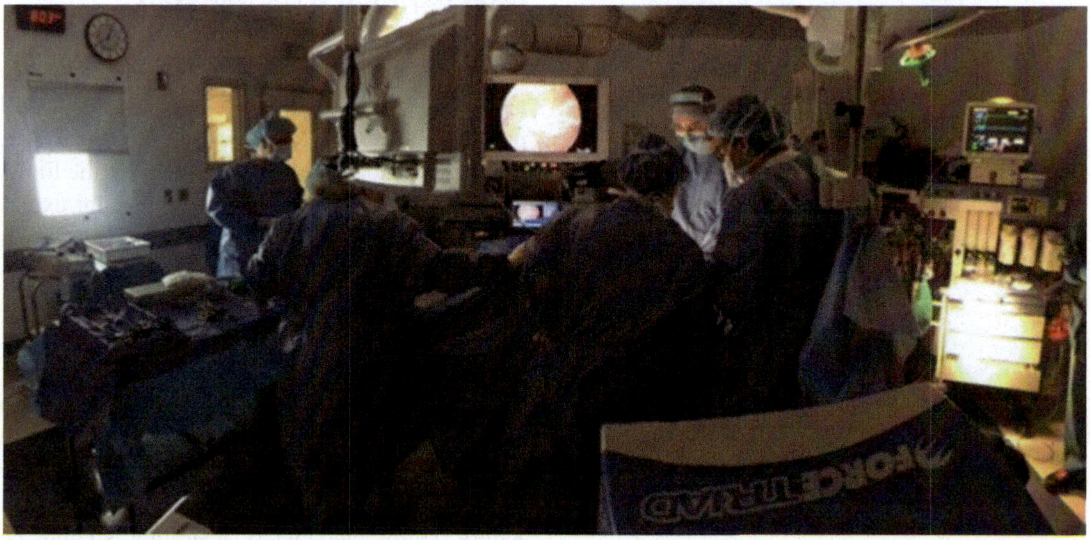

Fig. 5.6 Monitor positioning (side view)

CO_2 insufflator, camera boxes, light sources, insufflator, and recording/printing devices. The tower should be positioned opposite to the surgeon, so that it does not interfere with the assistant's position nor obstruct the surgeon's view of the insufflator and light source (Fig. 5.7) [4].

If robot-assisted laparoscopy is planned, prepare the robot for the procedure by draping it in a sterile manner. In order to maintain sterility, the robot should be positioned out of the way of OR traffic, preferably against the far wall (Fig. 5.8) [4].

In order to optimize OR space and functionality, the robotic console with or without the teaching console should be parked against the opposite OR wall. This should be accomplished while maintaining the surgeon's ability to easily communicate with their assistants at the bedside (Fig. 5.9) [4].

The robot will be docked in relation to the operating table depending on the surgeon's preference for the planned procedure. It can be docked parallel, perpendicular (90°), or at a 45° angle to the surgical table. If the patient is attached to a robot, caution should be taken before moving either the patient or the robot.

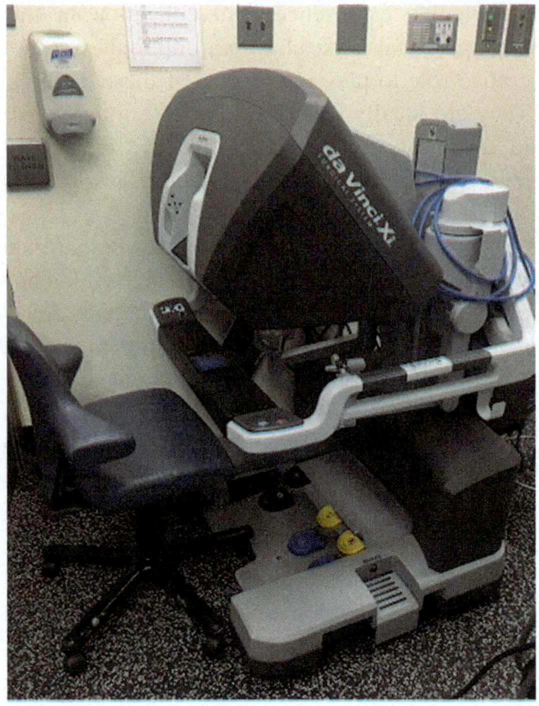

Fig. 5.8 Console is positioned against the far wall of the OR

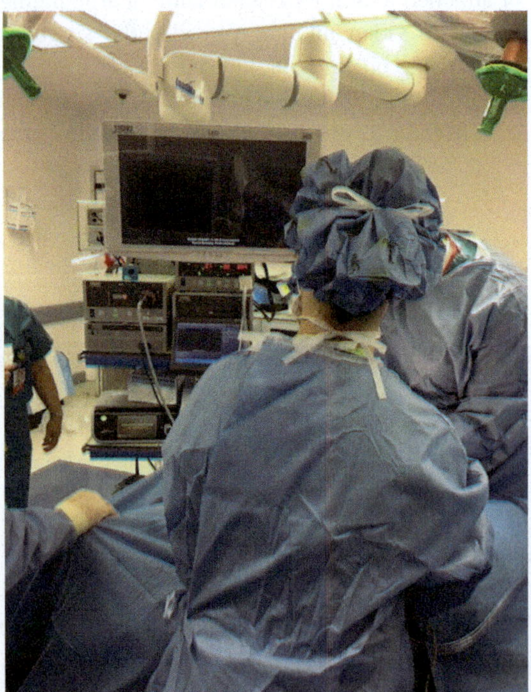

Fig. 5.7 The laparoscopic tower is positioned in direct view of the surgeons

Protecting the Patient from Peripheral Neuropathy

A patient safety goal is to maintain the body's natural alignment as much as possible while still providing adequate access to the surgical site. The surgical team needs to be aware of the limits to range of motion, refraining from joint extension beyond what is necessary. Improper positioning can lead to peripheral neuropathy of the upper and lower extremities [4]. Although rare and usually self-limited, the most common cause of injury is from compression or stretching of the nerves. These complications can be avoided with a few preventative measures while paying close attention to proper patient positioning in the planning and execution of the surgical procedure. Safety straps and wrist restraints should be applied carefully to avoid peripheral nerve

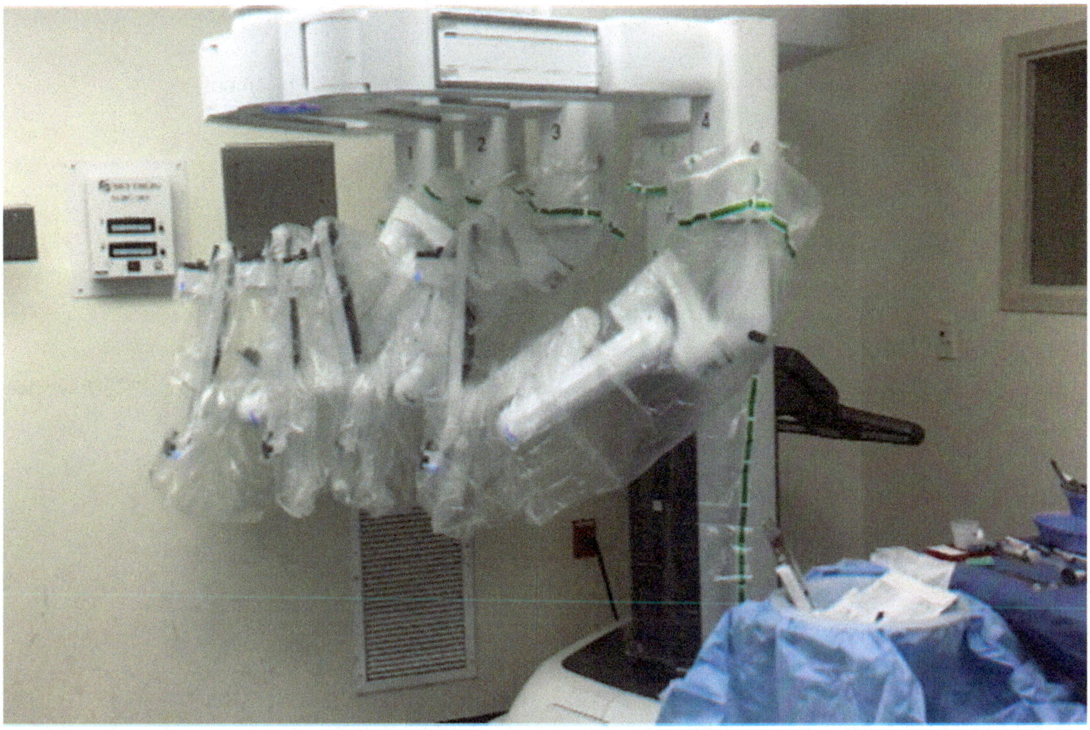

Fig. 5.9 Da Vinci Xi Robot is positioned in the far corner, optimizing OR space and decreasing risk of contamination

compression injury and compromised blood flow to deep and peripheral vessels from tight restraints. When peripheral nerves are injured during positioning, the result could be impaired sensory function, motor function, or both. Stretching and compression are avoidable position-induced nerve injuries [9].

Generally speaking, pregnant patients who are in the 20th week of gestation or greater should be placed in a left lateral recumbent position, created by placing a wedge under the patient's right hip to shift the abdominal contents away from the midline [9]. This position is used during transport and if possible during the procedure because it decreases the pressure caused by the enlarged uterus, the vena cava, or the aorta and also visceral compression on the diaphragm. The supine position may be modified into a sitting or semi-sitting position for access to the shoulder, posterior cervical spine, or posterior or lateral head.

Positioning the pregnant patient except in the semi-Fowler, sitting or reverse Trendelenburg positions could compromise the respiratory system [9]. While there is better lung excursion and diaphragmatic activity in these positions, there is increased risk for poor venous return from the lower extremities contributing to increased risk of thrombosis and pooling of blood in the patient's pelvis [2].

Upper Extremity Neuropathy

The patient's head should be in a neutral position and placed on a headrest. Unless necessary for surgical reasons, the patient's arms should not be tucked at her sides [2]. The left arm should be placed on an arm board at 90° to facilitate stabilization, and the right arm should be positioned to maintain proper alignment. If it is necessary to tuck the arms, the drawsheet should extend above the elbows and should be tucked between the patient and the surgical table mattress (Fig. 5.10) [2].

The patient's arms should be padded with special attention paid to cushioning the posteromedial aspect of the elbows, wrists, and hands

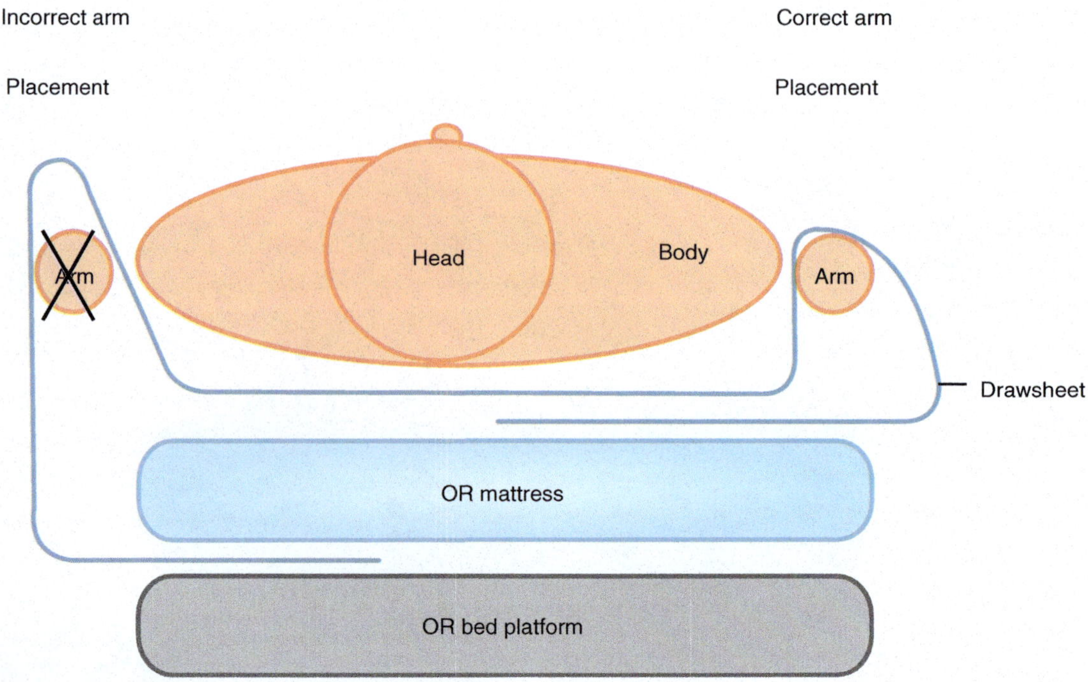

Fig. 5.10 Correct method for tucking arms in at patient's side

(Fig. 5.11). The location of the patient's fingers should be in a position that is clear of surgical table breaks or other hazards.

The ulnar nerve passes through the olecranon groove, close to the medial epicondyle of the humerus [4]. At this location, the superficial ulnar nerve is more susceptible to compression injury if the posteromedial portion of the elbow is not padded appropriately. The patient would present with complaints of sensory loss or paresthesia in the medial 1.5 fingers and loss of motor function of the small muscles of the hand. The radial nerve passes directly along the spiral groove of the humerus. The radial nerve can be injured by being compressed between the edge of the operating table and the humerus passing over the spiral groove. The patient would present with complaints of sensory loss or paresthesia to the lateral 3.5 fingers and loss of motor function in the extensor muscles in the wrist and the fingers, which may result in wrist drop [4]. Injury to the brachial plexus (C5-T1) is more likely to occur from an excessive stretching force. The upper nerve roots (C5–C6) are more likely to be injured

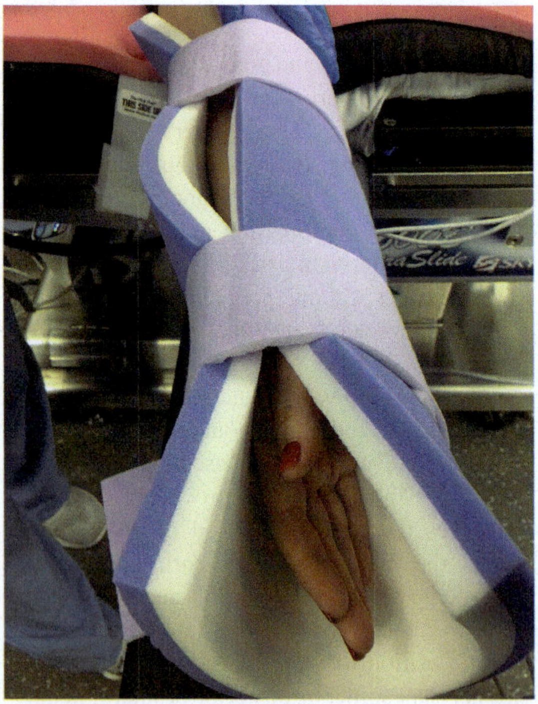

Fig. 5.11 Hand facing patients side with thumb pointing up

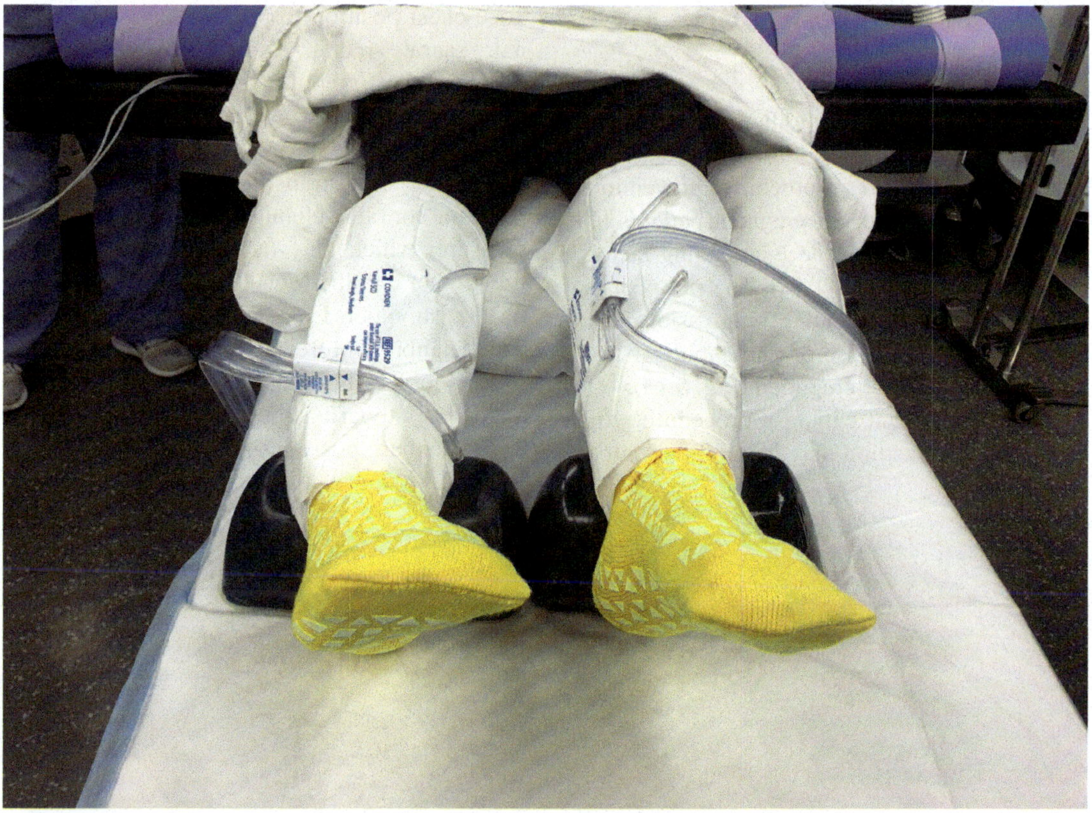

Fig. 5.12 Legs are parallel, ankles uncrossed, and heels elevated off the underlying surface

from hyperabducting the arms, when left on the arm boards at greater than 90°. The stretching trauma is further exacerbated if the arms are in a pronated position with the head turned to one side [4].

Lower Extremity Neuropathy

The patient's head and upper body should be aligned with the hips. The wedge will create a slight pronation of the right hip, knee, and ankle. The patient's legs should be parallel and the ankles uncrossed to reduce pressure to the occiput, scapulae, thoracic vertebrae, olecranon processes (elbows), sacrum/coccyx, calcaneus (heel), and ischial tuberosities. The patient's heels should be elevated off the underlying surface when possible, and her head should be in a neutral position and placed on a headrest (Fig. 5.12).

It is recommended to offload the heels from the table surface in patients undergoing supine and modified supine surgical procedures. However, studies also suggest that off-loading the heels can increase sacral pressure; therefore it is recommended to implement strategies to minimize sacral pressure [3].

The use of stirrups and the lithotomy position would be minimized whenever possible in the pregnant surgical patient. Lower extremity neuropathies result most frequently from prolonged, excessive sharp flexion (>120°) of the hip [9]. Patients could present with complaints of impaired sensation over the anterior medial thigh as well as the medial aspect of the calf in addition to weakness or inability to flex at the hip or to extend at the knee [4].

Deep Vein Thrombosis (DVT) Prevention

During pregnancy, the mother's blood is in a hypercoagulable state [10]. It is particularly vital that the organization's protocol for prevention of DVT is instituted for all pregnant patients [11]. The hypercoagulable state is a leading factor in the development of DVT [8]. The protocol may include the use of sequential compression devices with or without the use of antiembolism stockings and a medication regimen (Fig. 5.13).

For the pregnant patient a procedure requiring the prone position may be modified into the knee-chest position to provide exposure to spinal, sacral, rectal, and perineal areas [8]. Surgical staff should reposition the mother slowly when placing her into or out of the Trendelenburg or reverse Trendelenburg position. The slow transition will decrease the potential for rapid changes in the mother's blood pressure, which may have negative effects on the mother and the fetus [10]. To prevent injury of the shoulders, brachial plexus, or feet in Trendelenburg or reverse Trendelenburg positions, shoulder braces should be avoided, and a padded footboard should be used in reverse Trendelenburg positions [2].

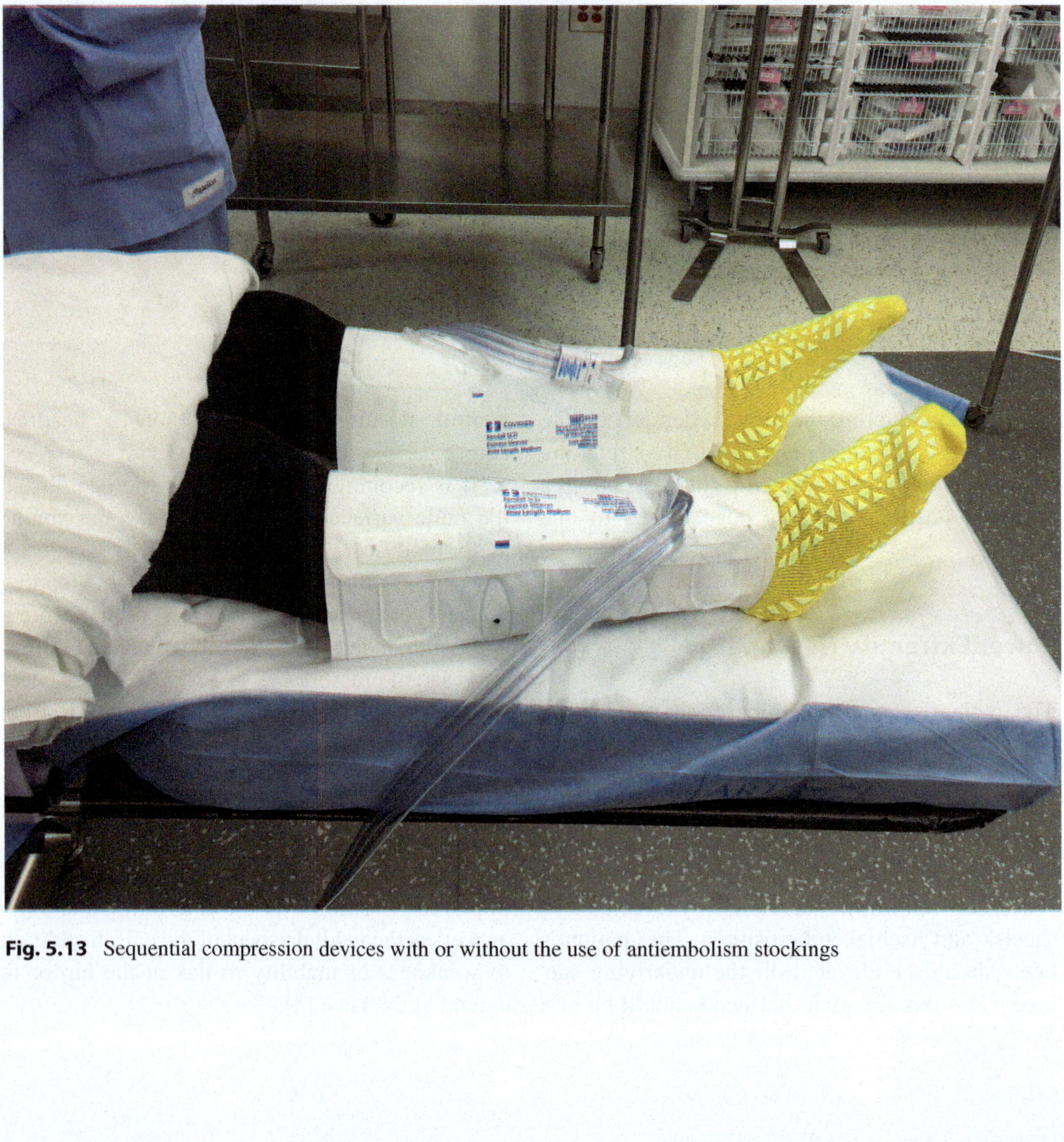

Fig. 5.13 Sequential compression devices with or without the use of antiembolism stockings

Document Assessments for Positioning-Related Outcomes

Document the patient's overall skin and extremity condition on arrival to the surgery area, at intervals during the procedure and at discharge from the operating room. It is important to note the type and location of positioning equipment used and any changes in position needed during the surgery [2]. Assess and describe pertinent information related to positioning or changes in condition to post anesthesia care providers upon arrival and admission to the next phase of perioperative care.

Conclusion

Configuring a safe and effective operating room, actively monitoring patient positioning throughout surgery, and adhering to appropriate protocols for prophylactic measures for peripheral neuropathy are vital components to keep in mind when preparing for non-obstetric surgery (Table 5.2).

Table 5.2 Step-by-step instructions for preparing the OR for non-obstetric surgeries

1. Equipment
2. Transportation
3. Positioning
4. Prophylaxis measures
(a) Decubitus ulcer or bed sore
(b) Antibiotics
(c) Deep vein thrombosis
(d) Nerve injury

References

1. Carzo SA, Viveiros JH. Gynecologic and obstetric surgery. In: Rothrock J, McEwen D, editors. Alexander's care of the patient in surgery. 15th ed. St. Louis, MO: Mosby/Elsevier; 2015. p. 405–60.
2. AORN Guideline for Positioning the Patient. Standards, recommended practices, and guidelines. Denver, CO: AORN, Inc.; 2007. p. 691–707.
3. National Pressure Ulcer Advisory Panel: Pressure Ulcer Stages/Categories. http://www.npuap.org/resources/educational-and-clinical-resources/npuap-pressure-injury-stages/. Accessed 26 Sept 2017.
4. Patient Positioning and Operating Room Setup. In: Nezhat C, Nezhat F, Nezhat C, editors. Nezhat's operative gynecologic laparoscopy and hysteroscopy. 3rd ed. New York, NY: Cambridge University Press; 2008. p. 9–35.
5. ACOG Committee on Obstetric Practice. ACOG Committee Opinion No. 474: non-obstetric surgery during pregnancy. Obstet Gynecol. 2011;117:420–1.
6. Graham G, Baxi L, Tharakan T. Laparoscopic cholecystectomy during pregnancy: a case series and review of the literature. Obstet Gynecol Surg. 1998;19:556–74.
7. Shaver SM, Shaver DC. Perioperative assessment of the obstetric patient undergoing abdominal surgery. J Perianesth Nurs. 2005;20:160–6.
8. Romanoski S. Management of the special needs of the pregnant surgical patient. Nurs Clin North Am. 2006;41:299–311.
9. Heizenroth PA. Positioning the patient for surgery. In: Rothrock J, McEwen D, editors. Alexander's care of the patient in surgery. 15th ed. St. Louis, MO: Mosby/Elsevier; 2015. p. 155–85.
10. Porteous J. Oh, by the way, the patient is pregnant! Can Oper Room Nurs J. 2008;26:35–42.
11. AORN guideline for prevention of venous stasis. Perioperative standards and recommended practices. Denver, CO: AORN, Inc.; 2008. p. 141–58.

Pneumoperitoneum for Laparoscopic Surgery During Pregnancy

6

Douglas E. Ott

When the need for non-obstetric surgery arises during pregnancy, does the choice between an open versus laparoscopic procedure matter? This chapter explores the following questions: Is the outcome different for the patient or fetus based on procedure? Are there different considerations for laparoscopy during pregnancy? What are the differences and consequences of either choice? Is the effect of surgery different for the patient based on route? What is the rate of spontaneous abortion and are there effects on the fetus? Is there a clinical benefit to either an open or laparoscopic approach, and what precautions are recommended? The variables that should be considered when choosing between open versus laparoscopic surgery for non-obstetric surgery during pregnancy include the stage of pregnancy, presence of a fetus, physiologic changes during pregnancy, and the non-obstetric surgical problem as it relates to pregnancy.

Pregnancy creates dynamic alterations to normal physiology. These changes may mimic medical disease, making it important to differentiate between a normal altered physiological condition and disease pathology. Drug metabolism and pharmacokinetic responses coupled with elevated concentrations of various hormones during pregnancy influence metabolism and a patient's response to surgery. Cardiac output, blood volume, red blood cell mass, heart rate, oxygen consumption, tidal volume, and minute ventilation all increase during pregnancy [1–4], causing compensated respiratory alkalosis, with the fetus normally having mild respiratory acidosis [5]. This requires increased oxygen concentration during anesthesia. The diaphragm is displaced due to the enlarging uterus, causing decreased residual lung volume and functional residual capacity. Changes in the coagulation system create a hypercoagulable state with fibrinogen, factor VII, and factor XII increasing but antithrombin III decreasing, causing an increased risk of venous thromboembolism.

Gastrointestinal motility slows during pregnancy due to increased progesterone, which delays drug absorption. Plasma volume is expanded, which dilutes plasma proteins and increases concentration(s) of unbound drugs. Glomerular filtration rate and renal plasma flow increase, which enhances renal drug excretion. Hepatic clearance, protein binding, and hepatic blood flow increase, which affects drug-metabolizing enzyme activity. Plasma concentrations of estrogens (estradiol, estrone, estriol, and estetrol) and progesterone dramatically increase. Placental growth hormone, human placental lactogen, and prolactin influence cellular responses and metabolism. Corticosteroid-binding globulin and free cortisol plasma levels increase [6]. Changes in the size of the uterus, kidneys, and

D. E. Ott
Biomedical Engineering, Mercer University, Macon, GA, USA

C. H. Nezhat (ed.), *Non-Obstetric Surgery During Pregnancy*, https://doi.org/10.1007/978-3-319-90752-9_6

other organs, along with metabolic and physiologic adaptations during pregnancy, are in flux as pregnancy progresses to term and through postpartum recovery [1]. The physiologic changes of pregnancy influence intraoperative and postoperative care for the patient and fetus. Knowledge of these physiologic changes can help the physician select a surgical approach and understand intraoperative and postoperative concerns and treatments. These physiologic changes of pregnancy are further affected by comorbidities, including diabetes, gestational diabetes, obesity, hypertension, preeclampsia, seizure disorders, asthma, renal disease, sickle cell disease, inflammatory bowel disease, hyperthyroidism, malignancy, heart disease, autoimmune disease, previous surgery, and substance abuse [7].

The abdomen behaves like a hydraulic system, with normal intra-abdominal pressure (IAP) of 5–7 millimeters of mercury (mmHg). Morbid obesity increases baseline IAP by 9–14 mmHg [8, 9]. Pregnant patients follow the laws of physics and formulas relevant to IAP: abdominal compliance, pressure calculation and differentials, flow dynamics, vector forces, Laplace's law, and hydraulic hydrostatic pressure laws of Pascal (Table 6.1). Intra-abdominal pressure gradually increases during pregnancy: "Factors causing increased intra-abdominal pressure in pregnancy include: progressive uterine expansion, obstetrical factors that increase intra-uterine volume excessively or acutely, maternal anthropometric measurements that affect intra-abdominal pressure thresholds, maternal postures that increase abdominal force direction, abdominal compliance that is decreased, diminished with advancing gestation, or has reached maximum expansion, habitation at high altitude, and rapid drops in barometric pressure" [10].

Pregnancy and the postpartum period create a continuum of biologic and mechanical alterations influenced by existing comorbidities. Creating a pneumoperitoneum for laparoscopy during pregnancy has different baseline parameters. What are the consequences for the patient and fetus and the differences from the nonpregnant state? The pregnancy puts the patient at higher risk due to mechanical and physiologic changes. For the pregnant patient undergoing laparoscopy, the challenges of creating a pneumoperitoneum include the overlapping pre-existing morbidities, the mechanical and physiologic adaptations caused by the pneumoperitoneum, the alterations caused by pregnancy, and the combination of all these factors. The principles governing increased IAP and carbon dioxide (CO_2) pneumoperitoneum during pregnancy are the same as for the nonpregnant state, but with an amplified effect and smaller margins of error. The majority of literature regarding laparoscopy and pregnancy was published between 2012 and 2017. This is due to laparoscopic surgical familiarity, safety, efficacy, experience, training, increased reporting, and shortened recovery time.

The abdominal wall is composed of viscoelastic tissues that predictably expand due to

Table 6.1 Physics principles for the pneumoperitoneum

Pressure	$P = F/A$ (pressure = unit force/unit of area)
Pascal's law	With an increase in pressure at any point in a contained fluid, there is an equal increase at every other point in the container—an incompressible fluid transmits applied pressure
Compliance	$C_{ab} = \Delta V/\Delta P$ (abdominal compliance = change in volume/change in pressure)
Vector force	VF = VM + D (vector force = volume magnitude + direction)
Darcy's law	$F = \Delta P/R$ (flow = pressure difference of a vessel/resistance) resistance (blood flow) has an inverse relationship proportional to the fourth power of the radius of the vessel, so even a small decrease in blood vessel diameter will lead to a significant decrease in blood flow and extreme elevation in vascular resistance
Laplace's law	Pressure = (2 × thickness × tension)/radius
	The greater the pressure differences between two sides of a wall (transmural pressure) and the larger the radius of the wall, the greater the tension on the wall. The tension within the wall of a sphere filled to a particular pressure depends on the thickness of the sphere

pneumoperitoneum pressure. The fascia has a lower compliance (higher stiffness) than the subcutaneous fat and muscle layers which have greater compliance (lower stiffness). The end result of creating and maintaining a pneumoperitoneum is uniform strain and stretch. At the final pressure attained, an equilibrium is reached between the expansion and contraction forces. The insufflation pressure applied over the internal surface of the abdominal wall equals the abdominal wall weight plus the elastic stress to contract back to its original shape. Most of the increase in laparoscopic working space is due to sagittal plane expansion because the rectus abdominis muscle is less rigid than transverse fascial fiber stiffness, with the stress force being almost double the sagittal plane [11–15].

Initiation of a pneumoperitoneum results in an initial elastic phase that has a direct linear relationship between the stress (IAP) on abdominal wall tissues and the strain created. During insufflation, the abdominal wall changes from a cylinder to a dome shape, expanding the working space on average by 20% [14]. Expansion continues until the stretch limit is reached. At this pressure, equilibrium occurs between the expansive and contractive forces. Any additional volume of gas past this point will not expand the intra-abdominal space but increases pressure. Once maximum expansion capacity is reached, IAP will increase acutely, rapidly, and logarithmically [16]. The absolute thickness of abdominal wall subcutaneous fat and the ratio of abdominal fat thickness to rectus abdominal muscle thickness have a statistically significant direct exponential correlation. Each patient will have her own specific maximum pressure, beyond which no additional volume gas creates more operating space. This may be different than the recommendation for nonpregnant patients of 12–15 mmHg pressure.

As pregnancy progresses, especially toward the end of the second trimester and the third trimester, diastasis recti can influence abdominal entry and the pneumoperitoneum. The optimal pressure for the operating space of the pneumoperitoneum is the lowest pressure that the surgeon can safely perform the surgery without compromising the best possible outcome. Patients with a higher abdominal fat thickness need a lower IAP to maintain adequate working space, but higher volume of gas; patients with less abdominal fat may need higher pressure and lower gas volume [13].

Intra-abdominal pressure increases during pregnancy, with standard values not defined and little studied [8]. The supine position is associated with a higher IAP compared to left lateral tilt (10.9 vs. 8.9 mmHg and as high as 25 vs. 23 mmHg) [17, 18]. To reduce aortocaval compression, a 10-degree left tilt is recommended. Normal IAP is defined as 5–7 mmHg [19]. Even though the IAP increase during pregnancy is not "abnormal" but a physiological accommodative steady-state process, the definition of intra-abdominal hypertension (IAH) is met in some patients (i.e., a sustained or repeated elevation of IAP over 12–15 mmHg) [10, 18, 19]. This increased IAP during pregnancy is a change in IAP being equal to the relationship between intra-abdominal volume and abdominal compliance, which results in a hydrodynamic shift decreasing visceral organ perfusion, ischemia reperfusion injury, and intestinal mucosal permeability translocation.

Laparoscopy is safe and feasible during pregnancy. The object is to maximize benefits of laparoscopic surgery for the pregnant person and the fetal occupant. Positioning, fetal monitoring and ultrasound assessments, sequential compression devices, modified trocar placement, attention to IAP, use of humidified warmed CO_2, appropriate IAP, and intraoperative monitoring of end expiratory CO_2 levels are benchmarks for laparoscopic surgery during pregnancy. Initial abdominal access can be safely accomplished by any method used by appropriately adjusting for fundal height [2, 3]. Use the lowest IAP you are able to tolerate to not compromise your surgical procedure for the best outcome without exceeding 12–15 mmHg [2, 3, 20]. You should prevent pressure peaks, not allow room-air introduction into the abdomen, and maintain stable gas inflow and pressure with a responsive insufflator [21]. Laparoscopic procedures performed during pregnancy for general surgical and gynecological indications appear to have no increase in fetal or maternal complications compared with laparotomy, and none were associated with the laparoscopic procedure itself [22, 23].

The gas used for a laparoscopic pneumoperitoneum is almost always CO_2 because it has the least undesirable consequences and effects on the patient. Chemistry, biochemistry, and physiology make CO_2 the gas of choice (Tables 6.2, 6.3, and 6.4) [24]. Carbon dioxide has a high diffusion coefficient (20:1 to oxygen and 25:1 to nitrogen) and is a normal metabolic end product that is rapidly cleared by the lungs. It is highly soluble in blood and tissues and does not support combustion. However, carbon dioxide is a drug; all laparoscopists should know its indications, effects, dosages, methods of administration, frequency and duration of administration, hazards, contraindications, side effects, and the precautions to be taken. Despite the benefits of creating an operating space, a pneumoperitoneum is not without physiological consequences. Insufflation reduces blood flow to organs within the peritoneal space due to pressure, not the chemistry of the gas. The reduction in blood flow promotes anaerobic metabolism, leading to lactic acidosis, postoperative alteration in liver enzymes, subclinical hepatic dysfunction, and increases in oxidative stress markers [25]. The release of vasoactive substances is stimulated, including vasopressin, angiotensin, cortisol, and adrenocorticotropin hormone (ACTH), which is not attributable to CO_2 chemistry [26]. Carbon dioxide causes vasodilatation and is counteracted by increased IAP, causing changes in blood flow within the pneumoperitoneum. The net effect of CO_2 and the pressure on tissues and organ blood flow is a combination of intrinsic and extrinsic mechanisms. Intrinsic factors include tissue metabolism, local reflexes, cell-induced vasoactive chemicals that influence vasodilatation, hypoxia, and flow regulation [26]. Extrinsic factors include systemic hemodynamics and circulating vasoactive chemicals, including anesthetic agents and sympathetic nerve response.

Regulatory agencies mandate that the gas be extremely dry (less than 200 parts per million of water vapor, 0.02% relative humidity [RH]) [2]. This makes it harsh and unphysiologic to the normal condition of the abdominal cavity. Without modification, the gas enters the abdomen at 20 °C, which is 15 °C below body temperature [27]. The pressurized gas flows at high velocities through constrictions from the insufflator to the abdomen. This circumstance of very dry, cool gas flowing over wet warm tissue surfaces in a high-moisture (>95% RH) environment causes rapid evaporation, tissue hypothermia, and peritoneal desiccation. Correcting CO_2 to more physiologic moisture and temperature parameters reduces peritoneal desiccation and damage, inflammatory response, hypothermia, and potential adhesion formation; improves postoperative pain; and shortens recovery time [28, 29].

Table 6.2 Physical + chemical + biologic effects = pneumoperitoneum

Physical effects	Chemical effects	Biologic effects
Mechanical effects Abdominal compliance Intra-abdominal pressure Time Patient position	Gas Desiccation Hypoxia Acidosis	Hypothermia Tissue disruption Increased peritoneal viscosity Acidosis Hypoxia

Table 6.3 Factors affecting the pneumoperitoneum independent of the gas used

Intra-abdominal pressure	Patient position
Dryness of the gas	Volume of gas used
Acidosis	Hypoxia
Length of exposure	Abdominal compliance

Table 6.4 Changes that occur due to a pneumoperitoneum regardless of the type of gas used

Increased		Decreased
Intra-abdominal pressure Neurohormonal vasoactivity Pulmonary vascular resistance Peripheral vascular resistance	Systemic blood pressure Mean arterial pressure Heart rate	Venous return Cardiac output Splanchnic blood flow Functional residual capacity

The insufflator is a gas throttling-down pressure-regulating device for flow rate and pressure [21]. Flow occurs until the preset pressure is reached. Insufflators comparatively have different performance characteristics for filling rates, and do not have the same performance characteristics even at the same settings. What is set and visualized on the dials does not always represent what is actually happening to the abdomen.

An abdominal wall will only stretch so much. Compliance and stretching occur with changes in volume per change in pressure. The volume of abdominal cavity insufflation has overlapping phases, reshaping with minimal changes from pressure and stretching with elastic expansion of the abdominal wall and pressure, which can be characterized by a pressure–volume relationship that produces maximum stretch [12]. When complete abdominal compliance is reached, adding another mmHg of gas pressure will not expand the abdominal wall any further; no more space is created in the pneumoperitoneum, but pressure is increased. This decreases capillary blood flow to the visceral splanchnic compartment and vessels under the abdominal fascia, increasing hypoxia and cellular inflammatory reactions [30, 31]. The chemical and biologic interactions of gas within the abdominal cavity are related to its surface characteristics, diffusion, local cellular and biochemical activities, and global responses to pressure and chemical changes [32, 33]. What matters is pressure, duration of pressure, and total volume of gas used. Therefore, IAP should be kept just below the limit of complete abdominal compliance to maintain sufficient operating space, improve perfusion, and reduce hypoxia.

Gas velocity delivered from an insufflator through a trocar cannula can reach 30 meters per second (m/s), becoming a "jet stream" [34]. The gas stream touches peritoneal surfaces, causing a circular hydraulic deflection. If the gas is dry and cool, it produces rapid tissue surface evaporative cooling, increased peritoneal fluid viscosity, changes in peritoneal fluid constituent concentration, and peritoneal tissue damage and disruption [35, 36]. The thin layer of peritoneal mesothelial cells can be damaged by dry gas, destroying microvilli, retracting and bulging cells, and exposing the basal lamina [28, 37–45]. When humidified warmed gas is used, these conditions are reduced [28, 38, 39, 44, 45]. Desiccation tissue damage is not possible when the gas is highly saturated with water vapor, keeping water at an elevated RH at the same temperature as the abdominal tissues [28]. Evaporative cooling, cell desiccation, and peritoneal fluid viscosity changes do not take place when the gas is hydrated and warmed [35, 36, 46]. Heating gas without humidification has no beneficial and some detrimental effects [47–50].

The rate of peritoneal gas absorption is determined by the inhibitor of apoptosis protein, IAP, partial pressure gradients influenced by tissue/gas permeability, tissue absorptive capacity, temperature, and the exposed surface area. The amount of CO_2 absorption through the peritoneum during laparoscopy is between 14 and 48 milliliters per minute (mL/min) [51–53], with 10–20% of CO_2 eliminated from peritoneal absorption variability due to different insufflation pressures. Carbon dioxide absorption reaches a plateau after 20–25 min of pneumoperitoneum and continues to be eliminated up to 30 min after desufflation [54]. Humidifying and warming CO_2 for insufflation leads to faster dissipation of residual gas after pneumoperitoneum desufflation [55].

The constancy of body temperature regulation is integral to the interior milieu required for health and proper functioning of cellular elements of warm-blooded animals, as recognized by Claude Bernard in 1854 [56, 57]. Bernard said that a healthy person does not exist with an internal body temperature much outside the normal range of 36°–38 °C. Internal stability of self-regulating homeostasis developed from this recognition [58].

Patients undergoing laparoscopy have a body temperature of approximately 37 °C with a peritoneal cavity high in humidity and a thin film of peritoneal fluid covering peritoneal tissues. Intentionally using gas that is 15–17 °C cooler and dry will cause problems. Thinking that this drastic difference will not matter nor has no detrimental biologic or physiologic effects is wrong, illogical, and incorrect. Hypothermia related to any surgical procedure is multifactorial, based on the patient age, sex, weight, anesthetic drugs, patient's original temperature, room temperature, length of operation, temperature of infused or irrigation fluids, volume of fluids used, temperature of skin cleansing solutions, and temperature and volume of irrigation left in the peritoneal cavity. However, there is irrefutable scientific evidence that humidifying and warming the gas for a pneumoperitoneum benefits the patient and improves outcomes.

Heat loss during surgery is due to radiation, convection, conduction, and evaporation. Reducing or preventing thermal losses from these situations is beneficial and desirable. The difference between laparoscopy and laparotomy is an open peritoneal cavity vs. a closed cavity. The ambient environment for laparotomy is 20 °C, 45–50% RH, and mild air current of 1–3 m/s. For laparoscopy, the ambient environment external to the peritoneal cavity is 20 °C, 45–50% RH, and mild air flow of 1–3 m/s on the patient's surface; inside the peritoneal cavity, there should be intermittent gas flow of 20 °C, 0.02% RH, and up to 30 m/s flow and hundreds of liters gas consumed [59–64].

The physiologic response to general anesthesia and anesthetic drugs is an increase in the threshold of warmth response and a decrease in the threshold of cold response [65]. Anesthetic drugs cause a chemical disconnect between the hypothalamic pituitary axis, suppressing control of afferent sensing and efferent responses for thermoregulation. During anesthesia, patients are at the mercy of their environment and what is done to them, which has an influence on the direction, rapidity, and how far their temperature will trend. Mild hypothermia is defined as a core body temperature below 35 °C. Intraoperative hypothermia alters pharmacodynamics and pharmacokinetics for each 0.1 °C below 35 °C, especially with inhalation agents (which are more soluble) and muscle relaxants (which have prolonged effects at lower internal temperatures). Intraoperative hypothermia also decreases respiratory volume and frequency per minute, decreases cerebral blood flow by 7% for each 1 °C decrease in core temperature, increases coagulopathy, prolongs recovery time, increases oxygen consumption, increases discomfort due to chill and shivering, delays wound healing, increases infection rates, increases immunosuppression for euthermic patients, and prolongs hospital stay.

Along with other contributing factors, general anesthesia contributes to hypothermia through three phases. In the first phase, central body heat is lost through thermal redistribution in the first 60 min with a temperature loss of 0.5–1.5 °C, mostly due to radiation. In the second phase, peripheral and central heat loss leads to clinical mild hypothermia with a temperature below 35 °C. In the third phase, peripheral vasoconstriction causes the core temperature to stay below 35 °C. All of these factors—anesthesia, drugs, the use of dry and cool gas for the pneumoperitoneum, rapid evaporation, and local cooling from the peritoneal tissue surface—contribute to the total hypothermia effect. Conditioning the CO_2 gas to just below body core temperature and humidifying to 95% RH can eliminate or reduce hypothermia, tissue desiccation, inflammation, adhesion formation, and postoperative pain; it also has clinical benefits and utility [28, 39, 66–79].

Peritoneal hypothermia causes vasoconstriction, which disrupts gastrointestinal peristalsis and myoelectric conduction. If a dry, cool gas is used for the pneumoperitoneum, a temperature gradient occurs, thus reducing myoelectric activity. A persistent ionic feedback response deforms and destabilizes the physiological enteric electrical activity due to intestinal surface cooling, which leads to intestinal arrhythmias and dysmotility and disrupts peristaltic activity. The interruption in velocity propagation and dynamics of intestinal electrophysiological wave propagation cause pain and temporary peristaltic dysfunction [80]. Intestinal hypothermia, disruption of gastrointestinal electrical activity and transit time, and postoperative bowel dysfunction are improved by preconditioning CO_2 gas.

Penetration of the abdominal wall to create and maintain a pneumoperitoneum sets in motion a cascade of normal cellular responses to repair the peritoneal injury. These healing processes are not abnormal. Any resulting adhesion or scarring distortions may create abnormalities in function and location, but the healing response to an insult is not abnormal.

The peritoneum is the body's largest serous membrane, with a surface area that is approximately equal to the integumentary system at 1.1–2.1 m^2 [26, 81]. The peritoneal surface is a continuous sheet of mesothelial cells overlying loose mesenchymal connective tissue, a basal lamina, and basement membrane attached to the abdominal wall and viscera well supplied with blood vessels, capillaries, and lymphatics [29, 82]. Peritoneal thickness ranges between 0.3 and 1.1 mm depending on the surface covered [83]. The visceral peritoneum represents 81.89% of the surface area, with the parietal making up 18.11%. The peritoneum contains microvilli, vessels and microcirculation that are most important for exchange [84].

The pneumoperitoneum affects the entire gas-exposed surface of the peritoneum; when damaged, it can uncover portions of the basal lamina [40, 85]. Characteristic alterations of the peritoneum caused by the use of cold, dry CO_2 for the pneumoperitoneum include mesothelial damage, desiccation, distorted and denuded peritoneal surfaces, and exposed areas of basal lamina [40–43, 45, 86–97]. Preconditioning CO_2 for laparoscopy by humidifying and warming the gas creates a physiologic pneumoperitoneum that enhances preservation of peritoneal integrity and has clinical benefits [37, 38, 98–101].

Mesothelial cells and peritoneal fluid protect and sustain peritoneal homeostasis. The apical surface of the mesothelium has a liquid film, the glycocalyx, which provides a slippery, nonadhesive, hydrodynamic boundary surface lubricant that protects the peritoneal viscera and mesothelial surfaces from abrasions and adhesions. The glycocalyx plays an important role in cell-cell contact, tissue hydration, regulation of inflammation, tissue remodeling, and flow of nutrients and growth factors across the peritoneal membrane [102–107]. The mesothelial cells synthesize cytokines, growth factors, and matrix protein components that are integral for the induction and resolution of inflammation and tissue repair.

There are four responses to peritoneal injury: repair and resurfacing with normal anatomic and functional location and three "adhesion processes," which are adhesion formation at locations with or without excess peritoneal attachments (adhesions formed at operative sites), de novo adhesion formation (adhesions formed at nonoperative sites), and adhesion reformation (adhesions formed after lysis of previous adhesions) [98–100, 108]. Regardless of how the insult occurred or its etiology, the peritoneum reacts with the same cellular response. Repairs are initiated in the same way no matter how the injury happened: scalpel, instrument, gauze pad, drying, scissors, cautery, laser, harmonic scalpel, freezing, and bacteria or body fluids.

Peritoneal drying, a desiccation injury, has long been recognized as a postoperative complication [101]. In 1918, it was suspected that "the amount of peritoneal drying" during laparotomy detrimentally influenced postoperative recovery; thus, it was recommended to "avoid peritoneal drying" [101]: "Peritoneal drying causes mesothelial desquamation" [109]. It was said "that the surgeon should try to avoid peritoneal drying" [110] and that "adhesions may be due to peritoneal drying, injury" [111]. Furthermore, "insufflations with heated, humidified CO_2 are the least likely to induce mesothelial damage" [44, 112] because "drying of tissue is a known cause of adhesion formation" [67, 82, 96] and that "due to the high flow rates, warming and moistening of the insufflated CO_2 are necessary" [113].

Because of peritoneal CO_2 absorption, minute respiratory, end-expiratory, or end-tidal CO_2 ($ETCO_2$) levels should be maintained throughout the procedure, adjusting to maintain normocapnia. Carbon dioxide causes reversible systemic and local acidosis, and the effect of IAP on parietal peritoneal pH has minor significance [114, 115]. Normal excretion of CO_2 is 100–200 mL/min, which is increased by 14–18 mL/min due to intraperitoneal CO_2 [54, 116–118]. A pneumoperitoneum decreases thoracopulmonary compliance by 30–50% in healthy patients (i.e., those classified as ASA I according to the American Society of Anesthesia) [119, 120]. Increased levels of CO_2 may help in detecting a CO_2

embolism and should not exceed 25% of original $ETCO_2$.

Cardiovascular effects during laparoscopy are usually due to hypercarbia, acidosis, and increased IAP [119]. Renal effects related to IAP and indirectly to CO_2 absorption include neuroendocrine and tissue damage from oxidative stress [121]. Transient oliguria is the most common due to activation of the renin-angiotensin-aldosterone system as a result of decreased renal perfusion [115]. During IAP, urine outflow decreases and creatinine increases. These levels normalize within 24 h after a pneumoperitoneum of less than 15 mmHg [122–124].

Oxidative stress is associated with surgery, whether the approach is open or laparoscopic [125]. This is influenced by the surgery performed, IAP, length of time, ischemia, reperfusion, and desufflation and is less severe with laparoscopy than open surgery [126–128]. Surgical response and recovery are measured by inflammatory markers and the immune response [129–133]. These are cytokines, lymphokines, and prostaglandins such as tumor necrosis factor alpha, interleukin-6, IL-8, C-reactive protein, and granulocuyte colony-stimulating factor [95, 129–133]. These immunologic factors are created by tissue damage. Laparoscopic surgery causes a decreased systemic immunologic response compared with open surgery [134, 135], especially when the distending gas is more physiologic by being humidified and warmed [136].

A pneumoperitoneum is safe during pregnancy. However, attention to detail is paramount because the margins of error are smaller, the physiology is more temperamental, and two persons are involved in the surgical event. The gas should be preconditioned by humidifying and warming to physiologic conditions to reduce hypothermia, decrease peritoneal damage, and improve outcomes. There should be continuous $ETCO_2$ monitoring. The patient should be in the left lateral decubitus position. IAP should not exceed 15 mmHg but should be less if abdominal compliance warrants; the procedure can be performed safely at lower pressure without compromising the outcome. Venous thrombosis prevention should be performed using intraoperative and postoperative compression devices with early ambulation. Perioperative fetal monitoring should be done when there is a viable fetus. Tocolytic prophylaxis may be required perioperatively if there are signs of preterm labor.

Summary

When the need for non-obstetric surgery arises during pregnancy, the choice between an open versus laparoscopic approach does matter. The effects that general anesthesia and surgical intervention have on a patient can influence the therapeutic choice. Reports on non-obstetric surgery (regardless of route) vary in indications, techniques, comorbidities, ages, lifestyles, and anesthesia choice, making comparison and evaluation of the literature difficult. The outcomes for patients undergoing laparoscopic procedures are better than those for open procedures. The miscarriage rate for laparoscopy compared with an open procedure is higher in the first trimester, but has only been reported for appendectomy. Fetal anomalies were not statistically significantly different. The variables to be considered in the selection of open versus laparoscopic surgery for non-obstetric surgery during pregnancy include stage of pregnancy, presence of a fetus, physiologic changes during pregnancy, and the non-obstetric surgical problem as it relates to pregnancy. Considerations for laparoscopic surgery compared with laparotomy during pregnancy include the type of procedure, the skill of the surgeon, and possibility of premature infant delivery.

References

1. Pillay P, Piercy C, Tolppanen H, Mebazaa A. Physiological changes in pregnancy. Cardiovasc J Afr. 2016;27:89–94.
2. Pearl J, Price R, Richardson W, Fanelli R. Guidelines for diagnosis, treatment and use of laparoscopy for surgical problems during pregnancy. Surg Endosc. 2011;25:3479–92. https://doi.org/10.1007/s00464-011-1927-3.
3. Pearl J, Price R, Tonkin A, Richardson W. SAGES guidelines for use of laparoscopy during pregnancy. Surg Endosc. 2017;31:3767–82.

4. Juhasz-Boss I, Solomayer E, Strik M, Raspe C. Abdominal surgery in pregnancy – an interdisciplinary challenge. Dtsch Arztebl Int. 2014;111:465–2.
5. Chun R, Kirkpatrick A. Intra-abdominal pressure, intra-abdominal hypertension, and pregnancy: a review. Ann Intensive Care. 2012;2(Suppl 1):55.
6. Jeong H. Altered drug metabolism during pregnancy: hormonal regulation of drug-metabolizing enzymes. Expert Opin Drug Metab Toxicol. 2010;6:689–99. https://doi.org/10.1517/17425251003677755.
7. Mhyre J, Bateman B, Leffert L. Influence of patient comorbidities on the risk of near-miss maternal morbidity or mortality. Anesthesiology. 2011;115:963–72. https://doi.org/10.1097/ALN.0b013e318233042d.
8. Fuchs F, Bruyere M, Senat M, Purenne E, Benhamou D, Fernandez H. Are standard intra-abdominal pressure values different during pregnancy? PLoS One. 2013;8(10):e77324. https://doi.org/10.1371/journal.pone.0077324.
9. DeKeulenaer B, De Waele J, Powell B, Malbrain M. What is normal intra-abdominal pressure and how it is affected by positioning, body mas and positive end-expiratory pressure? Intensive Care Med. 2009;35:969–76.
10. Sawchuck D, Wittman B. Pre-eclampsia renamed and reframed: intra-abdominal hypertension in pregnancy. Med Hypotheses. 2014;83:619–32. https://doi.org/10.1016/j.mehy.2014.08.001.
11. van Ramshorst G, Salih M, Hop W, van Waes O, Kleinrensink G, Goossens R, et al. Non-invasive. measurement of intra-abdominal pressure by assessment of abdominal wall tension. J Surg Res. 2011;171:240–4.
12. Blaser A, Bjorck M, De Keulenaer B, Regli A. Abdominal compliance: a bench-to-bedside review. J Trauma Acute Care Surg. 2015;78:1044–53.
13. Becker C, Plymale M, Wennergren J, Totten C, Stigall K, Roth H. Compliance of the abdominal wall during laparoscopic insufflation. Surg Endosc. 2017;31:1947–51.
14. Song C, Alijani A, Frank T, Hanna G, Cuschieri A. Elasticity of the living abdominal wall in laparoscopic surgery. J Biomech. 2006;39:587–91.
15. Forstemann T, Trzewik J, Holste J, Batke B, Konerding MA, Wolloscheck T, et al. Forces and deformations of the abdominal wall- a mechanical and geometrical approach to the linea alba. J Biomech. 2011;44:600–6.
16. Malbrain M, De Laet I, De Waele J, Kirkpatrick A. Intra-abdominal hypertension: definitions, monitoring, interpretation and management. Best Pract Res Clin Anaesthesiol. 2013;27:249–70.
17. Chung R, Kirkpatrick A. Intra-abdominal pressure, intra-abdominal hypertension, and pregnancy: a review. Ann Intensive Care. 2012;2(Suppl 1):85.
18. Sugerman H. Hypothesis: preeclampsia is a venous disease secondary to an increased intra-abdominal pressure. Med Hypotheses. 2011;77:841–9.
19. Kirkpatrick A, Roberts D, De Waele J, Jaeschke R, Malbrain M, De Keulenaer B, et al. Intra-abdominal hypertension and the abdominal compartment syndrome: updated consensus definitions and clinical practice guidelines from the world Society of the Abdominal Compartment Syndrome. Intensive Care Med. 2013;39:1190–11206.
20. Carter J, Soper D. Operative laparoscopy in pregnancy. JSLS. 2004;8:57–60.
21. Jacobs V, Morrison J. The real intraabdominal pressure during laparoscopy: comparison of different insufflators. J Minim Invasive Gynecol. 2007;14:103–7.
22. Reedy M, Kim U, Thompson E, Rayburn W. Laparoscopy during pregnancy. A safe alternative to laparoscopy? Contemp Ob Gyn 1998:75–91.
23. Hunter J, Swanstrom L, Thornberg K. Carbon dioxide pneumoperitoneum induces fetal acidosis in a pregnant ewe model. Surg Endosc. 1995;9:272–9.
24. Ott D. Pneumoperitoneum: production, management, effects and consequences. In: Prevention and management of laparoendoscopic surgical complications. 1st ed. Society of Laparoendoscopic Surgeons: Miami; 1999.
25. Awoniyi A, Belotte J, Abuanzeh S, Fletcher N, Diamond M, Saed G. Advances in the pathogenesis of adhesion development. The role of oxidative stress. Repro Sci. 2014;21:823–36.
26. Hatipoglu S, Akbultu S, Hatipoglu F, Abdullayev R. Effect of laparoscopic abdominal surgery on splanchnic circulation: historical developments. World J Gastroenerol. 2014;28:18165–76.
27. Ott D. The pneumoperitoneum. In: Prevention and management of laparoendoscopic surgical complications. 3rd ed. Society of Laparoendoscopic Surgeons: Miami; 2012.
28. Binda M. Humidification during laparoscopic surgery: overview of the clinical benefits of using humidified gas during laparoscopic surgery. Arch Gynecol Obstet. 2015;292:955–71.
29. Ott D. Laparoscopy and adhesion formation, adhesions and laparoscopy. Semin Reprod Med. 2008;26:322–30.
30. Balkin D, Duh Q, Kind G, Chang D, McGrath M. Failed pneumoperitoneum for laparoscopic surgery following autologous Deep Inferior Epigastric Perforator (DIEP) flap breast reconstruction: a case report. BMC Surg. 2016;27(16):28. https://doi.org/10.1186/s12893-016-0143-4.
31. Goldman J, Rose L, Morgan M, Denison D. Measurement of abdominal wall compliance in normal subjects and tetraplegic patients. Thorax. 1986;41:513–8.
32. Nguyen N, Wolfe BM. The physiologic effects of pneumoperitoneum in the morbidly obese. Ann Surg. 2005;241:219–26.
33. Srivastava A, Niranjan A. Secrets of safe laparoscopic surgery: anaesthetic and surgical considerations. J Minim Access Surg. 2010;6:91–4.

34. Lackey L, Ott D. Terminal gas velocity during laparoscopy. J Am Assoc Gynecolo Laparosc. 2002;9:297–305.
35. Gray R, Ott D, Henderson A, Cochran S, Roth C. Severe local hypothermia from laparoscopic gas evaporative jet-cooling; a mechanism to explain clinical observations. JSLS. 1999;3:171–7.
36. Ott D. Desertification of the peritoneum by thin-film evaporation during laparoscopy. JSLS. 2003;7:189–95.
37. Hazebroek E, Schreve M, Visser P, De Bruin R, Marquet R, Bonjer H. Impact of temperature and humidity of carbon dioxide pneumoperitoneum on body temperature and peritoneal morphology. J Laparoendosc Adv Surg Tech A. 2002;12:355–64.
38. Peng Y, Zheng M, Ye Q, Chen X, Yu B, Liu B. Heated and humidified CO2 prevents hypothermia, peritoneal injury, and intra-abdominal adhesions during prolonged laparoscopic insufflations. J Surg Res. 2009;151:40–7.
39. Mouton W, Bessell J, Pfitzner J, Dymock R, Brealey J, Maddern G. A randomized controlled trial to determine the effects of humidified carbon dioxide insufflation during thoracoscopy. Surg Endosc. 1999;13:382–5.
40. Volz J, Koster S, Spacek Z, Paweletz N. Characteristic alterations of the peritoneum after carbon dioxide pneumoperitoneum. Surg Endosc. 1999;13:611–4.
41. Suematsu T, Hirabayashi Y, Shiraishi N, Adachi Y, Kitamura H, Kitano S. Morphology of the murine peritoneum after pneumoperitoneum vs laparotomy. Surg Endosc. 2001;15:954–8.
42. Liu Y, Hou Q. Effect of carbon dioxide pneumoperitoneum during laparoscopic surgery on morphology of peritoneum. Zhonghua Yi Xue Za Zhi. 2006;86:164–6.
43. Ryan G, Grobety J, Majno G. Mesothelial injury and recovery. Am J Pathol. 1973;71:93–112.
44. Davey A, Hayward J, Marshall J, Woods A. The effects of insufflation conditions on rat mesothelium. Int J Inflam. 2013;2013:816283.
45. Erikoglu M, Yol S, Avunduk M, Erdemli E, Can A. Electron-microscopic alterations of the peritoneum after both cold and heated carbon dioxide pneumoperitoneum. J Surg Res. 2005;125:73–7.
46. Ott D. Laparoscopy and tribology: the effect of laparoscopic gas on peritoneal fluid. J Am Assoc Gynecol Laparosc. 2001;8:117–23.
47. Jacobs V, Keichle M, Morrison J. Carbon dioxide gas heating inside laparoscopic insufflators has no effect. JSLS. 2005;9:208–12.
48. Slim K, Bousquet J, Kwiatkowski F, Lescure G, Pezet D, Chipponi J. Effect of CO_2 gas warming on pain after laparoscopic surgery: a randomized double-blind controlled trial. Surg Endosc. 2000;13:1110–4.
49. Saad S, Minor I, Mohri T, Nagelschmidt M. The clinical impact of warmed insufflation carbon dioxide gas for laparoscopic cholecystectomy. Surg Endosc. 2000;14:787–90.
50. Wills V, Hunt D, Armstrong A. A randomized controlled trial assessing the effect of heated carbon dioxide for insufflation on pain and recovery after laparoscopic fundoplication. Surg Endosc. 2001;15:166–70.
51. Nunn J. Carbon dioxide. In: Applied respiratory physiology. London: Butterworth; 1987. p. 207–34.
52. Grzegorzewska A, Antoniewicz K. Effective peritoneal blood flow and patient characteristics. In: Khanna R, editor. Advances in peritoneal dialysis, vol. 10. Toronto, ON: Peritoneal Dialysis Publications; 1994. p. 27–9.
53. Kim M, Lofthouse J, Flessner M. A method to test blood flow limitation of peritoneal-blood solute transport. J Am Soc Nephrol. 1997;8:471–4.
54. Pacilli M, Pierro A, Kingsley C, Curry J, Herod J, Eaton S. Absorption of carbon dioxide during laparoscopy in children measured using a novel mass spectrometric technique. BJA. 2006;97:215–9.
55. Glew P, Campher M, Pearson K, Schofield B, Davey A. The effect of warm humidified CO2 on the dissipation of residual gas following laparoscopy in piglets. J Am Assoc Gynecol Laparosc. 2004;11:204–10.
56. Raffi A. Body temperature during surgery and anesthesia. MVC Quarterly. 1972;8:135–41.
57. Gross C. Claude Bernard and the constancy of the internal environment. Neuroscientist. 1998;4:380–5.
58. Cross S, Albury W. Walter B. Cannon, L.J. Henderson and the organic analogy. Osiris. 1987;3:165–92.
59. Cam R, Yonem H, Ozsoy H. Core body temperature changes during surgery and nursing management. Clin Med Res. 2016;5:1–5. https://doi.org/10.11648/j.cmr.s.2016050201.11.
60. Whelan R, Fleshman J, Fowler D. SAGES manual of perioperative care in minimally invasive surgery. New York: Springer; 2006.
61. Rosenthal R, Friedman R, Phillips E. The pathophysiology of pneumoperitoneum. In: Bessell J, Maddern G, editors. Influence of gas temperature during laparoscopic procedures. Heidelberg: Springer; 1998. p. 18–27.
62. Buhre W, Rossaint R. Perioperative management and monitoring in anaesthesia. Lancet. 2003;362:1839–46.
63. Sessler D. Complications and treatment of mild hypothermia. Anesthesiology. 2001;95:531–43.
64. Jacobs V, Morrison J, Mettler L, Mundhenke C, Jonat W. Measurement of CO_2 hypothermia during laparoscopy and pelviscopy: how cold it gets and how to prevent it. J Am Assoc Gynecol Laparosc. 1999;6(3):289–95.
65. Diaz M, Becker D. Thermoregulation: physiological and clinical considerations during sedation and general anesthesia. Anesth Prog. 2010;57:25–33.
66. Binda M, Molinas C, Mailova K, Koninckx P. Effect of temperature upon adhesion formation in a laparoscopic mouse model. Hum Reprod. 2004;19:2626–32.
67. Binda M, Molinas C, Hansen P, Koninckx P. Effect of desiccation and temperature during laparoscopy

on adhesion formation in mice. Fertil Steril. 2006;86:166–75.

68. Sajid M, Mallick A, Rimpel J, Bokari SA, Cheek E, Baig M. Effect of heated and humidified carbon dioxide on patients after laparoscopic procedures: a meta-analysis. Surg Laparosc Endosc Percutan Tech. 2008;18:539–46.
69. Sammour T, Kahokehr A, Hill A. Meta-analysis of the effect of warm humidified insufflation on pain after laparoscopy. Br J Surg. 2008;95:950–6.
70. Bessell J, Ludbrook G, Millard H, Baxter S, Ubhi S, Maddern G. Humidified gas prevents hypothermia induced by laparoscopic insufflation: a randomized controlled study in a pig model. Surg Endosc. 1999;13:101–5.
71. Bessell J, Karatassas A, Patterson J, Jamieson G, Maddern G. Hypothermia induced by laparoscopic insufflation. A randomized study in a pig model. Surg Endosc. 1995;9:791–6.
72. Ott D, Reich H, Love B, McCorvey R, Toledo A, Liu C, et al. Reduction of laparoscopic-induced hypothermia, postoperative pain and recovery room length of stay by pre-conditioning gas with the Insuflow device: a prospective randomized controlled multi-center study. JSLS. 1998;2:321–9.
73. Benavides R, Wong A, Nguyen H. Improved outcomes for lap-banding using the Insuflow device compared with heated-only gas. JSLS. 2009;13:302–5.
74. Beste T, Daucher J, Holbert D. Humidified compared with dry, heated carbon dioxide at laparoscopy to reduce pain. Obstet Gynecol. 2006;107:263–8.
75. Farley D, Greenlee S, Larson D, Harrington J. Double-blind, prospective, randomized study of warmed, humidified carbon dioxide insufflation vs standard carbon dioxide for patients undergoing laparoscopic cholecystectomy. Arch Surg. 2004;139:739–44.
76. Herrmann A, DeWilde R. Insufflation with humidified and heated carbon dioxide in short-term laparoscopy: a double-blinded randomized controlled trial. Biomed Res Int. 2015;2015:412618. https://doi.org/10.1155/2015/412618.
77. Klugsberger B, Schreiner M, Rothe A, Haas D, Oppelt P, Shamiyeh A. Warmed, humidified carbon dioxide insufflation versus standard carbon dioxide in laparoscopic cholecystectomy: a double-blinded randomized controlled trial. Surg Endosc. 2014;28:2656–60.
78. Mouton W, Bessell J, Millard S, Baxter P, Maddern G. A randomized controlled trial assessing the benefit of humidified insufflation gas during laparoscopic surgery. Surg Endosc. 1999;13:106–8.
79. Hamza M, Schneider B, White P, Recart A, Villegas L, Ogunnaike B, et al. Heated and humidified insufflation during laparoscopic gastric bypass surgery: effect on temperature, postoperative pain, and recovery outcomes. J Laparoendosc Adv Surg Tech A. 2005;15:6–12.
80. Gizzi A, Cherubini C, Migliori S, Alloni R, Portuesi R, Filippi S. On the electrical intestine turbulence induced by temperature changes. Phys Biol. 2010;7:1–12.
81. Hertzler AE. The peritoneum, vol. 1. St. Louis: C. V. Mosby Co.; 1919.
82. diZerega G, Rogers K. The peritoneum. New York: Springer-Verlag; 1992. p. 1–56.
83. Hanbidge A, Lynch D, Wilson S. Ultrasound of the peritoneum. Radiographics. 2003;23:663–384.
84. Albanese A, Albanese E, Mino J, Gomez E, Gomez M, Zandomeni M, Merlo A. Peritoneal surface area: measurements of 40 structures covered by peritoneum: correlation between total peritoneal surface area and the surface calculated by formulas. Surg Radiol Anat. 2009;31:369–77.
85. Volz J, Koster S, Schaeff B, Paolucci V. Laparoscopic surgery: the effects of insufflation gas on tumor-induced lethality in nude mice. Am J Obstet Gynecol. 1998;178:793–5.
86. Mutsaers S, Birnie K, Lansley S, Herrick S, Lim C, Prele C. Mesothelial cells in tissue repair and fibrosis. Front Pharmacol. 2015;6:113. https://doi.org/10.3389/fphar.2015.00113.
87. Ryan GB, Grobety J, Majno F. Postoperative peritoneal adhesions: a study of the mechanisms. Am J Pathol. 1971;65:117–48.
88. Raftery A. Regeneration of parietal and visceral peritoneum: an electron microscopical study. J Anat. 1973;115:375–92.
89. Raftery A. Regeneration of parietal and visceral peritoneum. A light microscopical study. Br J Surg. 1973;60:293–9.
90. Volz J, Koster S, Weiss M, Schmidt R, Urbaschek R, Melchert F, et al. Pathophysiologic features of a pneumoperitoneum at laparoscopy: a swine model. Am J Obstet Gynecol. 1996;174:132–40.
91. Volz J, Koster S, Leweling H. Surgical trauma and metabolic changes induced by surgical laparoscopy versus laparotomy. Gynaecol Endosc. 1997;6:1–6.
92. Holmdahl L, Risberg B, Beck D, Burns J, Chegini N, diZerega G, et al. Adhesions: pathogenesis and prevention-panel discussion and summary. Eur J Surg Suppl. 1997;577:56–62.
93. Rosario M, Ribeiro U, Corbett C, Ozaki A, Bresciani C, Zilberstein B, Gama-Rodrigues J. Does CO2 pneumoperitoneum alter the ultra-structure of the mesothelium? J Surg Res. 2006;133:84–8.
94. Grabowski J, Talamini M. Physiological effects of pneumoperitoneum. Gastrointest Surg. 2009;13:1009–16.
95. Brokelman W, Lensvelt M, Borel Rinkes I, Klinkenbijl J, Reijnen M. Peritoneal changes due to laparoscopic surgery. Surg Endosc. 2011;25:1–9.
96. Papparella A, Nino F, Coppola S, Noviello C, Paciello O, Papparella S. Peritoneal morphological changes due to pneumoperitoneum: the effect of intra-abdominal pressure. Eur J Pediatr Surg. 2013;24:322–7.

97. Mais V. Peritoneal adhesions after laparoscopic gastrointestinal surgery. World Gastroenterol. 2014;20:4917–25.
98. Arung W, Meurisse M, Detry O. Pathophysiology and prevention of postoperative peritoneal adhesions. World J Gastroenterol. 2011;17:4545–53. https://doi.org/10.3748/wjg.v17.i41.4545.
99. Diamond M, Freeman M. Clinical implications of post- surgical adhesions. Hum Reprod Update. 2001;7:567–76.
100. Ellis H. The clinical significance of adhesions: focus on intestinal obstruction. Eur J Surg Suppl. 1997;577:5–9.
101. Hawkins-Ambler G. What makes for success in abdominal surgery? In: Shrady G, editor. The British Gynaecological Society, 1892 Medical Record. New York: William Wood & Company; 1892.
102. Yung S, Chan T. Pathophysiological changes to the peritoneal membrane during PD-related peritonitis: the role of mesothelial cells mediators of inflammation. Mediat Inflamm. 2012;2012:484167. https://doi.org/10.1155/2012/484167.
103. Yung S, Chan T. Mesothelial cells. Perit Dial Int. 2007;27:110–5.
104. Flessner M. Endothelial glycocalyx and the peritoneal barrier. Perit Dial Int. 2008;28:6–12.
105. Anglani F, Forino M, Del Petre D, Ceol M, Favaro S. Molecular biology of the peritoneal membrane: in between morphology and function. Contrib Nephrol. 2001;131:61–73.
106. Molinas C, Binda M, Manavella G, Koninckx P. Adhesion formation after laparoscopic surgery: what do we know about the role of the peritoneal environment? Facts Views Vis Obgyn. 2010;2:149–60.
107. Bird S. Mesothelial primary cilia of peritoneal and other serosal surfaces. Cell Biol Int. 2004;28:151–9.
108. Pouly J, Seak-San S. Adhesions: laparoscopy versus laparotomy. In: DiZerega G, editor. Peritoneal surgery. New York: Springer-Verlag; 2000. p. 183–92.
109. Alvarez W. The cause and prevention of postoperative gas pains. Cal State J Med. 1918;16:338–41.
110. Nolph KD, editor. Chapter 4. Peritoneal dialysis. Boston: Martinus Nijhoff Publishers; 1985.
111. Howard F. Approach to the patient with chronic pelvic pain. In: Howard F, editor. Pelvic pain, diagnosis and management. Philadelphia, PA: Lippincott Williams & Wilkins; 2000.
112. Diamond M, Manvinder S, Puscheck E. Chronic pelvic pain and adhesions. In: Vercellini P, editor. Chronic pelvic pain. Singapore: Wiley-Blackwell; 2011.
113. Wildbrett P, Oh A, Naundorf D, Volk T, Jacobi C. Impact of laparoscopic gases on peritoneal microenvironment and essential parameters of cell function. Surg Endosc. 2003;17:78–82.
114. Wong Y, Shah P, Birkett D, Brams D. Peritoneal pH during laparoscopy is dependent on ambient gas environment. Surg Endosc. 2005;19:60–4.
115. Veekash G, Wei L, Su M. Carbon dioxide pneumoperitoneum, physiologic changes and anesthetic concerns. Ambulatory Surg. 2010;16:41–6.
116. Tan P, Lee T, Tweed W. Carbon dioxide absorption and gas exchange during pelvic laparoscopy. Can J Anaesth. 1992;39:677–81.
117. Muelett C, Viale J, Sagnard P, Miellet C, Ruynat L, Counioux H, et al. Pulmonary carbon dioxide elimination during surgical procedures using intra- or extraperitoneal CO2 insufflation. Anesth Analg. 1993;76:622–6.
118. Perrin M, Fletcher A. Laparoscopic abdominal surgery. Contin Educ Anaesth Crit Care Pain. 2004;4:107–10.
119. Martin-Cancho M, Celdran D, Lima J, Carrasco-Jimenez M, Sanchez-Margall F, Uson-Gargallo J. Anaesthetic considerations during laparoscopic surgery. Chapter 2. In: Darwish A, editor. Advanced gynecologic endoscopy. London: InTech; 2011. http://www.intechopen.com/books/advanced-gynecologic-endoscopy/anaesthetic-considerations-duringlaparoscopic-surgery.
120. Loring S, Behazin N, Novero A, Novack V, Jones S, O'Donnell C, et al. Respiratory mechanical effects of surgical pneumoperitoneum in humans. J Appl Physiol. 2014;117:1074–9.
121. Sodha S, Nazarian S, Adshead J, Vasdev N, Mohan-S G. Effect of pneumoperitoneum on renal function and physiology in patients undergoing robotic renal surgery. Curr Urol. 2016;9:1–4.
122. Wever J. Renal perfusion and function during pneumoperitoneum: a systematic review and meta-analysis of animal studies. PLoS One. 2016;11(9):e0163419. https://doi.org/10.1371/journal.pone.0163419.
123. Demyttenaere S, Feldman L, Fried G. Effect of pneumoperitoneum on renal perfusion and function: a systematic review. Surg Endosc. 2007;21:152–60.
124. Taskin O, Buhur A, Birincioglu M, Burak F, Atmaca R, Yilmaz I, et al. The effects of duration of CO2 insufflation and irrigation on peritoneal microcirculation assessed by free radical scavengers and total glutathione levels during operative laparoscopy. J Am Assoc Gynecol Laparosc. 1998;5:129–33.
125. Glantzounis G, Tselepis A, Tambaki A, Trikalinos T, Manataki A, Galaris D, et al. Laparoscopic surgery-induced changes in oxidative stress markers in human plasma. Surg Enndosc. 2001;15:1315–9.
126. Arsalani-Zadeh R, Ullah S, Khan S, MacFie J. Oxidative stress in laparoscopic versus open abdominal surgery: a systematic review. J Surg Res. 2011;169:59–68. https://doi.org/10.1016/j.jss.2011.01.038
127. Sammour T, Mittal A, Loveday B, Kahokehr A, Phillips A, Windsor J, Hill A. Systematic review of oxidative stress associated with pneumoperitoneum. Br J Surg. 2009;96:8366–50.
128. Yiannakopoulou E, Nikiteas N, Despina P, Tsigris C. Effect of laparoscopic surgery on oxidative stress

response: systematic review. Surg Laparosc Endosc Percutan Tech. 2013;23:101–8.
129. Cheong Y, Laird S, Li T, Shelton J, Ledger W, Cooke I. Peritoneal healing and adhesion formation/reformation. Hum Reprod Update. 2001;7:556–66.
130. Desborough J. The stress response to trauma and surgery. Br J Anaesth. 2000;85:109–17.
131. Sammour T, Kahokehr A, Soop M, Hill A. Peritoneal damage: the inflammatory response and clinical implications of the neuro-immuno-humoral axis. World J Surg. 2010;34:704–20.
132. Chegini N. Peritoneal molecular environment, adhesion formation and clinical implication. Front Biosci. 2002;1(7):e91–115.
133. Cheong Y, Laird S, Shelton J, Ledger W, Li T, Cooke I. The correlation of adhesions and peritoneal fluid cytokine concentrations: a pilot study. Hum Reprod. 2002;17:1039–45.
134. Yahara N, Abe T, Morita K, Tangoku A, Oka M. Comparison of interleukin-6, interleukin-8, and granulocyte colony-stimulating factor production by the peritoneum in laparoscopic and open surgery. Surg Endosc. 2002;16(11):1615–9.
135. Luk J, Tung P, Wong K, Chan K, Law S, Wong J. Laparoscopic surgery induced inerleukin-6 levels in serum and gut mucosa: implications of peritoneum integrity and gas factors. Surg Endosc. 2009;23:370–6.
136. Neuhaus S, Watson D. Pneumoperitoneum and peritoneal surface changes: a review. Surg Endosc. 2004;18:1316–22.

7 Anesthetic Considerations for the Gravid Patient for Non-obstetric Surgery

Laura E. Gilbertson, Milad Sharifpour, and Grant C. Lynde

Introduction

Over 75,000 pregnant patients each year undergo non-obstetric surgery [1], with the most common indications related to obstetric and gynecologic conditions, acute abdomen, and trauma. The vast majority of cases that are performed do so without complication.

Anesthesia plans must consider the needs of two patients. Maternal considerations will include the physiologic changes that accompany pregnancy, most significantly hemodynamic and pulmonary. Fetal considerations include the risk of birth defects as well as premature delivery. Careful consideration must be made for the entire perioperative care of the mother and fetus to ensure that each has the best possible outcome.

We will examine the maternal physiologic changes and fetal development during pregnancy. Additionally, we will discuss the intraoperative considerations that surgeons and anesthesiologists should have when performing non-obstetric surgery on the gravid patient. Finally, we will discuss national guidelines to consider when performing surgery on the gravid patient.

L. E. Gilbertson
Division of Pediatric Anesthesiology, Emory University, Atlanta, GA, USA
e-mail: laura.gilbertson@emory.edu

M. Sharifpour
Department of Anesthesiology and Critical Care, Emory University Hospital, Atlanta, GA, USA
e-mail: milad.sharifpour@emoryhealthcare.org

G. C. Lynde (✉)
Department of Anesthesiology, Practice and Process Improvement, Emory University, Atlanta, GA, USA
e-mail: glynde@emory.edu

Physiologic Changes During Pregnancy

The gravid patient undergoes many dramatic physiologic changes during pregnancy, the earliest of which are initiated by rising hormone levels and later are adaptations to resultant from maternal anatomical changes.

Cardiovascular

The cardiovascular system undergoes the most change during pregnancy for the mother and is the leading cause of maternal mortality [2]. Maternal blood volume, peripheral vascular resistance, and cardiac output all see changes of greater than 30% from preconception through birth. Understanding the cardiovascular changes will aid the physicians caring for the patient in predicting and identifying early stages of maternal distress.

Systemic vasodilation, cardiac output, and mean arterial pressure all drop by 6 weeks

C. H. Nezhat (ed.), *Non-Obstetric Surgery During Pregnancy*,
https://doi.org/10.1007/978-3-319-90752-9_7

post-gestation and are related to rapidly rising levels of hormones probably released from the corpus luteum [3]. Maternal blood volume increases approximately 15% by 6 weeks and between 30 and 50% by 34 weeks [3, 4]. Systemic vascular resistance will decrease by 33% by 6 weeks and remains at that level until delivery. And cardiac output will rise 30% by 6 weeks, where it will rise as high as 8.7 L/min in the third trimester. The maternal heart rate generally sees its greatest increase in the third trimester, rising to approximately 15% above baseline [4]. Concomitant with these physiologic changes, maternal hematocrit will generally fall from 39% to 35% at term [5]. Additional drops in hematocrit during pregnancy may signify inadequate maternal nutritional intake of iron or other macronutrients [6].

Dysrhythmias become more frequent during pregnancy. While pregnancy-related dysrhythmias are common, the need for aggressive treatment is rare and should be reserved for symptomatic patients or in situations where there is hemodynamic compromise affecting either the mother or fetus. There are two generally accepted mechanisms accounting for the increase in dysrhythmia during pregnancy. The first is a result of atrial stretching arising from increased intravascular volume, resulting in disturbances in cardiac conduction pathways. The second mechanism of dysrhythmia in gravid patients is a result of increased levels of estrogen, which lowers the threshold for arrhythmias. Additionally, estrogen increases the number of myocardial adrenergic receptors, increasing cardiac responsiveness to catecholamines [7].

Increased valve diameters result in regurgitant flows in all valves except the aortic valve. Pulmonary regurgitation is seen in 90% of healthy pregnant women, and almost 30% of all pregnancies experience mild mitral regurgitation [8]. While mild valvular regurgitation is typically well tolerated throughout pregnancy and delivery, new-onset murmurs should be evaluated by a cardiologist and an echocardiogram obtained to assess the severity of the valvular lesion.

Pulmonary

Changes in lung volumes precede increases in fetal metabolic demand, most likely due to rising levels of estrogen. From the nonpregnant state, minute ventilation rises 40% in the first trimester and maintains this increase throughout the duration of pregnancy. The expiratory reserve volume (ERV) decreases as the uterus displaces abdominal contents cephalad, decreasing by one-third while in a sitting position [9].

The reduction in ERV is most significant when performing general anesthesia on late-term pregnant patients. When inducing general anesthesia, the ERV is used as an oxygen reservoir to ensure that the patient maintains adequate blood oxygen saturation despite potentially prolonged apnea. The average nonpregnant patient consumes approximately 3 mL/kg/min of oxygen, while the average patient in their third trimester consumes approximately 4 mL/kg/min, rising to as high as 15 mL/kg/min when in labor [10]. The ERV in a nonpregnant patient is approximately 1.3 L, while in the third trimester, it is approximately 0.8 L [9]. Assuming adequate time was given to preoxygenate the patient, a nonpregnant patient may maintain blood oxygen saturation for as long as 6 min, while a pregnant patient in labor may begin to desaturate within 1 min of induction of general anesthesia.

Airway

The maternal airway undergoes significant change during pregnancy. Excessive weight gain can result in increased neck girth and size of oropharyngeal structures. Additionally, edema resulting from reduced oncotic pressure and increase in extracellular fluid results in engorgement of tissues in the mouth and pharynx. Physical examination of the posterior oropharynx is described using the Mallampati score, with a score of 1 indicating full visualization of the tonsillar pillars, soft palate, and uvula, and a score of 4 indicates that only the hard palate could be visualized [11]. An increase in Mallampati score reflects increasing difficulty intubating a patient.

The average pregnant patient has a 1 point increase in Mallampati score and a 1 cm increase in neck circumference [12], which may account for the disproportionate number of difficult and failed intubations noted in the obstetric population [13, 14].

Gastrointestinal

Aspiration is a rare, but serious, consequence of inducing general anesthesia prior to placement of the endotracheal tube. It is believed that the gastric reflux that many women experience during pregnancy is due to the upward displacement of the stomach and displacement of the intraabdominal esophagus into the thorax [15]. While pregnant patients were once believed to have lower gastric pH and increased residual volumes, consensus now believes that there is no significant difference between pregnant and nonpregnant patients [16, 17].

The American Society of Anesthesiologists practice guidelines do not provide specific recommendations for aspiration prophylaxis during pregnancy. However, in nonpregnant patients, they recommend a period of fasting of 2 h following the consumption of clear liquids, at least 6 h following a light meal (defined as toast and a clear liquid) and at least 8 h following the consumption of fatty and fried foods and meat [18]. Many of the techniques used to prevent aspiration in the gravid patient date to a retrospective review published in 1946 by Curtis Mendelson in which his main recommendation was to withhold oral feeding in the laboring patient [19]. As a result, some anesthesiologists advocate for longer fasting intervals as compared to the nongravid patient because the consequences of aspiration are high, while the risk of delaying an elective procedure as a result of eating a meal is low.

The approach to fasting times in nonlaboring pregnant patients is evolving. Two studies using ultrasound to evaluate antral cross-sectional area over time in both nonobese and obese pregnant patients revealed that subsequent to consumption of 300 mL of clear liquids, the gastric volumes returned to baseline values within 30 min [20, 21]. In a more recent study, 168 laboring women were randomized to drink a high-protein drink supplement or consume ice chips and water. The gastric volumes were compared in 18 of these patients, and both groups had statistically insignificant differences in emptying halftimes (25.5 vs. 20.0 min in the protein shake and ice chips groups, respectively) [22]. It would be a reasonable assumption that gastric emptying would be at least as efficient in the nonlaboring patient and that further studies will guide future consensus guidelines on fasting.

Renal

There is a 20% increase in renal blood flow and a 50% increase in glomerular filtration rate during pregnancy [23]. As a result, laboratory measurements of kidney function, including serum creatinine, urea, and uric acid, also decrease. Also resulting from this increase in GFR is the shorter half-life of renally cleared medications. Β-lactam antibiotics, atenolol, and digoxin all have more rapid serum clearances which may need to be accounted for when selecting the appropriate medication dose and frequency [24]. While the clearance of vecuronium is increased due to increases in GFR, the clinical duration of effect is prolonged due to a hypothesized increase in neuromuscular sensitivity to the medication [25]. Close monitoring of neuromuscular blocking agents should take place to ensure appropriate dosing intervals.

Coagulation

Pregnancy is a hypercoagulable state, characterized by an increase in levels of clotting factors, fibrinogen, and von Willebrand factor. Antithrombin III levels remain constant throughout pregnancy. In contrast, several anticoagulant factors are reduced [26]. Average platelet counts have significant variability, with studies demonstrating inconsistent changes in platelet counts [27–29]. What is clear, however, is that more than

10% of patients at term demonstrate platelet counts less than 150×10^9/L [27].

The hypercoagulability found in pregnancy results in increased rates of venous thromboembolism(VTE) [30] and stroke [31]. The risk of thrombotic complications can extend to 6 weeks postpartum. Due to the increased risk of these complications, the American College of Chest Physicians recommends early mobilization for all patients and the use of low-molecular-weight heparin in patients with either one major (including immobility for ≥1 week, history of VTE, and thrombophilia) or two minor risk factors (including BMI > 30, smoking > 10 cigarettes/day, and multiple gestation pregnancy) [32].

Fetal Development

In utero, the human brain and central nervous system develop from a small set of embryonic cells to a complex and efficient network of over 100 billion neurons. The process of neural development begins with proliferation from a neural stem cell, followed by migration and differentiation into a specialized neuron. By 4 weeks gestation, primary neuromodulation and neural tube formation ensues. Prosencephalon development is initiated between 8 and 12 weeks' gestation with neuronal proliferation and migration occurring simultaneously [33]. Beginning at 20 weeks gestation, there is a significant increase in cortical development, organization, and synapse formation. The cortical volume increases by fourfold in the third trimester alone with the size of the immature brain being one-third that of an adult at the time of birth [34, 35].

Cutaneous sensory receptors are present in the human fetus at approximately 7 weeks' gestation. By 20 weeks, a widespread network of cutaneous nociceptive receptors has been established [36]. Myelination of the pain pathways of the spinal cord and brain stem is then completed during the second and third trimesters of gestation [37]. As early as 18 weeks' gestation, human fetuses demonstrate pituitary-adrenal, sympathoadrenal, and circulatory stress responses to noxious stimuli [38]. In premature neonates studied at 25 weeks, near-infrared spectroscopy has demonstrated cortical activity in response to noxious stimuli [39]. Therefore, current evidence suggests that fetal nociception (the ability to feel pain) occurs after the midpoint of pregnancy (between 24 and 30 weeks).

Teratogenicity of Anesthetic Agents

While it still remains that maternal issues such as severe maternal hypoxia and hypotension pose the greatest risk to the fetus, there has now been considerable attention placed on the role of anesthetic agents on development. Teratogenicity involves any significant postnatal effect in function or form of a neonate brought about by prenatal treatment. Concern about the deleterious effects of anesthetics on the developing fetus has stemmed from animal studies, which have shown manifestations of teratogenicity associated with numerous anesthetic agents. There are a number of key factors that may influence teratogenicity, such as species susceptibility, dose of the teratogenic substance, duration and timing of the exposure, as well as genetic predisposition (Fig. 7.1).

Due to the substantial concern about the teratogenicity seen in animal models exposed to anesthetics, the US Food and Drug Administration (FDA) issued an extensive statement to the public on December 14, 2016. In the document, there are multiple warnings about the potential harmful effects of general anesthetics on the developing fetus. They state, "published studies in pregnant animals and young animals have shown the use of general anesthetic and sedation drugs for more than 3 h caused widespread loss of nerve cells in the brain. Studies in young animals suggest these changes result in long-term effects on the animals' behavior or learning …repeated or lengthy use of general anesthetic and sedation drugs during surgeries or procedures in pregnant women during their third trimester may affect the development of children's brain." The FDA felt that these concerns were valid enough to now place warnings on general anesthetic and sedation drug labels to this effect. As this statement is now in the public realm, it is even more important for

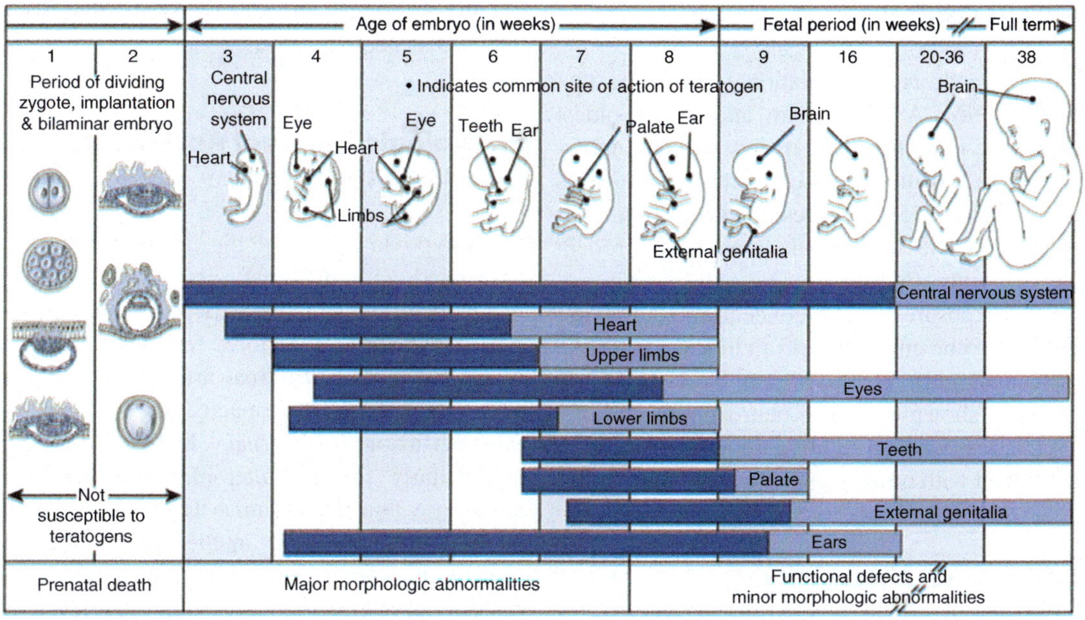

Fig. 7.1 This figure shows development of the fetus with critical periods for organ formation noted. The dark bars denote periods of high sensitivity to potential teratogens, while the lighter bars indicate periods of lesser sensitivity. Notice that during the first 2 weeks of development, there is an all-or-nothing phenomenon: where a substance either damages all of the cells resulting in death or it damages only a few cells allowing for the embryo to survive without complication. Reprinted with permission from Chestnut DH, Wong CA, Tsen LC, Kee WD, Beilin Y, Mhyre J. Chestnut's Obstetric Anesthesia: Principles and Practice E-Book, Chapter 17. Philadelphia: Elsevier Health Sciences; 2014 Feb 28: 362

physicians to stay knowledgeable on the most recent literature [40].

The contemporary belief is that anesthetics work by interfering with normal $GABA_A$ and NMDA receptor-mediated activity to produce effective amnesia and unconsciousness. GABA and NMDA modulation are also believed to be the essential mechanisms for central nervous system development in the fetus, making it plausible that anesthetic agents could affect normal neurodevelopment. The most widely studied deleterious consequence of exposure to sedatives or anesthetics in immature animals is apoptosis (programmed cell death). It currently remains unknown whether anesthesia-induced neuroapoptosis accelerates physiologic programmed cell death or whether it eliminates cells not destined to die, as in pathologic apoptosis. In order to provide a succinct overview, we will briefly review the potential teratogenicity of different classes of the major anesthetics.

Benzodiazepines

Benzodiazepines are GABA agonists that are frequently used for preoperative anxiolysis. Benzodiazepine therapy became controversial after an association between maternal diazepam ingestion during the first trimester and infants with cleft palate were reported. Subsequent prospective research showed that women who ingested diazepam during the first trimester did not demonstrate a higher risk of cleft palate associated with benzodiazepine therapy [41]. Studies have also consistently reported increased neuroapoptosis in neonatal rats after diazepam administration [42]. Although this neuroapoptosis has been described, two studies have shown no neurocognitive learning disabilities in adult mice after receiving sedation with diazepam as neonates [43]. In summary, no evidence suggests that a single dose of a benzodiazepine during the course of anesthesia is harmful to the fetus, but a risk benefit ratio should always be implemented prior to administration.

Nitrous Oxide

Nitrous oxide is an inhalational anesthetic that acts by NMDA antagonism and is the oldest anesthetic in clinical use. Its low potency necessitates the co-administration of other anesthetics to provide surgical anesthesia. Nitrous oxide has been shown to be a weak teratogen in rodent studies, with effects occurring only after a prolonged exposure to high concentrations that are unlikely to be encountered in clinical anesthesia in humans [44]. In rats, nitrous oxide alone has not been shown to induce neuroapoptosis; however, it does have an additive toxicity effect when combined with other anesthetic agents [45].

Inhalational Anesthetics

Volatile anesthetics such as isoflurane and sevoflurane exert their anesthetic properties predominantly by their agonistic effects on the $GABA_A$ receptor. Conflicting studies on the potential teratogenic risks of inhalational anesthetics have been published. Consistent findings in a variety of animal models have shown widespread apoptosis directly after exposure to inhalational anesthetics but have failed to show correlation with future developmental abnormalities. In one study, neonatal mice exposed to 6 h of isoflurane developed widespread neuronal degeneration immediately after exposure but failed to cause neurocognitive deficits or decreases in neuronal density in adulthood [46]. Long-term exposure to subanesthetic concentrations of halothane, an older inhalational anesthetic no longer currently popular in practice, caused fetal growth restriction in rats but no congenital abnormalities, while isoflurane, which is a more commonly used anesthetic, showed no adverse effects [47, 48].

Propofol

Propofol acts primarily via GABA and glycine receptor agonist properties and is often the IV induction agent of choice. Propofol has been shown to cause neuroapoptosis after doses exceeding 50 mg/kg in neonatal rats. However, there have been no consistent findings of neurocognitive deficits in adult animals that were exposed as neonates [49].

Physiologic Effects of Anesthetic Agents on the Fetus

Fetal hypoxia is one of the most serious risks associated with maternal surgery during pregnancy. Fetal oxygenation is dependent on maternal oxygenation; therefore, fetal well-being is reliant on normal maternal arterial oxygen tension, oxygen-carrying capacity, and uteroplacental perfusion. Maternal hypotension can significantly threaten uteroplacental perfusion and cause fetal hypoxemia. The most common sources of hypotension in the pregnant patient undergoing surgery include hypovolemia, hemorrhage, aortocaval compression, deep levels of general anesthesia, and sympathectomy from high levels of spinal or epidural anesthesia.

Volatile anesthetics can affect the fetus directly by depressing the fetal cardiovascular system or central nervous system and indirectly by causing maternal hypoxia or hypotension. Studies in animal models have shown maternal administration of moderate concentration volatile anesthetics produced minimal fetal effects. At normal concentrations of inhalational anesthetics, uterine vasodilation compensates for small decreases in maternal blood pressure to maintain uterine perfusion [50]. However, higher concentrations for prolonged periods can cause marked maternal hypotension which may result in reduced uteroplacental blood flow, fetal hypoxia, diminished fetal cardiac output, and fetal acidosis. Consequently, the avoidance of inhalational anesthetics in pregnant females is not supported provided that maternal hypotension is prevented.

Opioids and induction agents such as propofol may decrease fetal heart rate variability more than inhalational agents. In the absence of maternal hypotension or other abnormalities, the decrease in FHR variability is not cause for concern [51]. Fetal respiratory depression may also occur with administration of these medications; nonetheless this is only relevant if a cesarean section is to be performed in conjunction with the surgical procedure. The neonatologist should be informed of maternal administration of such agents to ensure that planning for neonatal respiratory support occurs.

Muscle relaxants and reversal agents have also been demonstrated to be safe to the fetus following maternal administration. Atropine and glycopyrrolate are anticholinergic medications administered with neuromuscular reversal agents. Atropine readily crosses the placenta and when given in large doses may potentially lead to fetal tachycardia and loss of fetal heart rate variability. Glycopyrrolate crosses the placenta less readily and therefore may result in mild fetal bradycardia when administered with acetylcholinesterase inhibitors for reversal. However, when standard clinical doses are administered neither atropine nor glycopyrrolate have been shown to significantly affect fetal heart rate variability [52].

National Standards

The American Society of Anesthesiologists (ASA) and the American College of Obstetricians and Gynecologists (ACOG) have jointly published ACOG Committee Opinion 696, "Nonobstetric Surgery During Pregnancy" [53]. It is felt by both organizations that indicated surgeries should be performed regardless of trimester with the second trimester being optimal for nonurgent procedures, while elective surgeries should be postponed until after delivery.

The joint statement further states that the primary obstetric care provider should be notified and, if that provider is not available, that another obstetric care provider should be involved with the perioperative care of the patient. Finally, the facility should be qualified to care for both the mother and fetus should they need delivery, including the ability to provide for neonatal and obstetric services.

Perioperative Fetal Monitoring

The joint ASA/ACOG Committee opinion recommends performing pre- and post-procedure fetal heart rate Doppler monitoring if the fetus is pre-viable. Once viability is obtained, pre- and post-procedure fetal heart rate and contraction monitoring should be performed [53]. Intraoperative monitoring is controversial, and there are no large randomized trials to guide recommendations. The ASA/ACOG joint statement recommends consideration of intraoperative monitoring when the fetus is viable, an obstetrician is present and available to intervene surgically, and the non-obstetric surgery is amenable to both intraoperative monitoring and interruption if an emergency delivery is necessary.

Proponents of intraoperative monitoring recommend using it to identify perturbations in maternal hemodynamics and to improve fetal oxygenation. Volatile anesthetic agents, such as sevoflurane, result in decreased fetal heart rate variability. However, significant fetal heart rate decelerations would only be expected in situations where there was inadequate oxygen delivery to the fetus. Options for correcting these decelerations include increasing left uterine displacement, optimizing maternal blood pressure and cardiac output, transfusing the mother when indicated, and decreasing insufflation pressures during abdominal laparoscopy. There is large regional variability in the adoption of continuous intraoperative fetal monitoring, and there are no widely accepted national standards for its use for the pre-viable fetus.

Specific Surgery Considerations

Patient Positioning

During the first trimester, pregnant women can be placed in supine position during surgery as the uterus is not large enough to compromise venous return [54]. However, after the first trimester, pregnant women should be placed in left lateral decubitus (LLD, 15-degree lateral tilt) position to avoid inferior vena cava (IVC) compression by the gravid uterus, which decreases venous return and leads to significant hypotension. Placing the patient in LLD will decompress the IVC and improve venous return to the heart and improves cardiac output [55]. Patients can be placed in partial LLD position if surgical access to abdominal cavity is compromised by full LLD.

Laparoscopy

Insufflation Pressures

Upward displacement of the diaphragm by CO_2 pneumoperitoneum further reduces the patient's FRC, increases the peak airway pressure, increases ventilation-perfusion mismatch, decreases thoracic cavity compliance, and may lead to significant hypoxia and difficulty with ventilation in pregnant patients [56]. The Society of American Gastrointestinal and Endoscopic Surgeons Guidelines for the Use of Laparoscopy During Pregnancy Guideline 12 states that CO_2 insufflation pressures of 10–15 mmHg can be safely used for laparoscopy; however, the level of insufflation should be adjusted to the patient's physiology [54].

Benefits of laparoscopy include reduced surgical pain, decreased postoperative opioid requirements, decreased incidence of postoperative ileus, and shorter length of hospital stay [57]. Benefits unique to pregnant patients include decreased risk of fetal respiratory depression as well as decreased postoperative maternal hypoventilation secondary to decreased opioid consumption, lower risk of wound complications, and decreased risk of thromboembolic events [58].

CO_2 Management

There are conflicting data from animal studies on the effects of CO_2 pneumoperitoneum on the fetus. While some studies report fetal tachycardia, hypertension, and hypercapnia, others refute these findings [54, 56]. There is a linear relationship between maternal arterial CO_2 ($PaCO_2$) and fetal $PaCO_2$. While there are no reports of fetal acidosis caused by CO_2 insufflation in humans, given the potentially detrimental consequences of fetal acidosis, the Society of American Gastrointestinal and Endoscopic Surgeons recommends intraoperative maternal end-tidal CO_2 monitoring to avoid maternal hypercapnia [54].

Other Perioperative Planning

Detailed planning should be undertaken prior to any pregnant patient undergoing surgery. This planning should include an evaluation of the facility and its available resources. It's vital to understand how any potential obstetric emergencies would be handled, whether or not there is a massive transfusion protocol available, and what other services exist for the care of a neonate and mother. Additionally, planning should include all potential providers caring for the patient: anesthesiology, neonatology, OB/GYN, nursing services, and surgical specialties. Finally, a risk assessment should be performed with consideration made to transferring the patient to a facility which may be more equipped to address any untoward outcomes that may be encountered in the perioperative period.

Conclusion

Careful attention to planning should occur prior to any surgery, and completely elective surgeries should be deferred until the fetus has been delivered. No anesthetic agents currently used have been demonstrated to have teratogenic effects, however, due to general concerns about the potential for teratogenicity and preterm labor, surgeries when necessary are ideally performed in the second trimester. Prior to viability, intraoperative fetal heart rate monitoring may be useful in the to help optimize maternal hemodynamics and may be necessary once viability has been achieved to help guide obstetric care. While performing non-obstetric surgery during pregnancy is not desirable, with proper planning and support, it may be performed safely for both the mother and fetus.

References

1. Goodman S. Anesthesia for nonobstetric surgery in the pregnant patient. Semin Perinatol. 2002;26(2):136–45.
2. Creanga AA, Berg CJ, Ko JY, Farr SL, Tong VT, Bruce FC, et al. Maternal mortality and morbidity in the United States: where are we now? J Women Health. 2014;23(1):3–9.
3. Chapman AB, Abraham WT, Zamudio S, Coffin C, Merouani A, Young D, et al. Temporal relationships between hormonal and hemodynamic changes in early human pregnancy. Kidney Int. 1998;54(6):2056–63.
4. Enriquez AD, Economy KE, Tedrow UB. Contemporary management of arrhythmias

during pregnancy. Circ Arrhythm Electrophysiol. 2014;7(5):961–7.

5. Abduljalil K, Furness P, Johnson TN, Rostami-Hodjegan A, Soltani H. Anatomical, physiological and metabolic changes with gestational age during normal pregnancy. Clin Pharmacokinet. 2012;51(6):365–96.
6. Steer PJ. Maternal hemoglobin concentration and birth weight. Am J Clin Nutr. 2000;71(5):1285s–7s.
7. Cox JL, Gardner MJ. Treatment of cardiac arrhythmias during pregnancy. Prog Cardiovasc Dis. 1993;36(2):137–78.
8. Campos O, Andrade JL, Bocanegra J, Ambrose JA, Carvalho AC, Harada K, et al. Physiologic multivalvular regurgitation during pregnancy: a longitudinal Doppler echocardiographic study. Int J Cardiol. 1993;40(3):265–72.
9. McAuliffe F, Kametas N, Costello J, Rafferty GF, Greenough A, Nicolaides K. Respiratory function in singleton and twin pregnancy. BJOG. 2002;109(7):765–9.
10. Pernoll M, Metcalfe J, Schlenker TL, Welch JE, Matsumoto JA. Oxygen consumption at rest and during exercise in pregnancy. Respir Physiol. 1975;25(3):285–93.
11. Mallampati SR, Gatt SP, Gugino LD, Desai SP, Waraksa B, Freiberger D, et al. A clinical sign to predict difficult tracheal intubation; a prospective study. Can Anaesth Soc J. 1985;32(4):429–34.
12. Leboulanger N, Louvet N, Rigouzzo A, de Mesmay M, Louis B, Farrugia M, et al. Pregnancy is associated with a decrease in pharyngeal but not tracheal or laryngeal cross-sectional area: a pilot study using the acoustic reflection method. Int J Obstet Anesth. 2014;23(1):35–9.
13. Barnardo P, Jenkins J. Failed tracheal intubation in obstetrics: a 6-year review in a UK region. Anaesthesia. 2000;55(7):690–4.
14. Pilkington S, Carli F, Dakin M, Romney M, De Witt K, Dore C, et al. Increase in Mallampati score during pregnancy. Br J Anaesth. 1995;74(6):638–42.
15. Ulmsten U, Sundström G. Esophageal manometry in pregnant and nonpregnant women. Am J Obstet Gynecol. 1978;132(3):260–4.
16. Van Thiel DH, Gavaler JS, Joshi SN, Sara RK, Stremple J. Heartburn of pregnancy. Gastroenterology. 1977;72(4):666–8.
17. O'Sullivan G, Bullingham R. The assessment of gastric acidity and antacid effect in pregnant women by a non-invasive radiotelemetry technique. BJOG. 1984;91(10):973–8.
18. Practice Guidelines for Preoperative Fasting and the Use of Pharmacologic Agents to Reduce the Risk of Pulmonary Aspiration: Application to Healthy Patients Undergoing Elective Procedures. An updated report by the American Society of Anesthesiologists Task Force on preoperative fasting and the use of pharmacologic agents to reduce the risk of pulmonary aspiration. Anesthesiology. 2017;126(3):376–93.
19. Mendelson CL. The aspiration of stomach contents into the lungs during obstetric anesthesia. Am J Obstet Gynecol. 1946;52(2):191–205.
20. Wong CA, Loffredi M, Ganchiff JN, Zhao J, Wang Z, Avram MJ. Gastric emptying of water in term pregnancy. J Am Soc Anesthesiol. 2002;96(6):1395–400.
21. Wong CA, McCarthy RJ, Fitzgerald PC, Raikoff K, Avram MJ. Gastric emptying of water in obese pregnant women at term. Anesth Analg. 2007;105(3):751–5.
22. Vallejo MC, Cobb BT, Steen TL, Singh S, Phelps AL. Maternal outcomes in women supplemented with a high-protein drink in labour. Aust N Z J Obstet Gynaecol. 2013;53(4):369–74.
23. Dunlop W. Serial changes in renal haemodynamics during normal human pregnancy. BJOG. 1981;88(1):1–9.
24. Anderson GD. Pregnancy-induced changes in pharmacokinetics. Clin Pharmacokinet. 2005;44(10):989–1008.
25. Guay J, Grenier Y, Varin F. Clinical pharmacokinetics of neuromuscular relaxants in pregnancy. Clin Pharmacokinet. 1998;34(6):483–96.
26. Katz D, Beilin Y. Disorders of coagulation in pregnancy. Br J Anaesth. 2015;115(Suppl_2):ii75–88.
27. Boehlen F, Hohlfeld P, Extermann P, Perneger TV, De Moerloose P. Platelet count at term pregnancy: a reappraisal of the threshold. Obstet Gynecol. 2000;95(1):29–33.
28. Tygart SG, McRoyan DK, Spinnato JA, McRoyan CJ, Kitay DZ. Longitudinal study of platelet indices during normal pregnancy. Am J Obstet Gynecol. 1986;154(4):883–7.
29. Ahmed Y, Iddekinge B, Paul C, Sullivan MH, Elder MG. Retrospective analysis of platelet numbers and volumes in normal pregnancy and in pre-eclampsia. BJOG. 1993;100(3):216–20.
30. Robertson L, Wu O, Langhorne P, Twaddle S, Clark P, Lowe G, et al. Thrombophilia in pregnancy: a systematic review. Br J Haematol. 2006;132(2):171–96.
31. Kittner SJ, Stern BJ, Feeser BR, Hebel JR, Nagey DA, Buchholz DW, et al. Pregnancy and the risk of stroke. N Engl J Med. 1996;335(11):768–74.
32. Bates SM, Greer IA, Middeldorp S, Veenstra DL, Prabulos A-M, Vandvik PO. VTE, thrombophilia, antithrombotic therapy, and pregnancy: antithrombotic therapy and prevention of thrombosis: American College of Chest Physicians evidence-based clinical practice guidelines. CHEST J. 2012;141(2_suppl):e691S–736S.
33. Kostovic I, Judas M, Rados M, Hrabac P. Laminar organization of the human fetal cerebrum revealed by histochemical markers and magnetic resonance imaging. Cereb Cortex. 2002;12(5):536–44.
34. Dobbing J. The later development of the brain and its vulnerability. J Inherited Metab Dis. 1982;5:88.
35. Kostovic I, Jovanov-Milosevic N. The development of cerebral connections during the first 20-45 weeks' gestation. Semin Fetal Neonatal Med. 2006;11(6):415–22.

36. Okado N. Onset of synapse formation in the human spinal cord. J Comp Neurol. 1981;201(2):211–9.
37. Benes FM. The development of prefrontal cortex: the maturation of neurotransmitter systems and their interactions. In: Handbook of developmental cognitive neuroscience. Cambridge, MA: MIT Press; 2001. p. 79–92.
38. Giannakoulopoulos X, Teixeira J, Fisk N, Glover V. Human fetal and maternal noradrenaline responses to invasive procedures. Pediatr Res. 1999;45(4 Pt 1):494–9.
39. Slater R, Cantarella A, Gallella S, Worley A, Boyd S, Meek J, et al. Cortical pain responses in human infants. J Neurosci. 2006;26(14):3662–6.
40. Andropoulos DB, Greene MF. Anesthesia and developing brains—implications of the FDA warning. N Engl J Med. 2017;2017(376):905–7.
41. Kanno K, Suzuki Y, Yamada A, Aoki Y, Kure S, Matsubara Y. Association between nonsyndromic cleft lip with or without cleft palate and the glutamic acid decarboxylase 67 gene in the Japanese population. Am J Med Genet Part A. 2004;127(1):11–6.
42. Bittigau P, Sifringer M, Genz K, Reith E, Pospischil D, Govindarajalu S, et al. Antiepileptic drugs and apoptotic neurodegeneration in the developing brain. Proc Natl Acad Sci U S A. 2002;99(23):15089–94.
43. Xu H, Liu ZQ, Liu Y, Zhang WS, Xu B, Xiong YC, et al. Administration of midazolam in infancy does not affect learning and memory of adult mice. Clin Exp Pharmacol Physiol. 2009;36(12):1144–8.
44. Mazze RI, Fujinaga M, Rice SA, Harris SB, Baden JM. Reproductive and teratogenic effects of nitrous oxide, halothane, isoflurane, and enflurane in Sprague-Dawley rats. Anesthesiology. 1986;64(3):339–44.
45. Head BP, Patel HH, Niesman IR, Drummond JC, Roth DM, Patel PM. Inhibition of p75 neurotrophin receptor attenuates isoflurane-mediated neuronal apoptosis in the neonatal central nervous system. Anesthesiology. 2009;110(4):813–25.
46. Loepke AW, Istaphanous GK, McAuliffe JJ 3rd, Miles L, Hughes EA, McCann JC, et al. The effects of neonatal isoflurane exposure in mice on brain cell viability, adult behavior, learning, and memory. Anesth Analg. 2009;108(1):90–104.
47. Wharton RS, Mazze RI, Baden JM, Hitt BA, Dooley JR. Fertility, reproduction and postnatal survival in mice chronically exposed to halothane. Anesthesiology. 1978;48(3):167–74.
48. Mazze RI. Fertility, reproduction, and postnatal survival in mice chronically exposed to isoflurane. Anesthesiology. 1985;63(6):663–7.
49. Coté CJ, Lerman J, Todres ID. A practice of anesthesia for infants and children E-book: expert consult: online and print. Philadelphia, PA: Elsevier Health Sciences; 2012.
50. Palahniuk RJ, Shnider SM. Maternal and fetal cardiovascular and acid-base changes during halothane and isoflurane anesthesia in the pregnant ewe. Anesthesiology. 1974;41(5):462–72.
51. Liu P, Warren T, Ostheimer G, Weiss J, Liu L. Fetal monitoring in parturients undergoing surgery unrelated to pregnancy. Obstet Anesth Dig. 1986;6(1):185.
52. Abboud T, Raya J, Sadri S, Grobler N, Stine L, Miller F. Fetal and maternal cardiovascular effects of atropine and glycopyrrolate. Anesth Analg. 1983;62(4):426–30.
53. Practice ACoO. ACOG Committee Opinion No. 696: nonobstetric surgery during pregnancy. Obstet Gynecol. 2017;129:777–8.
54. Pearl JP, Price RR, Tonkin AE, Richardson WS, Stefanidis D. SAGES guidelines for the use of laparoscopy during pregnancy. Surg Endosc. 2017;31(10):3767–82.
55. Reitman E, Flood P. Anaesthetic considerations for non-obstetric surgery during pregnancy. Br J Anaesth. 2011;107(suppl_1):i72–i8.
56. O'rourke N, Kodali B-S. Laparoscopic surgery during pregnancy. Curr Opin Anesthesiol. 2006;19(3):254–9.
57. Curet MJ, Allen D, Josloff RK, Pitcher DE, Curet LB, Miscall BG, et al. Laparoscopy during pregnancy. Arch Surg. 1996;131(5):546–51.
58. Williams J, Rosemurgy A, Albrink M, Parsons M, Stock S. Laparoscopic cholecystectomy in pregnancy. A case report. J Reprod Med. 1995;40(3):243–5.

Medical Complications in Pregnancy

8

Michael Franklin Neblett II, Shabnam Gupta, and Iris Krishna

Introduction

Two of the most commonly encountered medical complications in pregnancy are diabetes mellitus (DM) and hypertensive disorders. Diabetes mellitus in pregnancy is characterized as pregestational diabetes and gestational diabetes. Pregestational diabetes is diagnosed prior to pregnancy and affects approximately 1% of pregnancies [1]. Gestational diabetes is diagnosed during pregnancy and affects approximately 6–9% of pregnancies [1]. Hypertensive disorders affect approximately 10% of hospitalizations in the USA [2]. Hypertensive disorders of pregnancy have a wide spectrum of clinical manifestations, ranging from asymptomatic mild elevations in blood pressure to severely elevated pressures with concomitant laboratory abnormalities and dysfunction of numerous organ systems. Both diabetes mellitus and hypertension are associated with adverse perinatal, obstetric, and neonatal outcomes, and appropriate management of these conditions in pregnancy is key to ensuring a successful maternal and fetal outcome. This chapter will outline the management of these conditions in pregnancy.

M. F. Neblett II · S. Gupta
Department of Gynecology and Obstetrics, Emory University Hospital Midtown, Atlanta, GA, USA
e-mail: shabnam.gupta@emory.edu

I. Krishna (✉)
Division of Maternal-Fetal Medicine, Department of Gynecology and Obstetrics, Emory University Hospital Midtown, Atlanta, GA, USA
e-mail: iris.krishna@emory.edu

Pregestational Diabetes Mellitus

Pathophysiology

Pregestational diabetes is a metabolic abnormality characterized by elevated circulating glucose outside of pregnancy. The exact etiology of diabetes mellitus (DM) varies and can include a primary insulin production defect, insulin receptor abnormalities, end-organ insulin resistance, diabetes secondary to another disease process (e.g., cystic fibrosis), or drug-induced diabetes (e.g., steroid use) [3]. Type 1 DM, an insulin-deficient state, occurs secondary to an autoimmune destruction of the pancreatic islet beta cells [3]. This disease process typically occurs early in life, requiring insulin therapy for treatment and is more susceptible to ketoacidosis if no therapy is initiated [4]. Type 2 DM is more common than type 1 DM and is characterized by onset later in life, peripheral insulin resistance, relative insulin deficiency, and obesity [4]. These conditions can be further exacerbated by pregnancy itself as it is characterized by increased insulin resistance and reduced sensitivity to insulin action. Insulin

C. H. Nezhat (ed.), *Non-Obstetric Surgery During Pregnancy*,
https://doi.org/10.1007/978-3-319-90752-9_8

resistance increases throughout the pregnancy with the third trimester being the time of greatest insulin resistance. Insulin resistance is largely due to a result of a mixture of placental hormones: human placental lactogen, progesterone, prolactin, placental growth hormone, cortisol, tumor necrosis factor-α, and leptin [4].

Diagnosis

The diagnosis of diabetes mellitus prior to pregnancy is established on the basis of formal laboratory criteria (Table 8.1) [3, 5]. In general, patients are asymptomatic but can present with symptoms of hyperglycemia such as polyuria, polydipsia, and polyphagia [3, 5]. Women with long-standing DM may have microvascular disease (e.g., diabetic retinopathy, diabetic nephropathy), which may further complicate pregnancy. As a result, the evaluation of the pregnant woman with pregestational DM should include hemoglobin A1C, metabolic profile for evaluation of glucose and creatinine, urine culture, electrocardiogram (EKG), TSH for patients with type I diabetes, ophthalmologic exam, and 24-h urine collection for protein and creatinine clearance.

It is well recognized that adverse pregnancy complications related to diabetes are inversely proportional to the level of glucose control. Of utmost concern early in pregnancy, women with poorly controlled DM are at increased risk for congenital anomalies (most common cardiac and central nervous system anomalies) with rates as high as 20–25% with hemoglobin A1C concentrations near 10% [6, 7]. Poorly controlled DM has also been associated with preterm labor, polyhydramnios, preeclampsia, macrosomia, fetal growth restriction with microvascular disease, and cesarean delivery [8–10]. To improve overall pregnancy outcomes, the care of the pregnant woman with pregestational DM should begin early in pregnancy, and ideally women who are considering pregnancy should be counseled on improving blood glucose control prior to conception.

Table 8.1 Criteria for the diagnosis of diabetes mellitus in the nonpregnant state

Test	Diabetes mellitus
Fasting glucose[a]	≥ 126 mg/dL
75-g, 2-h OGTT[b]	≥ 200 mg/dL
Hemoglobin A1C	≥ 6.5%
Random glucose and symptoms of hyperglycemia	≥ 200 mg/dL

[a]No caloric intake for at least 8 h
[b]OGTT, oral glucose tolerance test

Antepartum Management

Management of pregestational DM consists of dietary modifications, exercise, and insulin therapy [4]. Dietary therapy consists of caloric intake of approximately 30 kcal/kg/day divided into three meals and three snacks [4, 11, 12]. Calories should be divided as 40–50% carbohydrates, 20% protein, and 30–40% unsaturated fat to help maintain a low glycemic index [4, 12]. Nutritional counseling should be offered to maximize dietary therapy, and a moderate weight training exercise program (increases lean muscle mass and improves tissue sensitivity to insulin) is recommended three times per week for a total of 20–45 min [12, 13].

All subcutaneous insulin types used for treatment of pregestational DM have been approved for use in pregnancy as they do not cross the placenta [4, 12]. Insulin requirements increase with increasing gestational age, and insulin should be adjusted accordingly throughout pregnancy. In general, insulin needs in the first trimester range from 0.7 to 0.8 U/kg/day, second trimester from 0.8 to 1 U/kg/day, and third trimester from 0.9 to 1.2 U/kg/day [14]. Capillary blood glucose monitoring should be performed at least four times a day, fasting, and 1 or 2 h postprandial with the goal of insulin therapy to maintain a fasting glucose level ≤95 mg/dL and 1-h level ≤140 mg/dL or 2-h level ≤120 mg/dL [4]. To achieve target glucose levels, a combination of short-acting and longer-acting insulins is administered. Generally, short-acting insulins (insulin lispro, insulin aspart, insulin regular) are administered before meals to reduce glucose elevations associated with eating, and longer-acting insulins (insulin

NPH, insulin detemir, insulin glargine) are used to restrain hepatic glucose production between meals and in the fasting state (Table 8.2) [4, 13]. Longer-acting insulins are usually administered before breakfast and/or bedtime [4, 13]. Close monitoring of glucose log at least weekly with provider is recommended to maximize care of the pregestational diabetic.

Women with pregestational DM are at an increased risk of birth defects and perinatal mortality [4]. Screening for birth defects is recommended by offering maternal serum alpha-fetoprotein testing at 16–18 weeks, detailed anatomy ultrasound at 18–20 weeks, and fetal echocardiogram at 20–22 weeks. Recommendations for antenatal testing for fetal well-being are generally accepted as serial growth scans throughout pregnancy and twice weekly nonstress test or biophysical profile starting at 32 weeks. The nature of this surveillance is by convention and expert consensus secondary to the increased risk of stillbirth [4].

Diabetic Ketoacidosis

Poorly controlled diabetes in pregnancy can result in diabetic ketoacidosis (DKA), an acute life-threatening complication for the mother and her fetus. Pregnancies complicated by DKA are associated with increased rates of perinatal morbidity and mortality and require a high index of suspicion as onset of DKA usually is at lower glucose levels and often progresses more rapidly as compared with nonpregnancy [4, 15]. Risk factors for DKA in pregnancy include new-onset diabetes, infections, poor patient compliance, and treatment with antenatal corticosteroids. Pregnant women may present with abdominal pain, nausea and vomiting, lethargy, and altered mental status. Laboratory evaluation will demonstrate acidosis with a low arterial pH <7.3, anion gap >12 mEq/L, serum bicarbonate level <15 mEq/L, and serum ketones. Fetal heart rate monitoring will demonstrate recurrent late decelerations which improve with treatment. Treatment is based on aggressive hydration with isotonic sodium chloride and intravenous insulin. Additionally, glucose and potassium concentrations should be monitored closely. A pregnant woman suspected of being in DKA is a medical emergency and requires multidisciplinary management by a maternal-fetal medicine specialist and endocrinologist [4, 15].

Table 8.2 Pharmacokinetics of commonly used insulin agents

Type	Onset	Peak	Duration
Lispro	1–15 min	1–2 h	4–5 h
Aspart	1–15 min	1–2 h	4–5 h
Regular	30–60 min	2–4 h	6–8 h
NPH[a]	1–3 h	5–7 h	13–18 h
Detemir	1–3 h	3–9 h	6–23 h
Glargine	1–2 h	No peak	24 h

[a]*NPH* neutral protamine hagedorn

Timing of Delivery

The optimal timing of delivery relies on balancing the risk of stillbirth with the risk of preterm birth in women with pregestational DM. Timing of delivery is usually recommended at 39 weeks of gestation unless maternal or fetal factors dictate earlier intervention [4]. Early delivery may be indicated in patient with microvascular disease, poor glucose control, or prior stillbirth [4]. With respect to mode of delivery, vaginal is preferred. Cesarean delivery may be considered to prevent a traumatic birth in patients with an estimated fetal weight >4500 g; patients, however, should be counseled regarding the risks and benefits of cesarean delivery as it has been estimated that up to 588 cesarean deliveries would be needed to prevent a single case of permanent brachial plexus palsy [4, 12, 13, 16].

Gestational Diabetes

Gestational diabetes mellitus (GDM) is defined as a state of hyperglycemia that results from carbohydrate intolerance that is first recognized or diagnosed during pregnancy [12]. The importance of screening for GDM and treatment is to optimize glycemic control to reduce complications associated with hyperglycemia. Universal screening for GDM is recommended at 24–28 weeks. The risk of developing GDM is directly associated with prepregnancy BMI, and women with risk factors (e.g., obesity, history of gestational diabetes, strong family history of diabetes, history of large for gestational age infant) should be screened preconception or at the first prenatal visit [3, 17]. If these women are identified early in pregnancy, they could benefit from receiving the diagnostic and therapeutic interventions routinely provided to women with pregestational diabetes. If the early screen is negative, a repeat screen should be performed at 24–28 weeks of gestation.

There is a two-step approach to screening in the USA. The first step involves a 50-g, 1-h oral glucose tolerance test (OGTT) given in the non-fasting state. A positive result on the first step is defined as a threshold of 130–140 mg/dL as there is insufficient data to support the ideal threshold value [12, 18]. Pregnant women who obtain a positive result then perform a 100-g, 3-h OGTT administered after an overnight fast. Two or more abnormal values on the 3-h OGTT using either the National Diabetes Data Group (NDDG) or Carpenter and Coustan criteria establish a diagnosis of GDM (Table 8.3) [3]. If initial screening value is greater than or equal to 200 mg/dL, it is considered diagnostic of GDM.

Woman with GDM have a higher risk of developing preeclampsia and undergoing a cesarean delivery during their pregnancy [19, 20]. Other complications include macrosomia, polyhydramnios, operative delivery, birth injury, delayed lung maturity, and stillbirth. Neonatal complications include respiratory distress syndrome, jaundice, and hypoglycemia [10, 21, 22]. Furthermore, women with GDM have an increased risk of developing diabetes later in life, and it has been estimated that up to 70% of woman with GDM will develop diabetes within 22–28 years after pregnancy [23]. Long-term adult disorders, such as glucose intolerance and obesity, have been demonstrated with fetal exposure to maternal diabetes [24].

Table 8.3 Diagnostic criteria for gestational diabetes mellitus

Status	Carpenter and coustan (mg/dL)	NDDG (mg/dL)
Fasting	95	105
1 h	180	190
2 h	155	165
3 h	140	145

Initial treatment of GDM involves nonpharmacological approaches with dietary modification and exercise [12]. If this approach fails to achieve target blood glucose levels (fasting <95 mg/dL and postprandial blood glucose values <140 mg/dL at 1 h or 120 mg/dL at 2 h), pharmacologic treatment should be initiated. Insulin is considered first-line treatment and should be dosed the same as pregestational diabetics. For women who decline insulin therapy or for those women who may not be able to safely administer insulin, oral hypoglycemic agents may be used with Metformin being the preferred second-line agent [12]. Metformin is a biguanide that inhibits hepatic gluconeogenesis and glucose absorption and stimulates glucose uptake in peripheral tissues [12]. Metformin does cross the placenta, and dosing usually starts at 500 mg nightly for a week and then increased to 500 mg twice daily due to common adverse side effects of abdominal pain and diarrhea. The maximum dose of metformin is 2500–3000 mg per day in two to three divided doses. Glyburide is another suggested oral hypoglycemic agent and is a sulfonylurea that binds to pancreatic beta cells to increase insulin secretion and insulin sensitivity of peripheral tissues [12]. Glyburide crosses the placenta, and the common dosage of glyburide is 2.5–20 mg daily in divided doses, but doses up to 30 mg may be necessary to achieve adequate glucose control [25]. When compared with insulin use, glyburide is associated with increased risks of respiratory distress syndrome, hypoglycemia, macrosomia, and birth injury [26].

Antepartum fetal testing is recommended for gestational diabetics on pharmacologic treatment similarly to pregestational diabetics [12]. Gestational diabetics who achieve target blood glucose control with nonpharmacological approaches should not be delivered prior to 39 weeks unless otherwise indicated. Delivery may be prolonged up to 40 6/7 weeks in setting of antenatal testing initiated at 40 0/7 weeks. Vaginal delivery is preferred for mode of delivery, but patients should be counseled regarding risks and benefits of cesarean delivery if the estimated fetal weight is >4500 g as in pregestational diabetics [12].

Surgery Considerations

Non-obstetric surgery during pregnancy requires a multidisciplinary team which should include surgeon, obstetrician, maternal-fetal medicine specialist, anesthesiologist, and neonatologist. In general, a pregnant woman should never be denied indicated surgery regardless of trimester; elective surgery should be postponed until after delivery, and if possible non-urgent surgery should be performed in the second trimester when preterm contractions and spontaneous abortion are least likely [27]. Surgery should be performed at an institution with access to pediatric services, obstetrician readily available for cesarean delivery, and with qualified staff readily available to interpret fetal heart rate tracings. Administration of antenatal corticosteroids for fetal benefit is recommended for non-obstetric surgery performed at viability. Antenatal corticosteroids will result in a transient hyperglycemia in diabetic patients which may require inpatient admission for blood glucose monitoring.

A diabetic woman whose blood glucose is well controlled before surgery is expected to have fewer complications [28]. Decisions regarding management depend on the patient's current regimen, which may include insulin, oral medications, or diet alone. Based on expert opinion, it is recommended to maintain glucose levels within target ranges of fasting <95 mg/dL and 1-h ≤140 mg/dL or 2-h postprandial ≤120 mg/dL. Ideally, surgery should be performed early in the day to avoid prolonged fasting. The patient should take full dose of insulin the night before surgery and take no insulin the morning of surgery. Even on a NPO regimen postoperatively, the patient should be advised to take one-half to two-thirds of their basal insulin regimen [28]. While inpatient, blood glucose levels can be drawn every 4–6 h, and sliding scale insulin can be used to maintain blood glucose levels at target ranges. Once home or eating, regular insulin regimen can be restarted. For diabetics on oral medication, the perioperative management depends on the length of the surgical case. If surgery is short or an anticipated same-day discharge, minimal change in medication is needed. Table 8.4 provides a guide to management of oral agents in the perioperative period [28].

Hypertensive Disorders of Pregnancy

Early identification and appropriate management of hypertensive disorders of pregnancy are important in preventing antepartum and postpartum complications, as well as development of future cardiovascular disease. This section will address hypertension in pregnancy and its management.

Classification

Elevated blood pressure (BP) in pregnancy can be characterized as mild range or severe range.

Table 8.4 Management of oral hypoglycemic medications in the perioperative period

	Metformin	Glyburide
Preoperative	Discontinue on day of surgery	Discontinue on day of surgery; if long acting consider discontinuing 24–36 h preoperatively
Intraoperative	Use short-acting insulin if needed	Use short-acting insulin if needed; monitor for hypoglycemia; use of IV dextrose acceptable
Postoperative	Resume postop; hold if renal function worsens or if contrast is used	Risk of hypoglycemia due to long half-life; monitor blood glucose; do not restart until eating regular diet

Mild range blood pressure is defined as systolic BP (SBP) ≥ 140 mmHg or diastolic BP (DBP) ≥ 90 mmHg. Severe range blood pressure is defined as SBP ≥ 160 mmHg or DBP ≥ 110 mmHg [29]. The most commonly encountered forms of hypertension in pregnant women are categorized as preeclampsia-eclampsia, chronic hypertension, chronic hypertension with superimposed preeclampsia, and gestational hypertension and defined as follows:

Preeclampsia-eclampsia refers to the syndrome of new-onset hypertension and proteinuria or new-onset hypertension without proteinuria in association with severe features defined as thrombocytopenia (platelet count < 100,000/μL), impaired liver function (liver transaminases at least twice the normal concentration or persistent right upper quadrant or epigastric pain), new development of renal insufficiency (serum creatinine > 1.1 mg/dL or doubling of serum creatinine in the absence of other renal disease), pulmonary edema, or new-onset cerebral or visual disturbances [29]. Hypertension is defined as elevated blood pressure on two occasions at least 4 h apart after 20 weeks gestation in a previously normotensive woman. Proteinuria is defined as the excretion of 300 mg or more in a 24-h urine collection, a protein to creatinine ratio of 0.3 mg/dL, or urine dipstick reading of 1 + [29]. Eclampsia is diagnosed when a seizure occurs.

Chronic hypertension (CHTN) is defined as SBP ≥ 140 mmHg and/or DBP ≥ 90 mmHg preceding pregnancy or present before the 20th week of pregnancy.

Chronic hypertension with superimposed preeclampsia is when a woman with CHTN develops worsening hypertension with new-onset proteinuria or other features of preeclampsia as noted above (e.g., thrombocytopenia, impaired liver function, renal insufficiency, pulmonary edema, cerebral or visual disturbances).

Gestational hypertension (GHTN) refers to new-onset elevated blood pressures after 20 weeks gestation, without proteinuria or severe features. This disorder is the most frequent type of hypertension during pregnancy.

Management of Chronic Hypertension

Physiologic changes in early pregnancy decrease blood pressure in the first and second trimester (increased blood volume and decreased colloid oncotic pressure). As a result, women with CHTN may have blood pressure < 140/90 mm/Hg early in pregnancy and may even discontinue antihypertensive drugs as a result of this physiologic lowering of blood pressure. Blood pressure will typically increase once again in the third trimester.

Evaluation of the pregnant woman with CHTN should include a baseline comprehensive metabolic panel (liver function, creatinine), complete blood count (platelets), and evaluation of proteinuria (24-h urine for total protein and creatinine clearance or protein to creatinine ratio). An EKG, echocardiogram, and ophthalmological examination in women with long-standing hypertension >4 years should be also be considered [29].

Antihypertensive medications are recommended in pregnancy in cases with severe range blood pressure defined as SBP ≥ 160 mmHg or DBP ≥ 110 mmHg [30]. The most commonly used antihypertensive drugs in pregnancy are labetalol, nifedipine, and methyldopa. Labetalol is the drug of choice for many experts [29]. It is an alpha- and beta-blocker with dosing typically started at 100 mg twice a day with a maximum dose of 2400 mg a day in two to three divided doses. Adverse effects include lethargy, fatigue, sleep disturbances, and bronchoconstriction. Nifedipine is a calcium channel blocker, and extended release formulations are typically used. Nifedipine XL is initiated at 30 mg a day and titrated up to a maximum of 120 mg a day. Methyldopa was historically used as a first-line agent, and onset of action is gradual over 6–8 h. Dosing is initiated at 250 mg two to three times a day with maximum dose of 2 g a day in divided doses. Serious adverse effects include hepatic dysfunction and hemolytic anemia. Current recommendations suggest that BP levels be maintained between 120/80 mmHg and 160/105 mmHg [29].

Maternal complications of CHTN include worsening hypertension and superimposed preeclampsia [31]. Superimposed preeclampsia develops in 13–40% of women with chronic hypertension. Home BP monitoring of women with CHTN is encouraged as gradual worsening of BP's can signal evolving preeclampsia. Fetal complications of CHTN include fetal growth restriction, placental abruption, preterm birth, and stillbirth. Women with CHTN are managed with serial ultrasounds to monitor fetal growth and antenatal testing for fetal well-being generally starting at 32 weeks. Women with uncomplicated CHTN should not be delivered prior to 38 0/7 weeks [29].

Management of Preeclampsia

Preeclampsia is the leading cause of maternal and perinatal morbidity and mortality with an estimated 50,000–60,000 preeclampsia related deaths per year worldwide [29]. The only known cure for preeclampsia is delivery. Women who present with severe preeclampsia typically have a progressive course with maternal and fetal clinical deterioration. Maternal complications of severe preeclampsia include pulmonary edema, stroke, myocardial infarction, acute respiratory distress, and renal failure [29, 32]. Fetal complications are the result of uteroplacental insufficiency or prematurity or both. Once the diagnosis has been made for women less than 34 0/7 weeks of gestation, they should be evaluated as to whether they require prompt delivery or are candidates for continued expectant management as clinical presentation and course may vary. Prompt delivery is recommended for women diagnosed with preeclampsia with severe features at 34 0/7 weeks or greater [29, 32].

Women with severe preeclampsia less than 34 0/7 weeks should be observed on labor and delivery for the first 24–48 h while undergoing further assessment. Magnesium sulfate prophylaxis should be initiated and antihypertensives administered to women with severe range blood pressures (systolic > 160 or diastolic > 110). Magnesium sulfate is typically administered as a 4–6 g IV loading dose administered over 20–30 min, followed by a 2–3 g/h IV maintenance dose. The fetus should undergo ultrasound evaluation for growth, amniotic fluid, and fetal well-being. Antenatal corticosteroids should be administered for fetal benefit. The pregnant woman that demonstrates any of the following features requires prompt delivery after maternal stabilization: eclampsia, pulmonary edema, uncontrollable severe hypertension, disseminated intravascular coagulopathy, placental abruption, abnormal fetal testing, nonviable fetus, or fetal demise. For women with severe preeclampsia at 33 6/7 weeks or less with preterm premature rupture of membranes, labor, platelet count <100,000/μL, abnormal hepatic enzymes, fetal growth restriction, oligohydramnios, reversed end-diastolic flow on umbilical artery Doppler, or new-onset renal dysfunction, delivery may be deferred to allow for antenatal corticosteroid administration if maternal and fetal condition remains stable with delivery at 48 h. Women with severe preeclampsia at less than 34 0/7 weeks who meet criteria for continued expectant management should remain inpatient with serial evaluation of vital signs, symptoms, and blood tests with delivery occurring if abnormal maternal/fetal tests, new contraindications to expectant management, or achievement of 34 0/7 weeks [29, 32].

For women who are diagnosed with mild GHTN or preeclampsia without severe features and not delivered, management may continue in the hospital or at home with modified activity and close maternal and fetal surveillance. Maternal surveillance should include regular BP monitoring, in clinic and home, and serial evaluation of platelets, serum creatinine, and liver enzymes at least once a week [29]. Women with GHTN should have weekly assessment of proteinuria. Women should be counseled to report symptoms that may suggest severe features: persistent, severe headache, blurred vision or scotoma, and right upper quadrant or epigastric pain. Fetal evaluation should include serial ultrasounds for growth every 3 weeks, daily fetal kick counts, and amniotic fluid assessment at least once weekly. Additionally, it is recommended that women with GHTN have a NST or biophysical profile weekly and women with preeclampsia

Table 8.5 Drugs used in the management of acute-onset severe hypertension

Drug	Onset (min)	Mechanism of action	Starting dose	Maximum dose (mg)	Side effects
Hydralazine	10–20	Vasodilator, relaxes arterial smooth muscle	5–10 mg IV q 20 min	30	Avoid with tachycardia, persistent headaches
Labetalol	10–15	Alpha- and beta-receptor blocker	20 mg IV and then 40–80 mg q 10 min	300	Avoid with asthma, CHF
Nifedipine	5–10	Calcium channel blocker	10–20 mg PO q 30 min	240	Avoid with tachycardia, palpitations

have twice weekly NSTs or biophysical profiles. Timing of delivery in women with preeclampsia without severe features or GHTN is recommended at 37 0/7 weeks, if not delivered sooner for worsening maternal or fetal condition [29]. If women are 34 0/7 weeks or greater with labor or rupture of membranes, abnormal maternal or fetal test results, ultrasound estimate of fetal weight less than 5%tile, or suspected placental abruption, then delivery is recommended [29]. It is important to note that women with gestational hypertension may progress to severe gestational hypertension or preeclampsia over the span of 1–3 weeks, conversely women with preeclampsia may progress to severe preeclampsia within days [33]. Mode of delivery for the woman with preeclampsia should be based on gestational age, fetal presentation, cervical status, and maternal/fetal condition.

Management of Acute-Onset Severe Hypertension

A hypertensive emergency is diagnosed when the pregnant woman presents with acute-onset severe range blood pressures that persist for more than 15 min. Severe hypertension can result in neurologic injury; therefore the use of antihypertensives is recommended to reduce risk [34]. Antihypertensives used for acute management include labetalol, nifedipine, and/or hydralazine (Table 8.5). The goal of treatment is to reduce blood pressure to 140–150/90–100 mmHg. Any of these drugs may be used as first-line agents as some pregnant women may respond to one drug and not another. Although each of these medications can successfully be used to manage a hypertensive emergency, each can be associated with adverse effects. Administration of parenteral labetalol has been associated with bradycardia and should be avoided among women with asthma or congestive heart failure. The use of parenteral hydralazine can cause tachycardia and maternal hypotension (systolic BP < 90 mmHg). Oral nifedipine can also cause tachycardia and overshoot hypotension. In rare instances, labetalol or nicardipine infusions may be used to improve severe hypertension. Sodium nitroprusside should be reserved for extreme cases out of concern for possible cyanide toxicity for mother/fetus and potential worsening of maternal cerebral edema [34]. Management of the pregnant woman with acute-onset severe hypertension resistant to first-line agents should include maternal-fetal medicine specialist, anesthesia, or critical care specialist.

References

1. Lawrence JM, Contreras R, Chen W, Sacks DA. Trends in the prevalence of preexisting diabetes and gestational diabetes mellitus among a racially/ethnically diverse population of pregnant women, 1999–2005. Diabetes Care. 2008;31(5):899–904.
2. Mogos MF, Salemi JL, Spooner KK, McFarlin BL, Salihu HH. Hypertensive disorders of pregnancy and postpartum readmission in the United States: national surveillance of the revolving door. J Hypertens. 2018;36(3):608–18.
3. Classification and diagnosis of diabetes. Diabetes Care. 2017;40(Suppl 1):S11–24.
4. ACOG Practice Bulletin. Clinical Management Guidelines for Obstetrician-Gynecologists. Number 60, March 2005. Pregestational diabetes mellitus. Obstet Gynecol. 2005;105(3):675–85.
5. Report of the expert committee on the diagnosis and classification of diabetes mellitus. Diabetes Care. 2003;26(Suppl 1):S5–20.
6. Kitzmiller JL, Wallerstein R, Correa A, Kwan S. Preconception care for women with diabetes and

prevention of major congenital malformations. Birth Defects Res A Clin Mol Teratol. 2010;88(10):791–803.
7. Greene MF, Hare JW, Cloherty JP, Benacerraf BR, Soeldner JS. First-trimester hemoglobin A1 and risk for major malformation and spontaneous abortion in diabetic pregnancy. Teratology. 1989;39(3):225–31.
8. Modanlou HD, Komatsu G, Dorchester W, Freeman RK, Bosu SK. Large-for-gestational-age neonates: anthropometric reasons for shoulder dystocia. Obstet Gynecol. 1982;60(4):417–23.
9. Reece EA, Sivan E, Francis G, Homko CJ. Pregnancy outcomes among women with and without diabetic microvascular disease (White's classes B to FR) versus non-diabetic controls. Am J Perinatol. 1998;15(9):549–55.
10. Galerneau F, Inzucchi SE. Diabetes mellitus in pregnancy. Obstet Gynecol Clin North Am. 2004;31(4):907–33. xi–xii
11. Gabbe SG, Graves CR. Management of diabetes mellitus complicating pregnancy. Obstet Gynecol. 2003;102(4):857–68.
12. Practice Bulletin No. 180: gestational diabetes mellitus. Obstet Gynecol. 2017;130(1):e17–37.
13. Management of diabetes in pregnancy. Diabetes Care. 2015;38(Suppl):S77–9.
14. Langer O, Anyaegbunam A, Brustman L, Guidetti D, Levy J, Mazze R. Pregestational diabetes: insulin requirements throughout pregnancy. Am J Obstet Gynecol. 1988;159(3):616–21.
15. Sibai BM, Viteri OA. Diabetic ketoacidosis in pregnancy. Obstet Gynecol. 2014;123(1):167–78.
16. Rouse DJ, Owen J, Goldenberg RL, Cliver SP. The effectiveness and costs of elective cesarean delivery for fetal macrosomia diagnosed by ultrasound. JAMA. 1996;276(18):1480–6.
17. Torloni MR, Betran AP, Horta BL, Nakamura MU, Atallah AN, Moron AF, et al. Prepregnancy BMI and the risk of gestational diabetes: a systematic review of the literature with meta-analysis. Obes Rev. 2009;10(2):194–203.
18. Rumbold AR, Crowther CA. Women's experiences of being screened for gestational diabetes mellitus. Aust N Z J Obstet Gynaecol. 2002;42(2):131–7.
19. Yogev Y, Xenakis EM, Langer O. The association between preeclampsia and the severity of gestational diabetes: the impact of glycemic control. Am J Obstet Gynecol. 2004;191(5):1655–60.
20. Ehrenberg HM, Durnwald CP, Catalano P, Mercer BM. The influence of obesity and diabetes on the risk of cesarean delivery. Am J Obstet Gynecol. 2004;191(3):969–74.
21. Wu ET, Nien FJ, Kuo CH, Chen SC, Chen KY, Chuang LM, et al. Diagnosis of more gestational diabetes lead to better pregnancy outcomes: Comparing the International Association of the Diabetes and Pregnancy Study Group Criteria, and the Carpenter and Coustan Criteria. J Diabetes Investig. 2016;7(1):121–6.
22. Rosenstein MG, Cheng YW, Snowden JM, Nicholson JM, Doss AE, Caughey AB. The risk of stillbirth and infant death stratified by gestational age in women with gestational diabetes. Am J Obstet Gynecol. 2012;206(4):309.e1–7.
23. Kim C, Newton KM, Knopp RH. Gestational diabetes and the incidence of type 2 diabetes: a systematic review. Diabetes Care. 2002;25(10):1862–8.
24. Clausen TD, Mathiesen ER, Hansen T, Pedersen O, Jensen DM, Lauenborg J, et al. Overweight and the metabolic syndrome in adult offspring of women with diet-treated gestational diabetes mellitus or type 1 diabetes. J Clin Endocrinol Metab. 2009;94(7):2464–70.
25. Lehmann ED, Tarin C, Bondia J, Teufel E, Deutsch T. Incorporating a generic model of subcutaneous insulin absorption into the AIDA v4 diabetes simulator. 3. Early plasma insulin determinations. J Diabetes Sci Technol. 2009;3(1):190–201.
26. Tieu J, McPhee AJ, Crowther CA, Middleton P, Shepherd E. Screening for gestational diabetes mellitus based on different risk profiles and settings for improving maternal and infant health. Cochrane Database Syst Rev. 2017;8:Cd007222.
27. Committee Opinion No. 696: nonobstetric surgery during pregnancy. Obstet Gynecol. 2017;129(4):777–8.
28. Johnson BE, Porter J. Preoperative evaluation of the gynecologic patient: considerations for improved outcomes. Obstet Gynecol. 2008;111(5):1183–94.
29. Hypertension in pregnancy. Report of the American College of Obstetricians and Gynecologists' Task Force on Hypertension in Pregnancy. Obstet Gynecol. 2013;122(5):1122–31.
30. SMFM Statement: benefit of antihypertensive therapy for mild-to-moderate chronic hypertension during pregnancy remains uncertain. Am J Obstet Gynecol 2015;213(1):3–4.
31. Sibai BM, Lindheimer M, Hauth J, Caritis S, VanDorsten P, Klebanoff M, et al. Risk factors for preeclampsia, abruptio placentae, and adverse neonatal outcomes among women with chronic hypertension. National Institute of Child Health and Human Development Network of Maternal-Fetal Medicine Units. N Engl J Med. 1998;339(10):667–71.
32. Sibai BM. Evaluation and management of severe preeclampsia before 34 weeks' gestation. Am J Obstet Gynecol. 2011;205(3):191–8.
33. Barton JR, O'Brien JM, Bergauer NK, Jacques DL, Sibai BM. Mild gestational hypertension remote from term: progression and outcome. Am J Obstet Gynecol. 2001;184(5):979–83.
34. Committee Opinion No. 692: emergent therapy for acute-onset, severe hypertension during pregnancy and the postpartum period. Obstet Gynecol. 2017;129(4):e90–e5.

Part II

General Surgery During Pregnancy

Trauma and Surgical Management During Pregnancy

9

Morgan Schellenberg and Travis M. Polk

Introduction

Trauma is the leading cause of maternal death, accounting for approximately 50% of deaths during pregnancy [1]. Approximately 7% of pregnant women will experience physical trauma during pregnancy [2–3], and trauma is associated with increases in both maternal and fetal mortality.

In this chapter, both maternal and fetal outcomes in the short and long term after trauma will be presented, along with mechanisms of injury and the anatomic and physiologic changes of pregnancy. Key aspects of assessment, evaluation, and management of a pregnant woman and her fetus after trauma are highlighted. Indications for emergent cesarean section after trauma and the management of non-traumatic causes of intra-abdominal bleeding are described.

M. Schellenberg
Division of Trauma and Surgical Critical Care, LAC+USC Medical Center, University of Southern California, Los Angeles, CA, USA
e-mail: morgan.schellenberg@med.usc.edu

T. M. Polk (✉)
Division of Trauma and Surgical Critical Care, LAC+USC Medical Center, Keck School of Medicine, University of Southern California, Los Angeles, CA, USA
e-mail: travis.polk@usc.edu

Maternal and Fetal Outcomes After Trauma

There are important sequelae for both the pregnant woman and her fetus after trauma, both in the short and long term. In the short term, there is a high risk for premature delivery, a risk that is doubled when compared to a pregnant woman who has not sustained trauma [4]. The risk of fetal death is increased by 4.6-fold after a pregnant woman sustains trauma [4], with 1 large case series documenting a fetal survival rate of only 56% after maternal trauma [5]. Interestingly, the consequences of maternal trauma on the fetus persist after delivery. In one study, the rate of neonatal death among children of women who sustained traumatic injuries while pregnant was three times higher than the neonatal death rate among the general population [4]. Low birth weight is also more common among neonates born to women who sustained trauma during pregnancy [6].

From the mother's perspective, the rate of maternal death is also greatly increased after traumatic injury, with a mortality rate that is 69 times higher than that of pregnant women without a history of trauma [4]. Both maternal and fetal mortality are higher after penetrating than blunt trauma, with maternal mortality 7% and 2%, respectively, and fetal mortality 73% and 10%, respectively [7]. Studies comparing mortality rates between pregnant and nonpregnant

C. H. Nezhat (ed.), *Non-Obstetric Surgery During Pregnancy*,
https://doi.org/10.1007/978-3-319-90752-9_9

women after trauma are conflicting. Some studies show that, after adjusting for Injury Severity Score (ISS) and other confounders, pregnant women have almost twice the mortality rate of nonpregnant female trauma patients [8]. Other studies have demonstrated lower mortality rates among pregnant trauma patients compared to nonpregnant trauma patients, citing differences in hormonal factors as a potential explanation [9]. At the present time, the effect of pregnancy on mortality after trauma is unclear.

Mechanism of Injury

In pregnancy, traumatic injuries can be broadly considered to occur after blunt trauma, penetrating trauma, or intimate partner violence. The incidence of blunt trauma far outweighs penetrating trauma [7]. Among causes of blunt trauma, motor vehicle collisions (MVCs) are most common (55–70%), followed by assaults (12–22%) [10–11]. The most common mechanism of injury that causes fetal mortality is MVCs [7]. Because of the frequency of MVCs as a mechanism of injury during pregnancy, proper seat belt use for pregnant women, in which the lap belt is placed across the hips instead of across the uterus (Fig. 9.1), has been an important public health intervention. Although studies on seat belt use during pregnancy are limited, there are case studies that demonstrate that incorrect seat belt placement contributes to fetal death [12]. Overall, blunt trauma results in a 2% risk of maternal mortality and a 10% risk of fetal mortality [7].

Penetrating trauma is most commonly caused by gunshot wounds (GSWs) [1, 7]. Both maternal and fetal mortality are higher after penetrating

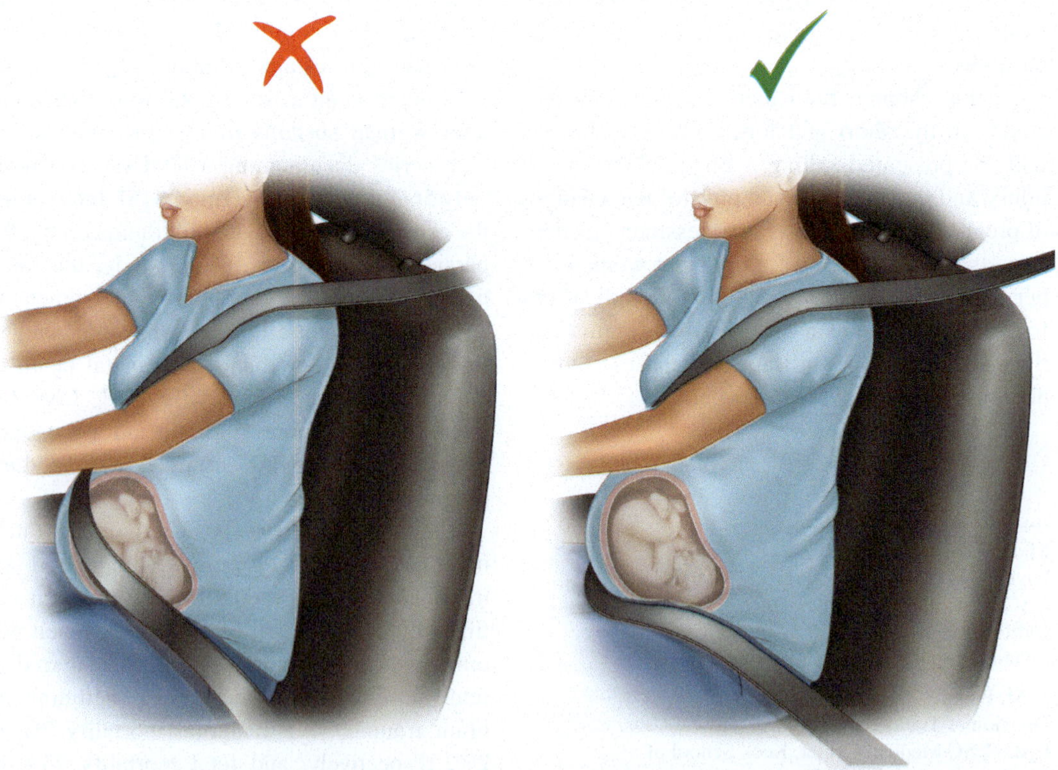

Fig. 9.1 Proper seat belt use during pregnancy. The lap belt should be placed across the maternal hips, below the gravid uterus. The lap belt should not be worn across the gravid uterus as this results in the transfer of force to the fetus if a collision occurs. This has become an important public health education topic

than blunt trauma, with maternal mortality of 7% and fetal mortality of 73% [7]. As the fetus grows out of the maternal pelvis, it becomes particularly vulnerable to penetrating trauma while offering a degree of protection to maternal organs by the displacement and shielding that occur from the gravid uterus. Interestingly, fetal mortality rates are much higher than maternal mortality rates after the same trauma [13], reflecting the sensitivity of the fetus to catecholamine-induced vasoconstriction of the placenta after maternal trauma.

Pregnancy is a high-risk time for intimate partner violence, and this must be considered in the assessment of any injured pregnant patient. Intimate partner violence involves physical violence, sexual violence, or psychological aggression toward a person by someone with a close emotional and/or physical relationship to that person [14]. Rates of intimate partner violence during pregnancy vary widely according to geographical location, age and race of the woman, and socioeconomic status but have been reported to be as high as 40% [14]. For this reason, the American College of Surgeons' Advanced Trauma Life Support (ATLS) course recommends that all pregnant women who present with traumatic injuries be screened for intimate partner violence [15].

Anatomic and Physiologic Changes in Pregnancy

Anatomic

The anatomic changes in pregnancy, as they relate to maternal and fetal trauma, are best considered by trimester. As the fetus grows and its relationship to the maternal pelvis changes, it is at risk for injury after different forms of trauma and imparts different degrees of protection to various maternal organs.

In the first trimester, the fetus is confined to the maternal pelvis. This confers protection to the fetus, as the strength of the pelvic ring shields the fetus from both blunt and penetrating trauma. However, this enclosure within the pelvis also places the fetus at high risk for direct injury after maternal pelvic fractures [15–16]. There is also a risk of fetal loss, even after seemingly minor trauma.

In the second trimester, the fetus grows out of the maternal pelvis, increasing the risk of injury after penetrating trauma. It remains vulnerable to injury after maternal pelvic trauma, and the risk of fetal loss persists throughout pregnancy. As the volume of amniotic fluid increases, the risk of amniotic fluid embolism grows. Through the first and second trimesters, the maternal organs remain in similar locations to their nonpregnant states, and therefore maternal injury patterns tend to be similar, although some data suggest a 25% increased risk of hepatic and splenic injury after blunt trauma due to changes in vascularity and displacement of other intra-abdominal contents [17].

In the third trimester, as the fetus occupies an increasingly larger proportion of the maternal abdomen, the maternal viscera are displaced up under the costal margins and are relatively protected (Fig. 9.2). The fetus, meanwhile, is exposed and vulnerable to injury.

Physiologic

While the anatomic changes in pregnancy are best considered by trimester, the physiologic changes a pregnant woman experiences are most clearly described by organ system. The physiologic changes of pregnancy merit an entire chapter of their own, but the changes critical to the trauma patient are discussed here.

Neurologic

Neurological conditions of pregnancy can be confused with signs and symptoms of neurological injury after trauma and must be considered. For example, eclampsia, which occurs in a woman with preeclampsia once she has the onset of seizures, can mimic head or spinal cord injury in the polytrauma patient with seizures and hyperreflexia. Although neurological abnormalities in a trauma patient are the result of trauma until proven otherwise, the physician must consider non-traumatic causes in the differential as the treatment can be dramatically different.

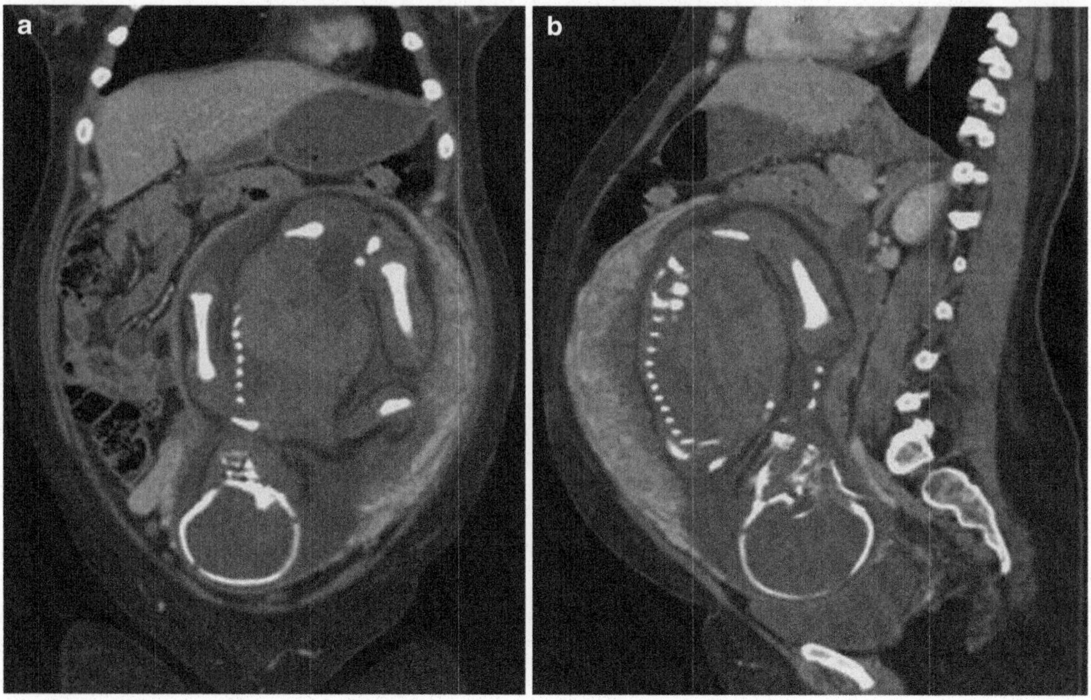

Fig. 9.2 CT scan of a pregnant trauma patient. Especially in the third trimester, displacement of maternal organs occurs as the gravid uterus enlarges. Photo credit: Lee Myers, MD

Respiratory

Particularly as the fetus grows, the respiratory changes from pregnancy can be dramatic. Diaphragm elevation occurs with the growth of the fetus, which must be considered when placing a chest tube into a trauma patient with a pneumo- or hemothorax. Tidal volume and minute ventilation increase in pregnancy, and because of this, a $PaCO_2$ of 30 mmHg is normal for these patients [15]. Blood gas interpretation in the pregnant trauma patient must be done with this in mind, as a "normal" $PaCO_2$ of 40 mmHg may reflect hypoventilation and respiratory failure in a pregnant woman.

Cardiovascular

Although heart rate increases in pregnancy, the change is subtle and is generally not clinically significant. It is typically in the range of 5–10 beats per minute higher than in the nonpregnant state by term. Cardiac output increases by about 20% to allow for perfusion of the high-capacitance placenta. Even with the increase in cardiac output, pregnant women experience a lowering of both the systolic and diastolic blood pressures, which reaches a nadir in the second trimester. In trauma, one of the important considerations when evaluating a pregnant woman's circulatory status during the primary survey is her body positioning. In later stages of pregnancy, compression of the IVC by the gravid uterus and fetus is most significant with the woman in the supine position and can result in hemodynamically significant decreases in venous return and hypotension as a result. This is overcome by tilting the woman slightly to the right, which can be accomplished while maintaining full spinal precautions by placing a wedge below the right side of the spine board (Fig. 9.3).

Hematologic

Pregnant women have an increased blood volume as compared to their nonpregnant counterparts. Although the volume of red blood cells increases, the plasma volume increases to a greater extent. This produces a dilutional physiologic anemia of

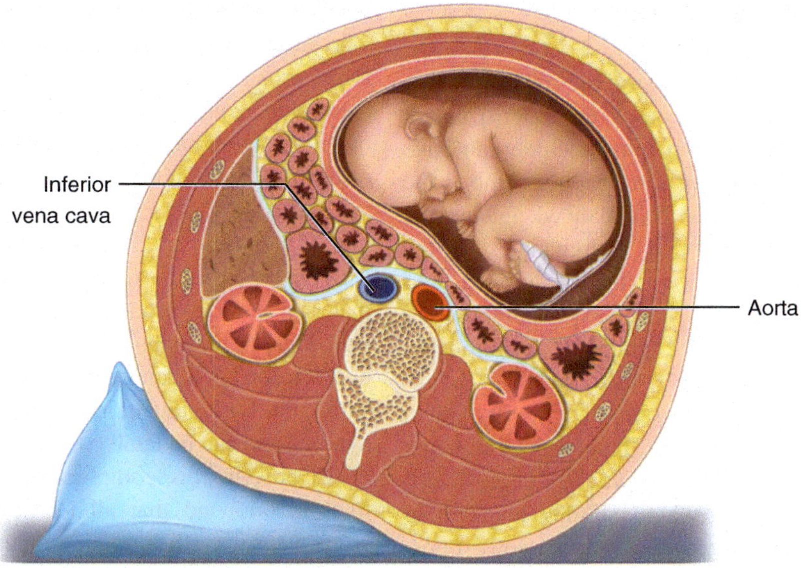

Fig. 9.3 Inferior vena cava compression (IVC) may cause supine hypotension syndrome. In later stages of pregnancy, the gravid uterus compresses the mother's IVC when she is supine, resulting in decreased venous return and hypotension. Rolling the patient toward the left can help mitigate this effect (as seen in this figure). If necessary, spine precautions can be maintained by stacking several blankets under the spine board near the woman's right flank, which shifts the uterus off of the IVC and allows uncompromised venous return

pregnancy, with a typical hematocrit of 32–34% [18]. This process begins toward the end of the first trimester and increases thereafter. In contrast to the hematocrit, a mild leukocytosis occurs in pregnancy as the result of hormonal changes. Platelets tend to remain unchanged. In terms of coagulation, pregnant women are notably hypercoagulable. This occurs by a number of mechanisms, including an increase in fibrinogen and coagulation factors combined with a decrease in fibrinolysis. This manifests clinically as an increased rate of venous thromboembolic events among pregnant women.

Evaluation of the Pregnant Trauma Patient

Initial Assessment

An in-depth description of the primary and secondary survey for a pregnant trauma patient is detailed elsewhere [15]. In brief, the primary survey of the pregnant patient should proceed as it does for the nonpregnant patient. The optimal treatment of the fetus is the optimal treatment of the mother. The anatomic and physiology changes of pregnancy outlined above must be considered. Once life-threatening maternal injuries have been excluded or managed, the maternal secondary survey ensues and should include fetal assessment, the details of which depend upon signs and symptoms of injury as well as fetal gestational age. In addition to the usual components of the secondary survey, the secondary survey in a pregnant woman must include physical examination for signs of uterine rupture and placental abruption, presented in detail in the sections that follow.

In addition to the history and physical exam, the diagnostic work-up of any injured pregnant patient consists of both radiographic and nonradiographic investigations, discussed in detail below. The selection of each test depends upon the magnitude of the trauma sustained as well as gestational age and signs and symptoms of injury. After assessing the mother for injury, the fetus may require individual assessment as well, depending on the gestational age.

Radiographic Evaluation

The recommended radiographic investigations for injured pregnant women are controversial. The risks of missing an injury, which can have particularly devastating consequences among the pregnant patient, must be balanced against the risk of radiation-induced malignancies in the fetus. Common sense must be employed, and only investigations that have the potential to alter management should be pursued. Additionally, increased effort should be made to avoid redundancy in imaging. For example, a stable patient who will proceed to the CT scan does not first require chest and pelvic x-rays [19]. Fetal shielding should be used when imaging areas other than the abdomen and pelvis, and the lowest possible doses of radiation possible to achieve appropriate CT scan quality should be employed.

Radiation exposure of <5 rad appears to be safe at any point in pregnancy, although there is no high-quality evidence [19]. For reference, an abdominal CT scan is roughly 3 rads, but this depends upon the CT scanner used and the protocol employed. The increased malignancy risk imparted by fetal radiation is very small. The absolute risk increase of developing a childhood cancer is on the order of 0.00002 times greater for every mGy of radiation exposure [19].

In summary, the clinician should not hesitate to perform radiologic investigations in pregnant women following trauma if suspicion for injury exists. The increased fetal malignancy risk imparted by imaging is very small but does exist. Therefore, every effort should be made to limit the imaging required, to perform it with the lowest radiation doses possible, and to use fetal shielding.

Non-radiographic Evaluation

Standard trauma labs, including a complete blood count, serum creatinine, and coagulation profile including a fibrinogen level, should be obtained in all pregnant trauma patients. Fibrinogen levels may be helpful in predicting placental abruption. Major trauma society guidelines also recommend a Kleihauer-Betke (KB) test for all pregnant patients who are >12 weeks in gestation [19]. The KB test is important in the assessment for maternal-fetal hemorrhage, one of the most well-known sequelae of maternal trauma. Maternal-fetal hemorrhage can result in isoimmunization of Rh-negative women as fetal blood gains access to the maternal circulation. If this occurs in a Rh-negative woman with a Rh-positive fetus, this mixing of blood can result in maternal antibody production against fetal Rh antigen. This, in turn, can produce immune-mediated hydrops fetalis, a condition where dramatic interstitial fluid accumulation in the fetus leads to hypoxia and can be fatal.

To prevent this complication, current guidelines recommend that all Rh-negative pregnant women receive Rh immune globulin within 72 h of any type of maternal trauma, however minor, because mixing of as little as 0.001 cc of fetal blood into the maternal bloodstream can be sufficient to cause isoimmunization [20]. The typical dose is 300 mg, which provides coverage against 30 cc of fetal blood that has accessed the maternal circulation. In the vast majority of women (>90%), this dose is sufficient [20]. However, if greater amounts of fetal blood have accessed the maternal circulation, higher doses will be required. In this situation, the KB test is useful. This test, performed on a maternal blood sample, quantifies the extent of the maternal-fetal hemorrhage and will alert the clinician if additional dosing of Rh immune globulin is required [20]. Although the KB test's principal utility in the trauma patient is to guide the administration of Rh immune globulin to Rh-negative mothers, its ability to quantify the extent of maternal-fetal hemorrhage may also be clinically useful in Rh-positive women since the extent of transplacental hemorrhage has been shown to be associated with poorer fetal outcomes [20–21]. Therefore, the KB test has potential utility in any pregnant trauma patient.

Fetal Monitoring

The indications, type, and duration of fetal monitoring following maternal trauma are controversial. In general, any pregnant woman with a gestation >10 weeks should undergo some form of fetal monitoring. Prior to 10 weeks, fetal heart tones are generally undetectable, and therefore fetal monitoring devices are not useful. For gestations between 10 and 20 weeks, periodic fetal heart rate assessment with a Doppler ultrasound is sufficient and should be repeated following any significant changes in maternal condition or major interventions. For gestations >20 weeks, continuous fetal heart rate monitoring and external tocometry is typically the standard method of fetal assessment. Major trauma society guidelines conservatively recommend 6 h of continuous fetal heart rate monitoring for fetuses >20 weeks, based upon the limited existing studies that recommend between 2 and 6 h of monitoring [19]. Fetal monitoring should be continued for 24 h if there are any signs of fetal distress, uterine contractions, signs/symptoms of placental abruption or uterine rupture, serious maternal injuries, or a high-risk mechanism of injury [19–20].

Management of the Pregnant Trauma Patient

Surgical Considerations

When preparing for a trauma laparotomy on a pregnant patient, many of the considerations are the same as for a nonpregnant patient. An appropriate surgical retractor must be on the field, and the operating surgeon should wear a head lamp. Particularly in the pregnant patient, longer instruments may be needed, depending on the trimester of pregnancy. If time permits, a wedge should be placed under the woman's right side in order to tilt the gravid uterus off her IVC to avoid hypotension from caval compression.

In terms of selection of surgical incision, the authors recommend a standard vertical laparotomy incision for trauma patients undergoing laparotomy. Although a Pfannenstiel incision can provide proper exposure in some cases, it takes longer to complete, is not extensile, and does not allow thorough evaluation of the upper abdomen.

In general, laparoscopy is used infrequently in the treatment of trauma patients due to concerns for missed injuries, longer operative times, and the hemodynamic consequences of pneumoperitoneum. However, it may occasionally serve as a useful tool in the diagnosis and treatment of delayed injuries, abdominal lavage, or repair of the diaphragm. While there is ample evidence to support the safety of laparoscopy in the pregnant patient, concerns for fetal compromise due to maternal instability usually preclude its use in the acute trauma patient. A very limited role may exist for repair of certain injuries (diaphragm/splenectomy) in a delayed fashion in the most stable of gravid patients. However, the reported experience is limited to only a few case reports or small case series [22]. Therefore, in the absence of strong evidence to guide its use, the use of laparoscopy in the pregnant trauma patient should be guided by the astute clinical judgment of an attending traumatologist.

Non-obstetric Injuries

Blunt Trauma

In general, blunt trauma in the pregnant patient is managed as it is in the nonpregnant patient. As previously mentioned, the incidence of solid organ injury is higher in pregnancy by about 25%. Solid organ injuries in pregnancy are generally managed as they are in nonpregnant states, with operative intervention reserved for hemodynamically unstable patients. However, angioembolization, a common intervention for solid organ injury and pelvic fractures in nonpregnant patients, is used more sparingly because of the significant radiation exposure. Therefore, management options are more limited. Another important consideration after blunt abdominal and pelvic trauma is the association with uterine and fetal pathology, including direct fetal injury, uterine rupture, placental abruption, and premature induction of labor, discussed further below.

Penetrating Trauma

The pregnant trauma patient can sustain any injury that a nonpregnant trauma patient sustains.

However, the anatomic changes that occur during pregnancy must be considered when examining weapon trajectory for consideration of resultant injuries. As the fetus enlarges during pregnancy and grows out of the maternal pelvis, it becomes increasingly vulnerable to penetrating injury due to its anterior position in the maternal abdomen. Conversely, it confers protection to the maternal organs, which are relatively shielded by the gravid uterus or displaced under the costal margin or into the pelvis and protected by these bony structures. Therefore, the clinician must be cautious about correlating penetrating wound tracts with injuries that would be expected in nonpregnant patients.

Obstetric Injuries

Direct Fetal Injury

Direct fetal injury is rare and can occur following either blunt or penetrating abdominopelvic trauma. In blunt trauma, maternal pelvic fracture can cause severe fetal head trauma [23]. Additionally, any force that compresses the maternal abdomen or pelvis can be transmitted to the more vulnerable fetus, and catastrophic injuries to the fetus can occur in the absence of any significant maternal injuries. Improper seat belt use [12] and even airbag deployment [23] have been known to cause direct fetal injury. In most cases, penetrating injury to the uterus results in fetal mortality.

Uterine Rupture

Uterine rupture occurs after significant blunt force trauma. It is associated with high rates of maternal mortality and is nearly uniformly fatal for the fetus [24]. Uterine rupture presents with abdominal pain, uterine tenderness, vaginal bleeding, and fetal distress. The diagnosis should be considered in any pregnant woman who sustains blunt trauma and has suggestive features on physical examination and is typically confirmed at laparotomy with visualization of full-thickness uterine disruption. If the diagnosis is suspected, a fetal nonstress test (NST) should be obtained. Any evidence of fetal distress is an indication for emergent cesarean section.

Placental Abruption

Placental abruption, in which the placenta is separated from the uterine wall as a result of bleeding from maternal vessels, impedes the ability of the placenta to sustain the fetus and may occur after blunt trauma. Abruption is suggested clinically by abdominal pain, vaginal bleeding, uterine tenderness, or premature labor, and therefore all pregnant trauma patient should be examined for these signs and symptoms. Vaginal bleeding should be investigated with a sterile speculum examination, and not with a digital vaginal exam, in order to avoid potentially exacerbating bleeding from a placenta previa. If suspected, a fetal NST should be performed immediately, and a cesarean section should be performed if fetal distress is present. Ultrasound can be helpful to distinguish placental abruption from uterine rupture, which presents similarly, and from other placental disorders such as placenta previa. Fibrinogen levels can be instructive as a fibrinogen of $\leq$200 mg/dL on presentation has a positive predictive value of 1.00 in predicting severe maternal hemorrhage [25]. Placental abruption results in fetal loss in up to 60% of cases [24, 26].

Premature Labor

Maternal trauma can result in premature labor, in which uterine contractions and cervical dilation occur. This should be suspected on the basis of the physical examination, and urgent obstetrical consultation should be obtained. A fetal NST is warranted. The management depends on a number of factors, including the gestational age, maternal injuries, and stability of the fetus. In the presence of premature labor or significant contractions, the administration of tocolytics should be considered, along with cortico steroids to assist in fetal lung maturation prior to delivery, but these management decisions are complex after trauma and require joint input from the trauma surgeon, obstetrician, and patient.

Amniotic Fluid Embolism

Amniotic fluid embolism (AFE) is a rare but potentially devastating consequence of maternal trauma. In AFE, amniotic fluid gains access to the maternal circulation as a result of uterine trauma and can precipitate cardiovascular collapse. There is no definitive method of confirming the diagnosis of AFE, and therefore it must be suspected clinically in any pregnant trauma patient with the sudden development of hypotension and hypoxemia with an appropriate inciting factor. There is no specific treatment for AFE, and management consists of hemodynamic and respiratory support. Urgent obstetrical consultation should be obtained for consideration of delivery.

Indications for Cesarean Section

Cesarean section (c-section) in the trauma setting can be considered under three different circumstances. First, there is fetal distress requiring emergent c-section with or without a maternal indication for an operation. Second, a woman pregnant with a viable fetus requires emergent laparotomy without signs of fetal distress. Third, the mother has had cardiac arrest or is peri-arrest, and a perimortem c-section is being considered.

The first scenario, in which fetal distress after maternal trauma occurs in the absence of maternal indications for laparotomy, should be managed as it is in the nonpregnant patient, with emergent obstetrics consultation and c-section through a Pfannenstiel incision.

In the second scenario, c-section at maternal trauma laparotomy in the absence of fetal distress has been considered for pregnancies in the third trimester. However, there is no high-quality evidence to support this practice, and avoidance of the additional blood loss associated with c-section may be best in some situations. In general, the absence of fetal distress precludes the need for c-section, regardless of maternal injuries or need for maternal trauma laparotomy.

Most dramatically, perimortem c-sections are considered when the mother is moribund or undergoing CPR. One early study attempted to define features that made a fetus salvageable after catastrophic maternal trauma and found that there were no survivors when c-section was performed for fetuses less than 26 weeks in gestation or for those who had no fetal heart tones immediately prior to section [27]. These authors therefore recommend that perimortem c-section not be undertaken unless the fetus is $\geq$26 weeks and fetal heart tones are present. Since the gestational age may not be known, and the perimortem clinical setting may not lend itself to an ultrasound to assess fetal gestational age, the clinician can estimate viability on the basis of gestational age by palpating a uterine fundus a few fingerbreadths above the maternal umbilicus [27] (Fig. 9.4).

Other studies have demonstrated the importance of performing this procedure expeditiously, with improved fetal outcomes if the fetus is delivered within 5 min of maternal cardiac arrest [28–33]. Interestingly, perimortem cesarean section with evacuation of the uterus has been shown in some cases to help achieve return of spontaneous circulation (ROSC) in the mother, especially when the section is performed within 4 min of maternal cardiac arrest [30]. Although this study did not examine trauma patients exclusively, trauma was the cause for cardiac arrest in 21% of patients. It is possible that the increased venous return permitted by relieving pressure on the IVC with c-section helps achieve ROSC. Therefore, we recommend perimortem c-section after maternal trauma if the mother is in cardiac arrest with a uterine fundal height above the umbilicus if it can be performed expeditiously, in order to potentially salvage the fetus and additionally for potential resuscitative benefit to the mother.

The steps of a perimortem c-section include rapid skin preparation with Betadine followed by a generous midline laparotomy incision. Once access to the peritoneal cavity is gained, a full-thickness vertical incision is made in the uterus, and the fetus is delivered. Appropriate neonatal resuscitation should be administered by a separate team, while the surgical team continues to focus on maternal resuscitation. After delivery of the fetus, if ROSC is achieved, the placenta is delivered, and the uterus is closed in the standard two-layer fashion (Fig. 9.5).

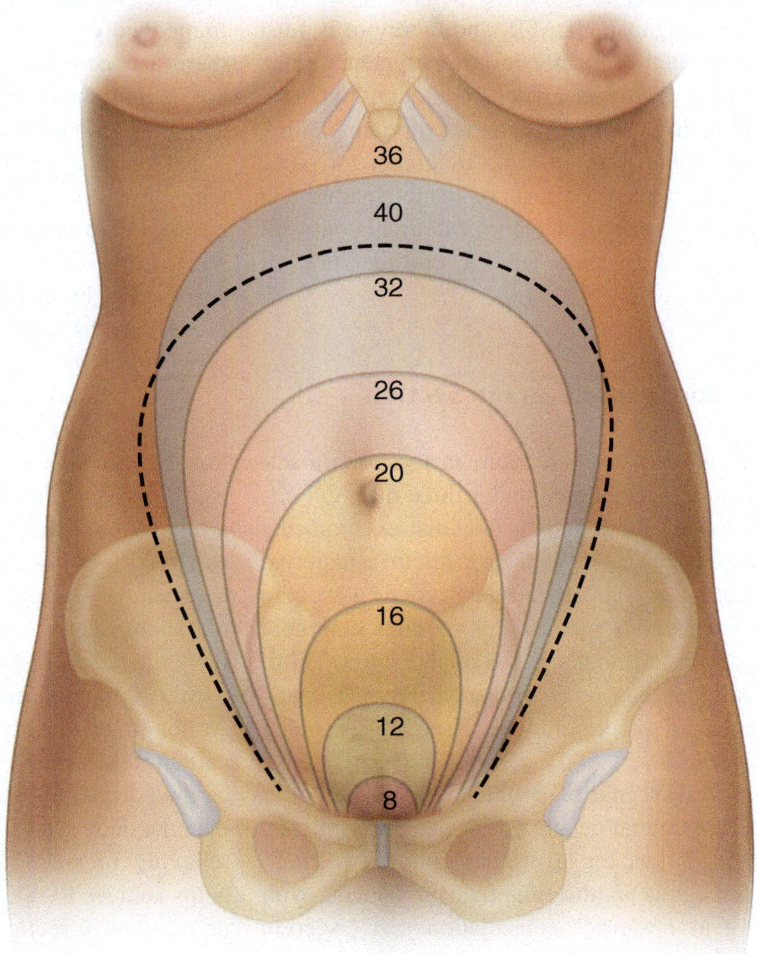

Fig. 9.4 Uterine fundal height. Palpation of the uterine fundus in a pregnant woman allows the estimation of gestational age on the basis of physical examination findings

Non-traumatic Causes of Intra-abdominal Bleeding in Pregnancy

A number of non-traumatic surgical emergencies may also present during pregnancy. While non-bleeding surgical emergencies are covered elsewhere in this textbook, two pregnancy complications associated with significant intra-abdominal bleeding are described here.

HELLP Syndrome

HELLP is an acronym that stands for hemolysis, elevated liver enzymes, and low platelets, describing the intravascular sequelae and resultant laboratory abnormalities that occur with this condition. HELLP syndrome can lead to spontaneous subcapsular hematomas of the liver, which can rupture and cause catastrophic

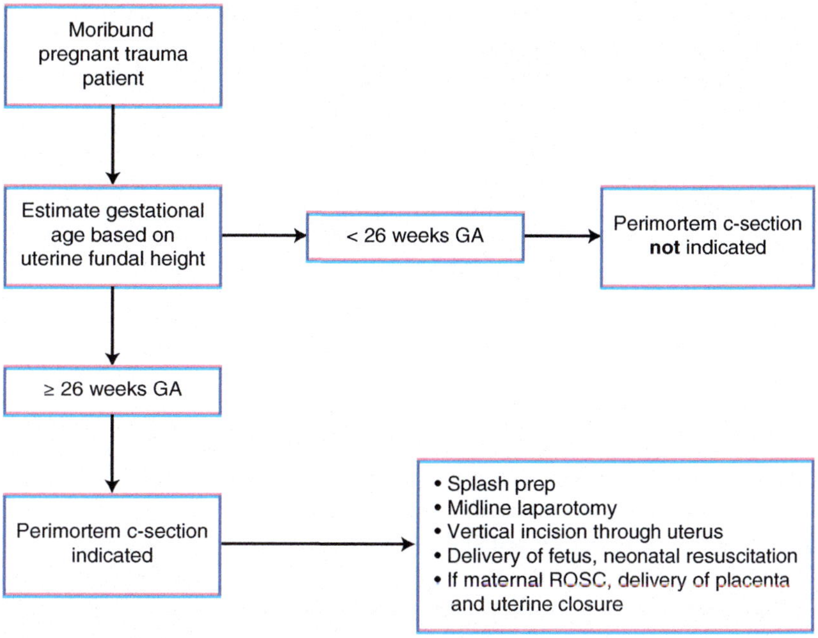

Fig. 9.5 Steps and considerations in perimortem c-section. *GA* gestational age, *C-section* cesarean section, *ROSC* return of spontaneous circulation

intra-abdominal bleeding. It affects less than 1% of pregnant women, particularly those with pre-eclampsia or eclampsia [34]. Its etiology is not entirely understood, but it is generally considered to be related to abnormal development of the placenta, which results in abnormal activation of the coagulation system and subsequent systemic inflammation, particularly within the liver. Some believe HELLP is a severe form of preeclampsia, while others consider it a distinct disease of the placenta.

Patients with HELLP generally present in the third trimester with abdominal pain and hypertension, but symptoms can be nonspecific, and therefore clinical suspicion should remain high. Diagnosis is confirmed with laboratory tests demonstrating a microangiopathic hemolytic anemia with schistocytes, platelet count ≤100,000 cells/μL, bilirubin ≥1.2 mg/dL, and AST more than double the upper limit of normal [35]. Delivery of the placenta is curative. Therefore, management decisions must involve an obstetrician and account for gestational age and overall maternal stability.

Intraparenchymal bleeding and subcapsular hematomas of the liver are severe complications of HELLP syndrome. These can rupture and bleed significantly. When rupture occurs, maternal and fetal mortality both exceed 50% [36]. Clinically, ruptured liver hematomas should be suspected among patients with HELLP who present with markedly elevated transaminases and evidence of bleeding. These patients should be managed with aggressive blood product resuscitation and should be brought expeditiously to the OR for liver packing if they are unstable. If stable, interventional radiology for embolization should also be considered. The development of a subcapsular hematoma or intraparenchymal hemorrhage of the liver among patients with HELLP is generally considered an indication for delivery of the fetus in order to remove the causative agent, the placenta [37].

Splenic Artery Aneurysms

Aneurysms of the splenic artery are uncommon among the general population but increase in incidence among pregnant women. In fact, multiparous women are at four times the risk of developing these aneurysms as compared to nulliparous women [38]. The hormonal changes in pregnancy may cause arterial dilatation with resultant development or worsening of splenic artery aneurysms [39–40]. Although they are rare, they are important causes of mortality for both the mother (75%) and fetus (>95%) when rupture occurs [38]. The risk of rupture exists at any size of aneurysm but is especially marked with aneurysms >2.5 cm in diameter [41].

Rupture of a splenic artery aneurysm in a pregnant woman presents with abdominal pain, nausea, vomiting, and signs of bleeding, especially sudden circulatory collapse. Digital subtraction angiography (DSA) is the imagine technique of choice to diagnose these aneurysms in nonpregnant patients but is avoided in pregnancy because of risks to the fetus [38]. Ultrasound and MRI may be better options among pregnant patients but should only be performed if the patient is stable.

If the diagnosis of ruptured splenic artery aneurysm is suspected in a pregnant woman in hemorrhagic shock, it should be treated with prompt maternal resuscitation and laparotomy with splenectomy. If the fetus is viable, strong consideration of delivery via c-section at the time of laparotomy should be made [38].

Conclusion

Pregnancy is a high-risk time for trauma. Clinicians who manage trauma patients must be aware of the anatomic and physiologic changes that occur in pregnancy, especially as they relate to the types of traumatic injuries that occur and to the maternal response to trauma. The optimal treatment of the fetus after maternal trauma is prompt resuscitation and management of maternal injuries, followed by fetal assessment and monitoring appropriate for gestational age. Early involvement of both a trauma surgeon and an obstetrician in the management of any injured pregnant patient is most prudent.

References

1. Fildes J, Reed L, Jones N, Martin M, Barrett J. Trauma: the leading cause of maternal death. J Trauma. 1992;32(5):643–5.
2. Knudson MM, Yeh DD. Trauma in pregnancy. In: Mattox KL, Moore EE, Feliciano DV, editors. Trauma. 7th ed. New York: The McGraw Hill Companies; 2013. p. 709–24.
3. Lavery J, Staten-McCormick M. Management of moderate to severe trauma in pregnancy. Obstet Gynecol Clin North Am. 1995;22:69–90.
4. El Kady D, Gilbert WM, Anderson J, Danielsen B, Towner D, Smith LH. Trauma during pregnancy: an analysis of maternal and fetal outcomes in a large population. Am J Obstet Gynecol. 2004;190:1661–8.
5. Battaloglu E, McDonnell D, Chu J, Lecky F, Porter K. Epidemiology and outcomes of pregnancy and obstetric complications in trauma in the United Kingdom. Injury. 2016;47:184–7.
6. Sperry JL, Casey BM, McIntire DD, Minei JP, Gentilello LM, Shafi S. Long-term fetal outcomes in pregnant trauma patients. Am J Surg. 2006;192:715–21.
7. Petrone P, Talving P, Browder T, Teixeira PG, Fisher O, Lozornio A, et al. Abdominal injuries in pregnancy: a 155-month study at two level 1 trauma centers. Int J Care Injured. 2011;42(1):47–9.
8. Deshpande NA, Kucirka LM, Smith RN, Oxford CM. Pregnant trauma victims experience nearly 2-fold higher mortality compared to their nonpregnant counterparts. Am J Obstet Gynecol. 2017;217(5):590.e1–9.
9. John PR, Shiozawa A, Haut ER, Efron DT, Haider A, Cornwell EE, et al. An assessment of the impact of pregnancy on trauma mortality. Surgery. 2011;149:94–8.
10. Ikossi DG, Lazar AA, Morabito D, Fildes J, Knudson MM. Profile of mothers at risk: an analysis of injury and pregnancy loss in 1,195 trauma patients. J Am Coll Surg. 2004;200(1):49–56.
11. Weiss H. Pregnancy-associated injury hospitalizations in Pennsylvania, 1995. Ann Emerg Med. 1995;34:626–36.
12. Bunai Y, Nagai A, Nakamura I, Ohya I. Fetal death from abruptio placentae associated with incorrect use of a seatbelt. Am J Forensic Med Pathol. 2000;21(3):207–9.
13. Prokop A, Swol-Ben J, Helling HJ, Neuhaus W, Rehm KE. Trauma in the last trimester of pregnancy. Unfallchirurg. 1996;99:450–3.
14. Chisholm CA, Bullock L, Ferguson JE. Intimate partner violence and pregnancy: epidemiology and impact. Am J Obstet Gynecol. 2017;217(2):141–4.
15. American College of Surgeons Committee on Trauma. Advanced Trauma Life Support (ATLS). 10th ed. Chicago, IL: American College of Surgeons; 2017.
16. Pape HC, Pohlemann T, Gansslen A, Simon R, Koch C, Tscherne H. Pelvic fractures in pregnant multiple trauma patients. J Orthop Trauma. 2000;14(4):238–44.

17. Shah KH, Simons RK, Hollbrook T, Fortlage D, Winchell RJ, Hoyt DB. Trauma in pregnancy. Maternal Fetal Outcomes J Trauma. 1998;45(1):83–6.
18. Hill CC, Pickinpaugh J. Physiologic changes in pregnancy. Surg Clin North Am. 2008;88:391–401.
19. Barraco RD, Chiu WC, Clancy TV, Como JJ, Ebert JB, Hess LW, et al. Practice management guidelines for the diagnosis and management of injury in the pregnant patient: the EAST practice management guidelines work group. J Trauma. 2010;69(1):211–4.
20. Jain V, Chari R, Maslovitz S, Farine D. Maternal Fetal Medicine Committee. Guidelines for the management of a pregnant trauma patient. J Obstet Gynaecol Can. 2015;37(6):553–71.
21. Muench MV, Baschat AA, Reddy UM, Mighty HE, Weiner CP, Scalea TM, et al. Kleihauer-Betke testing is important in all cases of maternal trauma. J Trauma. 2004;57(5):1094–8.
22. Latic F, Delibegovic S, Latic A, Miskic D, Pitlovic V, Koluh A. Laparoscopic splenectomy in blunt trauma: is the procedure safe in pregnant patient? Med Arh. 2010;64(1):51–2.
23. Bard MR, Shaikh S, Pestaner J, Newell MA, Rotondo MF. Direct fetal injury due to airbag deployment and three-point restraint. J Trauma. 2009;67(4):E98–E101.
24. Tsuei BJ. Assessment of the pregnant trauma patient. Injury. 2006;37:367–73.
25. Charbit B, Mandelbrot L, Samain E, Baron G, Haddaoui B, Keita H, et al. The decrease of fibrinogen is an early predictor of the severity of postpartum hemorrhage. J Thromb Haemost. 2007;5(2):266–73.
26. Henderson SO, Mallon WK. Trauma in pregnancy. Emerg Clin North Am. 1998;16:209–28.
27. Morris JA, Rosenbower TJ, Jurkovich GJ, Hoyt DB, Harviel JD, Knudson MM, et al. Infant survival after caesarean section for trauma. Ann Surg. 1996;223(5):481–91.
28. Healey ME, Kozubal DE, Horn AE, Vilke GM, Chan TC, Ufberg JW. Care of the critically ill pregnant patient and perimortem caesarean delivery in the emergency department. J Emerg Med. 2016;51(2):172–7.
29. Katz VL. Perimortem caesarean delivery: its role in maternal mortality. Semin Perinatol. 2012;36:68–82.
30. Katz V, Balderston K, DeFreest M. Perimortem caesarean delivery: were our assumptions correct? Am J Obstet Gynecol. 2005;192:1916–20.
31. Boyd R, Teece S. Towards evidence-based emergency medicine: best BETs from the Manchester Royal Infirmary: Perimortem caesarean section. Emerg Med J. 2002;19:324–235.
32. Strong THJ, Lowe RA. Perimortem caesarean section. Am J Emerg Med. 1989;7:489–94.
33. Oates S, Williams GL, Rees GA. Cardiopulmonary resuscitation in late pregnancy. BMJ. 1988;297:404–5.
34. Abildgaard U, Heimdal K. Pathogenesis of the syndrome of hemolysis, elevated liver enzymes, and low platelet count (HELLP): a review. Eur J Obstet Gynecol Reprod Biol. 2013;166(2):117–23.
35. Sibai BM, Ramadan MK, Usta I, Salama M, Mercer BM, Friedman SA. Maternal morbidity and mortality in 442 pregnancies with hemolysis, elevated liver enzymes, and low platelets (HELLP syndrome). Am J Obstet Gynecol. 1993;169(4):1000.
36. O'Brien JM, Barton JR. Controversies with the diagnosis and management of HELLP syndrome. Clin Obstet Gynecol. 2005;48(2):460–77.
37. American College of Obstetricians and Gynecologists; Task Force on Hypertension in Pregnancy. Hypertension in Pregnancy: Report of the American College of Obstetricians and Gynecologists' Task Force on Hypertension in Pregnancy. Obstet Gynecol. 2013;122(5):1122–31.
38. Sadat U, Dar O, Walsh S, Varty K. Splenic artery aneurysms in pregnancy - a systematic review. Int J Surg. 2008;6:261–5.
39. Selo-Ojeme DO, Welch CC. Review: spontaneous rupture of splenic artery aneurysm in pregnancy. Eur J Obstet Gynecol Reprod Biol. 2003;109(2):124–7.
40. Mattar SG, Lumsden AB. The management of splenic artery aneurysms: experience with 23 cases. Am J Surg. 1995;169:580–5.
41. Salo JA, Salmenkivi K, Tenhunen A, Kivilaakso EO. Rupture of splanchnic artery aneurysms. World J Surg. 1986;10:123–7.

10 Acute Appendicitis During Pregnancy

Hakan Orbay, Christine M. Kariya, and Stephen M. Kavic

Introduction

Appendicitis is the most common non-obstetric condition requiring surgery during pregnancy [1–3]. It accounts for 25% of all non-obstetric surgical procedures performed on gravid women and complicates every 1 in 1500–2000 pregnancies [1–3]. The risk of appendicitis peaks during the second trimester of pregnancy [2, 4, 5]. The overall risk of appendicitis is equal in pregnant and nonpregnant women, but the incidence of perforated appendicitis in pregnant women is greater (43% vs. 4–19%) [1, 2]. The increased incidence of perforation may indicate a delay in diagnosis or a reluctance to operate on pregnant women [1].

The first report on the operative management of appendicitis in pregnancy was in 1848. Henry Hancock performed a laparotomy on a pregnant woman to drain an appendiceal abscess [6], although this is disputed by some historians [7]. Early series that followed this case report described very high maternal and fetal mortality rates, especially in the cases of perforated or gangrenous appendicitis. Babler reported an early literature review in 1908 that included 235 pregnant women with appendicitis, with 103 perforated or gangrenous appendices and 104 non-perforated appendices and an overall maternal mortality of 24% and fetal mortality of 40% [8]. Based on his observations, Babler concluded "the mortality of appendicitis complicating pregnancy is the mortality of delay," which continues to be one of the main principles today [9].

Complications of Appendicitis During Pregnancy

Since Babler's report in 1908, there has been a dramatic decline in maternal and fetal mortality due to appendicitis, which can be attributed to the advancements in diagnostic and surgical tools as well as the use of antibiotics and improved supportive care (e.g., fluid resuscitation, hemodynamic and fetal monitoring, earlier recognition of sepsis, improved anesthesia, etc.) [10]. Current maternal mortality rate is less than 0.4% [10–12] and is almost always associated with perforation [10]. Perforation occurs more than twice as often in the third trimester compared to the first and second trimesters [3, 13]. Fetal loss has likewise decreased from 40% in 1908 to 1.5% to 8.7% in recent retrospective studies [12]. However, the fetal loss rate increases to 10.9% when peritonitis

H. Orbay · C. M. Kariya
Department of Surgery, University of Maryland Medical Center, Baltimore, MD, USA
e-mail: ckariya@som.umaryland.edu; horbay@som.umaryland.edu

S. M. Kavic (✉)
Department of Surgery, University of Maryland School of Medicine, Baltimore, MD, USA
e-mail: skavic@som.umaryland.edu

C. H. Nezhat (ed.), *Non-Obstetric Surgery During Pregnancy*,
https://doi.org/10.1007/978-3-319-90752-9_10

Table 10.1 Complications of appendicitis during pregnancy

Maternal and fetal morbidity
Peritonitis
Preterm labor
Unexplained antepartum hemorrhage Abruptio placenta
Sepsis and septic shock
Pneumonia
Bowel obstruction
Postoperative infection
Increased hospital length of stay
Primary microcephaly
Intrauterine growth retardation
Low birth weight

Table 10.2 Differential diagnosis of acute abdomen during pregnancy[a]

Non-obstetric	Obstetric
Acute appendicitis	Labor
Cholecystitis	Preterm labor
Inflammatory bowel disease	Placental abruption
Pancreatitis	Uterine rupture
Gastritis	Preeclampsia with liver involvement
Mesenteric adenitis	
Diverticulitis	
Urinary tract calculi	
Urinary tract infection	
Ovarian torsion	
Ovarian cyst rupture	
Ectopic pregnancy	
Pelvic inflammatory disease	
Adnexal mass	
Degenerating fibroid	
Ligamentalgia	
Pulmonary embolism	
Right lower lobe pneumonia	

[a]Adapted from [3]

is present, making the perforated appendicitis the most common surgical cause of fetal loss during pregnancy [12, 14, 15]. Despite the decreased mortality in recent decades, pregnant women with appendicitis are more likely to deliver preterm and have a fourfold [11] increased risk of unexplained antepartum hemorrhage and abruptio placenta. The increased risk of preterm delivery does not continue beyond the first week after appendectomy in uncomplicated cases [16]. However, in cases complicated with appendiceal rupture and peritonitis, there is increased risk of preterm delivery and of cesarean sections (C-sections) throughout the remainder of the pregnancy [11].

In addition to abovementioned common complications, appendicitis in pregnancy is also associated with increased risks of sepsis and septic shock, transfusion requirement, pneumonia, bowel obstruction, postoperative infection, increased hospital stay, primary microcephaly, intrauterine growth retardation, and low fetal birth weight (Table 10.1) [4, 11, 17, 18].

Diagnosis of Appendicitis During Pregnancy

The diagnosis of appendicitis during pregnancy begins with a thorough history and complete physical examination. Often the patient will give a history of nausea (71%), vomiting (54%), and anorexia (51%) [10], which are all common complaints during pregnancy [3]. The elevation in body temperature is not considered helpful in diagnosing acute appendicitis but may predict perforation [19]. The most reliable symptom of appendicitis is right lower quadrant pain (Table 10.2) [1, 3, 10, 20]. Other abdominal signs, such as rebound tenderness and guarding, are not very specific during pregnancy, being present in 55%–77% and 50%–68% of patients, respectively, as a result of the distension of the abdominal wall muscles and the interposition of the uterus between the appendix and the anterior abdominal wall [1, 3, 10, 20–23]. Flank and back pain can represent a urinary tract infection (UTI), especially pyelonephritis, or a retrocecal inflamed appendix. Psoas irritation (i.e., psoas sign) is observed less frequently during pregnancy compared to nongravid women [20].

Laboratory studies should consist of a complete blood count, urinalysis, aspartate aminotransferase and alanine transaminase levels, and amylase and lipase levels to exclude UTI, hepatitis, and pancreatitis. Urinalysis is performed to rule out pyelonephritis or nephrolithiasis, but it should be kept in mind that pyuria can also be present in appendicitis [24]. Leukocytosis ranging from 10,000 to 20,000/mm^3 is also a common finding during normal pregnancy and is thus not very helpful as a diagnostic sign [1, 3, 19, 22, 23, 25]. On the contrary, the presence of granulocytosis (i.e., a left shift) is more specific for an infectious etiology such as appendicitis or UTI and may be of some utility in narrowing the differential diagnosis. Clinical scoring systems such as the Alvarado scale have been designed in order to simplify the diagnosis of appendicitis in the general population [26]. However, Alvarado scale is not widely used, and there is currently no validated scoring system for use in pregnancy [3].

Other diseases that should be considered in the differential diagnosis of abdominal pain during pregnancy are listed in Table 10.3. Fetal assessment is essential and involves ultrasound (US) for viability and confirmation of gestational age and biophysical profile and/or nonstress test, depending on the gestational age. Abdominal imaging studies may include US, magnetic resonance imaging (MRI), and computerized tomography (CT) [2].

Abdominal Imaging Studies

Abdominal imaging is an important part of the diagnostic work-up of appendicitis during pregnancy. However, the vulnerability of the fetus and teratogenic effects of conventional x-rays necessitates careful consideration. Because of concerns for ionizing radiation, graded compression US has been the initial diagnostic imaging modality of choice because of its long record safety specifically in pregnant women [2, 20, 27]. More recently, MRI and CT have also become important techniques in improving diagnostic accuracy beyond that which is provided by US alone [2, 28]. The American College of Radiology published *Appropriateness Criteria* guidelines that recommend that US should be used first, followed by MRI (sensitivity 80%, specificity 99%) if the US is inconclusive [29]. In general, US and MRI can be used throughout gestation, but CT imaging is reserved for those patients beyond the first trimester [2, 30]. Fetuses between 2 and 15 weeks gestation are the most at risk for adverse events from ionizing radiation, so special care should be taken to minimize radiation exposure during these gestational weeks. An algorithmic approach to the imaging of appendicitis during pregnancy based on the most recent data can be seen in Fig. 10.1.

Ultrasound

Graded compression US remains the preferred initial imaging test for suspected appendicitis in pregnancy [31, 32]. This preference is largely because there are no documented adverse fetal effects of US in humans by either thermal or

Table 10.3 Comparison of imaging methods in diagnosis of appendicitis during pregnancy

	US	MRI	CT
Sensitivity	46.1–100%[a] [35, 49, 86]	80–100% [28, 43, 80, 87]	85.7–100% [48, 49, 87]
Specificity	83–96% [35, 86]	92–99% [28, 43, 80, 87]	97.4% [48, 87]
Ionizing radiation	–	–	+
Interference by uterine size	+	–	–
Cost	+	+++	++
Duration	+	+++	++
Availability	+++	+	++
Diagnostic criteria	Incompressible fluid-filled appendix, measuring >6 mm in diameter, and a calcified appendicolith	Enlarged, fluid-filled appendix measuring >7 mm in diameter accompanied by periappendiceal fat stranding	Tubular, fluid-filled appendix measuring >7 mm with an enhancing wall, which may or may not contain a fecalith

[a]The sensitivity of US decreases to 28.5% in case of perforated appendicitis [20, 88]

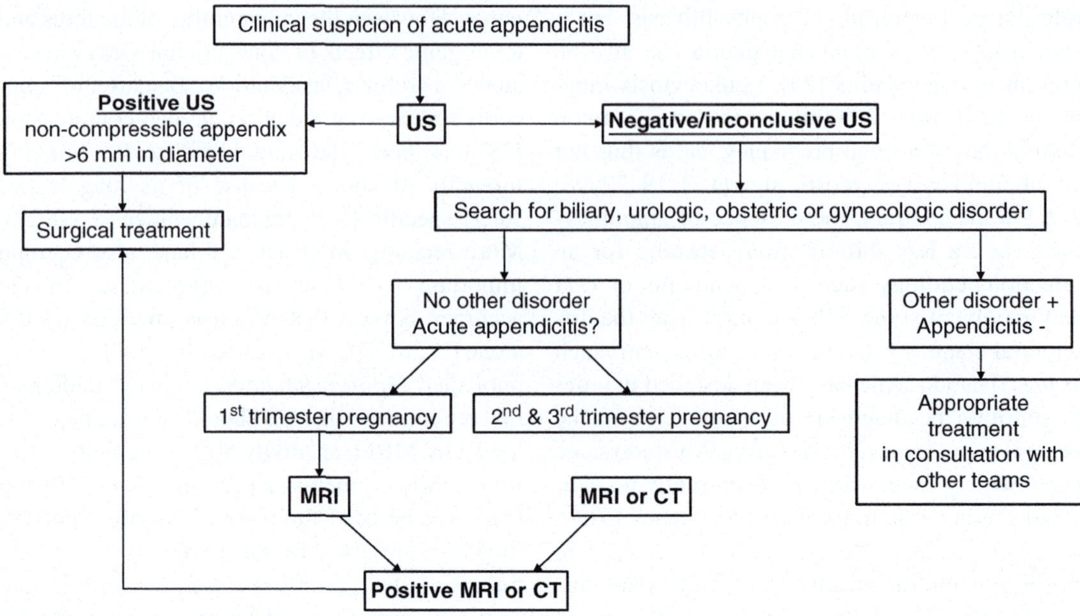

Fig. 10.1 The algorithmic approach to the abdominal imaging in a pregnant patient for the diagnosis of acute appendicitis. Adapted from [82]

nonthermal mechanisms, and thus there are no contraindications to its use during pregnancy [33]. The major limitations of US in pregnant patients are primarily related to impaired visualization of the appendix due to the enlarged uterus, especially in the later stages of pregnancy [31, 32], and the need for an experienced ultrasonographer. The typical diagnostic criteria are incompressible fluid-filled appendix, appendix diameter >6 mm, and a calcified appendicolith [2, 31, 34, 35]. Moreover, the presence of loculated periappendiceal fluid collection in conjunction with an inflamed appendix indicates appendiceal perforation (Fig. 10.2) [35]. The sensitivity and specificity of US in the diagnosis of appendicitis during pregnancy range between 67% and 100% and 83% and 96%, respectively [32, 35, 36], but is operator-dependent, as with all other US studies [28]. If US is inconclusive and no clear alternative diagnosis is identifiable, then MRI is the next step in the imaging ladder [31].

Magnetic Resonance Imaging

The American College of Radiology White Paper on MRI Safety states that pregnant patients may undergo MRI at any stage of pregnancy if the benefits outweigh the risks [37]. Recent studies have shown MRI to be safe in pregnancy and has a higher specificity and sensitivity for diagnosing appendicitis than US [38–41]. MRI is also a reasonable alternative to CT in pregnancy since it does not use ionizing radiation [28, 38, 42], but it should always be remembered that the safety of MRI in pregnancy has not been conclusively proven [30, 37, 43]. Disadvantages of MRI include its high cost, poorer spatial resolution compared to CT, increased sensitivity to motion artifacts, longer acquisition time, and limited compatibility with other patient monitoring equipment which may be necessary for an acutely ill patient [43]. Findings on MRI consistent with appendicitis include an enlarged, fluid-filled (not contrast-filled) appendix measuring more than 7 mm in diameter (Fig. 10.3) [39, 44] that is frequently accompanied with periappendiceal fat stranding [45].

Computed Tomography

CT has traditionally been avoided during pregnancy because of ionizing radiation and its risk of

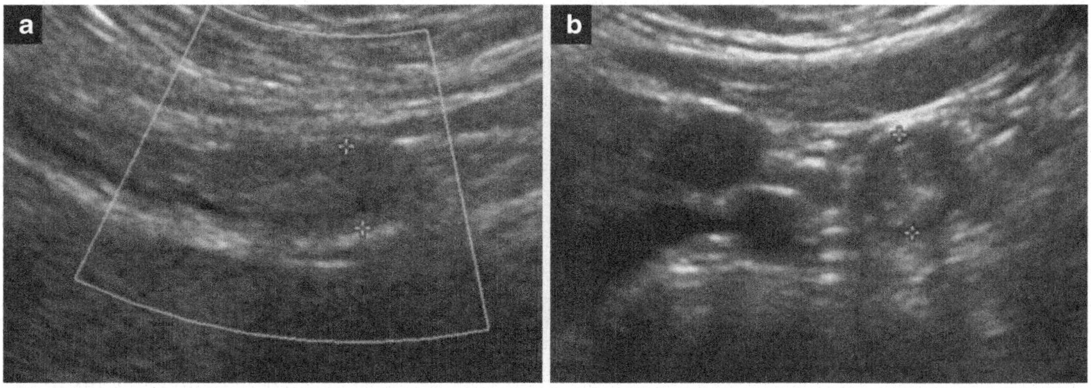

Fig. 10.2 Transverse (**a**) and sagittal (**b**) sonograms show an inflamed appendix (between cursors). European Radiology, Added value of ultrasound re-evaluation for patients with equivocal CT findings of acute appendicitis: a preliminary study, 23(7), 2013, 1882–90, Sim JY, Kim HJ, Yeon JW, Suh BS, Kim KH, Ha YR, et al. With permission of Springer [83]

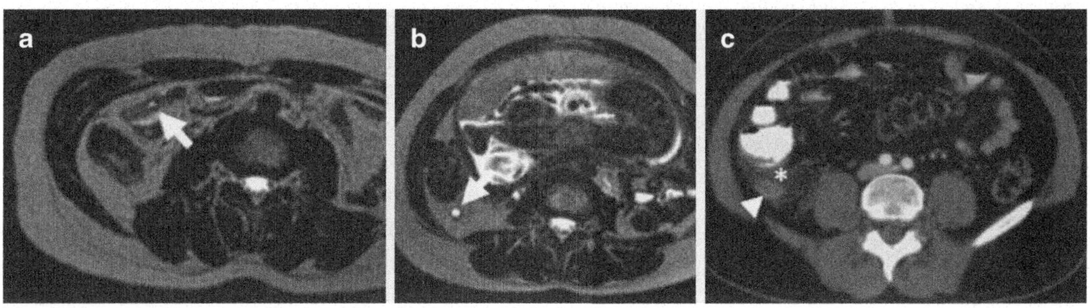

Fig. 10.3 (**a**) Axial MRI view of the normal appendix (*white arrow*). The appendix contains no intraluminal fluid. (**b**) Axial MRI shows a dilated appendix with wall edema and fluid in the lumen (*white arrow*). (**c**) Axial contrast-enhanced CT image shows a prominent appendix with periappendiceal rim enhancement due to inflammation (*arrowhead*). Periappendiceal fat stranding is also visible and marked with asterisk. Adapted from European Radiology, T1 bright appendix sign to exclude acute appendicitis in pregnant women, 27(8), 2017, 3310–6, Shin I, An C, Lim JS, Kim MJ, Chung YE, and European Radiology, Evaluation of a low-dose CT protocol with oral contrast for assessment of acute appendicitis, 19(2), 446–54, Platon A, Jlassi H, Rutschmann OT, Becker CD, Verdun FR, Gervaz P, et al. With permission of Springer [84, 85]

teratogenesis and carcinogenesis [30]. Radiation from an abdominal CT scan ranges from 10 to 20 millisievert (mSv), which is comparable to 500 to 1000 chest radiographs [3]. A newer CT technique, helical CT, has a rapid imaging time of under 15 min [21], and it also decreases the radiation exposure to one third of the average abdominal-pelvic CT, approximately 3 mSv, which is well below the accepted safe level of fetal exposure (50 mSv) [21]. Current consensus is that when US findings are inconclusive and further imaging is deemed necessary, CT can be considered for pregnant women in their second and third trimesters [21] and is the preferred second-line imaging modality if an MRI would risk a significant delay in diagnosis [46]. The combination of clinical examination, US, and CT decreases the negative appendectomy rates significantly (from 54% to 8% in one series of 86 patients) with high diagnostic accuracy [47–49]. The typical finding of appendicitis in CT is an enlarged (>7 mm), tubular, fluid-filled appendix with an enhancing wall, which may or may not contain a fecalith and may be surrounded by inflammatory changes such as fat stranding, fluid collections, and extraluminal air (see Fig. 10.3) [21, 46]. Table 10.4 shows a comparison of the abdominal imaging methods used in pregnancy.

Table 10.4 Symptoms and signs of appendicitis during pregnancy

Common	
Right lower quadrant pain	Most reliable sign of appendicitis in pregnant patient
Direct abdominal tenderness	Observed in most of the patients
Uncommon/not specific	
Rebound tenderness	Not specific, present in 55%–75% of patients
Abdominal guarding	Not specific, present in 50%–65% of patients
Flank or back pain	Present in case of retrocecal appendix
Right upper quadrant pain	Questionably due to displaced appendix
Psoas sign	Less frequent during pregnancy
Anorexia and vomiting	Not specific, common in the first trimester of pregnancy
Leukocytosis (10,000–20,000/mm^3)	Not specific, very common in pregnancy
Granulocytosis	Suggests an infectious etiology such as appendicitis
Elevated body temperature	May predict perforation
Pyuria	Also present in urinary tract infections
Positive Bryan's sign[a]	First described by Kurtz et al. [89]
Diarrhea	

[a]Abdominal pain produced by shifting the gravid uterus to the right

Pregnancy-Related Diagnostic Challenges

Delayed diagnosis of appendicitis is unfortunately not unusual during pregnancy [21–23, 50]. The diagnosis of appendicitis during pregnancy can be difficult due to:

1. The upward displacement of the appendix by the gravid uterus
2. Absence or blunting of usual signs and symptoms of appendicitis such as abdominal guarding and rebound
3. Physiological leukocytosis during pregnancy

The progressive upward displacement of the appendix during pregnancy was first described by Baer et al. [51]. They claimed that the appendix reaches to the level of the iliac crest at the end of the fifth month and continues to rise above this level during the last trimester and returns to its normal position by postpartum day 10 [51]. This displacement accounts for the abnormal localization of pain and tenderness in patients in their second and third trimester to the right upper quadrant and flank whenever inflammation spreads to the parietal peritoneum [1, 10, 22]. However, this hypothesis was challenged by a recent study that failed to detect upward displacement of appendicitis in 114 pregnant patients [52]. Therefore, whether the appendix migrates during pregnancy and whether the surgeon should adjust abdominal incisions accordingly remains a controversial issue.

Treatment of Appendicitis During Pregnancy

If appendicitis is suspected in a pregnant woman, careful diagnostic work-up and immediate antibiotic administration with surgical intervention are indicated within the first 24 h [10, 17, 22, 53] since the incidence of perforation and related complications increases dramatically if surgery is delayed more than 24 h [22, 53]. The only indication to delay appendectomy is active labor, and in these cases the surgery should be performed immediately after delivery [1].

If appendiceal perforation and peritonitis are suspected, the patient should be adequately fluid resuscitated and given IV antibiotics. Antibiotics should cover normal colonic flora, i.e., a second-generation cephalosporin (e.g., cefuroxime) or extended-spectrum penicillin (e.g., ampicillin), combined with an anti-anaerobe antibiotic (e.g., metronidazole). In a series of 50 appendicitis patients, 94% of appendectomy pathologic specimens grew *Escherichia coli*, and there were more anaerobic bacteria, especially members of the *Bacteroides fragilis* group, than aerobic bacteria, which underscores the need for anaerobic and gram-negative antibiotic coverage [54]. Antibiotics should be continued until the patient is afebrile, normal bowel function has returned, and the leukocytosis has improved [1, 55]. Appropriate fluid resuscitation should be administered in cases of hypovolemia and should have continuous fetal heart rate (FHR) monitoring if the gestational age is in the range of fetal viability, since FHR may be the best sign of fetal hypoxia [1, 56, 57]. In the case of perforation, fetal loss rate can be up to 20–36%, so a C-section may be recommended depending on the gestational age of the fetus. Regardless of whether a C-section is performed, the definitive treatment of acute appendicitis is appendectomy. Intraoperatively, the peritoneal cavity should be irrigated copiously, and an intraperitoneal drain may be placed to prevent abscess formation. If an appendiceal abscess occurs, it may be managed using parenteral antibiotics and percutaneous drainage followed by an interval appendectomy after delivery. In the absence of appendiceal perforation or sepsis, a C-section is not recommended since the risk of fetal loss is significantly lower. Thus, the treatment is only appendectomy [22, 23, 57]. Treatment with tocolytics is recommended if there are perceived or documented contractions, but they have not been shown to be helpful in most cases and should be discontinued after 48 h [58].

Surgical Treatment

Medical management of appendicitis has been reported with favorable outcomes [59–61], but the widely accepted standard of care treatment for appendicitis during pregnancy is surgical appendectomy [17, 62]. The second trimester is generally the safest time to perform surgery because of the lower spontaneous abortion rate (5.6% compared with 12% in the first trimester), low rate of preterm labor, better surgical visibility due to the smaller uterus, and the very low risk of teratogenesis [63].

The surgery can be open (i.e., laparotomy) or minimally invasive (i.e., laparoscopy). The choice of surgical procedure is largely based on uterine size and operator experience, although laparoscopy is generally contraindicated in cases of generalized peritonitis because of a significantly higher complication rate [1]. Laparotomy incisions can be a muscle-splitting incision over the point of maximal tenderness, a right paramedian, or a midline vertical incision [10, 22]. A vertical midline incision is advised by some authors in the late second trimester and beyond when the uterus grows larger [1], while some others stated that the incision in all trimesters can be successfully made over McBurney's point [52].

Laparoscopy in pregnancy was once considered contraindicated due to fear of damage to the gravid uterus, fetal acidemia, and decreased maternal venous return secondary to pneumoperitoneum. There is now sufficient evidence to demonstrate that diagnostic/operative laparoscopy is reasonable and as safe as laparotomy in adult patients [1, 64–66]. The trocar placement poses unique perils in the pregnant patient as there is risk of damage to the uterus during blind insertion. In this situation, open insertion of the first trocar (Hasson technique) is recommended [1, 20]. Alternatively, some surgeons inserted Veress needle in the midclavicular line approximately 2 cm below the inferior costal margin to minimize the risk of uterine injury [63, 64]. Intraoperative fetal monitoring is recommended during laparoscopy, and an intraperitoneal pressure of 10–15 mmHg is generally well tolerated by the fetus [63, 64, 67]. Additionally, maternal end tidal CO_2 should be followed closely, and systolic blood pressure should be kept within 20% of baseline since inadequate perfusion to the fetus results in fetal hypoxia [46]. When creating the CO_2-pneumoperitoneum, maternal arterial CO_2 partial pressure ($paCO_2$) may mildly increase secondary to increased transperitoneal absorption of CO_2. This increase can lead to hypercapnia and respiratory acidosis which in turn may cause stimulation of the sympathetic nervous system, cardiac arrhythmias, and fetal acidosis [58]. Surgical positioning is also important; rolling the patient approximately 30° to the left helps prevent occlusion of the inferior vena cava by the enlarged uterus and facilitates visualization of the essential structures [22, 23, 67, 68]. A head-down lateral positioning also improves the view of the contralateral adnexal structures [58]. The surgeon should avoid uterine manipulation as much as possible during appendectomy to decrease the risk of uterine irritability and preterm labor [23]. The Society

Table 10.5 The Society of American Gastrointestinal and Endoscopic Surgeons recommendations for laparoscopy during pregnancy[a]

Patient selection	Laparoscopic treatment of acute abdominal processes has the same indications in pregnant and nonpregnant patients
Patient positioning	Gravid patients should be placed in the left lateral recumbent position to minimize compression of the vena cava and the aorta
Initial port placement	Initial access can be safely accomplished with an open or Hasson, Veress needle, or optical trocar if the location is adjusted according to fundal height, previous incisions, and experience of the surgeon
Insufflation pressure	CO2 insufflation of 10–15 mmHg can be safely used for laparoscopy in the pregnant patient Intra-abdominal pressure should be sufficient to allow for adequate visualization
Intraoperative CO_2 monitoring	Intraoperative CO_2 monitoring by capnography should be used during laparoscopy in the pregnant patient
Venous thromboembolic prophylaxis	Intraoperative and postoperative pneumatic compression devices and early postoperative ambulation are recommended prophylaxis for deep venous thrombosis in the gravid patient
Fetal heart monitoring	Fetal heart monitoring should occur pre- and postoperatively in the setting of urgent abdominal surgery during pregnancy
Obstetrical consultation	Obstetric consultation can be obtained pre- and/or postoperatively based on the acuteness of the patient's disease and availability
Tocolytics	Tocolytics should not be used prophylactically but should be considered perioperatively when signs of preterm labor are present in coordination with obstetric consultation

[a]Adapted from [46, 67]

of American Gastrointestinal and Endoscopic Surgeons recommend laparoscopic method for appendectomy during pregnancy, and they published a series of recommendations that should be followed by all surgeons (Table 10.5) [67].

Laparoscopy vs. Laparotomy

Laparoscopic appendectomy is the standard treatment of acute appendicitis for the general population; however, there is still some doubt regarding its risks and benefits for pregnant patients [62]. One of the first large studies that examined the impact of laparoscopic surgery on fetal or neonatal outcome was performed using the Swedish Health Registry from 1973 to 1993 [69]. In this study, outcomes of 2181 laparoscopies and 1522 laparotomies performed between 4 and 20 weeks gestation were compared. Overall the women who underwent laparoscopic appendectomy had a statically significant increased risk of low birth weight (<2500 g), delivery before 37 weeks, and increased incidence of growth restriction compared with the pregnant patients in the open surgery group. However, there was no difference in the rate of fetal malformations or infant survival at 1 year. Although the risks of preterm delivery and growth restriction increased after both open and laparoscopic appendectomy, there was no difference between the operative approaches in terms of birth weight, gestational duration, intrauterine growth restriction, congenital malformations, stillbirths, and neonatal deaths [69]. A more recent study that examined the US National Health Insurance Research Database from 2005 to 2010 examined pregnant patients with appendicitis that were treated with nonoperative management, open appendectomy, and laparoscopic appendectomy and concluded laparoscopic and open appendectomy were not statistically different in terms of preterm labor, abortion, and need for C-section but that open surgery was associated with a reduced length of hospital stay [62]. Contrary to these studies, a large retrospective database study including 3133 pregnant women in California documented a higher fetal loss rate after laparoscopic appendectomy compared to open appendectomy [70]. A large meta-analysis found no significant difference in preterm delivery, birth weight, Apgar score of the newborn, postoperative wound infection, and duration of operation between laparoscopy and laparotomy groups [71]. Increased fetal loss after laparoscopic appendectomy was consistently reported by other large review papers [58, 72] leading some surgeons to favor and choose open appendectomy over laparoscopic appendectomy. Despite these controversial results and since it is unlikely a randomized trial will be conducted in this pregnant population, the Society of American Gastrointestinal and Endoscopic Surgeons recommend a laparoscopic approach to the pregnant patient with suspected appendicitis [67].

Laparoscopic surgery has numerous advantages over open surgery, such as (1) less invasive surgery, (2) a better postoperative course and shorter hospital stay, and (3) the ability to visualize the entire abdomen and diagnose other possible causes of acute abdominal pain in case of a normal appendix [3, 10, 62, 65, 66, 73–75]. A complete list of the advantages and disadvantages of laparoscopic appendectomy can be found in Table 10.6. Once a feared complication, fetal congenital anomalies are unlikely to occur after laparoscopy with an incidence less than 0.5% and are likely due to the underlying pathologic condition rather than the surgical approach itself [50, 63]. Appendectomy during pregnancy is not associated with any other developmental delays in children, regardless of which trimester the procedure was performed [76]. The modification of gasless laparoscopy was introduced in 1993 that avoids the effects of carbon dioxide insufflation and high intra-abdominal pressure [77]; however, it provides a much narrow operative field and causes retraction pain [50]. Although gasless and conventional laparoscopic appendectomy have been retrospectively compared and found to be comparable, there have not been any studies specifically conducted in the pregnant population, and as a result, fetal outcomes have not been properly evaluated [78].

Table 10.6 Pros and cons of laparoscopic appendectomy[a]

Pros	Cons
• Early mobilization, rapid postoperative recovery, and early return to normal activities[b] • Decreased postoperative morbidity • Small scars and few incisional hernias • Short or no hospital stay • Low rate of fetal depression due to decreased pain and less narcotic use • Decreased incidence of wound infections • The ability to perform a differential diagnosis in case of negative appendicitis	• Technical difficulty due to the gravid uterus • Possible injury to the pregnant uterus • Potential decrease in uteroplacental blood flow • Risk of CO_2 pneumoperitoneum • A potential risk of fetal exposure to smoke, especially carbon monoxide generated by electrocautery or lasers • A theoretical risk of uterine irritation by the use of electrocautery in the proximity of the uterus • Longer operation times • Higher operation costs • Increased risk of preterm delivery • Increased risk of fetal loss

[a]Adapted from [63, 66, 71]
[b]This is an important advantage due to the relatively higher incidence of thromboembolism in the pregnant patients

Negative Appendectomy

The need for prompt surgical intervention in appendicitis during pregnancy must be balanced with the need for additional diagnostic information, especially advanced imaging (i.e., CT or MRI) to enhance preoperative diagnostic accuracy to avoid unnecessary surgical intervention (i.e., negative appendectomy) [79]. Reported negative appendectomy rates in pregnant women range between 4 and 50%, which is significantly higher compared with nonpregnant women [53, 70, 72, 80, 81]. The diagnostic accuracy in the first trimester is greater than the second and third trimesters [53, 80]. This is important because surgical interventions are not riskless procedures as illustrated by the higher rate of fetal morbidity in negative appendectomies compared to normal pregnancies [70–72, 81]. If there is no appendicitis upon surgical exploration despite the best diagnostic efforts, it is recommended to leave a macroscopically noninflamed appendix in situ, contrary to the recommendations in nonpregnant women [81].

Conclusion

Acute appendicitis in pregnancies remains the most common non-obstetric surgical condition that requires immediate attention. Proper diagnostic work-up includes a thorough physical exam, bloodwork, and diagnostic imaging, which should include abdominal US but may also include CT or MRI. After diagnosis and fluid resuscitation and IV antibiotics have been started, definitive treatment with appendectomy, preferably via laparoscopy, should follow. Appendectomy should only be delayed in case of active labor. Although there may be significant complications to both the patient and the fetus, the diagnosis and treatment of appendicitis in pregnancy continues to improve with better technology, more accurate diagnoses, and better supportive care.

References

1. Dietrich CS 3rd, Hill CC, Hueman M. Surgical diseases presenting in pregnancy. Surg Clin North Am. 2008;88(2):403–19. vii–viii
2. Gilo NB, Amini D, Landy HJ. Appendicitis and cholecystitis in pregnancy. Clin Obstet Gynecol. 2009;52(4):586–96.
3. Flexer SM, Tabib N, Peter MB. Suspected appendicitis in pregnancy. Surgeon. 2014;12(2):82–6.
4. Wei PL, Keller JJ, Liang HH, Lin HC. Acute appendicitis and adverse pregnancy outcomes: a nationwide population-based study. J Gastrointest Surg. 2012;16(6):1204–11.
5. Hee P, Viktrup L. The diagnosis of appendicitis during pregnancy and maternal and fetal outcome after appendectomy. Int J Gynaecol Obstet. 1999;65(2):129–35.
6. Hancock H. Disease of the appendix caeci cured by operation. Lancet. 1848;2:380–2.
7. Easton AL. Acute appendicitis in pregnancy. Postgrad Med J. 1957;33(380):272–7; passim
8. Babler EA. Perforative appendicitis complicating pregnancy. JAMA. 1908;51:1310–3.
9. McGee TM. Acute appendicitis in pregnancy. Aust N Z J Obstet Gynaecol. 1989;29(4):378–85.
10. Gomez A, Wood M. Acute appendicitis during pregnancy. Am J Surg. 1979;137(2):180–3.
11. Abbasi N, Patenaude V, Abenhaim HA. Evaluation of obstetrical and fetal outcomes in pregnancies complicated by acute appendicitis. Arch Gynecol Obstet. 2014;290(4):661–7.
12. Babaknia A, Parsa H, Woodruff JD. Appendicitis during pregnancy. Obstet Gynecol. 1977;50(1):40–4.
13. Weingold AB. Appendicitis in pregnancy. Clin Obstet Gynecol. 1983;26(4):801–9.
14. Cohen-Kerem R, Railton C, Oren D, Lishner M, Koren G. Pregnancy outcome following non-obstetric surgical intervention. Am J Surg. 2005;190(3):467–73.
15. Affleck DG, Handrahan DL, Egger MJ, Price RR. The laparoscopic management of appendicitis and cholelithiasis during pregnancy. Am J Surg. 1999;178(6):523–9.
16. Mazze RI, Kallen B. Appendectomy during pregnancy: a Swedish registry study of 778 cases. Obstet Gynecol. 1991;77(6):835–40.
17. Abbasi N, Patenaude V, Abenhaim HA. Management and outcomes of acute appendicitis in pregnancy-population-based study of over 7000 cases. BJOG. 2014;121(12):1509–14.
18. Acs N, Banhidy F, Czeizel AE. Primary microcephaly in two children born to mothers with complicated appendicitis or late appendectomy during pregnancy. Birth Defects Res A Clin Mol Teratol. 2009;85(7):655–6.
19. Maslovitz S, Gutman G, Lessing JB, Kupferminc MJ, Gamzu R. The significance of clinical signs and blood indices for the diagnosis of appendicitis during pregnancy. Gynecol Obstet Invest. 2003;56(4):188–91.
20. Augustin G, Majerovic M. Non-obstetrical acute abdomen during pregnancy. Eur J Obstet Gynecol Reprod Biol. 2007;131(1):4–12.
21. Ames Castro M, Shipp TD, Castro EE, Ouzounian J, Rao P. The use of helical computed tomography in pregnancy for the diagnosis of acute appendicitis. Am J Obstet Gynecol. 2001;184(5):954–7.
22. Horowitz MD, Gomez GA, Santiesteban R, Burkett G. Acute appendicitis during pregnancy. Diagnosis and management. Arch Surg. 1985;120(12):1362–7.
23. Sharp HT. The acute abdomen during pregnancy. Clin Obstet Gynecol. 2002;45(2):405–13.
24. Wise GJ, Schlegel PN. Sterile pyuria. N Engl J Med. 2015;372(24):2373.
25. Williams R, Mackway-Jones K. Towards evidence based emergency medicine: best BETs from the Manchester Royal Infirmary. White cell count and diagnosing appendicitis in pregnancy. J Accid Emerg Med. 2000;17(5):365.
26. Alvarado A. A practical score for the early diagnosis of acute appendicitis. Ann Emerg Med. 1986;15(5):557–64.
27. Hiersch L, Yogev Y, Ashwal E, From A, Ben-Haroush A, Peled Y. The impact of pregnancy on the accuracy and delay in diagnosis of acute appendicitis. J Matern Fetal Neonatal Med. 2014;27(13):1357–60.
28. Blumenfeld YJ, Wong AE, Jafari A, Barth RA, El-Sayed YY. MR imaging in cases of antenatal suspected appendicitis—a meta-analysis. J Matern Fetal Neonatal Med. 2011;24(3):485–8.
29. Rosen MP, Ding A, Blake MA, Baker ME, Cash BD, Fidler JL, et al. ACR Appropriateness Criteria® right lower quadrant pain—suspected appendicitis. J Am Coll Radiol. 2011;8(11):749–55.
30. Jaffe TA, Miller CM, Merkle EM. Practice patterns in imaging of the pregnant patient with abdominal pain:

a survey of academic centers. AJR Am J Roentgenol. 2007;189(5):1128–34.
31. Katz DS, Klein MA, Ganson G, Hines JJ. Imaging of abdominal pain in pregnancy. Radiol Clin North Am. 2012;50(1):149–71.
32. Drake FT, Kotagal M, Simmons LE, Parr Z, Dighe MK, Flum DR. Single institution and statewide performance of ultrasound in diagnosing appendicitis in pregnancy. J Matern Fetal Neonatal Med. 2015;28(6):727–33.
33. Abramowicz JS. Benefits and risks of ultrasound in pregnancy. Semin Perinatol. 2013;37(5):295–300.
34. Coleman MT, Trianfo VA, Rund DA. Nonobstetric emergencies in pregnancy: trauma and surgical conditions. Am J Obstet Gynecol. 1997;177(3):497–502.
35. Lim HK, Bae SH, Seo GS. Diagnosis of acute appendicitis in pregnant women: value of sonography. AJR Am J Roentgenol. 1992;159(3):539–42.
36. Williams R, Shaw J. Ultrasound scanning in the diagnosis of acute appendicitis in pregnancy. Emerg Med J. 2007;24(5):359–60.
37. Kanal E, Borgstede JP, Barkovich AJ, Bell C, Bradley WG, Felmlee JP, et al. American College of Radiology White Paper on MR Safety. AJR Am J Roentgenol. 2002;178(6):1335–47.
38. Pedrosa I, Levine D, Eyvazzadeh AD, Siewert B, Ngo L, Rofsky NM. MR imaging evaluation of acute appendicitis in pregnancy. Radiology. 2006;238(3):891–9.
39. Pedrosa I, Zeikus EA, Levine D, Rofsky NM. MR imaging of acute right lower quadrant pain in pregnant and nonpregnant patients. Radiographics. 2007;27(3):721–43. discussion 43–53
40. Cobben LP, Groot I, Haans L, Blickman JG, Puylaert J. MRI for clinically suspected appendicitis during pregnancy. AJR Am J Roentgenol. 2004;183(3):671–5.
41. Birchard KR, Brown MA, Hyslop WB, Firat Z, Semelka RC. MRI of acute abdominal and pelvic pain in pregnant patients. AJR Am J Roentgenol. 2005;184(2):452–8.
42. Spalluto LB, Woodfield CA, DeBenedectis CM, Lazarus E. MR imaging evaluation of abdominal pain during pregnancy: appendicitis and other nonobstetric causes. Radiographics. 2012;32(2):317–34.
43. Singh A, Danrad R, Hahn PF, Blake MA, Mueller PR, Novelline RA. MR imaging of the acute abdomen and pelvis: acute appendicitis and beyond. Radiographics. 2007;27(5):1419–31.
44. Beddy P, Keogan MT, Sala E, Griffin N. Magnetic resonance imaging for the evaluation of acute abdominal pain in pregnancy. Semin Ultrasound CT MR. 2010;31(5):433–41.
45. Dewhurst C, Beddy P, Pedrosa I. MRI evaluation of acute appendicitis in pregnancy. J Magn Reson Imaging. 2013;37(3):566–75.
46. Kilpatrick CC, Orejuela FJ. Management of the acute abdomen in pregnancy: a review. Curr Opin Obstet Gynecol. 2008;20(6):534–9.
47. Wallace CA, Petrov MS, Soybel DI, Ferzoco SJ, Ashley SW, Tavakkolizadeh A. Influence of imaging on the negative appendectomy rate in pregnancy. J Gastrointest Surg. 2008;12(1):46–50.
48. Lazarus E, Mayo-Smith WW, Mainiero MB, Spencer PK. CT in the evaluation of nontraumatic abdominal pain in pregnant women. Radiology. 2007;244(3):784–90.
49. Shetty MK, Garrett NM, Carpenter WS, Shah YP, Roberts C. Abdominal computed tomography during pregnancy for suspected appendicitis: a 5-year experience at a maternity hospital. Semin Ultrasound CT MR. 2010;31(1):8–13.
50. Al-Fozan H, Tulandi T. Safety and risks of laparoscopy in pregnancy. Curr Opin Obstet Gynecol. 2002;14(4):375–9.
51. Baer JL, Reis RA, Arens RA. Appendicitis in pregnancy with changes in position and axis of the normal appendix in pregnancy. JAMA. 1932;52:1359–64.
52. de Moya MA, Sideris AC, Choy G, Chang Y, Landman WB, Cropano CM, et al. Appendectomy and pregnancy: gestational age does not affect the position of the incision. Am Surg. 2015;81(3):282–8.
53. Tamir IL, Bongard FS, Klein SR. Acute appendicitis in the pregnant patient. Am J Surg. 1990;160(6):571–5. discussion 5–6
54. Pieper R, Kager L, Weintraub A, Lindberg AA, Nord CE. The role of Bacteroides fragilis in the pathogenesis of acute appendicitis. Acta Chir Scand. 1982;148(1):39–44.
55. Malangoni MA. Gastrointestinal surgery and pregnancy. Gastroenterol Clin North Am. 2003;32(1):181–200.
56. Steer PJ. Has electronic fetal heart rate monitoring made a difference. Semin Fetal Neonatal Med. 2008;13(1):2–7.
57. Sharp HT. Gastrointestinal surgical conditions during pregnancy. Clin Obstet Gynecol. 1994;37(2):306–15.
58. Juhasz-Boss I, Solomayer E, Strik M, Raspe C. Abdominal surgery in pregnancy—an interdisciplinary challenge. Dtsch Arztebl Int. 2014;111(27–28):465–72.
59. Young BC, Hamar BD, Levine D, Roque H. Medical management of ruptured appendicitis in pregnancy. Obstet Gynecol. 2009;114(2 Pt 2):453–6.
60. Liu K, Fogg L. Use of antibiotics alone for treatment of uncomplicated acute appendicitis: a systematic review and meta-analysis. Surgery. 2011;150(4):673–83.
61. Varadhan KK, Neal KR, Lobo DN. Safety and efficacy of antibiotics compared with appendicectomy for treatment of uncomplicated acute appendicitis: meta-analysis of randomised controlled trials. BMJ. 2012;344:e2156.
62. Cheng HT, Wang YC, Lo HC, Su LT, Soh KS, Tzeng CW, et al. Laparoscopic appendectomy versus open appendectomy in pregnancy: a population-based analysis of maternal outcome. Surg Endosc. 2015;29(6):1394–9.
63. Bisharah M, Tulandi T. Laparoscopic surgery in pregnancy. Clin Obstet Gynecol. 2003;46(1):92–7.
64. Upadhyay A, Stanten S, Kazantsev G, Horoupian R, Stanten A. Laparoscopic management of a

nonobstetric emergency in the third trimester of pregnancy. Surg Endosc. 2007;21(8):1344–8.
65. Croce E, Olmi S, Azzola M, Russo R. Laparoscopic appendectomy and minilaparoscopic approach: a retrospective review after 8-years' experience. JSLS. 1999;3(4):285–92.
66. Sauerland S, Jaschinski T, Neugebauer EA. Laparoscopic versus open surgery for suspected appendicitis. Cochrane Database Syst Rev. 2010;(10):Cd001546.
67. Pearl JP, Price RR, Tonkin AE, Richardson WS, Stefanidis D. Guidelines for the use of laparoscopy during pregnancy. Surg Endosc. 2017;31:3767–82.
68. Anderson RE, Pontius GV, Witkowski LJ. A modified technic for the removal of the appendix during pregnancy. Am J Surg. 1957;93(1):117–8.
69. Reedy MB, Kallen B, Kuehl TJ. Laparoscopy during pregnancy: a study of five fetal outcome parameters with use of the Swedish Health Registry. Am J Obstet Gynecol. 1997;177(3):673–9.
70. McGory ML, Zingmond DS, Tillou A, Hiatt JR, Ko CY, Cryer HM. Negative appendectomy in pregnant women is associated with a substantial risk of fetal loss. J Am Coll Surg. 2007;205(4):534–40.
71. Wilasrusmee C, Sukrat B, McEvoy M, Attia J, Thakkinstian A. Systematic review and meta-analysis of safety of laparoscopic versus open appendicectomy for suspected appendicitis in pregnancy. Br J Surg. 2012;99(11):1470–8.
72. Walsh CA, Tang T, Walsh SR. Laparoscopic versus open appendicectomy in pregnancy: a systematic review. Int J Surg (London, England). 2008;6(4):339–44.
73. Gaitan HG, Reveiz L, Farquhar C, Elias VM. Laparoscopy for the management of acute lower abdominal pain in women of childbearing age. Cochrane Database Syst Rev. 2014;(5):Cd007683.
74. Chung JC, Cho GS, Shin EJ, Kim HC, Song OP. Clinical outcomes compared between laparoscopic and open appendectomy in pregnant women. Can J Surg. 2013;56(5):341–6.
75. Cox TC, Huntington CR, Blair LJ, Prasad T, Lincourt AE, Augenstein VA, et al. Laparoscopic appendectomy and cholecystectomy versus open: a study in 1999 pregnant patients. Surg Endosc. 2016;30(2):593–602.
76. Choi JJ, Mustafa R, Lynn ET, Divino CM. Appendectomy during pregnancy: follow-up of progeny. J Am Coll Surg. 2011;213(5):627–32.
77. Smith S, Organ CH Jr. Gasless laparoscopy with conventional instruments: the next phase in minimally invasive surgery. San Francisco, CA: Jeremy Norman Co; 1993.
78. Ge B, Zhao H, Chen Q, Jin W, Liu L, Huang Q. A randomized comparison of gasless laparoscopic appendectomy and conventional laparoscopic appendectomy. World J Emerg Surg. 2014;9(1):3.
79. Aggenbach L, Zeeman GG, Cantineau AE, Gordijn SJ, Hofker HS. Impact of appendicitis during pregnancy: no delay in accurate diagnosis and treatment. Int J Surg (London, England). 2015;15:84–9.
80. Pedrosa I, Lafornara M, Pandharipande PV, Goldsmith JD, Rofsky NM. Pregnant patients suspected of having acute appendicitis: effect of MR imaging on negative laparotomy rate and appendiceal perforation rate. Radiology. 2009;250(3):749–57.
81. Ito K, Ito H, Whang EE, Tavakkolizadeh A. Appendectomy in pregnancy: evaluation of the risks of a negative appendectomy. Am J Surg. 2012;203(2):145–50.
82. Patel SJ, Reede DL, Katz DS, Subramaniam R, Amorosa JK. Imaging the pregnant patient for nonobstetric conditions: algorithms and radiation dose considerations. Radiographics. 2007;27(6):1705–22.
83. Sim JY, Kim HJ, Yeon JW, Suh BS, Kim KH, Ha YR, et al. Added value of ultrasound re-evaluation for patients with equivocal CT findings of acute appendicitis: a preliminary study. Eur Radiol. 2013;23(7):1882–90.
84. Shin I, An C, Lim JS, Kim MJ, Chung YE. T1 bright appendix sign to exclude acute appendicitis in pregnant women. Eur Radiol. 2017;27(8):3310–6.
85. Platon A, Jlassi H, Rutschmann OT, Becker CD, Verdun FR, Gervaz P, et al. Evaluation of a low-dose CT protocol with oral contrast for assessment of acute appendicitis. Eur Radiol. 2009;19(2):446–54.
86. Barloon TJ, Brown BP, Abu-Yousef MM, Warnock N, Berbaum KS. Sonography of acute appendicitis in pregnancy. Abdom Imaging. 1995;20(2):149–51.
87. Basaran A, Basaran M. Diagnosis of acute appendicitis during pregnancy: a systematic review. Obstet Gynecol Surv. 2009;64(7):481–8. quiz 99
88. Puylaert JB, Rutgers PH, Lalisang RI, de Vries BC, van der Werf SD, Dorr JP, et al. A prospective study of ultrasonography in the diagnosis of appendicitis. N Engl J Med. 1987;317(11):666–9.
89. Kurtz GR, Davis RS, Sproul JD. Acute appendicitis in pregnancy and labor, a report of 41 cases. Obstet Gynecol Clin North Am. 1964;23:528–32.

Cholelithiasis, Cholecystitis, and Cholecystodochotomy During Pregnancy

11

Raymond J. Lanzafame

Introduction

The relationship between gallbladder disease and gender, parity, body weight, and other characteristics such as age and ethnicity has long been known and oft repeated as the four (or five) "Fs" of gallstone disease mnemonic recited by medical students for decades [1]. The classic four Fs include "female," "fat," "fertile," and "forty," with "fair" representing a fifth F. This classic demographic is changing as a result of the use of contraceptives, increasing incidence of obesity and type 2 diabetes, and the so-called Western diet, all of which have dramatically reduced the age of incidence to the second and third decades and to nulliparous or primigravida women [1–3].

It is also known that certain ethnic groups including North American Indians, and the Pima in particular, as well as Mexican populations have a higher incidence of gallstones, whereas black Africans consuming a high-fiber diet have a low incidence [1, 2]. It is estimated that 10–15% of the US population has gallstones, including some 14 million women [1, 2]. Approximately 10–20% of patients develop symptoms related to gallstone disease, and 25% of those will develop complications within 10–20 years of diagnosis if they remain untreated [2, 3].

Gallstones can be detected in 1–3.5% of pregnant women, and symptomatic biliary tract disease has been reported to occur in 0.05–8% of pregnancies [2, 4–6]. Acute cholecystitis is the second most frequent non-obstetric cause of an acute abdomen during pregnancy occurring at a frequency of 1–6 per 10,000 pregnancies [2, 4–6]. Acute appendicitis by comparison is the most frequent non-obstetric surgical emergency of pregnancy with an incidence of 1 per 1600 to 1 per 1000 pregnancies [5, 7]. Cholelithiasis accounts for >90% of cases of acute cholecystitis during pregnancy, and approximately 40% of acute cases will require surgery during pregnancy [4–9].

Biliary and Gallbladder Pathophysiology

The gallbladder is a pear-shaped hollow organ that has both sympathetic and parasympathetic innervation. Motor stimulation for contraction of the gallbladder is controlled via the vagus nerve and the celiac ganglion. Pain sensation is relayed via visceral sympathetic fibers [2, 10–12]. The gallbladder primarily functions to concentrate, store, and release bile.

The normally functioning gallbladder reduces hepatic bile volume by 80–90% by the absorption of sodium and water. Sodium trans-

R. J. Lanzafame
School of Dental Medicine, State University of New York at Buffalo, Buffalo, NY, USA

Society of Laparoendoscopic Surgeons, Rochester, NY, USA

C. H. Nezhat (ed.), *Non-Obstetric Surgery During Pregnancy*,
https://doi.org/10.1007/978-3-319-90752-9_11

port is the greatest contributor to the resorption of gallbladder fluid [2, 3, 10]. Evidence suggests that bile normally flows in a continuous fashion and that the gallbladder is continuously emptying to some degree, irrespective of the ingestion of food and cholecystokinin (CCK) release, which are the major stimuli for gallbladder emptying. Duodenal CCK release is stimulated by food, with fat being the most potent stimulator [2, 3, 10, 13]. Motilin, secretin, prostaglandins, histamine, and progesterone also affect gallbladder contraction. Progesterone inhibits gallbladder smooth muscle contraction and impairs the response to CCK stimulation, which reduces gallbladder emptying [2, 3, 8, 13, 14]. It has been proposed that progesterone receptors within the gallbladder increase their binding potential which results in direct inhibition of gallbladder contraction during pregnancy [2, 12, 13]. Rates of gallbladder emptying and contraction are not different between pregnant and nonpregnant women [13]. However, the gallbladder fasting volumes and residual volumes are increased during the second and third trimesters of pregnancy [3, 13, 14]. The fasting gallbladder volume doubles in the second trimester. This reduced gallbladder ejection fraction promotes biliary stasis, which promotes the formation of biliary sludge and gallstones [2, 3, 6–8, 13, 14]. These contractility deficits resolve and normalize within the first week postpartum [2].

Bile is secreted by hepatocytes and is a solution containing organic lipids, electrolytes, and water. Cholesterol, phospholipids, and bile salts comprise 80% of the dry weight of bile, and these, along with bile acids, represent the major lipid components of bile [2, 3]. Biliary cholesterol is synthesized de novo by the liver rather than being a result of absorption of ingested cholesterol. HMG-CoA reductase is the rate-limiting enzyme in the cholesterol production pathway and is inhibited by statins and other drugs used to alter bile composition [2, 3]. Lecithin accounts for >90% of human biliary phospholipids.

The enterohepatic circulation is a highly efficient negative feedback mechanism that regulates the hepatic synthesis of bile acids. Approximately 95% of the bile acid pool synthesized by the liver is actively absorbed in the terminal ileum as conjugated bile acids or is passively reabsorbed in the colon due to colonic bacterial enzymatic dehydroxylation as deoxycholic or lithocholic acid [2, 3].

Cholesterol is insoluble in bile but forms micelles when it is in the presence of a sufficiently high concentration of bile acids. Lecithin incorporated in the micelles allows them to absorb water, swell, and transport greater amounts of cholesterol [2, 3]. Unilamellar cholesterol-phospholipid vesicles account for a significant portion of cholesterol transport and are found in both hepatic and gallbladder bile. Total bile acid and total lipid concentrations and the degree of cholesterol saturation determine the amount of cholesterol that is solubilized in micelles or vesicles. Interference with the equilibrium between vesicles and micelles leads to crystal formation, which subsequently results in the formation of cholesterol gallstones [2, 3, 13, 14].

The mean rate of secretion of biliary lipids is unaltered during pregnancy. However, the rate of secretion of cholesterol increases relative to bile acids and phospholipids during the second and third trimesters, which increases the saturation index of fasting hepatic and gallbladder bile, making them more lithogenic [3, 13]. Weight gain during pregnancy may also increase hepatic cholesterol secretion and increase the cholesterol saturation index. The percentage of chenodeoxycholic acid progressively decreases while cholic acid increases. The rate of chenodeoxycholic acid synthesis decreases linearly during the first 20 weeks of pregnancy [3]. The size of the pool of the major bile acids expands in the first trimester. The fractional turnover rate of the primary bile acids is slower during pregnancy due to altered hepatic metabolism and reduced enterohepatic cycling due to alterations in the biliary-intestinal portion of the system [3].

Pregnancy-induced gallbladder stasis causes bile acid accumulation in the gallbladder lumen, which alters bile salt kinetics and enterohepatic circulation [3, 13]. Gallbladder stasis promotes the formation of biliary sludge and cholesterol gallstones [3, 13, 14]. Ultrasound studies performed immediately postpartum demonstrated the presence of biliary sludge in 25% of cases, which is present in only 4% of cases at 1 year postpartum [14]. Another study noted the presence of biliary sludge in up to 31% of pregnant patients and gallstone formation in 2% of cases [15].

Gallstones in humans are most commonly composed of cholesterol, with pigment stones occurring less frequently [2, 3]. Pigment stones occur in patients with hemolytic disorders or cirrhosis. Gallstones tend to grow for the first 2–3 years of their formation and stabilize in size thereafter, with more than 85% being <2 cm diameter [2, 3].

Cholesterol gallstone formation occurs in stages beginning with the hepatic secretion of cholesterol supersaturated bile, followed by the accelerated nucleation and precipitation of cholesterol monohydrate crystals and agglomeration and growth of cholesterol crystals into gallstones [1–3]. Gallbladder stasis and gallbladder dismotility provide the time required for these processes to occur and progress [3]. It can be readily appreciated that pregnancy induces physiologic changes that influence each of these conditions, thereby promoting the formation of gallstones and biliary sludge.

Biliary Colic and Acute Cholecystitis

Symptomatic cholecystitis with severe episodes of abdominal pain is generally more common during the puerperium and early months postpartum than during pregnancy per se [2, 4–9, 14]. Approximately 40% of patients presenting with symptomatic cholelithiasis during pregnancy will require surgery during pregnancy [2, 4, 5, 7–9, 13–16]. Patients will have a history of biliary colic prior to pregnancy in approximately 50% of the cases [14].

The clinical symptoms and features of biliary colic and acute cholecystitis are similar in both nongravid and pregnant patients. Mid-epigastric and right upper quadrant (RUQ) pain is the most frequent symptom of biliary colic, is present in 60–90% of cases, and is present in more than 95% of cases of acute cholecystitis [2, 4–9, 12–16]. Nausea, vomiting, fatty food intolerance, and bloating may occur but can be associated with other conditions and are less helpful in establishing a diagnosis, occurring in 30–50% of patients [14]. Biliary causes of jaundice account for 5% of patients presenting with jaundice during pregnancy [2, 5, 8, 9, 13, 14].

The differential diagnosis for the gravid patient presenting with RUQ pain includes acute viral hepatitis, acute alcoholic hepatitis, duodenal ulcer, acute pancreatitis, pulmonary embolus, acute myocardial infarction, right lower lobe pneumonia, acute appendicitis, acute fatty liver of pregnancy, preeclampsia, and the HELLP syndrome (i.e., hemolysis, elevated liver enzymes, and low platelets) [2, 4, 5, 7–9, 14–16] (Table 11.1).

RUQ tenderness is the most common physical finding on clinical examination of the gravid patient with severe biliary colic or acute cholecystitis. However, Murphy's sign, which is defined as the inability of a patient to take a deep breath when the RUQ is palpated deeply at the hepatic (costal) margin, is less commonly present in the pregnant patient [2, 4, 5, 7–9, 14–16]. Fever and tachycardia may also be present [2, 4, 5, 7–9, 14–16]. It should be noted that acute appendicitis is more common, occurring 4–5 times more frequently than acute cholecystitis during pregnancy [2, 4, 5, 7, 9, 14–16]. The pain of acute appendicitis may also localize to the right upper quadrant due to upward shifting of the viscera by the gravid uterus, particularly in the latter stages of pregnancy [2, 4, 7, 9, 14–16].

Table 11.1 Differential diagnosis of acute right upper quadrant abdominal pain in pregnancy

Acute appendicitis
Acute fatty liver of pregnancy
Acute viral hepatitis
Acute alcoholic hepatitis
Duodenal ulcer
Acute pancreatitis
Pulmonary embolus
Right lower lobe pneumonia
Myocardial infarction
Preeclampsia
HEELP syndrome (hemolysis, elevated liver enzymes, and low platelets)

Imaging Studies and Diagnostic Testing

Laboratory values are of limited help in establishing a diagnosis, since they tend to be nonspecific. Leukocytosis and elevated alkaline phosphatase levels are seen but are often normally elevated during pregnancy [2, 5, 7–9, 14, 15]. Elevations of bilirubin may indicate the presence of choledocholithiasis, with the caveat that nonbiliary causes of jaundice are much more likely [2, 5, 8, 9, 13, 14]. Elevations of serum amylase or lipase indicate the presence of acute pancreatitis and when coupled with elevations of the serum bilirubin are consistent with a diagnosis of biliary pancreatitis [4, 5, 8, 9, 13–15].

Ultrasonography is the procedure of choice for determining the presence of gallstones in the gravid patient, with a sensitivity >95%. It is also capable of visualizing the pancreas, the intrahepatic and extrahepatic bile ducts, and other structures [2, 4, 7–9, 13–20].

Concerns regarding the effects of ionizing radiation on the developing fetus are understandable, and the decision to undertake diagnostic testing must be weighed carefully. Expeditious and accurate diagnosis, particularly in the evaluation of the acute abdomen, should take precedence over concerns for ionizing radiation [17, 19, 20]. Exposure to <50 milligray (mGy) has not been associated with an increase in fetal anomalies or pregnancy loss [17]. The risk of malformations significantly increases over control only at doses >150 mGy [17]. The cumulative radiation dosage should be limited to 50–100 mGy [17, 19].

CT scan is of limited use in the diagnosis of cholelithiasis but may be useful in the workup of the patient with jaundice. Contemporary multidetector CT protocols deliver a low radiation dose to the fetus and may be used judiciously [19]. Magnetic resonance imaging without the use of intravenous gadolinium is considered to be safe and may be performed at any stage of pregnancy [19].

Radionucleotide imaging may be helpful in the diagnosis of acute cholecystitis by delineating cystic duct obstruction or in ruling out common duct obstruction in the nongravid patient. These techniques are also useful in the workup of postoperative complications such as bile leaks or biliary injuries. The use of these agents is currently considered to generally be safe for mother and fetus [19]. However, the use of these modalities should always be weighed carefully.

Pre- or postoperative ERCP and intraoperative cholangiography have well-defined roles in the diagnosis and treatment of patients with cholelithiasis and suspected choledocholithiasis or other pathologies of the common duct. The lower abdomen should be shielded to decrease fetal radiation exposure and fluoroscopy should be used judiciously [6, 13, 17, 19].

Medical Management of Biliary Colic

The management of biliary colic has traditionally been conservative, with an attempt to delay surgery to the postpartum period [2, 4, 5, 14, 20, 21]. Proponents argue that up to 84% of patients can be successfully managed without surgical intervention for an initial episode of biliary colic [14]. The decision to perform cholecystodochotomy is based on persistent pain, the inability to maintain hydration and oral intake, or the presence of complications such as choledocholithiasis or acute pancreatitis.

This strategy is supported by data demonstrating that 5% of women incur adverse obstetrical outcomes after appendectomy or cholecystodochotomy during pregnancy including cervical incompetence, preterm labor, vaginitis, vulvovaginitis, or sepsis [21]. There is also an elevated risk of low birth weight and intrauterine growth retardation (IUGR) associated with surgery during pregnancy [6, 16]. Others have argued that early surgical intervention and laparoscopic approaches have in fact reduced overall morbidity and maternal and fetal complications, as well as decreasing hospitalization and emergency room visits [6, 16, 19].

The classic features of medical management include the use of analgesics to control discomfort, bed rest, intravenous fluids, and limited or no oral intake [2, 4, 5, 14]. Medications known to cross the placenta are avoided. Nasogastric suction is reserved for cases of severe, uncontrolled emesis. Some advocate the use of antibiotics "to prevent sequelae of acute cholecystitis" [6, 14]. However, this is controversial at best. The patients are followed closely during the course of their pregnancy, and surgery is planned for the postpartum period. Patients failing these measures are referred for surgical intervention.

Surgical Management of Biliary Colic and Acute Cholecystitis

Laparoscopic cholecystodochotomy has become the standard method for elective cholecystodochotomy in the management of cholecystitis and cholelithiasis in the nongravid patient. This procedure can be performed with an acceptably low incidence of complications and morbidity but is certainly capable of resulting in devastating or life-threatening injuries when it is performed improperly. Laparoscopic cholecystodochotomy has similarly become the procedure of choice for cholecystodochotomy during pregnancy with more than 600 successful cases having been reported to date [4, 6–9, 13–16, 19–21].

Advocates for surgery propose early, aggressive surgical therapy in order to reduce high-risk complications and fetal death in particular [6–9, 13–16, 19–21]. The decision to proceed with surgery must be individualized, and close interdisciplinary communication and cooperation between the surgeon, the anesthesiologist, and the obstetrician is essential in order to provide optimal perioperative care. The safety of non-obstetric surgery and anesthesia during pregnancy is well-documented for nearly every operative procedure [21].

The SAGES guidelines on surgery in the pregnant patient [19] have affirmed that this is the procedure of choice, regardless of the trimester of pregnancy. That said, procedures performed in the second trimester procedures are the most common [4, 6–9, 13–21]. Procedures performed during the third trimester are more challenging as a result of the uterine size and the limitations imposed on space within the abdominal cavity.

Surgery is typically performed under general anesthesia. DVT prophylaxis should be implemented and should include the use of pneumatic sequential compression devices [19]. The additional use of heparin is suggested by some authors, although data regarding its additive benefit is lacking [14, 19]. It is noted that heparin does not cross the placenta and pregnancy may predispose the patient to venous thromboembolic disease for a variety of reasons [14]. Early ambulation should be encouraged [19].

Standard noninvasive monitoring is considered to be sufficient for healthy parturients undergoing laparoscopic surgery. Hypoxemia, hypotension, acidosis, hypoventilation, and hyperventilation must be avoided. Pneumoperitoneum during pregnancy results in more pronounced restrictive lung physiology. CO_2 insufflation of 10–15 mmHg can be used safely. Intraoperative CO_2 monitoring by capnography should be used during laparoscopy [14–16, 18–20]. The fetal heart rate and uterine activity should be monitored pre- and postoperatively. There is increased risk of aspiration due to hormonally induced decreased LES tone and mechanical effects of the gravid uterus. Steps should therefore be taken to decompress the stomach. The supine hypotensive syndrome can occur due to aortocaval compression. Patients should be placed in the left lateral decubitus position or rotated and positioned so as to minimize vena cava and pelvic venous compression. Tocolytics should not be used prophylactically but should be considered perioperatively when signs of preterm labor are present [4, 6–9, 13–16, 18–21]. The routine use of prophylactic antibiotics is controversial [4, 6–9, 13–16, 18–21]. There is an argument against the use of prophylactic antibiotics in low-risk biliary surgery based on current guidelines [19]. However, most surgeons opt to give antibiotics since acute cholecystitis and pregnancy increase surgical risk. A plan for open conversion must be understood in advance, and the necessary equipment must be readily available prior to beginning the operation.

Trocar placement should be planned in relation to body habitus, uterine size, fundal height, and the location of any prior incisions. Modified trocar placements relative to the typical locations used in the nongravid patient are usually required in late third trimester in order to avoid injury to or restricted motion due to the presence of the gravid uterus. Initial abdominal access can be safely performed using Hasson (open) trocar, Veress needle, or optical trocar [4, 6, 14, 16, 19]. Many authors prefer the use of open access techniques for initial entry and establishing pneumoperitoneum. However, the Veress needle can be used safely, and initial entry at alternative puncture sites such as Palmer's point (LUQ) or the right upper quadrant (RUQ) can be considered [4, 6, 14, 16, 19]. It is advisable to avoid placing the trocars too low on the abdomen since the uterus will significantly reduce the ability to safely maneuver instruments. The presence of a thick abdominal wall in the obese patient should also be taken into consideration since this will further reduce instrument maneuverability. The right lateral trocar should be positioned below the liver edge at the lateral fat stripe.

The procedure then commences using standard techniques. The gallbladder is grasped and careful traction is applied to lift the gallbladder and expose the infundibulum. The tensely distended or acutely inflamed gallbladder should be decompressed to increase maneuverability. The infundibulum is reflected downward and laterally to expose and open the triangle of Calot. The investing peritoneum is carefully opened and dissected to expose and identify the cystic duct, cystic artery, and the neck of the gallbladder. Use of energy sources should be minimized or avoided in order to reduce potential iatrogenic injuries [22]. Structures should not be ligated or divided until their identity is certain.

The role of intraoperative cholangiography is controversial in cholecystodochotomy and is no less so in the management of cholecystitis and cholelithiasis in the gravid patient. Some authors routinely perform cholangiography on both pregnant and nonpregnant patients [4–6, 13–16, 18, 19]. Cholangiography can be performed safely by shielding the pelvis and with judicious use of fluoroscopy [4, 13, 14, 19]. If the procedure is performed, it is advisable to make a lateral cholecystodochotomy to facilitate placement of the catheter. Any abnormalities should be assessed and managed appropriately. Any injuries or common duct stones are dealt with using sound surgical principles.

Choledocholithiasis may be managed with preoperative ERCP with sphincterotomy followed by lap chole, laparoscopic common bile duct exploration (LCBDE), or postoperative ERCP [6, 13, 14, 19]. Translaparoscopic stone retrieval can be accomplished via the cystic duct or common duct. Conversion to an open procedure is always an acceptable option. The laparoscopist should be capable of using stents, drains, balloons, and other techniques if common duct exploration is contemplated. Lithotripsy with lasers and intraluminal devices is helpful when available. Extracorporeal shockwave lithotripsy (ESWL) is contraindicated during pregnancy. Fluoroscopy and vascular access techniques facilitate instrumentation of the common duct. As has already been noted, the pelvis must be adequately shielded.

The dissection of the gallbladder from the gallbladder bed can be safely accomplished with electrosurgical devices, lasers, the harmonic scalpel, and other energy sources [2, 4, 6, 8–10, 13–16, 19]. Structures should be carefully identified and controlled prior to their division. Injuries due to stray energy are avoided by with careful technique. It is important to remember that many of these devices remain hot for variable periods after they have been deactivated and contact with adjacent structures can result in thermal injuries [22].

Compression of tissues at bleeding sites, irrigation, and frequent aspiration of blood and fluid improves visualization and control during the procedure. Aspiration of the vaporized tissue plume (smoke) is advisable in order to enhance visualization and to reduce maternal and fetal absorption of noxious substances present in the plume [4, 22]. Placement of oxidized regenerated cellulose or other topical hemostatic agents can enhance hemostasis in the liver bed.

Removal of the gallbladder after it has been completely dissected from the liver bed is facilitated by placing the gallbladder on the right lobe surface. A grasper is then inserted under direct vision, and the gallbladder is grasped. The use of a bag or pouch is advisable if the gallbladder is necrotic or if its wall is tenuous. The degree of insufflation is reduced, and the trocar site wound is carefully enlarged. The gallbladder is decompressed as needed. Any loose stones and debris should be removed as can be safely accomplished. The operative area should be irrigated and remaining fluid should be aspirated. The operative site and abdomen should be carefully inspected to verify that hemostasis is good and that there is no evidence of bile staining, injury, or other untoward event.

Perioperative care should focus on managing the patient's discomfort, reducing anxiety, and promoting early ambulation. Preemptive analgesia enhances patient comfort, reduces stays, and reduces complications. Postoperative nausea and vomiting (PONV) can be addressed by pretreatment with metoclopramide and/or ondansetron or other agents approved for use in the gravid patient. Oral analgesics should be started early. The use of NSAIDS such as indomethacin or ketorolac in the gravid patient is controversial, especially in third-trimester patients. Bupivacaine wound infiltration is helpful in reducing trocar site and abdominal wall discomfort [2, 4, 5, 14].

Biliary Pancreatitis

The incidence of acute pancreatitis in pregnancy ranges from 1 in 1066 live births to 1 in 3000 pregnancies [8, 13]. It appears to be more prevalent with advancing gestational age and occurs more commonly in the third trimester and during the postpartum period [8]. Significant maternal morbidity can occur including metabolic disturbances, sepsis, pancreatic necrosis, hypovolemic shock, and the need for intensive care unit admission and care [8, 13]. Acute pancreatitis increases the observed rates of preterm delivery, fetal distress, and fetal demise [13].

The majority of pancreatitis cases occurring during pregnancy are secondary to biliary sludge or gallstones, with alcohol-induced pancreatitis representing the second most common etiology [8, 13]. Conservative management of biliary pancreatitis has a high relapse rate in gravid patients and occurs in as many as 70% of cases [8].

The signs and symptoms of pancreatitis, including severe epigastric pain, are the same in the gravid and nongravid patient. Serum amylase and lipase levels are not normally altered by pregnancy, making the presence of significant elevations of these enzymes diagnostic for pancreatitis [8, 13]. Diagnostic imaging can be accomplished with ultrasound, CT scan, or MRI [13]. CT scan is not recommended for this purpose in pregnancy due to the degree of radiation exposure required and its inability to identify early indicators of necrotizing pancreatitis and since other modalities are available [13]. Endoscopic ultrasound (EUS) can be used under sedation to document the presence of CBD stones and sludge and can be combined with ERCP as both a diagnostic and therapeutic procedure [13]. MRCP is also useful in defining common duct pathology [13]. However, it should be noted that gravid patients with abdominal pain and elevated amylase and lipase do not require imaging in order to confirm a diagnosis of pancreatitis [8, 13].

The initial management of pancreatitis during pregnancy includes fluid resuscitation, nutrition, and pain control, as is generally the case for patients with pancreatitis. Cholecystodochotomy is the treatment of choice in biliary pancreatitis and is generally accomplished once the amylase and lipase levels have normalized with laparoscopic cholecystodochotomy as is described in the preceding section. It is advisable to verify that the common duct is free from stones, sludge, or other abnormalities using cholangiography, choledochoscopy, or ERCP [6–9, 13–16, 19–21]. Patients with severe pancreatitis and those with suspected cholangitis may be managed with ERCP and sphincterotomy to decompress the common duct and remove the obstructing stone or stones [13]. As with the milder case of pancreatitis, a subsequent cholecystodochotomy is performed.

Summary

Cholelithiasis and cholecystitis are common during pregnancy. Biliary sludge is present in 25–30% of pregnant women, and gallstone formation is detectable in 2% of cases. Asymptomatic cholelithiasis occurs in 3.5% of pregnancies. Acute cholecystitis is the second most common non-obstetric surgical emergency of pregnancy with 40% of acute cholecystitis cases requiring surgery. Current recommendations state that pregnant patients with biliary colic have better outcomes and fewer hospitalizations and emergency department visits if they undergo cholecystodochotomy. Patients with biliary pancreatitis during pregnancy should undergo cholecystodochotomy and management of common duct stones with their initial presentation. Laparoscopic cholecystodochotomy appears to be safe in the gravid patient with gallbladder symptoms and is considered to be the procedure of choice in the symptomatic pregnant patient regardless of trimester. The decision to commence, continue, or abort a laparoscopic cholecystodochotomy must be based on sound surgical principles.

References

1. Pak M, Lindseth G. Risk factors for cholelithiasis. Gastroenterol Nurs. 2016;39(4):297–309.
2. Lanzafame RJ. Gallstones and cholecystitis. In: Howard FM, Leppert P, editors. Primary care for women. Philadelphia, PA: Lippincott-Raven; 1997. p. 427–32.
3. Nakayama F. Cholelithiasis causes and treatment. New York: Igaku-Shoin; 1997. 298
4. Lanzafame RJ. Laparoscopic cholecystodochotomy during pregnancy. Surgery. 1995;118(4):627–33.
5. Lanzafame RJ, Barada C. Acute abdominopelvic pain. In: Howard FM, Leppert P, editors. Primary care for women. Philadelphia, PA: Lippincott-Raven; 1997. p. 162–70.
6. Nasioudis D, Tsilimigras D, Economopoulos KP. Laparoscopic cholecystodochotomy during pregnancy: a systematic review of 590 patients. Int J Surg. 2016;27:165–75.
7. Gilo NB, Amini D, Landy HJ. Appendicitis and cholecystitis in pregnancy. Clin Obstet Gynecol. 2009;52(4):586–96.
8. Angelini DJ. Gallbladder and pancreatic disease during pregnancy. J Perinatl Neonat Nurs. 2002;15(4):1–12.
9. Sharp HT. The acute abdomen during pregnancy. Clin Obstet Gynecol. 2002;45(2):405–13.
10. Nahrwold DL. The biliary system. In: Sabiston DC, Lyerly HK, editors. Textbook of surgery: the biological basis of modern surgical practice. 15th ed. Philadelphia, PA: WB Saunders; 1997. p. 1117–25.
11. Nahrwold DL. Chronic cholecystitis and cholelithiasis. In: Sabiston DC, Lyerly HK, editors. Textbook of surgery: the biological basis of modern surgical practice. 15th ed. Philadelphia, PA: WB Saunders; 1997. p. 1132–9.
12. Nahrwold DL. Acute cholecystitis. In: Sabiston DC, Lyerly HK, editors. Textbook of surgery: the biological basis of modern surgical practice. 15th ed. Philadelphia, PA: WB Saunders; 1997. p. 1126–32.
13. Cain MA, Ellis J, Vengrove MA, Wilcox B, Yankowitz J, Smulian JC. Gallstone and severe hypertriglyceride-induced pancreatitis in pregnancy. Obstet Gynecol Surv. 2015;70(9):577–83.
14. Comitalo JB. Laparoscopic cholecystodochotomy during pregnancy. In: Lanzafame RJ, editor. Prevention and management of complications in minimally invasive surgery. New York: Igaku-Shoin; 1996. p. 95–103.
15. Chohan L, Kilpatrick CC. Laparoscopy in pregnancy a literature review. Clin Obstet Gynecol. 2009;52(4):557–69.
16. Sedaghat N, Cao AM, Eslick GD, Cox MR. Laparoscopic versus open cholecystodochotomy in pregnancy a systematic review and meta-analysis. Surg Endosc. 2017;31:673–9.
17. Melnick DM, Wahl WL, Dalton VK. Management of general surgical problems in the pregnant patient. Am J Surg. 2004;187(2):170–80.
18. Kilpatrick CC. Orejuela. Management of the acute abdomen in pregnancy: a review. Curr Opin Obstet Gynecol. 2008;20:534–9.
19. Pearl JP, Price RR, Tonkin AE, Richardson WS, Stefanidis D. Guidelines for the use of laparoscopy during pregnancy. Surg Endosc. 2017;31:3767–82.
20. Kizer NT, Powell MA. Surgery in the pregnant patient. Clin Obstet Gynecol. 2011;54(4):633–41.
21. Sachs A, Guglieminotti J, Miller R, Landau R, Smiley R, Li G. Risk factors and risk stratification for adverse obstetrical outcomes after appendectomy or cholecystodochotomy during pregnancy. JAMA Surg. 2017;152(5):436–41.
22. Lanzafame RJ. Chapter 12: laser energy and minimally invasive surgery. In: Wetter PA, Kavic MS, Nezhat C, Winfield H, editors. Prevention and management of laparoendoscopic surgical complications. 4.0 ed: Society of Laparoendoscopic Surgeons Press, iBooks, www.apple.com; 2012. p. 285–309.

Upper and Lower Endoscopy for Gastrointestinal (GI) Bleeding in Pregnancy

12

Atoosa Rabiee and Baharak Moshiree

Introduction

Each year, more than 12,000 US pregnant women are in need of upper endoscopy, and around 6000 have conditions that may require lower endoscopy for evaluation. Despite this large number of endoscopic procedures performed in the USA in pregnant women, research in this area is limited, and the safety of their performance needs further review. Of note, the spectrum of gastrointestinal disease in the pregnant patient is very similar to that in nonpregnant women, but common causes of gastrointestinal bleeding (GIB) in the acute setting may be different.

In general, gastroenterologists and obstetricians agree that endoscopic procedures during pregnancy should be performed with great caution and with weighing of risks and potential benefits given their risk of maternal hypoxemia and hypotension resulting in harm to the mother as well as fetal hypoxia and even fetal death. This risk involves both the procedure itself and the risk of the actual sedatives required during the various endoscopic procedures as we outline below. Other risks include but are not limited to intrauterine exposure of the fetus to radiation with risk of premature birth, malformations, mutations, and even intrauterine fetal death. Despite the risk of endoscopic procedures, however, there are instances where various endoscopic therapies and procedures are indicated, and these are discussed below and categorized by type of procedure performed by gastroenterologists.

A. Rabiee (✉)
Washington DC VA Medical Center, Washington, DC, USA

B. Moshiree
Department of Gastroenterology, Carolinas Healthcare System, Charlotte, NC, USA
e-mail: baha.moshiree@carolinashealthcare.org

Indications by Procedure

Upper Endoscopy

The most common indications for an endoscopic gastroduodenoscopy (EGD) of the upper GI tract in pregnant patients include GI hemorrhage, dysphagia, and refractory nausea and vomiting (hyperemesis gravidarum or gastroparesis). In fact, over 12,000 pregnant women in the USA present annually with complaints that have an indication for upper endoscopy [1]. An ASGE survey in 1986 studied 73 endoscopies in pregnant patients with the most common indication being nausea and vomiting in 56% of cases with finding of esophagitis in 34% of cases. Among patients who presented with the indication of upper GI bleeding, the most common findings were esophagitis, followed by Mallory-Weiss tear, a tear in the mucous membrane of the esophagus, and ulcers of various locations [2].

C. H. Nezhat (ed.), *Non-Obstetric Surgery During Pregnancy*,
https://doi.org/10.1007/978-3-319-90752-9_12

The causes of GI bleeding may be different in pregnant versus nonpregnant females. In one population-based study of non-variceal upper GI bleeding (NVUGIB), for example, 1210 pregnant women and 6050 nonpregnant patients were identified who had upper endoscopy performed. The most common cause of NVUGIB was found to be a Mallory-Weiss tear in pregnant patients; however, peptic ulcer disease (PUD) and gastritis were more commonly seen in nonpregnant patients [3]. The proportion of upper endoscopic procedures that led to therapeutic intervention was similar for pregnant and nonpregnant women (8.9% vs. 7.2%). In this study, the frequency of maternal mortality and fetal loss was <1%. The authors concluded that given the self-limiting nature of Mallory-Weiss tears with often spontaneous healing and such low rates of necessary therapeutic intervention, perhaps endoscopy can be deferred in most patients who were hemodynamically stable and with self-limited NVUGIB.

The case may be different however for variceal GIB. Although cirrhotic women are less likely to become pregnant, the exact incidence is not known, and in rare cases of GIB, an upper endoscopy should be performed given a high mortality associated with variceal bleeding. Women with non-cirrhotic portal hypertension have normal fertility and will have 45% incidence of variceal bleed during pregnancy with 18–50% associated mortality. Variceal bleeding in this setting typically occurs in the second or third trimester. This could be attributed to increased fluid retention and cardiac output in pregnancy. Given the risk associated with variceal bleeding in cirrhotic women during pregnancy, and mortality associated with such bleed, the benefits of screening and preemptive intervention outweigh the risk. Timing of screening for esophageal varices appears to be best in the second trimester [4].

Complications related to performance of upper endoscopy in pregnant women have been explored in a study of 83 women with follow-up of fetal outcomes [5]. The mean gestational week when endoscopy was performed was 19.8 ± 8.9. Despite the early performance of upper endoscopy, no significant immediate complications were seen in the patients. Ninety-five percent of patients went on to deliver healthy babies, with four poor outcomes recorded; however, none of these poor outcomes (three stillbirths and one abortion) were related to upper endoscopy performance. Nine of the infants had low birth weight, but this was not significantly higher than the national control rates. Mean Apgar score was also similar to the national control groups. No congenital malformations were reported in any of the infants. Diagnostic yield of upper endoscopy in these patients approached 95% for acute GI bleeding and ranged from 50% to 82% for the other indications.

The safety of upper endoscopy in the first trimester has been demonstrated when looking at other retrospective studies of 60 pregnant patients who underwent upper endoscopy showing no significant difference in gestational age at delivery, fetal weight, and mean Apgar score. No fetal malformations were observed [6]. Although performance of the upper endoscopy was useful for treatment of upper GIB, for those with indications of nausea, vomiting, or suspected hyperemesis gravidarum, the endoscopic findings did not change the treatment. Despite the low risk associated with performance of upper endoscopy in pregnant patients, we propose holding its performance until after delivery in those patients with nausea, vomiting, and abdominal pain as predominant symptoms and reserving its performance for those with upper GIB and hemodynamic instability who would benefit most from endoscopic therapies as mentioned above.

Procedure Description

Once the above considerations are first discussed with the patient and their obstetrician, an upper endoscopy can be performed with cautious use of the minimal amount of sedation necessary and with monitoring of the fetus throughout the procedure. An upper gastrointestinal endoscopy (esophagogastroduodenoscopy, EGD) involves the visualization and assessment of the oropharynx, esophagus, stomach, and proximal duodenum, with interpretation of the findings for purposes mainly of diagnosing the cause of gastrointestinal bleeding in a pregnant patient. An appropriate patient selection as discussed above is paramount to performance of the upper endoscopy with clear indications for this procedure outlined by the American Society for Gastrointestinal Endoscopy (ASGE) (2012) [7]. In general, an upper endoscopy is indicated if the results cannot be otherwise obtained by less invasive methods such as radiographic evaluation or if a therapeutic strategy is needed to treat a patient's condition, for example, in case of coagulation in a patient with GI bleeding. If results do not alter management decisions, then an upper endoscopy is not warranted. Once the decision is made to perform an upper endoscopy, considerations for patient preparation are made, and these include diet (no solid food until 4 h prior and no clear liquids up to 2 h prior to testing) [8]. Most other medications can be continued up to the time of the endoscopy with small sips of water. No other routine preprocedure testing is required unless the patient is taking anticoagulation. Hemoglobin or hematocrit should be checked if the patient is having bleeding with appropriate coagulation studies. Appropriate sedation management in the pregnant patient also will include evaluation of the airway to make sure the airway is not difficult to manage (i.e., the uvula is visible) or that airway obstruction is not a risk due to patients' obesity. Prior to the procedure, a topical pharyngeal anesthesia may be applied with an agent such as benzocaine spray. Patients are typically placed on their left side with the neck flexed forward [9]. The endoscope is then passed from the mouth above the tongue with limited visualization of the oropharynx and then above the hypopharynx. The endoscopist can often view the epiglottis, the vocal cords, both the piriform sinuses, and the arytenoid cartilages, but that is not a part of the usual upper endoscopy. Once these are visualized, the endoscopist makes sure not to intubate the trachea and enters posterior at the piriform sinuses into the upper esophageal sphincter with the use of air insufflation from the endoscope and with use of mild pressure. The rest of the upper GI tract, the esophagogastric junction, the stomach, and the duodenum are all visualized using air insufflation and visual inspection with the endoscope. Photographs of any abnormal findings such as a diverticulum, hernia, tumor, or polyp can be made during the procedure. To better inspect the proximal portion of the stomach called the cardia and fundus, the scope is retroflexed by the endoscopist during the procedure. Rotation of the endoscope and forward and backward movements allow for visualization of different segments of the upper GI tract including the pylorus, incisura, antrum, and duodenal bulb. These are all areas where ulcers or erosions may be seen. If a biopsy is needed, it is obtained through the accessory channel located on the endoscope and advance to the lesion; then a pinch biopsy is obtained using the forceps.

Therapeutic Endoscopy

Endoscopic hemostatic techniques for non-variceal hemorrhage include injection (epinephrine, sclerosing agents), ablation (electrocoagulation, thermocoagulation, photocoagulation, or argon plasma), and compression (hemoclips, snares, graspers, or sutures). In the few reports available regarding safety of these techniques in pregnancy, all patients had successful outcomes except one patient who had to undergo surgery due to ongoing GIB. Fetal outcomes were all favorable without any malformation or fetal deaths reported [5, 6, 10, 11]. Of note, each therapeutic technique is chosen from expert opinion based on studies in nonpregnant patients. Data is not available for all therapeutic techniques in the pregnant population.

Epinephrine

Epinephrine is considered safe although it is a category C medication and may theoretically cause a decrease in uterine blood flow through its vasoconstricting effects. However, no adverse events have been reported to date with the use of epinephrine in pregnancy [12, 13].

Thermoablation

In terms of thermoablation techniques, the potential risk includes the electrical current conducting through amniotic fluid to the fetus [14]. Proposed techniques are to place a grounding pad in a way that the uterus is not located between the electrical catheter and the pad. Bipolar cautery should be used as much as possible. Although electrocautery is relatively safe when used for sphincterotomy and hemostasis, in cases of polyp removal, this should be postponed until after delivery.

Band Ligation

Although the data for pregnant patients with variceal GIB is very limited, prophylactic band ligation is generally thought of as safe during pregnancy. When bleeding cannot be stopped in cirrhotic patients post-band ligation, transjugular intrahepatic portosystemic shunt (TIPS) is indicated [15–20].

This procedure allows for creation of a connection between the hepatic vein and the intrahepatic portal vein which would allow blood to flow from portal vein to the inferior vena cava and back to systemic circulation with little resistance. These procedures are high risk and performed only in tertiary care settings, and given their rare occurrence in pregnancy, no conclusions can be made as far as their efficacy and safety.

Sigmoidoscopy and Colonoscopy

Although upper endoscopies appear to be fairly safe during pregnancy, colonoscopies and sigmoidoscopies may lead to potential harm to the fetus. More than 6000 pregnant women have conditions requiring colonoscopy per year in the USA [1].

In a study of 46 patients, 48 sigmoidoscopies and 8 colonoscopies were done during pregnancy. Of these, 18 patients were in their second trimester (N = 18), 13 patients in their first trimester, and 15 in their third trimester. Ninety-three percent of these patients delivered healthy babies, but there were four voluntary abortions and one unknown outcome. Mean Apgar scores were not significantly different from controls. Although fetal demise occurred in the high-risk pregnancies, this was not related to the performance of sigmoidoscopy or colonoscopy [10]. Sigmoidoscopy was diagnostic in 59% of 46 patients, specifically when the reason for its performance was lower gastrointestinal bleeding (hematochezia). Among 17 patients undergoing sigmoidoscopy for other indications, diagnoses included ulcerative colitis (2), non-specific colitis/proctitis (2), and postsurgical anastomotic ulcer (1).

Similarly, another retrospective study of 20 pregnant patients who underwent colonoscopy also showed no evidence of fetal distress during colonoscopy as assessed by fetal heart rate monitoring, and patients even had similar or lower rates of unfavorable outcomes than healthy controls [10].

In a more recent study, 42 pregnant patients with inflammatory bowel disease underwent lower GI endoscopies. Two spontaneous abortions were found and were temporally related to endoscopy; however, the rates of spontaneous abortion were not more frequent than in controls. Median birth weight was significantly lower in patients with IBD than in controls, but no significant difference in terms of gestational age at birth, congenital malformation, or Apgar score was observed [21].

Overall lower endoscopy, specifically sigmoidoscopy, can be safely performed in pregnant patients. However, the procedure should be limited to patients with appropriate indications such as hematochezia or significant diarrhea or abdominal pain. The procedure should be deferred for elective indications such as change in bowel habits or colon cancer screening.

Procedure Description

If a colonoscopy or sigmoidoscopy needs to be performed in a pregnant patient for evaluation of ongoing and significant diarrhea with weight loss, abdominal pain without other etiology found, or hematochezia, several considerations should be made first. The joint American Society for Gastrointestinal Endoscopy/American College of Gastroenterology Taskforce on Quality in Endoscopy has advocated several quality indicators before, after, and during a colonoscopy. In summary some of these include adequate patient preparation with a laxative prior to the procedure for purposes of adequate visualization of the mucosa examined; adequate assessment of sedation as with upper endoscopy above, bleeding risk assessment, and a detailed review of risks and benefits; and adequate skills including with withdrawal time, documentation, and assessments post-procedure [22–24]. Several validated scoring systems can be used to assess the adequacy of the preparation. Adequate preparation means no fiber or high residue diet (only clears) the day prior to endoscopy and several laxatives that are administered to obtain a clear stool. Patients cannot eat for 4–8 h prior to the procedure. The same recommendations are made with regard to medications, sedation issues, and laboratory data prior to performing the procedure. One option for sedation for colonoscopy and sigmoidoscopy which is unique to lower endoscopy may be no sedation if this can be tolerated by the patient as it does provide for less risk to the fetus. In most cases, either moderate or deep sedation is necessary to complete the procedure.

The colonoscope and sigmoidoscopic procedures involve a high-definition white-light colonoscope, usually with a diameter of 11 mm, which is flexible and has variable stiffness. The scope is then advanced with the patient in the left lateral decubitus position, unless the patient has an ostomy or a postsurgical anatomy, and is advanced into the anal canal after a digital rectal examination. A standard gel lubricant can be used for examination of the perianal region and digital examination. The tip of the colonoscope is then inserted into the rectum with air insufflation, suctioning of residual fluid, and pulling back of the colonoscope to enable visualization. An insertion and withdrawal method is used to advance through the rectum to the sigmoid, descending, transverse, ascending colon and then cecum and even the terminal ileum. Several techniques are used to advance the scope including turning the knobs left and right while filling the colon with either air or water for insufflation and better visualization, aspirations of air and fluid, and further intubation with stiffening of the colonoscope. Typical maneuvers used in the nonpregnant patient such as changing patient's position to prone positioning and use of abdominal pressure should *not* be performed in the pregnant patient given the obvious risks to the fetus with increased abdominal tension. Minimal air insufflation should be done to adequately examine the mucosa for any abnormalities that may lead to patient's bleeding. Excessive air insufflation could result in patient discomfort with need for more sedation which is not optimal in this patient setting.

One known risk of colonoscopy is the risk of perforation which occurs in varying rates of 0.01–0.1% for screening, not diagnostic colonoscopy as what would be done in this setting.

If perforation is suspected in a patient with severe abdominal pain or fevers after the procedure or during the procedure, an immediate abdominal radiograph (plain and upright or lateral decubitus) and an upright chest radiograph should be obtained [25]. If plain films are normal but there is a high suspicion of perforation, an abdominopelvic computed tomography scan with water-soluble contrast should be obtained. All patients with perforations should receive intravenous fluids and broad spectrum antibiotics. Although some perforation can be repaired endoscopically, many patients with perforations will require surgery; therefore, colonoscopy and flexible sigmoidoscopy should only be done in the pregnant patient if absolute indications as noted above exist and not for screening purposes.

Endoscopic Retrograde Cholangiopancreatography

Endoscopic retrograde cholangiopancreatography (ERCP) is a therapeutic and diagnostic procedure performed most commonly in pregnant patients for suspected cholangitis when a gallstone is suspected to be obstructing the bile duct. Indications of ERCP include biliary pancreatitis, choledocholithiasis, and cholangitis which can themselves lead to fetal demise if left untreated.

This procedure normally carries more risk even in the nonpregnant individual with risk of pancreatitis seen in 3–5%, bleeding risk of 2%, and perforation risk of less than 1%. ERCP is not uncommonly done in pregnant patients. In one study of 23 pregnant patients who had 29 ERCPs, most of which were done in the first trimester ($N = 15$), investigators found pancreatitis in one patient, spontaneous abortion in another patient (3 months post-ERCP), and one neonatal death with no apparent causal relationship to ERCP. Authors concluded that diagnostic and therapeutic ERCP can be done in a reasonably safe and effective way in pregnancy [26].

Radiation exposure to the fetus given the need to use fluoroscopy with ERCP performance is another risk of ERCP which is often used as the reason for delay of procedure unless it is absolutely indicated. In 1 study of 17 ERCPs in pregnant patients, the mean fluoroscopy time was 14 s. Estimated fetal radiation exposure was 40 mrad. Complications included post-sphincterotomy bleed in one patient and post-ERCP pancreatitis in another patient. Two women developed third trimester preeclampsia, in both of which labor had to be subsequently induced [27]. Radiation remains a major concern during ERCPs, and exposure depends on patient body size, gestational age, and exposure technique [28]. Although external shielding is common practice, a majority of radiation exposure still affects the pregnant patient. The most effective way is to reduce fluoroscopy time and overall radiation exposure as well as collimating the beam to the area of interest.

A larger study of 65 pregnant patients undergoing 68 ERCPs with median fluoroscopy time of 1.45 min showed no procedure related to maternal or fetal death. Post-ERCP pancreatitis was diagnosed in 11 patients. Almost 90% of patients carried to term, with patients having ERCP in their first trimester with lowest percentage of term pregnancy (73.3%) and highest risk of preterm delivery and low birth weight. None of these patients had spontaneous fetal loss, perinatal death, stillbirth, or malformation [29].

ERCP can also be done without use of fluoroscopy and by using wire-guided cannulation technique. Cannulation then can be confirmed by bile aspiration or visualization of bile around the guidewire [30–32]. If possible, ERCP should be performed after the first trimester when organogenesis is complete. It is also important that an experienced advanced endoscopist performs the procedure with consultation from an obstetrician.

Procedure Description

ERCP is a technically advanced endoscopic procedure which requires advanced training by a gastroenterologist or surgeon. A specialized side-viewing upper endoscope is guided through the oropharynx and into the esophagus, stomach, and then the duodenum, allowing for examination of the bile and pancreatic ducts. A contrast medium is utilized in visualizing the anatomy of the bile ducts using radiologic visualization and for purposes of therapies such as stone removal and dilation of the small-sized bile ducts using balloons and other specialized instruments [33]. As noted above, the considerations for an ERCP are few in the pregnant patient. Similar considerations with regard to preparation, diet and patient assessment should be performed prior to the procedure much like with upper endoscopy; however, patients having an ERCP may require more sedation.

Most ERCP complications are apparent during the first 6 h after the procedure; therefore, post-procedure recovery of patients is paramount in ensuring lack of adverse post-procedure events such as post-ERCP pancreatitis, bleeding, sepsis, or perforation and for continued monitoring of the fetus [34, 35]. Other causes of abdominal pain following ERCP include discomfort due to air insufflation and perforation.

Differentiating pain due to air insufflation versus post-ERCP pancreatitis can be difficult especially as even the pancreatic enzymes are often elevated in a majority of patients without post-ERCP pancreatitis. In general, if the serum lipase is less than three times the upper limit of normal, pancreatitis is unlikely (specificity of 85–98%). However, although immediately after the ERCP pancreatic enzyme levels may be elevated, if suspicion for pancreatitis is high, amylase and lipase should be repeated after at least 4 h post-procedure for adequate diagnosis of acute post-procedure pancreatitis [36].

Medications Used for Sedation During Endoscopic Procedures

Narcotics for Sedation

Category B and C medications can be used during endoscopic procedures to provide sedation. Meperidine is considered a category B medication and is a preferred medication over morphine which is category C during pregnancy. Meperidine however has been associated with loss of fetal beat-to-beat cardiac variability, but this finding is not associated with fetal distress [37, 38]. Another class of narcotics, fentanyl, is also considered category C and is embryocidal in rats [39] and therefore is seldom used in the pregnant population. Overall, meperidine is preferred over fentanyl and morphine in pregnant patients undergoing endoscopy.

Benzodiazepines

The preferred benzodiazepine in pregnancy is midazolam, and its use has not been associated with congenital anomalies. If possible, midazolam should be avoided in the first trimester due to concern for congenital malformations [1]. Diazepam is a long-acting benzodiazepine and should not be used for sedation in pregnant patients due to its association with cleft palate and neurobehavioral disorders [40–42].

Barbiturate-Like Sedatives

Propofol is a short-acting barbiturate-like agent used for general anesthesia and procedural sedation such as during ERCPs and can be administered by a trained anesthesia provider given its narrow therapeutic index and need for close monitoring. Safety in the first trimester is not well studied [43]. Propofol use is associated with nausea, cough, burning in IV site, skin rash, numbness or tingling, agitation/anxiety, and muscle pain in the general population.

Topical Anesthesia

Topical anesthetics such as lidocaine can be used to decrease gag reflex during an upper endoscopy, and this is considered a category B medication. No fetal malformations have been associated with its use in the first trimester [39].

Overall, none of the above currently used anesthetic agents in standard concentrations at any gestational age have been associated with any teratogenic effect in humans [44].

Colonic Preparation

A common colonic preparation given prior to colonoscopic evaluations is polyethylene glycol which is an osmotic laxative. Polyethylene glycol solutions are considered category C in pregnancy. Sodium phosphate preparations are also considered category C but should be used with great caution due to the potential fluid and electrolyte abnormality [45]. We advocate use of PEG formulation in pregnant patients who need to undergo lower endoscopy.

Proton Pump Inhibitors

Fetal safety of proton pump inhibitors has been studied in pregnancy. In a large meta-analysis [46], a total of 1530 exposed patients were compared to 133,410 not exposed pregnancies. There was no increased risk for major congenital birth defect, spontaneous abortion, or preterm labor. In another nationwide cohort study of 840,968 live births with 5082 infants exposed to PPI during pregnancy, there was no significant association between the use of PPI in the first trimester and major birth defects. There was also no significant association between the use of any specific PPI and the risk of birth defect. This study followed the children for 1 year after birth [47]. These results provide reassurance that PPIs can be safely used during pregnancy for reflux symptoms or peptic ulcer disease.

Summary and Recommendations

Risks of upper and lower endoscopy and ERCP have to be weighed against their benefit; however, in general, based on the body of existing evidence in pregnant patients, upper endoscopies are relatively safe during pregnancy. If these procedure can be delayed until after delivery, we often propose that they should be. In case of ERCPs, given risk of post-ERCP pancreatitis and radiation exposure to the fetus, these should only be done during pregnancy when therapeutic intervention is indicated and not for diagnostic purposes. Otherwise, this can be done after delivery.

Due to lack of evidence in the pregnant population and based on ASGE guidelines, endoscopy should be deferred to the second trimester and in those with strong indications after a careful assessment of risk versus benefits. Only patients with the greatest therapeutic benefit should have endoscopy performed, and in those with hemodynamic stability and GIB, perhaps watchful waiting may be optimal given the most common causes of UGIB are Mallory-Weiss tear and PUD. Decision to monitor fetal heart rate and uterine contractions should be made with an obstetrician and would depend on gestational age [48].

In a recent study, 1,592,225 pregnancies in 1,002,604 women, 0.19% (3052) were exposed to endoscopy during pregnancy (upper 2025, lower 1109, ERCP 58). Any endoscopic procedure during pregnancy was associated with increased risk of preterm labor or small for gestational age. There was no increase in congenital malformation or stillbirth. These results were independent of trimester of pregnancy. Restricting the data to women without a diagnosis of IBD, celiac disease, or liver disease, endoscopy during pregnancy was not associated with preterm birth. This nationwide population-based cohort study showed that the risk of endoscopy during pregnancy was small and likely due to intra-familial or disease activity [49].

A few suggestions have been made regarding patient positioning during anesthesia and other pulmonary risks related to their positioning. Patients in the second or third trimester should not be positioned on their back before, during, or after the procedure to avoid maternal hypotension and decreased placental perfusion. There is also higher chance of aspiration in pregnant patients compared to nonpregnant controls; therefore, patients should be strictly NPO for at least 6 h prior to endoscopy.

Based on guidelines from gastrointestinal endoscopy (GIE) [50], endoscopists should always have a strong indication when proceeding to endoscopy. Endoscopy should be postponed to the second trimester if at all possible when the organogenesis is complete. When sedation is needed, the lowest effective dose of sedative medication should be used. Procedure time should be very short to minimize sedation exposure and aspiration. To avoid vena caval or aortic compression, pregnant women should be positioned in left pelvic tilt or left lateral position. Fetal heartbeat should be detected before sedation as well as after the endoscopic procedure. Obstetric support should be available whenever pregnancy-related complications occur. Placenta abruption, imminent delivery, ruptured membranes, and eclampsia are defined as obstetric complications of endoscopy; however, these are not seen commonly and may be theoretical risks.

When adherence to above risk assessments is made, however, any of the endoscopic procedures are safe for the fetus and the mother with positive outcomes that outweigh risks of the procedures. Finally, endoscopy remains an important diagnostic and therapeutic procedure for evaluation of gastrointestinal symptoms in pregnant patients. Overall, endoscopy appears to be safe, especially if performed after the first trimester. The presence of an experienced endoscopist working closely with the patient's obstetrician is of utmost importance.

References

1. Cappell MS. The fetal safety and clinical efficacy of gastrointestinal endoscopy during pregnancy. Gastroenterol Clin N Am. 2003;32(1):123–79.
2. Rustgi VK, Cooper JN, Colcher H. Gastrointestinal and hepatic complications in pregnancy. New York: Churchill Livingstone; 1986. p. 104–23.
3. Nguyen GC, Dinani AM, Pivovarov K. Endoscopic management and outcomes of pregnant women hos-

pitalized for nonvariceal upper GI bleeding: a nationwide analysis. Gastrointest Endosc. 2010;72:954–9.
4. Tran TT, Ahn J, Reau NS. ACG clinical guideline: liver disease and pregnancy. Am J Gastroenterol. 2016;111(2):176–94.
5. Cappell MS, Colon VJ, Sidhom OA. A study of eight medical centers of the safety and clinical efficacy of esophagogastroduodenoscopy in 83 pregnant females with follow-up of fetal outcome with comparison control groups. Am J Gastroenterol. 1996;91(2):348–54.
6. Debby A, Golan A, Sadan O, Glezerman M, Shirin H. Clinical utility of esophagogastroduodenoscopy in the management of recurrent and interactable vomiting in pregnancy. J Reprod Med. 2008;53(5):347–51.
7. ASGE Standards of Practice Committee, Early DS, Ben-Menachem T, Decker GA, Evans JA, Fanelli RD, et al. Appropriate use of GI endoscopy. Gastrointest Endosc. 2012;75:1127.
8. American Society of Anesthesiologists Committee. Practice guidelines for preoperative fasting and the use of pharmacologic agents to reduce the risk of pulmonary aspiration: application to healthy patients undergoing elective procedures: an updated report by the American Society of Anesthesiologists Committee on Standards and Practice Parameters. Anesthesiology. 2011;114:495.
9. Faigel DO, Eisen GM, Baron TH, Dominitz JA, Goldstein JL, Hirota WK, et al. Preparation of patients for GI endoscopy. Gastrointest Endosc. 2003;57:446.
10. Cappell MS, Fox SR, Gorrepati N. Safety and efficacy of colonoscopy during pregnancy: an analysis of pregnancy outcome in 20 patients. J Reprod Med. 2010;55(3–4):115–23.
11. Brunner C, Meyer H, Athmann C. Omeprazole for peptic ulcer disease in pregnancy. Digestion. 1998;59(6):651–4.
12. Bruno JM, Kroser J. Efficacy and safety of upper endoscopy procedures during pregnancy. Gastrointest Endosc Clin N Am. 2006;16(1):33–40.
13. Marcus MA, Vertommen JD, Van Aken H, Wouters PF. Hemodynamic effects of intravenous isoproterenol versus epinephrine in the chronic maternal-fetal sheep preparation. Anesth Analg. 1996;82(5):1023–6.
14. Einarson A, Bailey B, Inocencion G. Accidental electric shock in pregnancy: a prospective cohort study. Am J Obstet Gynecol. 1997;176(3):678–81.
15. Russell MA, Craigo SD. Cirrhosis and portal hypertension in pregnancy. Semin Perinatol. 1998;22(2):156–65.
16. Lodato F, Cappelli A, Montagnani M, Colecchia A, Festi D, Azzaroli F, et al. Transjugular intrahepatic portosystemic shunt: a case report of rescue management of unrestrainable variceal bleeding in a pregnant woman. Dig Liver Dis. 2008;40(5):387–90.
17. Starkel P, Horsmans Y, Geubel A. Endoscopic band ligation: a safe technique to control bleeding esophageal varices in pregnancy. Gastrointest Endosc. 1998;48(2):212–4.
18. Dhiman RK, Biswas R, Aggarwal N, Sawhney H, Chawla Y. Management of variceal bleeding in pregnancy with endoscopic variceal ligation and N-butyl-2-cyanoacrylate: a report of three cases. Gastrointest Endosc. 2000;51(1):91–3.
19. Iwase H, Morise K, Kawase T, Horiuchi Y. Endoscopic injection sclerotherapy for esophageal varices during pregnancy. J Clin Gastroenterol. 1994;18(1):80–3.
20. Ghidirim G, Mishin I, Dolghii A, Lupashcu A. Prophylactic endoscopic band ligation of esophageal varices during pregnancy. J Gastrointestin Liver Dis. 2008;17(2):236–7.
21. De Lima A, Zelinkova Z, van der Woude CJ. A prospective study of the safety of lower gastrointestinal endoscopy during pregnancy in patients with inflammatory bowel disease. J Crohns Colitis. 2015;9(7):519–24.
22. Rex DK, Schoenfeld PS, Cohen J, Pike IM, Adler DG, Fennerty MB, et al. Quality indicators for colonoscopy. Gastrointest Endosc. 2015;81:31.
23. Appropriate use of gastrointestinal endoscopy. American Society for Gastrointestinal Endoscopy. Gastrointest Endosc. 2000;52:831.
24. Williams JE, Faigel DO. Colonoscopy reports and current state of performance measures. Gastrointest Endosc Clin N Am. 2010;20:685.
25. ASGE Standards of Practice Committee, Fisher DA, Maple JT, Ben-Menachem T, Cash BD, Decker GA, et al. Complications of colonoscopy. Gastrointest Endosc. 2011;74:745.
26. Jamider PA, Beck GJ, Hoffman BJ, Lehman GA, Hawes RH, Agrawal RM, et al. Endoscopic retrograde cholangiopancreatography in pregnancy. Am J Gastroenterol. 1995;90(8):1263–7.
27. Kahaleh M, Hartwell GD, Arseneau KO, Pajewski TN, Mullick T, Isin G, et al. Safety and efficacy of ERCP in pregnancy. Gastrointest Endosc. 2004;60(2):287–92.
28. Samara ET, Stratakis J, Enele Melono JM, Mouzas IA, Perisinakis K, Damilakis J. Therapeutic ERCP and pregnancy: is the radiation risk for conceptus trivial? Gastrointest Endosc. 2009;69(4):824–31.
29. Tang SJ, Mayo MJ, Rodriguez-Frias E, Armstrong L, Tang L, Sreenarasimhaiah J, et al. Safety and utility of ERCP during pregnancy. Gastroitest Endosc. 2009;69(3 Pt 1):453–61.
30. Akcakaya A, Ozkan OV, Okan I, Kocaman O, Sahin M. Endoscopic retrograde cholangiopancreatography during pregnancy without radiation. World J Gastroenterol. 2009;15(29):3649–52.
31. Shelton J, Linder JD, Rivera-Alsina ME, Tarnasky PR. Commitment, confirmation, and clearance: new techniques for nonradiation ERCP during pregnancy (with videos). Gastrointest Endosc. 2008;67(2):364–8.
32. Chong VH, Jalihal A. Endoscopic management of biliary disorders during pregnancy. Hepatobiliary Pancreat Dis Int. 2010;9(2):180–5.
33. ASGE Standards of Practice Committee, Chandrasekhara V, Khashab MA, Muthusamy VR, Acosta RD, Agrawal D, et al. Adverse events associated with ERCP. Gastrointest Endosc. 2017;85:32.
34. Rabenstein T, Schneider HT, Nicklas M, Ruppert T, Katalinic A, Hahn EG, et al. Impact of skill and

experience of the endoscopist on the outcome of endoscopic sphincterotomy techniques. Gastrointest Endosc. 1999;50:628.

35. Freeman ML, Nelson DB, Sherman S, Haber GB, Herman ME, Dorsher PJ, et al. Complications of endoscopic biliary sphincterotomy. N Engl J Med. 1996;335:909.
36. Pieper-Bigelow C, Strocchi A, Levitt MD. Where does serum amylase come from and where does it go? Gastroenterol Clin N Am. 1990;19:793.
37. Briggs GG, Freeman RK, Yaffe SJ. Drugs in pregnancy and lactation: a reference guide to fetal and neonatal risk. Philadelphia: Lippincott Williams and Wilkins; 2011.
38. Heinonen OP, Slone D, Shapiro S. Birth defects and drugs in pregnancy. Littleton, MA: Publishing Sciences Group; 1977.
39. Martin LV, Jurand A. The absence of teratogenic effects of some analgesics used in anesthesia. Additional evidence from a mouse model. Anaesthesia. 1992;47(6):473–6.
40. Ornoy A, Armon J, Schechtman S, Moerman L, Lukashova I. Is benzodiazepine use during pregnancy really teratogenic? Reprod Toxicol. 1998;12(5):511–5.
41. Dolovich LR, Addis A, Vaillancourt JM, Power JD, Koren G, Einarson TR. Benzodiazepine use in pregnancy and major malformations or oral cleft: meta-analysis of cohort and case-control studies. BMJ. 1998;317(7162):839–43.
42. Laegreid L, Olegard R, Walstrom J, Conradi N. Teratogenic effects of benzodiazepine use during pregnancy. J Pediatr. 1989;114(1):126–31.
43. Gin T, Chan MT. Decreased minimum alveolar concentration of isoflurane in pregnant humans. Anesthesiology. 1994;81(4):829–32.
44. ACOG Committee on Obstetric Practice. ACOG Committee Opinion No. 474: nonobstetric surgery during pregnancy. Obstet Gynecol. 2011;117(2 Pt 1):420–1.
45. Ell C, Fischbach W, Keller R, Dehe M, Mayer G, Schneider B, et al. A randomized, blinded, prospective trial to compare the safety and efficacy of three bowel cleansing solutions for colonoscopy. Endoscopy. 2003;35:300–4.
46. Gill SK, O'Brien L, Einarson TR, Koren G. The safety of proton pump inhibitors (PPIs) in pregnancy: a meta-analysis. Am J Gastroenterol. 2009;104(6):1541–5.
47. Pasternake B, Hviid A. Use of proton-pump inhibitors in early pregnancy and the risk of birth defects. N Engl J Med. 2010;363(22):2114–23.
48. ASGE standard of practice committee. Guidelines for endoscopy in pregnant and lactating women. Gastrointest Endosc. 2012;76(1):18–24.
49. Ludvigsson JF, Lebwohl B, Ekbom A, Kiran RP, Green PH, Höijer J, et al. Outcomes of pregnancies for women undergoing endoscopy while they are pregnant: a nationwide cohort study. Gastroenterology. 2017;152(3):554–63.
50. Qureshi WA, Rajan E, Adler DG, Davila RE, Hirota WK, Jacobson BC, et al. ASGE guideline: guidelines for endoscopy in pregnant and lactating women. Gastrointest Endosc. 2005;61(3):357–62.

Small Bowel Obstruction and Volvulus During Pregnancy

13

James M. Bardes and Daniel Grabo

Introduction

Bowel obstructions are one of the most common causes of surgical admissions in the pregnant patient. In pregnancy, only acute appendicitis and acute cholecystitis are more common [1]. Rates vary from 1 in 1,500 to 1 in 16,000 and increase as the pregnancy progresses [2]. Similar to the general surgery population, adhesive small bowel disease causes the majority of cases, up to 70% in some series. Volvulus, however, is much more common in the obstetric population than in the general surgical population. Cecal volvulus causes 25–40% of mechanical bowel obstructions in pregnant patients [1]. Bowel obstruction that progresses to bowel ischemia and necrosis puts the developing fetus at risk. Estimates of fetal loss range from 17–26% after the development of bowel necrosis. Maternal mortality can also be high in this setting, and risk appears to worsen as the pregnancy progresses. Maternal mortality may be as low as 2% in the first trimester but increases to 10–20% in the third [1, 3]. Because of this serious risk, the physician must maintain a high index of suspicion to rapidly diagnose and treat this condition.

Presentation and Initial Evaluation

Most patients with small bowel obstruction will present similarly with cramping, intermittent abdominal pain, accompanied by nausea and vomiting. Patients will frequently complain of diffuse pain with a feeling of bloating and abdominal distension. Obstipation will be an additional key complaint. Unfortunately, these are similar symptoms to normal pregnancy in many women, and a high index of suspicion is necessary to identify a bowel obstruction. A thorough past medical history should be taken focusing on a history of abdominal surgeries including cesarean section, history of pelvic inflammatory disease, and any history of hernia.

Physical exam will reveal a distended and tympanic abdomen. Classically, the description of high-pitched bowel sounds has been associated with small bowel obstruction; however, the absence of this finding should not be reassuring. The physician should carefully examine the abdomen for prior surgical scars, as well as check the umbilicus and groin for hernias. Sites of tenderness should be identified, and the patient evaluated for signs of peritonitis. A digital rectal exam should be performed to rule out distal obstruction or impaction. Fevers and tachycardia

J. M. Bardes
Department of Trauma and Acute Care Surgery, LAC+USC Medical Center, Los Angeles, CA, USA
e-mail: james.bardes@med.usc.edu

D. Grabo (✉)
Department of Surgery, West Virginia University, Morgantown, WV, USA
e-mail: Daniel.grabo@hsc.wvu.edu

C. H. Nezhat (ed.), *Non-Obstetric Surgery During Pregnancy*,
https://doi.org/10.1007/978-3-319-90752-9_13

are concerning signs for bowel ischemia and should prompt further evaluation.

Initial management includes laboratory analysis of blood chemistry panels as electrolyte abnormalities are commonly due to the poor oral intake and vomiting often associated with bowel obstructions. Renal function and volume status should be checked and patients given intravenous (IV) fluids for hydration as needed. A hypochloremic, hypokalemic, metabolic alkalosis is common after prolonged vomiting. This same pattern can be seen with prolonged nasogastric tube (NGT) drainage. Complete blood counts should be sent as well to evaluate for leukocytosis. Similarly lactate should be checked, as elevations in these labs can be a sign of bowel ischemia.

Imaging will be required to diagnose a bowel obstruction and may assist with identifying the etiology. Plain abdominal X-ray should be the first imaging modality ordered. Bowel dilation and air-fluid levels are diagnostic for the presence of an obstruction (Fig. 13.1). Often no gas will be seen in the rectum (Fig. 13.2). Plain X-ray is generally non-specific as to the etiology of an obstruction; however, volvulus will have a distinct X-ray finding. Cecal volvulus will be seen extending to the left upper quadrant and have a coffee bean shape (Fig. 13.3). Sigmoid volvulus will extend toward the right upper quadrant and have an omega shape (Fig. 13.4).

Computed tomography (CT) imaging with IV contrast is considered superior to plain X-ray imaging for bowel obstruction and has been shown to be up to 93% accurate at diagnosing an obstruction [4, 5]. A CT can often provide the location of the obstruction, evaluate for ischemia, and may be able to differentiate between complete and partial small bowel obstructions. Signs of ischemia will include free fluid, decreased bowel wall enhancement, bowel wall thickening, swirling of the mesentery, and mesenteric venous congestions (Fig. 13.5). Portal venous gas is a late finding and should raise concern for bowel necrosis. A CT will provide additional information on the severity of bowel distension and can show high-risk factors such as a transition point or fecalization of the small bowel (Figs. 13.6 and 13.7). The addition of oral contrast can be beneficial during CT imaging. The use of gastrografin will be discussed in the section on adhesive small bowel disease, but this agent can be both diagnostic and therapeutic in the treatment of a small bowel obstruction. Given the high risk for maternal and fetal mortality from an untreated obstruction, imaging will likely outweigh the potential risk of radiation exposure. Guidelines published in 2008 indicate the standard abdominal and pelvic CT likely delivers a radiation dose below the threshold for teratogenesis. However, these same guidelines do note the risk for carcinogenesis

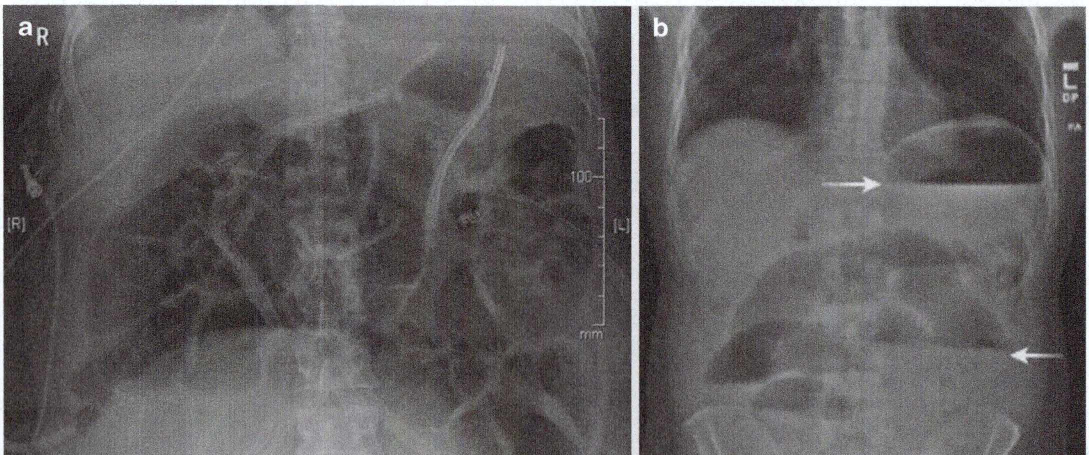

Fig. 13.1 (**a**) Plain X-ray of a 27-week pregnant female with multiple dilated loops of small bowel secondary to adhesive small bowel disease. (**b**) Plain X-ray of a small bowel obstruction with multiple air fluid levels (*white arrows*)

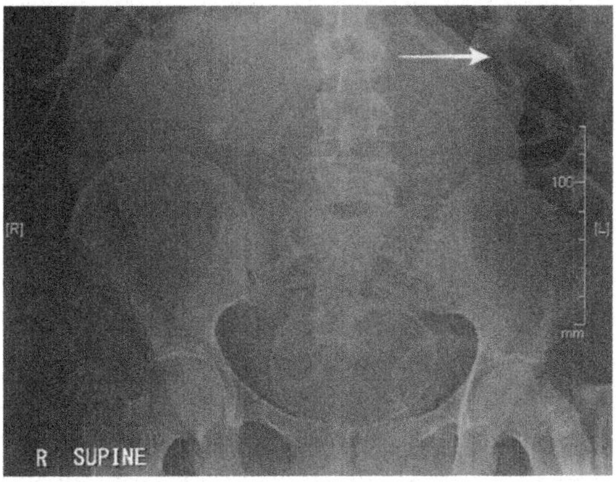

Fig. 13.2 Plain X-ray of a 27-week pregnant female with adhesive small bowel obstruction. Note the lack of air in the rectum inferior to the visualized fetus. Dilated small bowel loops (*white arrow*) can be partially visualized in the upper abdomen

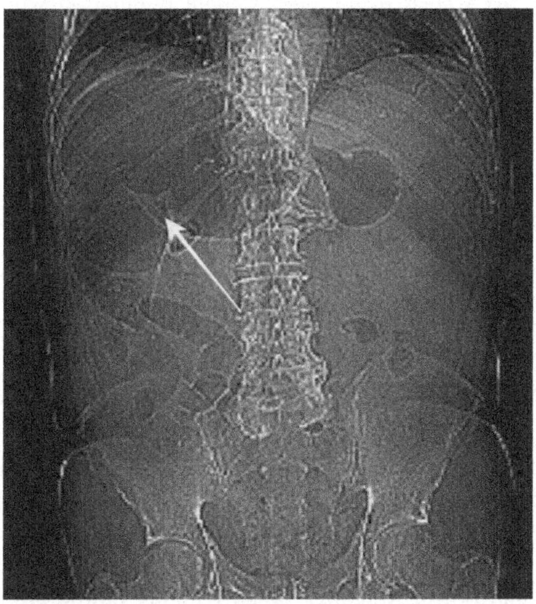

Fig. 13.3 X-ray of cecal volvulus (*white arrow*)

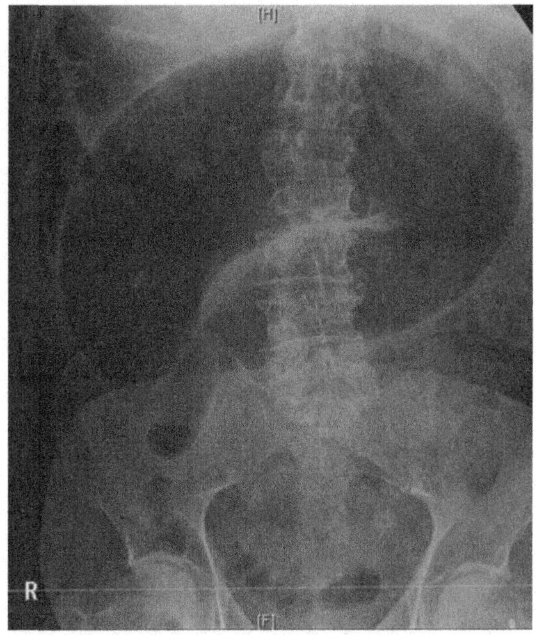

Fig. 13.4 X-ray of Sigmoid volvulus with classic omega shape

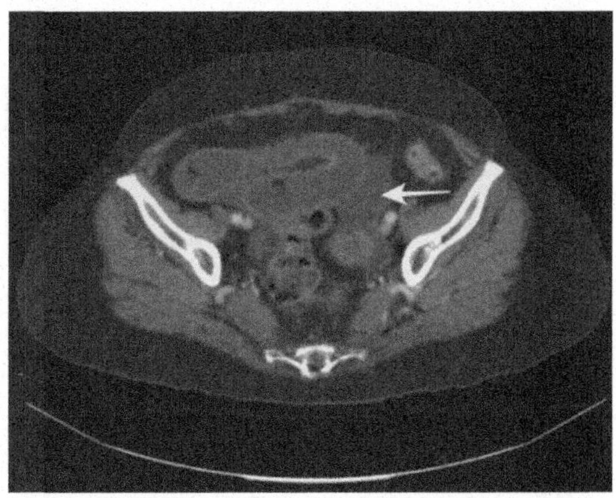

Fig. 13.5 CT imaging of a patient with a small bowel obstruction. Note the fluid-filled dilated loops of bowel. The mucosa can be seen enhancing symmetrically. However, there is free fluid, concerning for ischemia (*white arrow*)

does increase from a baseline of 1 in 2000 to 2 in 2000 [6]. The physician should counsel patients on the risks and benefits of imaging.

To avoid ionizing radiation, some physicians will use alternative imaging modalities such as magnetic resonance imaging (MRI) or ultrasound (U/S). MRI is infrequently used in the setting of a bowel obstruction. MRI takes significantly longer than plain X-ray and CT imaging. MRI also requires patients to lay flat for prolonged periods of time; this can be problematic in the severely nauseated patient and place them at risk for an aspiration event. Despite these limitations, for patients early in pregnancy, or those with significant radiation concerns, MRI is a reliable alternative to diagnose bowel obstruction.

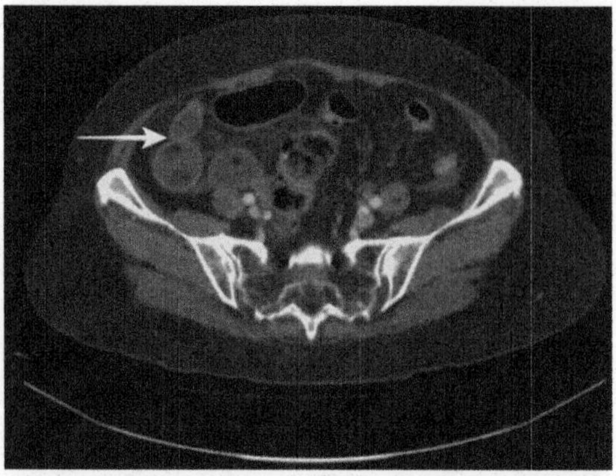

Fig. 13.6 CT imaging of a transition point in the right lower quadrant (*white arrow*)

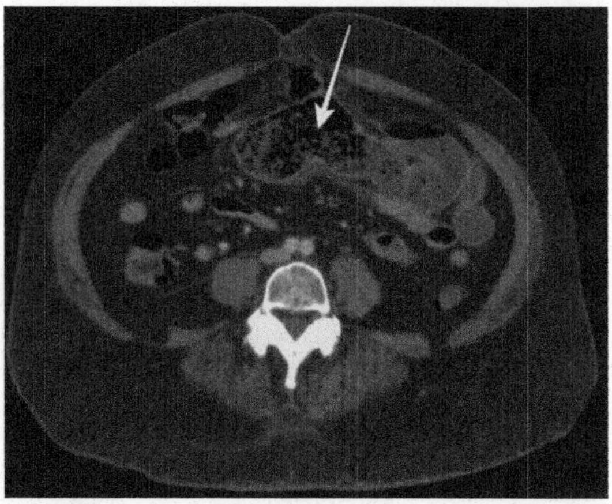

Fig. 13.7 CT imaging of a small bowel obstruction. The fecalization of the small bowel (*white arrow*) represents a patient at higher risk for failing conservative management

The accuracy of MRI has been reported as high as 92% for diagnosis of bowel obstruction [7]. U/S is another imaging modality that is not commonly used for bowel obstruction. While it can identify bowel dilation and free fluid, there is limited experience with its use.

Overall, the treatment algorithm for pregnant patients is similar to nonpregnant patients. After the initial evaluation, if there is no concern for acute bowel ischemia, most patients are managed nonoperatively. Treatment begins with insertion of an NGT, correction of electrolyte abnormalities, and IV hydration. Serial abdominal exams and laboratory tests are important to detect signs of worsening obstruction and potentially ischemia. Specific causes of bowel obstruction and their differing treatments are discussed below.

Adhesive Small Bowel Disease

Adhesive disease causes the majority of small bowel obstructions in both the general surgical population and obstetric patients. Any previous abdominal or pelvic surgery puts a patient at risk for adhesive small bowel obstruction. Repeated episodes of pelvic inflammatory disease can also lead to pelvic adhesions forming and causing obstruction. The majority of patients, 80%, with adhesive disease are treated successfully nonoperatively. The use of gastrografin as a diagnostic and therapeutic contrast agent has been repeatedly trialed in the nonpregnant population with positive results [8–10]. Several different protocols exist, but the general principles are the same (Fig. 13.8). The hyperosmolar contrast is given via the NGT after the stomach has been decompressed. Serial abdominal X-rays are taken to evaluate for contrast progress through the small bowel and into the colon (Figs. 13.9 and 13.10). The contrast is felt to decrease bowel wall edema, which assists with resolution of small bowel obstructions related to adhesive disease. Failure for the contrast to pass into the colon, or to cause a bowel movement, within 8–24 h has been associated with the need for operative intervention. These protocols are generally successful in relieving small bowel obstructions or identifying patients that require an operation sooner. Trials have shown a decreased rate of bowel necrosis, and bowel ischemia, when patients failing conservative management are identified earlier in their care.

For patients with repeated admissions for small bowel obstruction, or those that fail a gastrografin challenge, operative intervention is needed. If the bowel can be adequately decompressed with an NGT, and the abdomen is not severely distended, a laparoscopic approach can be considered. Frequently, there is one adhesive band causing an obstruction, and simply releasing this band will relieve the obstruction. However

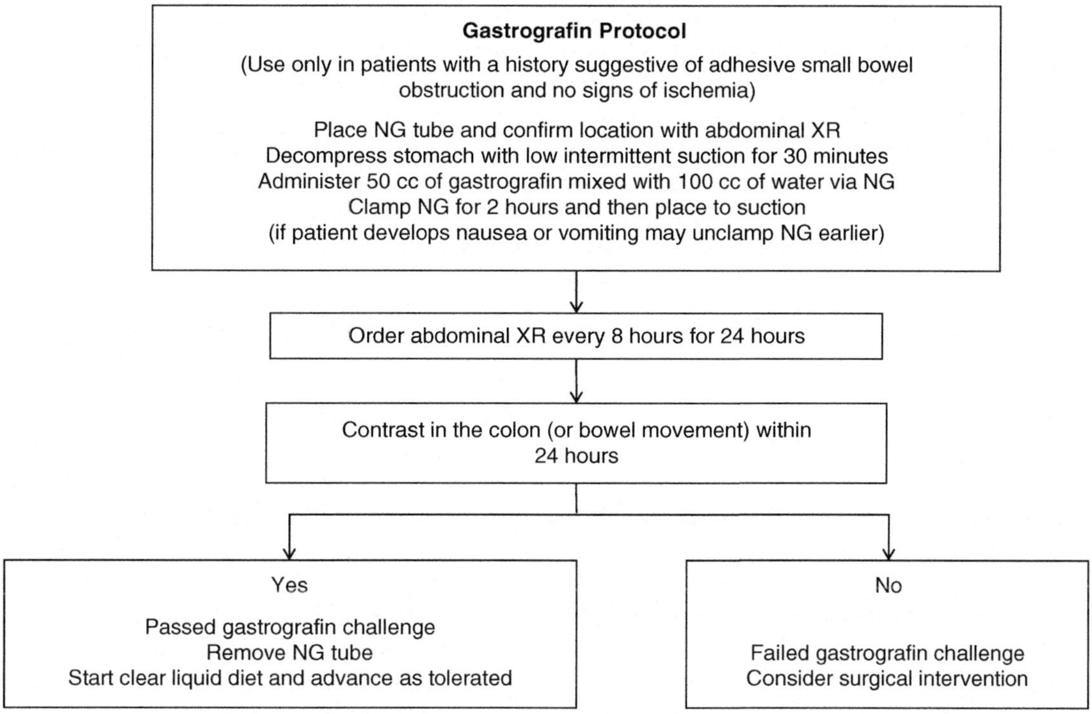

Fig. 13.8 Gastrografin protocol for adhesive small bowel disease

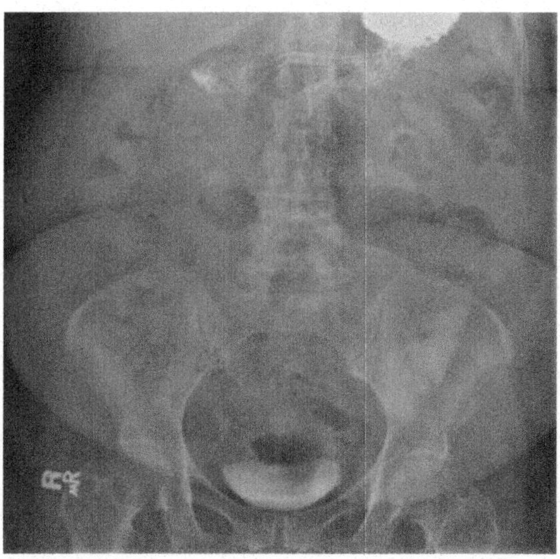

Fig. 13.9 X-ray of gastrograffin protocol with contrast agent in the stomach and first portions of the duodenum

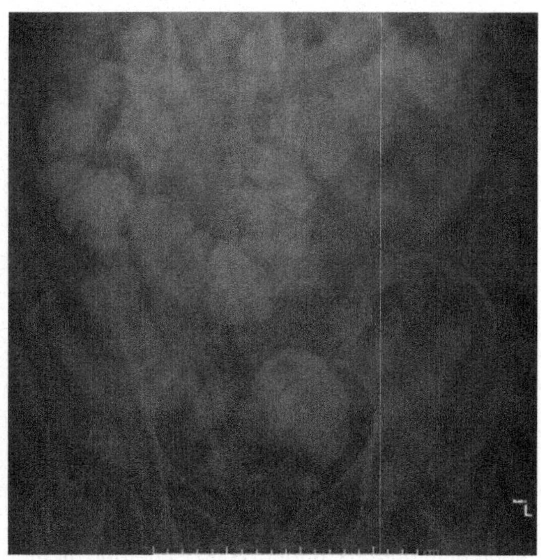

Fig. 13.10 X-ray of gastrografin protocol. Same patient 8 h later with contrast in the colon

the surgeon must have the technical skills to evaluate the bowel completely to ensure no additional bands exist. This can be challenging laparoscopically given the bowel dilation and is even more difficult in the presence of a gravid uterus. Most patients will be managed with a laparotomy, identification of the site of obstruction, and release of the adhesive band. The entire bowel can then easily be evaluated for additional sites of obstruction.

Volvulus

Volvulus is much more common in the pregnant patient than the general surgical population. It most frequently presents during times of rapid uterine growth as the cecum is pushed out of the pelvis [11]. The presence of a colonic volvulus will generally require surgical intervention. However the type of volvulus should be identified preoperatively, as the timing of surgery can be different. In the absence of signs of ischemia or peritonitis, a sigmoid volvulus can be reduced with a colonoscope. By reducing the volvulus, the bowel can be properly prepped, and the patient planned for a single-stage sigmoid colectomy with anastomosis. Sigmoid volvulus during pregnancy is however very rare.

Cecal volvulus is much more common and may represent 25–44% of all bowel obstructions in the pregnant patient [1]. Colonoscopic approaches are unlikely to detorse a cecal volvulus. While colonoscopy can be used to evaluate for mucosal ischemia, it is an unnecessary and potentially dangerous procedure. The patient will ultimately require surgery, and the colon will be edematous and friable, making colonoscopic perforation more likely. These patients should be prepped for laparotomy as soon as possible. Once in the operating room, the surgeon should again evaluate the patient for an ischemic- or necrotic-appearing bowel. If ischemia is found, the surgeon must proceed with bowel resection. Treatment options, if there is no ischemia, include cecopexy or resection with primary anastomosis. Cecopexy can be accomplished laparoscopically, or performed open, and is a rapid procedure with a low complication rate. However recurrence rates after cecopexy range up to 40% [12, 13]. In most cases resection is favored. The resulting ileocolonic anastomosis is low risk and the patient's risk for recurrence has been eliminated.

Hernia

When examining a patient with signs and symptoms of a bowel obstruction, the physician must evaluate for hernias. While rare in females, umbilical and inguinal hernias can cause bowel obstructions. Data on pregnant patients with hernias is limited to small case series. Inguinal hernias appear to be the most common type of hernia, up to 60% [14]. The majority of patients will not require operative intervention and can be observed with a "watchful waiting" strategy. These patients can then be scheduled electively in the postpartum period. Patients will frequently describe a symptomatic bulge, which may worsen with straining and lifting. Some patients will have a known hernia and may have been managing it conservatively prior to becoming pregnant.

There are several indications for surgical repair of a hernia. Strangulation is a surgical emergency and requires rapid evaluation and operative intervention. Incarceration of the bowel with resulting obstruction is another indication for surgical intervention. The repair of hernia defects is similar to the nonpregnant patient. The type of repair should be guided by the surgeon's skill and the patient's clinical condition.

Rare Causes

Numerous other, rare, causes of obstruction have been reported in pregnant patients. One specific type of hernia that must be considered is the internal hernia. Several reports have been published describing cases in pregnant patients [15, 16]. Patients who have undergone laparoscopic Roux-en-Y gastric bypass surgery are at risk for internal hernia after significant weight loss. The risk is usually the highest within the first 2 years after surgery. The true rate in pregnancy is unknown; however, the increased abdominal pressure and cephalad displacement of the bowel are believed to play a role. In a review of published cases, the mean gestational age for hernia was 28 weeks. Any patient who has undergone bypass surgery, and presents with fever and leukocytosis, should be evaluated for internal hernia. Consultation with a bariatric surgeon may assist with treatment, as these patients will require surgical intervention. Some may be repaired laparoscopically by reducing the hernia and closing the mesenteric defect. More severe cases may require small bowel resection and anastomosis. This may be performed openly or laparoscopically depending on the surgeon's skillset.

Intussusception is an additional cause of bowel obstruction reported in the literature [1, 2]. When involving the small bowel, these require operation. Intussusception can be caused by adhesive disease or a lead point from viral infection. Simple reduction may be adequate; however, bowel resection is frequently required when the bowel has become edematous and cannot easily be reduced.

Patients with Concern for Ischemia

Patients with concern for bowel ischemia, either initially or after failure of conservative management, need to be urgently taken to the operating room. Signs associated with bowel ischemia include fever, tachycardia, progressive leukocytosis, worsening lactic acidosis, and peritonitis on exam. Most will benefit from beginning with a midline laparotomy. The only exception is some inguinal hernias, which can be managed entirely through the groin. However for many surgeons, a bowel resection will be much easier through a midline incision. After entering the abdomen, the bowel should be run in its entirety to evaluate for a site of obstruction. Depending on the etiology, the obstruction should be released or resected as indicated.

Any necrotic sections of bowel will need to be resected. Often a section will demonstrate ischemic changes but not be frankly necrotic. Blood flow can be evaluated in these segments of bowel in several ways. The surgeon should look for peristalsis and evaluate the color of the wall. Placing the bowel within a warm, wet lap pad may improve the bowel viability. The surgeon can then feel the mesentery for pulsatile flow; the use of a Doppler is recommended as well as checking for pulsatile flow at the mesenteric edge and on the antimesenteric side of the bowel wall. Fluorescein dye can also be injected, and the bowel evaluated with a woods lamp to confirm flow within the bowel. Fluorescein dye is pregnancy category C and is noted to cross the placenta. One large ophthalmology case series reviewed outcomes after fluorescein angiography [17]. This series identified a low rate of complications, but the physician should weigh the risks and benefits of its use. If areas of ischemia are present, and will not be resected at the initial operation, the surgeon should consider placing a temporary abdominal closure device and returning to the operating room in 24 h for a second look. At that second operation, either the bowel can be resected and anastomosed, or if the bowel appears viable, the abdomen is closed.

Conclusion

Bowel obstruction in the obstetric population can present very similarly to the normal symptoms of pregnancy. The physician must maintain a high index of suspicion to avoid missing the diagnosis. Most bowel obstructions are caused by adhesive disease, similarly to the nonpregnant population. However, cecal volvulus is much more common in this special population, causing up to 40% of obstructions. A thorough history and physical exam, with laboratory analysis and imaging, are useful in diagnosing a bowel obstruction. X-ray and CT imaging are frequently used with minimal risk to the fetus. Management for each condition is no different in the pregnant patient, and most are managed nonoperatively. Decompression with a nasogastric tube, fluid resuscitation, and repletion of electrolytes are critical first steps. In the event of bowel ischemia, the physician must intervene immediately to avoid the risk of fetal loss.

References

1. Augustin G, Majerovic M. Non-obstetrical acute abdomen during pregnancy. Eur J Obstet Gynecol Reprod Biol. 2007;131(1):4–12.
2. Parangi S, Levine D, Henry A, Isakovich N, Pories S. Surgical gastrointestinal disorders during pregnancy. Am J Surg. 2007;193(2):223–32.
3. Webster PJ, Bailey MA, Wilson J, Burke DA. Small bowel obstruction in pregnancy is a complex surgical problem with a high risk of fetal loss. Ann R Coll Surg Engl. 2015;97(5):339–44.
4. Maung AA, Johnson DC, Piper GL, Barbosa RR, Rowell SE, Bokhari F, et al. Evaluation and management of small-bowel obstruction: an Eastern Association for the Surgery of Trauma practice management guideline. J Trauma Acute Care Surg. 2012;73(5):S362–9.
5. Suri S, Gupta S, Sudhakar PJ, Venkataramu NK, Sood B, Wig JD. Comparative evaluation of plain films, ultrasound and CT in the diagnosis of intestinal obstruction. Acta Radiol. 1999;40(4):422–8.
6. Chen MM, Coakley FV, Kaimal A, Laros RK Jr. Guidelines for computed tomography and magnetic resonance imaging use during pregnancy and lactation. Obstet Gynecol. 2008;112(2, Part 1):333–40.
7. Matsuoka H, Takahara T, Masaki T, Sugiyama M, Hachiya J, Atomi Y. Preoperative evaluation by magnetic resonance imaging in patients with bowel obstruction. Am J Surg. 2002;183(6):614–7.
8. Zielinski MD, Haddad NN, Cullinane DC, Inaba K, Yeh DD, Wydo S, et al. Multi-institutional, prospective, observational study comparing the Gastrografin challenge versus standard treatment in adhesive small bowel obstruction. J Trauma Acute Care Surg. 2017;83(1):47–54.
9. Branco BC, Barmparas G, Schnüriger B, Inaba K, Chan LS, Demetriades D. Systematic review and meta-analysis of the diagnostic and therapeutic role of water-soluble contrast agent in adhesive small bowel obstruction. Br J Surg. 2010;97(4):470–8.
10. Choi HK, Chu KW, Law WL. Therapeutic value of gastrografin in adhesive small bowel obstruction after unsuccessful conservative treatment: a prospective randomized trial. Ann Surg. 2002;236(1):1.
11. Ballantyne GH, Brandner MD, Beart RW Jr, Ilstrup DM. Volvulus of the colon. Incidence and mortality. Ann Surg. 1985;202(1):83.
12. Madiba TE, Thomson SR, Church JM. The management of cecal volvulus. Dis Colon Rectum. 2002;45(2):264–7.
13. Hiltunen KM, Syrjä H, Matikainen M. Colonic volvulus. Diagnosis and results of treatment in 82 patients. Eur J Surg. 1992;158(11–12):607–11.
14. Buch KE, Tabrizian P, Divino CM. Management of hernias in pregnancy. J Am Coll Surg. 2008;207(4):539–42.
15. Kakarla N, Dailey C, Marino T, Shikora SA, Chelmow D. Pregnancy after gastric bypass surgery and internal hernia formation. Obstet Gynecol. 2005;105(5, Part 2):1195–8.
16. Anthony C, Shirley D, Aaron G, Jason F, Richard L, Robert M. Small bowel ischemia after Roux-en-Y gastric bypass complicated by pregnancy: a case report. Am Surg. 2005;71(3):231–4.
17. Halperin LS, Olk RJ, Soubrane G, Coscas G. Safety of fluorescein angiography during pregnancy. Am J Ophthalmol. 1990;109(5):563–6.

Surgical Management of Inflammatory Bowel Disease in Pregnancy

14

Wayne L. Ambroze Jr
and Bradley Paul Champagne

Introduction

Inflammatory bowel disease (IBD) is a collective term encompassing two distinct disorders wherein the immune system targets the bowel as a foreign entity and induces varying degrees of inflammation and tissue damage. Inflammatory bowel disease includes both Crohn's disease (CD) and ulcerative colitis (UC). The inflammation associated with these pathologies can cause a variety of problems including diarrhea, pain, bleeding, fistula formation, abscess, bowel obstruction, as well as toxic megacolon and bowel perforation. The treatment algorithm of these diseases has changed substantially in recent years with the introduction of new and more specific immunosuppressants. The development of these immunosuppressants has led to a decreased use of chronic steroids, thereby reducing the risks associated with long-term use of corticosteroids. Changes in the treatment algorithm have been carried over to management of pregnant patients with inflammatory bowel disease.

Pregnancy has not been empirically associated with an increased risk for developing IBD. However, patients with a history of IBD at the time of conception have an increased risk of active flairs or exacerbations of active disease during pregnancy. Theories exist that this increased risk may be due to hormonal changes during the pregnancy or could represent a misunderstanding of the maintenance medications safety when used during pregnancy. This misunderstanding can cause a discontinuation of maintenance medications either by physician recommendation or voluntary discontinuation by the patient [1]. At this time, there is no literature consensus regarding any association with an acute flair of UC or CD or their medical management during pregnancy leading to an increased risk to the fetus including preterm delivery, low birth weight, small size for gestational age, or an increase in miscarriage or abortion [2–5]. This ambiguity in the literature can present a problem for the patient and the practitioner in developing a treatment strategy for IBD during pregnancy. Current thinking favors aggressive medical management over the deleterious effects of disease progression during pregnancy.

Medical management and maintenance therapy are the cornerstones of treatment for inflammatory bowel disease and have been shown to be safe for expectant mothers and fetuses with the exceptions of methotrexate and thalidomide, which are proven to be teratogenic [6–9]. In light of more recent medications becoming available, surgery for inflammatory bowel disease has

W. L. Ambroze Jr (✉)
Department of Surgery, Northside Hospital, Atlanta, GA, USA
e-mail: wayne.ambroze@northside.com

B. P. Champagne
Department of Surgery, Our Lady of Lourdes Regional Medical Center, Lafayette, LA, USA

C. H. Nezhat (ed.), *Non-Obstetric Surgery During Pregnancy*,
https://doi.org/10.1007/978-3-319-90752-9_14

moved out of the algorithm for initial management of noncomplicated disease and is used primarily for controlling septic sources, severe bleeding, bowel obstruction, and progressive intractable disease. When surgery is indicated for IBD, it is important to distinguish between UC and CD as the procedure performed may have long-term ramifications.

Understanding the etiology of IBD, the distinction between UC and CD, the available medical options during pregnancy, as well as the indications and surgical options for each disease is critical for maximizing outcomes to both the mother and fetus.

Incidence and Etiology

Inflammatory bowel disease is characterized by a chronic and relapsing inflammatory reaction of the GI tract as an effect of inappropriate immunologic targeting of the bowel antigens. The two subcategories of IBD are ulcerative colitis and Crohn's disease. These entities, while distinct, can present with similar symptoms and can be difficult to differentiate. The exact etiology of IBD remains unknown, although it is thought to be multifactorial in nature. The prevailing theory is that environmental factors act as triggers for patients with a genetically predisposed impaired immunity. The environmental factors that have been suggested as playing a role in the disease process include living in an industrialized country, infectious entities, smoking, NSAID usage, previous appendectomy, and the patient's own microbiome of the colon. There are likely more environmental factors at work that may become apparent as our knowledge and testing of these diseases increase. Genetic compiling associated with the human genome project has revealed a number of alleles associated with IBD. Most of the identified genes are associated with both CD and UC; however, some have been associated with a singular entity. The vast variability in the genetic cascade associated with inflammatory bowel may suggest a reason for the wide variability of the physiology phenotypes that can manifest in patients with IBD.

The incidence of UC in North America is estimated at 8–15 cases per 100,000 persons per year, while the incidence for CD ranges from 3 to 15 patients per 100,000 per year [1]. The incidence of both diseases has been on the rise for the past 50 years, and both incidence curves show a peak around the second and third decades of life. While UC has an equal female-to-male ratio, CD has a slight female predominance with a 1.3:1 incidence. Given these statistics, it is easy to see that a significant portion of female patients may have or develop IBD during their fertility years. Approximately 25% of female patients with IBD will become pregnant subsequently to their diagnosis. This association with IBD and pregnancy can create clinical difficulties for the patient and complex treatment decisions for the providers caring for them.

Crohn's vs. Ulcerative Colitis

Inflammatory bowel disease can present with a broad spectrum of complaints and may offer significant challenges to the physician tasked with diagnosing and treating these diseases. Differentiation between CD and UC is important when making medical and surgical management decisions. Although both UC and CD are disease entities that may cause similar symptoms, there are several ways to help to differentiate the two disease entities.

UC tends to present as new onset cramping and bloody diarrhea. Because of this presentation, it can sometimes be mistaken for infectious colitis. The inflammatory effects of UC are usually limited to the mucosa but can extend into the superficial submucosa. UC is also limited to only the colon and rectum. It tends to spread distally to proximally with the rectum always being the first point of involvement. While the inflammation is limited to the colon, occasionally with severe cecal disease, you can have "backwash ileitis," which can mimic CD. Also with anti-inflammatory suppository or enema regimens, you can have apparent rectal sparing due to local therapeutic effect. The stereotypical gross appearance of UC is of a continuous diffusely inflamed mucosa with ulcerations and sometimes pseudopolyps starting in the rectum and continuing proximally with sparing of the terminal ileum (Fig. 14.1). Histologically, UC biopsies will show crypt distortion, mucosal limitation of inflammation, crypt abscesses, mucin depletion, and basal plasmacytosis.

CD is more variable in its presentation, and while it can produce cramping and bloody diarrhea, it may also present as fistula disease, aphthous ulcers, strictures with obstruction, watery diarrhea, and abdominal abscesses and can sometimes mimic appendicitis in patients with terminal ileal disease. CD can also present with debilitating perianal ulcers, abscesses, and fistulas (Fig. 14.2). This variability in clinical presentation is secondary to the transmural inflammation associated with CD and its ability to affect the entire GI tract from mouth to anus. CD can further be divided into three subgroups including inflammatory, stricturing, and penetrating disease based on the phenotype present in the patient. The most common site of disease is the terminal ileum. The classic colonoscopic appearance of colonic CD consists of aphthous ulcers, skip lesions, inflammation, deep linear ulcers, "cobblestone" appearance of the mucosa, and occasional strictures. The terminal ileum is commonly associated with disease and the rectum may be spared (Fig. 14.3). Histologically, CD presents with local crypt destruction, granulomatous lesions, lymphoid aggregates, plasma cells, and muscular hypertrophy. On gross examination of the external bowel wall, you may see stereotypical fat wrapping (Fig. 14.4).

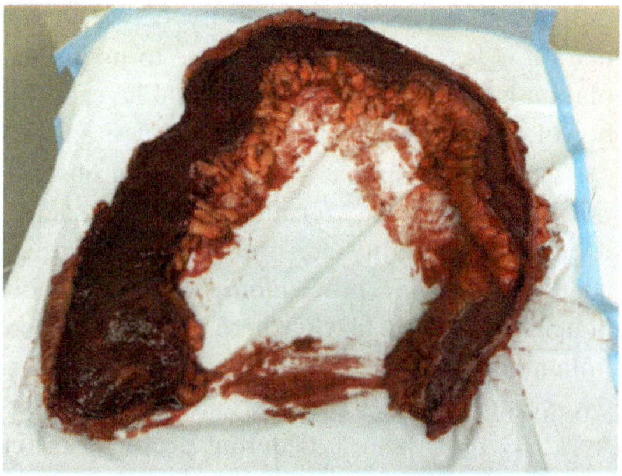

Fig. 14.1 Ulcerative colitis with continuous disease throughout the colon

Serology studies can assist in the differentiation between CD and UC. Perinuclear anti-neutrophil cytoplasmic antibodies (pANCA) and anti-saccharomyces cerevisiae antibodies (ASCA) are the most studied of the serologic markers in IBD. However, given their presence in other inflammatory conditions including rheumatoid arthritis, vasculitis, and glomerulonephritis, they are not appropriate as screening tests. The presence of pANCA in CD ranges from 2 to 28%, while UC has a range of 20–85%. pANCA, therefore, has a sensitivity of 56% and specificity of 89% for UC when evaluating an IBD patient.

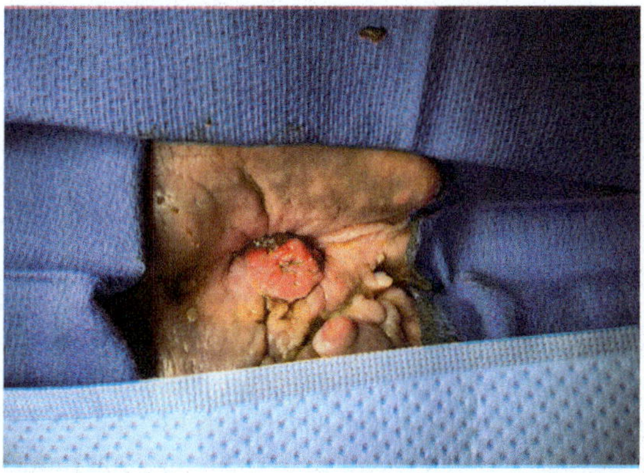

Fig. 14.2 Severe perianal Crohn's disease with multiple abscesses and fistulae

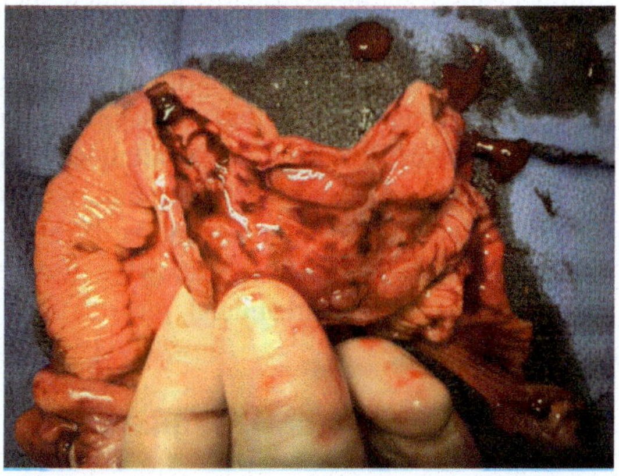

Fig. 14.3 The most common site of Crohn's disease is the terminal ileum

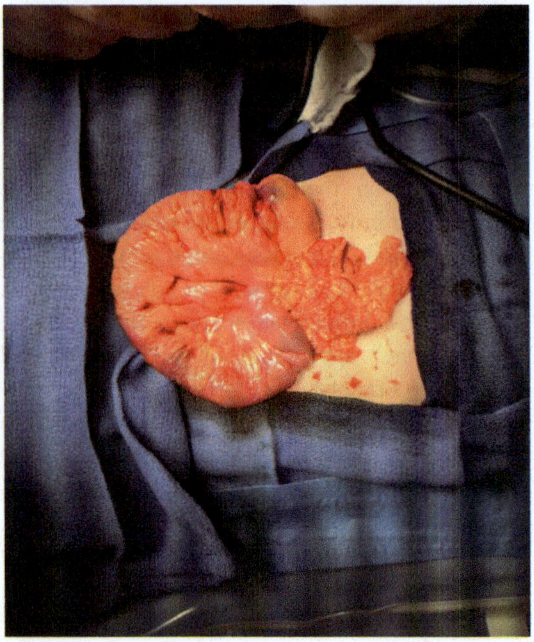

Fig. 14.4 Fat wrapping of the small bowel in Crohn's disease

ASCA is essentially the reverse with a positive incidence in CD of 39–69%, while UC has a positivity of 5–15% [10]. These can be helpful in cases where biopsies and workups have returned as indeterminate colitis. Other serum markers to follow the disease activity include serum albumin, C-reactive protein (CRP), and erythrocyte sedimentation rate (ESR). While these will not help differentiate CD from UC, they can assist in following disease activity as the inflammation of the GI tract caused by these diseases will often alter the acute phase markers. Pregnancy, however, may cause hemodilution and an artificial lowering of the serum albumin, as well as a baseline rise in ESR making these less helpful in trending disease activity during pregnancy. CRP remains within normal limits during pregnancy and is therefore the serum marker of choice for following disease activity and response to treatment.

Effects on Fertility and Pregnancy

IBD can cause issues with fertility in a number of different ways including real reductions in fertility from disease-related pelvic scarring and prior surgery or perceived reductions in fertility or voluntary childlessness. Both UC and CD can cause patients to have a change in their perception of sexual desire which can cause a decrease in attempts at sexual intercourse, thereby decreasing reproductive attempts and perceived fertility. UC and CD can cause pelvic inflammation, which can cause discomfort and dyspareunia also decreasing sexual attempts and perceived fertility. There can also be concern by the patient about IBD causing complications in pregnancy, fetal harm while in utero, and fear of passing on IBD to their offspring that can lead to voluntary childlessness. A study in 2016 by Ellul et al. showed this had an effect on >60% of IBD patients [1]. Furthermore, the transmural inflammation of CD can cause abscesses and fistulas in the pelvis leading to PID or pelvic scarring of the fallopian tubes decreasing fertility. Pelvic inflammation is less common in UC due to its inflammation being limited to the mucosal layer of the bowel. Surgery in the pelvis for both UC and CD can cause scarring that may cause tubal obstruction and decrease fertility. For UC actual decreases in fertility are limited to postsurgical changes following proctectomy with or without pouch formation. In UC there is little external inflammation of the bowel, so female reproductive ability is essentially unchanged from baseline. CD represents a different problem as the transmural inflammation can directly impair fertility [2–4].

Medical Management of Ulcerative Colitis and Crohn's Disease

The general medical approach to therapy for UC and CD is often similar and can be categorized by two different treatment strategies referred to as a "top-down" approach or a "bottom-up" approach. The medications used during these two strategies are similar, but the approach is dictated by the patient's symptoms and disease state. The "top-down" approach is for severe disease states with the early use of aggressive therapy including antitumor necrosis factor immunomodulators and pulse high-dose steroids until control of symptoms has been reached with subsequent maintenance therapy initiated. The "bottom-up" approach is the reverse and utilized for more quiescent and less symptomatic disease states. This strategy uses low-dose steroids and other first-line therapies such as aminosalicylates, azathioprine, and methotrexate to begin with and medications are titrated up or added until control is achieved, and maintenance therapy is continued. Both arms of therapy can utilize multiple different medical therapies including steroids, aminosalicylates, cyclosporine, tacrolimus, methotrexate, and biologic medications including TNF inhibitors. Each of the above medications has risks associated with its usage, including collectively increasing the risk of infectious complications. The choice of approach is a complex issue and is normally tailored to the patient's presentation and should be dictated and directed by a gastroenterologist who is knowledgeable about IBD management.

The pregnant patient has similar options as the nonpregnant IBD patient when it comes to medications with a few exceptions. Methotrexate and thalidomide have been labeled category X signifying great risk to the fetus with increases in fetal abnormalities and should not be used in pregnant patients (Table 14.1). Azathioprine and 6-MP are category D medications showing a risk to the fetus and fetal abnormalities but can be used if the benefit outweighs the risks of usage. Of note, anti-TNF inhibitors are labeled a class B medication showing no risks in animal studies but without well controlled studies in pregnant women. There are studies showing the efficacy of treatment into the third trimester of pregnancy with recommendations to avoid vaccination of neonates for 8 weeks after birth secondary to placental crossing of these medications in the second trimester [5–9, 11, 12]. There have not been any reports of fetal abnormalities with the biologic agents; however, there have been occurrences of premature labor or miscarriages, but these have not reached statistical significance in the literature [6, 7, 11]. Early removal of these agents has shown an increase in relapse of disease states, and discontinuation during pregnancy in patients with severe disease is not recommended [8, 9]. In patients with mild disease, the continuation of these medications during pregnancy remains a difficult decision as there are no well-designed studies delineating the risk benefit curve [3]. In patients with moderate or severe disease, the benefit of remaining in remission and avoiding disease-related complications seems to outweigh the low risk of these medications [3].

Surgical Management in the Pregnant Patient

Surgical management of CD and UC is as much about timing of the procedure as it is about the technique used. This becomes more important in surgical management of the pregnant patient. It has been shown that surgery with general anesthesia in the first trimester is associated with an increase in miscarriage, while surgery in the third trimester is associated with a high risk of preterm labor. Sedation with endoscopy does not appear to carry a high a risk to the fetus during these time periods and is generally considered safe [1, 13]. The surgical timing and management of UC and CD is dictated by the different presenting complications associated with these diseases.

Indications for surgical intervention for UC are reserved for medically refractory disease, uncontrolled bleeding, and for toxic megacolon either with or without perforation. Since UC is

Table 14.1 Safety of IBD medications during pregnancy [5]

Category B	Category C	Category D	Category X
Loperamide Mesalamine Balsalazide Corticosteroids Sulfasalazine Anti-TNG agents Metronidazole[a]	Ciprofloxacin Cyclosporine Diphenoxylate Olsalazine Tacrolimus Natalizumab	Azathioprine 6-Mercaptopurine	Methotrexate Thalidomide

[a]Safe for use after first trimester

limited to the colon and rectum, surgical excision of the entire colon and rectum is curative. While a permanent ileostomy is an option, most younger patients prefer a restorative ileal pouch-anal anastomosis (IPAA) procedure to preserve perineal defecation and avoid a permanent ileostomy. The most common pouch performed is the J-shaped pouch (Fig. 14.5). In a nonpregnant patient for medically refractory disease, this can be accomplished in a two-stage procedure where the total proctocolectomy and IPAA are performed at the initial surgery combined with a diverting loop ileostomy. At a later date, normally 6–12 weeks after the initial surgery, the loop ileostomy is reversed after the pouch has been inspected with a contrast imaging study. For unstable patients with toxic megacolon with or without perforation, or for patients with severe malnutrition from chronic disease, a three-stage procedure is performed removing the bulk of the disease with a total colectomy and end ileostomy followed at a later date after full recovery with a J-pouch and temporary loop ileostomy. Subsequent loop ileostomy takedown is the final stage. The pregnant patient requiring surgical management for UC should undergo a three-stage approach to IPAA. This is due to the multiple issues associated with the pregnant patient. Manipulation of the large gravid uterus with a pelvic dissection can cause premature labor or put the fetus in extremus. Another consideration is that IPAA with pouch creation is associated

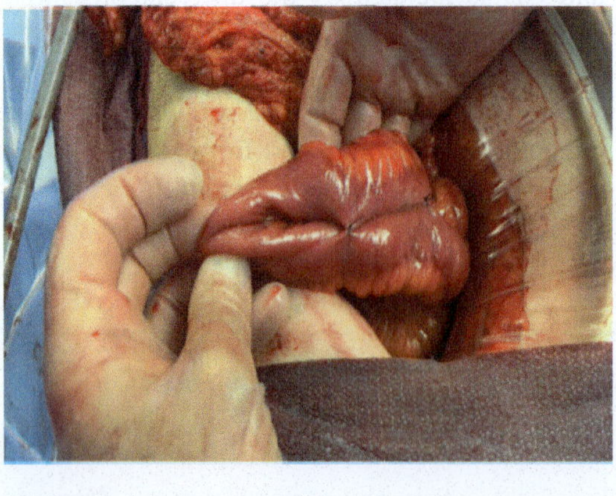

Fig. 14.5 A J-shaped pouch is created from the terminal 30 cm of ileum

with a significant leak rate, and that is why most surgeons performing IPAA surgeries create a loop ileostomy as a precautionary step. If the patient has a leak with a pelvic abscess or develops pelvic sepsis, the rate of premature labor and a nonviable baby is increased significantly. For these reasons, if a pregnant patient with UC requires a colectomy, a three-stage procedure is indicated with the second and third stages being performed after delivery [13].

Lower gastrointestinal bleeding in the pregnant patient with IBD is slightly more complex. For a nonpregnant patient, bleeding is initially assessed with either a CT angiography or a nuclear medicine bleeding scan to locate the area of bleeding. Once the bleeding is located, interventional radiology can attempt embolization of the offending blood vessel. If the bleeding cannot be localized or cannot be stopped with embolism, an attempt at endoscopic therapy and intervention with cautery, epinephrine injection, or clip application is done. If these procedures fail and bleeding persists, then colectomy is indicated. In patients who are pregnant, these first two steps are reversed. The first-line treatment should be endoscopic intervention. This limits exposure of the fetus to radiation. If this step fails, then IR embolization can be attempted. Again, if these fail then surgical intervention is warranted. For acute refractory bleeding in the pregnant patient with UC, a total abdominal colectomy and end ileostomy leaving a short rectal stump is the procedure of choice. Performing the remaining two stages to restore GI continuity can take place after the pregnancy and the patient has fully recovered.

The indications for surgical intervention in CD can be variable and more complex. Surgical intervention may be indicated for perianal fistulas or abscesses, bowel strictures with obstruction, intra-abdominal abscesses, perforations, and medically refractory disease with bleeding being a less common indication. Unlike UC, CD cannot be cured surgically which compounds the complexity of the approach to surgical therapy. Since surgery is not curative in the CD patient, it is generally reserved for those with acute complications or those who have failed aggressive medical therapy. An attempt to avoid surgical intervention is enhanced in the pregnant patient due to the added risk of harm to the fetus [1, 13]. Similar to the management of UC, initial management of CD in pregnancy focuses on maximizing medical therapy [1]. If surgery is indicated, the choice of procedure and quick recognition of any acute distress in the mother or the fetus is key. Surgery in the pregnant patient with CD can be indicated for either perianal or intra-abdominal manifestations of the disease.

Perianal abscess and fistula are a bothersome and complex problem in the CD patient. The presentation of this problem can range from a simple chronic draining sinus to signs of sepsis with large complex abscesses surrounding the sphincter apparatus. The initial management of these abscesses follows the long-standing surgical tradition of "find pus, drain pus." Adequate drainage of the purulence and addition of IV or oral antibiotics if the patient is significantly immune suppressed or showing signs of sepsis will usually alleviate the acute problem. Unlike non-CD-associated perianal abscesses which show a roughly 50% chance of spontaneous closure with drainage alone, CD-associated abscesses will seldom close spontaneously. Given the predisposition of fistulization and recurrence, it is appropriate to allow for long-term drainage to avoid recurrent abscess formation. Seton placement should be considered in the pregnant patient to avoid recurrent abscess formation and subsequent surgeries. Multiple setons are often necessary in CD (Fig. 14.6). Seton material choice is variable, and the number of setons placed is dictated by the extent of disease and the need to insure appropriate control of the perineal sepsis. This intervention of incision and drainage coupled with non-cutting seton placement will allow for long-term drainage of the perineal fistula while medical treatment of the CD is initiated or enhanced. Many of the CD-associated fistulas will heal with anti-TNF therapy and seton placement. If improvements with medical therapy are demonstrated, then the setons can be removed in the office after the pregnancy is complete. However, if failure to close with medical therapy or extensive perianal disease with loss of function of the sphincter complex occurs in the patient, then this may necessitate further surgical interventions ranging from local procedures such as LIFT, cutting setons, fistula plugs, or fibrin glue to total proctectomy with end colostomy. Given that pregnancy is temporally limited, the recommendation at this time is that surgical management of perianal abscess and fistula in the pregnant patient with CD be limited to drainage and seton placement followed with appropriate medical therapy. Any further indicated procedures to attempt closure can be safely postponed until after the patient has given birth [13].

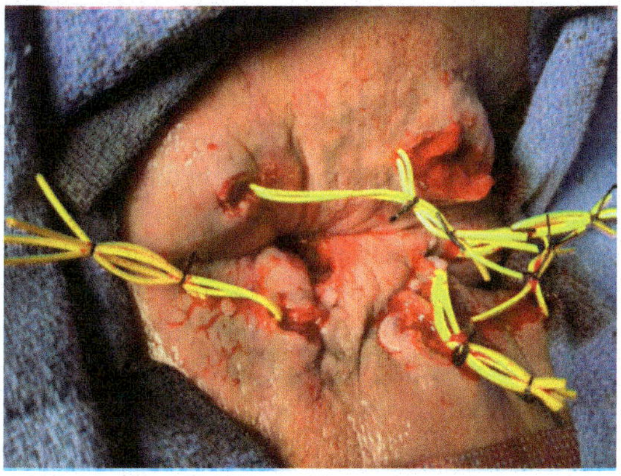

Fig. 14.6 Seton drainage of multiple abscesses and fistulae in a patient with severe perianal Crohn's disease

There are multiple different clinical presentations for patients with intra-abdominal CD, including strictures with obstruction. Management of stricturing bowel disease in patients who have failed medical therapy remains dependent on the length of the stricture and its location in the GI tract. There have been reports of successful management of small bowel and colonic strictures with endoscopic balloon dilation. The success rate remains higher for shorter segment strictures and is dependent on the strictures being able to be reached with the endoscope. The relief experienced from balloon dilation may be short lived with return of symptoms often within 2 years. There is no data available on the use of endoscopic dilation of bowel strictures in the pregnant patient with CD. While it is tempting to choose this less invasive approach over surgical intervention, this must be tempered by the possibility of iatrogenic bowel perforation which is not insignificant. If this approach is used, it should be done in consultation with a surgeon who is available to do an emergency resection should a perforation occur. Surgical management for obstructing bowel stricture consists of either resection of the segment or stricturoplasty. Resection and primary anastomosis tends to be utilized for long-segment strictures where a stricturoplasty is not feasible. Stricturoplasty is used primarily for short-segment strictures. Stricturoplasty consists of making a full-thickness transverse incision along the bowel wall through the stricture and then closing it vertically to open the stricture. These techniques can be applied singularly or in combination to appropriately address multiple strictures. Bypass of the stricture has been used in the past but is associated with a number of negative sequelae and as such used in limited situations.

Intra-abdominal abscesses and perforations in CD are severe complications and of greater concern in the pregnant patient as it increases the stress on the fetus. The standard approach for an abscess is drainage, preferentially CT-guided, with a course of intravenous antibiotics. If the abscess is not amenable to percutaneous drainage due to its location, multi-loculation, or if it is associated with a free perforation, then surgical management will be needed. Whether or not to place a diverting ostomy at surgery is dictated by the stability of the patient, the overall condition of the patient, and the condition of the bowel to be included in the anastomosis. A pregnant patient with a stable fetus and a small abscess can undergo an attempt with conservative treatment via drain placement and antibiotics. There needs to be close monitoring of the mother and fetus and a low threshold to convert to surgical management. If the patient does require surgical intervention, then the patient should undergo washout and resection. In the pregnant patient, however, there has been shown to be a higher rate of leak and anastomotic failure, so in this situation, the creation of an end ostomy with plans to reverse the ostomy after the pregnancy may be the preferred approach [13]. Episodes of dehydration with hypotension during pregnancy as well as possible tension on an anastomosis placed by a gravid uterus may predispose to an anastomotic leak. An anastomotic leak in an already stressed pregnancy could be catastrophic for the mother or fetus, and a bias toward avoiding an anastomosis is warranted [1, 13]. In the pregnant patient with a low perforation where a pelvic dissection would be needed to resect the involved segment of the rectum, a diverting ostomy with washout and drain placement may be preferable to avoid a pelvic dissection with a gravid uterus.

For medically refractory disease with progressive deterioration or toxic megacolon, resection is the management option of choice. Toxic megacolon is a rare complication of CD compared to UC, though it can occur. In this case total colectomy and end ileostomy is the initial management with potential reversal with an ileorectal anastomosis at a later date once the patient has fully recovered and the rectal disease is under control. Medically refractory severe progressive disease warrants resection with the intent to remove all visible macroscopic disease at the time of the operation. This can be paired with primary anastomosis or placement of ostomy depending on the clinical status of the patient and fetus. Again, a bias toward a temporary ostomy is appropriate for the reasons mentioned above [1, 13].

Finally, bowel obstruction is one of the more common indications for surgery in the pregnant patient with CD. The gravid uterus pushing on an inflamed segment of bowel may account for this. An attempt with NGT decompression, IV hydration, and a bolus dose of steroids to decrease the bowel inflammation and open the swollen lumen is appropriate. If this fails, then diverting ostomy is appropriate. If the focus of obstruction is associated with an abscess, then resection would be necessary. The same considerations with regard to temporary diversion as discussed above apply here as well.

Conclusion

Inflammatory bowel disease in pregnancy is a complicated issue that presents many difficult decisions for the patient and the treatment team. The pregnant patient will require education specific to the treatment of their disease and its effect on both the mother and fetus. Education is key regarding the continuation or appropriate changes to medications during pregnancy to minimize their risk for flair or complications of disease. The need for surgical intervention in the pregnant patient with IBD is relatively uncommon, but when indicated the pregnancy presents unique challenges. To properly manage the issues presented and the possible complications of the disease and the pregnancy, there should be a management team of physicians including the obstetrician, as well as a gastroenterologist, and surgeon experienced in treating IBD. This group of physicians should be well versed in the care of these complex patients and communicate with the patient and each other to bring the best short-term and long-term outcome for both the patient and fetus.

References

1. Ellul P, Zammita S, Katsanos K, Cesarini M, Allocca M, Danese S, et al. Perception of reproductive health in women with inflammatory bowel disease. J Crohns Colitis. 2016;10(8):886–91.
2. de Lima-Karagiannis A, Zelinkova-Detkova Z, van der Woude C. The effects of active IBD during pregnancy in the era of novel IBD therapies. Am J Gastroenterol. 2016;111(9):1305–12.
3. Bröms G, Granath F, Stephansson O, Kieler H. Preterm birth in women with inflammatory bowel disease—the association with disease activity and drug treatment. Scand J Gastroenterol. 2016;51(12):1462–9.
4. Kokoszko-Bilska A, Sobkiewicz S, Fichna J. Inflammatory bowel diseases and reproductive health. Pharmacol Rep. 2016;68(4):859–64.
5. Minami N, Matsuura M, Koshikawa Y, Yamada S, Honzawa Y, Yamamoto S, et al. Maternal and fetal outcomes in pregnant Japanese women with inflammatory bowel disease: our experience with a series of 23 cases. Intest Res. 2017;15(1):90.
6. Gaidos J, Kane S. Overcoming challenges of treating inflammatory bowel disease in pregnancy. Expert Rev Clin Immunol. 2016;12(8):871–8.
7. Mahadevan U, Vermeire S, Lasch K, Abhyankar B, Bhayat F, Blake A, et al. Vedolizumab exposure in pregnancy: outcomes from clinical studies in inflammatory bowel disease. Aliment Pharmacol Ther. 2017;45(7):941–50.
8. Gaidos J, Kane S. Managing IBD therapies in pregnancy. Curr Treat Option Gastroenterol. 2017;15(1):71–83.
9. Cortes X, Borrás-Blasco J, Antequera B, Fernandez-Martinez S, Casterá E, Martin S, et al. Ustekinumab therapy for Crohn's disease during pregnancy: a case report and review of the literature. J Clin Pharm Ther. 2016;42(2):234–6.
10. Philip MM, Ross HM. IBD diagnosis and evaluation. In: Steele S, Hull T, Reed T, Saclarides T, Senegore A, Whitlow C, editors. The ASCRS textbook of surgery. Third Edition. New York: Springer; 2016. p. 771–86. Print.
11. Poturoglu S, Ormeci A, Duman A. Treatment of pregnant women with a diagnosis of inflammatory bowel disease. World J Gastrointest Pharmacol Ther. 2016;7(4):490.
12. Protic M, Markovic S, Tarabar D. Case report: acute flair of ulcerative colitis during pregnancy is still a major problem. Dig Dis. 2017;35(1–2):134–8.
13. Killeen S, Gunn J, Hartley J. Surgical management of complicated and medically refractory inflammatory bowel disease during pregnancy. Color Dis. 2017;19(2):123–38.

Colorectal Cancer in Pregnancy

15

Cici Zhang and Marion Schertzer

Introduction

Since the first reported case of rectal adenocarcinoma in pregnancy in 1842 by Cruveilhier [1], colorectal cancer (CRC) incidence has been estimated at approximately 0.002–0.008% of pregnancies [2–5]. It is the seventh most common type of cancer diagnosed in pregnancy [6], and only about 200 cases have been reported in literature. Despite paucity in published material, the rise in incidence of CRC among young women and delay in maternal age have brought renewed attention to CRC in pregnancy.

Just as obstetricians and general practitioners are well informed of the possibility that a breast lump or vaginal bleeding can signify malignancy in pregnancy, rectal bleeding should generate a high index of suspicion for colorectal cancer. A family history of colorectal malignancy should raise index of suspicion, especially if a patient experience changes in bowel habits or bleeding. The most common presenting symptom of colon and rectal cancer is rectal bleeding. Nearly half (47%) of all patients with CRC in pregnancy experience rectal bleeding as the initial presenting symptom. Other concerning findings are abdominal pain (38%) and constipation (14%). Table 15.1 demonstrates the most common presenting symptoms of CRC in pregnancy after a review of 119 published cases [7].

C. Zhang (✉) · M. Schertzer ·
Department of Colon and Rectal Surgery,
Northside Hospital, Atlanta, GA, USA
e-mail: marion.schertzer@northside.com

Evaluation

Similar to the evaluation of nonpregnant CRC patients, initial diagnosis should be followed by staging of disease. This requires an endoscopic examination of the colon and evaluation for potential metastatic disease. A complete colonoscopy is necessary to screen for synchronous lesions, as with serum carcinoembryonic antigen (CEA) levels, and liver ultrasound and/or magnetic resonance imaging (MRI) for the detection of metastatic disease. In addition, an endorectal ultrasonography or MRI is necessary for adequate examination of rectal tumor size and depth of invasion. When advanced rectal cancer is diagnosed in the latter stages of pregnancy, careful assessment of the tumor location in relation to surrounding structures is necessary to evaluate for potential obstruction during vaginal delivery [8].

Sigmoidoscopy and Colonoscopy

Pregnant patients who experience rectal bleeding should elicit a high index of suspicion for colorectal pathology and be evaluated initially with flexible sigmoidoscopy. Flexible sigmoidoscopy can frequently be performed in an office setting

C. H. Nezhat (ed.), *Non-Obstetric Surgery During Pregnancy*,
https://doi.org/10.1007/978-3-319-90752-9_15

Table 15.1 Common presenting complaints of patients with pregnancy-associated colorectal cancer[a]

Rectal bleeding	47%
Abdominal pain	37.6%
Constipation/obstipation	14.1%
Bowel obstruction	6.7%
Diarrhea	5%

[a]Data extrapolated from Pellino et al. (2017) pooled analysis of 119 published cases of CRC in pregnancy

Table 15.2 Colonoscopy general principles in pregnancy

Evaluation for imminent high-risk pregnancies (i.e., abruption, ruptured membranes, or eclampsia)
Use lowest effective dosage of sedative
Use category A or B drugs when possible
Minimize procedure time
Position patient in left laterally and avoid vena caval compression
Fetal heart monitoring before and after procedure

without sedation; it can often identify a source of bleeding; and it has demonstrated a high safety profile regardless of gestational age. In a case-controlled study of 48 patients undergoing sigmoidoscopy during pregnancy, 93% of women experienced normal, healthy births. All three poor outcomes occurred in high-risk pregnancies and markedly ill mothers, thus unlikely to be related to the sigmoidoscopy [9].

The theoretical risk of mechanical pressure on the gravid uterus is minimal during sigmoidoscopy and its impacts are unsubstantiated. Of more significant concern is the safety of drugs used in endoscopic procedures on the developing fetus. The US Food and Drug Administration (FDA) has identified five categories of drugs during pregnancy. Although there are no category A drugs used in endoscopic procedures, most anesthetic and sedative agents used in colonoscopy fall into the B category, which are determined to be safe for pregnancy. The most common agent used for anesthesia during endoscopy, propofol, is a category B drug and has demonstrated no risk in well-controlled human studies [10]. The preferred analgesia agent is meperidine (category B), over benzodiazepines such as midazolam and diazepam (category D), which has a better documented fetal safety profile [11]. Fentanyl (category C), another frequently used analgesic during endoscopy, appears to be safe when used in low doses during pregnancy in clinical experiences [11].

There is limited data regarding the safety and adverse events of colonoscopy during pregnancy. The largest case-controlled study included 20 patients who underwent complete colonoscopy for evaluation of various gastrointestinal complaints. Eighteen patients experienced healthy births, one elected for termination for an unrelated reason, and one gave birth to an infant with a cardiac defect thought to be developed earlier in gestation [12]. Despite the insufficiency of large-scale, well-controlled human studies, colonoscopy is recommended for preoperative evaluation of synchronous lesions and obtaining pathologic diagnosis [13].

Nonetheless, precautions and modifications should be employed to optimize safety when performing colonoscopy during pregnancy (Table 15.2). When performed late in pregnancy, patients should not be placed in the decubitus or prone position [10]. External abdominal pressure should be limited to a minimum and directed away from the uterus. The majority of the available laxatives and bowel preparations are without documented side effects; however, castor oil carries an absolute contraindication for use in pregnancy (category X) due to its associated risk of uterine rupture. For flexible sigmoidoscopies, both Fleets enemas and tap water enemas appear to be safe options, although Fleets appear to be more effective in a review of surveyed endoscopists [14].

Ultrasonography

The safe utilization of ultrasound has been long established in pregnancy. Its safety profile, wide availability, and low cost have made ultrasonography the mainstay of diagnosing abdominal complaints during pregnancy. In evaluating pregnant patients with CRC, ultrasonography is an important modality for detection of metastatic disease. Early investigators have demonstrated focused ultrasonography has a sensitivity of 85–90% for detecting hepatic metastases [15–17].

With growing interest in endoluminal approaches and technological advances, ultrasonography has regained purpose in the evaluation of rectal cancer. The treatment and prognosis of rectal cancer are highly influenced by primary tumor (T) and regional lymph node (N) stage of disease at the time of diagnosis. Initial staging is crucial for the decision-making process of rectal cancer treatment, especially in pregnant patients. Endoluminal transrectal ultrasonography (TRUS) has demonstrated notable accuracy for the initial staging and evaluation of tumor infiltration [18, 19]. In experienced hands, detection of tumor infiltration can be achieved with an accuracy of 78–85.5% [18–21]. The accuracy for detection of malignant lymph nodes ranges between 64% and 84% [21–23]. Large bodies of evidence are building for the reliability and accuracy of TRUS in high-volume centers. Particularly in pregnant patients who are wary of the risks associated with MRI, TRUS is emerging as a valuable modality for the evaluation of rectal malignancy.

Despite its wide availability, long accepted safety profile and utility, ultrasonography has several limitations. The lack of patient cooperation, unfavorable body habits, especially in later stages of pregnancy, and intraluminal bowel gas can all hinder visualization and decrease sensitivity. Although useful and highly predictive of hepatic metastatic disease when visualized, negative results do not exclude metastatic disease in pregnant patients with CRC.

Computed Tomography

The use of computed tomography (CT) as an imaging modality during pregnancy is fraught with trepidation and misconceptions. Teratogenesis occurs largely in early fetal development, and the risk decreases through the second and third trimesters. The developing brain between the 8th and 15th weeks of gestation is especially vulnerable to radiation damage. Fetal exposure up to 100–200 mGy is unlikely to substantially increase fetal anomalies [24, 25]. The lower threshold of hazardous exposure, 100 mGy of radiation, is roughly reached by 20 conventional diagnostic radiographs or 3 pelvic CT scans. Significant radiation exposure, however, can be associated with neurological and developmental malformations. Fetal doses in the range of 1000 mGy can result in severe mental retardation and microcephaly, particularly during 8–15 weeks and to a lesser extent at 16–25 weeks [25]. Nonetheless, ionizing radiation should be limited to the lowest amount of exposure and only be utilized for essential testing during staging investigations in CRC patients during pregnancy.

Magnetic Resonance Imaging

Magnetic resonance imaging (MRI) has become the imaging modality of choice in determining tumor stage and predicting resectability for rectal cancer [26]. The accurate identification of circumferential margin is paramount for planning an effective therapeutic strategy, especially in the complex management of rectal cancer in pregnancy. MRI can accurately measure tumor invasion beyond the muscularis propria (T3), providing crucial information in determining whether neoadjuvant chemotherapy is advisable or complete surgical resection is feasible [27, 28]. Several studies have demonstrated the valuable potential of MRI in predicting the distance between the tumor and the fascial plane. Meta-analysis of nine studies demonstrated the overall sensitivity and specificity for detecting circumferential margin involvement preoperatively to be 94% and 85%, respectively [29]. Despite its clear advantage in the preoperative evaluation of rectal cancer, several factors regarding safety specific to pregnancy have challenged its utilization.

One safety concern of MRI arises from its emission of radiofrequency pulses, which results in energy deposition and potential tissue heating [30]. The unit of energy deposited is referred to as the specific absorption rate (SAR), and no adverse fetal effects have been documented from MR imaging by using routine sequences, even at relatively high SAR [30]. The effects of MR exposure in the prenatal period have not been fully determined, but the predicted fetal temperature rise associated with MR imaging is below the expected teratogenic levels. Despite this, the potential heating to the fetus and amniotic fluid should be considered especially during the first trimester, when the fetus is the most vulnerable [31].

Intravenous gadolinium is another source of controversy during pregnancy. Gadolinium is considered a pregnancy category C drug by the US Food and Drug Administration (FDA). Gadolinium can cross the placenta and can accumulate in the fetal gastrointestinal and genitourinary systems. Several investigators reported mutagenic affects in animal models, but no adverse effects have been found on small human studies in first, second, and third trimester of pregnancy [32–34]. Current recommendations suggest cautionary usage of gadolinium, especially in the first trimester, since the risks of teratogenic fetal effects have not been clearly established [35].

Disease Management

Patients diagnosed with CRC during pregnancy face particularly difficult decisions regarding the therapeutic options. Confronted with treatments that may require termination, iatrogenic prematurity, or intentional delay in treatment, patients should be provided with all the relevant information regarding the ramifications of operative management, chemotherapy, and radiation therapy. Gestational age and assessment of fetal viability is critical for both emergency and elective presentation of CRC. A fetus between 24 and 28 weeks is considered extremely preterm and is associated with increased infant morbidity [7]. Delivery after 30–34 weeks is generally advised [7, 36]. Because of the potential for obstruction during delivery, cesarean section is to be preferred to vaginal delivery in patients with rectal cancers. Figures 15.1 and 15.2 demonstrate a therapeutic algorithm for the treatment of colon and rectal cancer presented in the elective setting.

Chemotherapy

Unfortunately, all chemotherapeutic agents cross the placental barrier [36]. The teratogenicity of any drug depends on the gestation age at exposure, the dose, and the specific characteristics affecting placental transfer. This affect is most clinically significant in the first 12 weeks of gestation, during which organogenesis is completed. In the first trimester, exposure to chemotherapeutic drugs can result in congenital malformations and/or spontaneous abortions [37, 38]. Approximately 10–20% of infants exposed to cytotoxic agents during the first trimester have major malformations as compared with a rate of 3% in the general population [39]. Exposure to chemotherapy during the second and third trimester increases the risk of low birth weight, although this has been attributed to the influence of maternal cancer on fetal growth and the tendency to elect for iatrogenic prematurity [37, 40].

The mainstay of CRC chemotherapy is FOLFOX therapy which consists of leucovorin, fluorouracil (5-FU), and oxaliplatin. Fortunately, FOLFOX has demonstrated significant tolerability and safety profile when administered during the second and third trimesters [41]. Leucovorin is rated category A by the FDA, representing no known risk of fetal harm based on human data. Oxaliplatin and 5-FU during pregnancy are category D drugs and are recommended to be avoided during the first trimester. Both have demonstrated teratogenicity in animal models and human case reports [42]. Irinotecan is FDA approved for first-line treatment of metastatic CRC as part of the FOLFIRI (leucovorin, fluorouracil, and irinotecan) regimen. It is also a category D drug because of its theoretical risk of teratogenicity during organogenesis based on rat and rabbit models. However, case reports of irinotecan use during later stages of gestation have demonstrated no untoward affects [43].

Newer chemotherapy drugs used as adjuvant treatments for metastatic or locally advanced CRC include bevacizumab (Avastin®, Genentech, San Francisco, CA) and capecitabine (Xeloda®, Hoffmann-La Roche, Nutley, NJ). Both have evidence of fetotoxicity and teratogenicity in animal studies and are classified as category D drugs [44, 45]. Bevacizumab is also associated with reduced placental perfusion and is not recommended throughout pregnancy [43].

Although few studies shine light onto the long-term sequelae of children exposed to chemotherapy for colorectal cancer in utero, studies

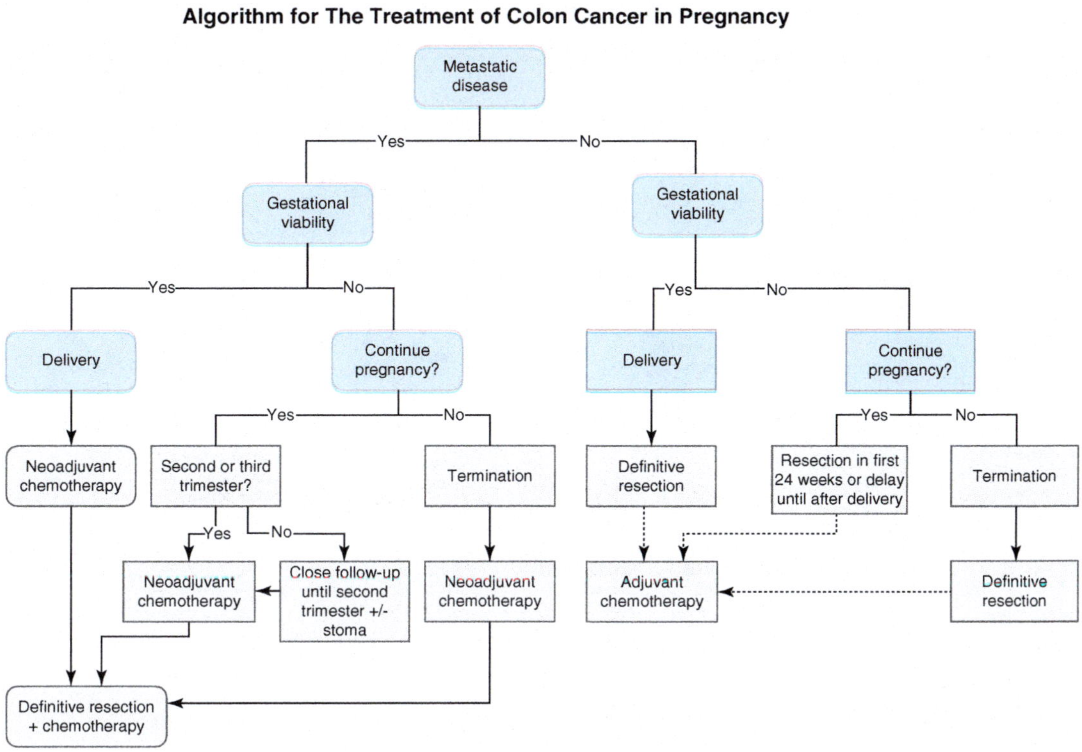

Fig. 15.1 Algorithm for treatment pathway of colon cancer in pregnancy, not including emergent operative management. Gestational viability is determined as 30–34 weeks. Cesarean section is the preferable delivery method in rectal cancer. Dotted arrows demonstrate possible treatment options after definitely staging

investigating chemotherapy agents for breast and hematological malignancies have not reported significant learning impairment and hematologic or immunologic abnormalities [46]. While most chemotherapeutic agents cross the placental barrier, they often do not have the ability to pass into breast milk. However, little information regarding breastfeeding during chemotherapy is available, and breastfeeding is not recommended while undergoing chemotherapy [37, 47].

Surgical Intervention

Surgical resection can be offered before 24 weeks of gestation when appropriate [48]. Fetal heart monitoring should be performed before and after any surgical intervention. Patients in the third trimester of gestation should delay operative management until after delivery unless tumor complications such as bowel obstruction, perforation, or bleeding warrant immediate surgical intervention. Manipulation of the gravid uterus in last gestation can promote premature labor, and all published cases of colectomy in the third trimester have resulted in premature delivery. This ubiquitous finding has led several investigators to recommend a synchronous cesarean section and colectomy in the emergent and elective setting [49–51]. In the later stages of the second trimester, the gravid uterus may obstruct exposure to the pelvis, especially during low rectal cancer resections. In such cases, gentle elevation and stabilization throughout the case is recommended. If technical difficulty is encountered during the creation of colorectal continuity, a diverting stoma should be created rather than attempting to create an anastomosis. Fetal heart monitoring should be performed before and after surgery. Delivery is recommended at the earliest fetal maturity. If cesarean delivery is indicated, as in the case of rectal cancer, concomitant resection

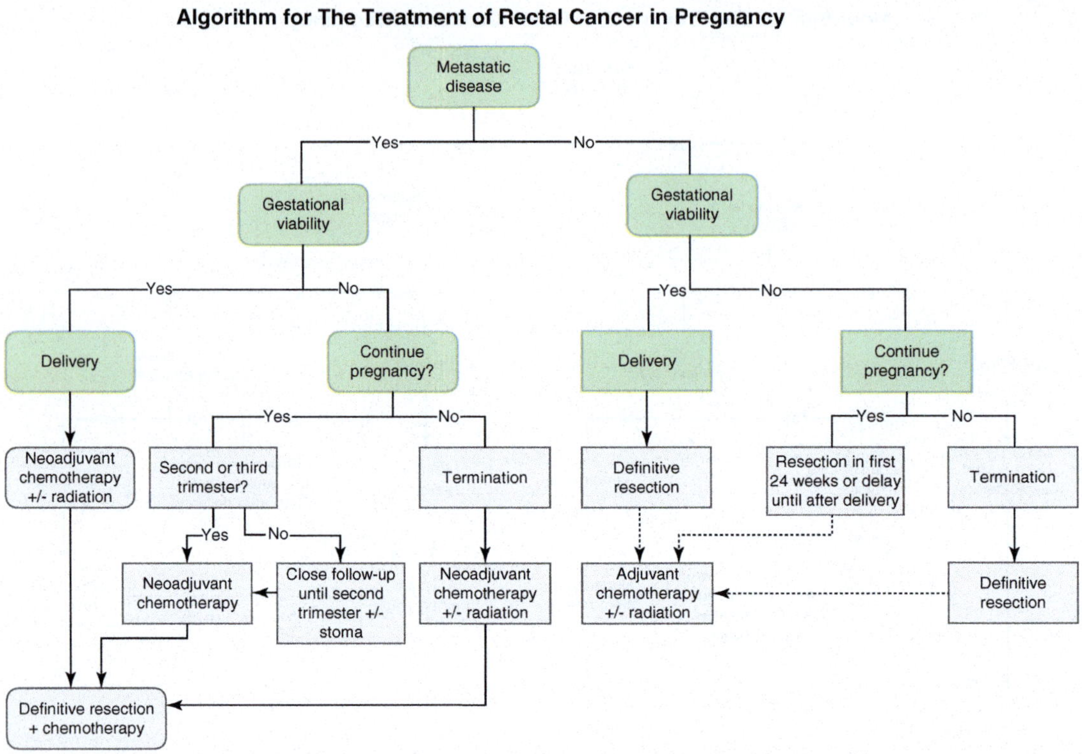

Fig. 15.2 Algorithm for treatment pathway of rectal cancer in pregnancy, not including emergent operative management. Gestational viability is determined as 30–34 weeks. Cesarean section is the preferable delivery method in rectal cancer. Dotted arrows demonstrate possible treatment options after definitely staging

of tumor is recommended. In cases of metastatic disease, surgical treatment should follow neoadjuvant chemoradiation therapy when appropriate and possible.

Depending on the location of the tumor and size of the gravid uterus, considerations for surgical approach must be individualized to prevent unnecessary manipulation of the uterus. Figure 15.3 demonstrates uterine size based on weeks of gestation. Operative incision should be tailored as to avoid injuring the uterus upon entering the peritoneal cavity. Care also should be taken to minimize anesthesia time. For this reason, laparoscopy, which introduces increased intra-abdominal pressure and is associated with increase operative time, is not recommended. Much of what is known regarding the effects of laparoscopy on maternal and fetal morbidity is extracted from literature on laparoscopic cholecystectomy and appendectomy. Maternal complications following laparoscopic procedures occur at an estimated rate of 0.006% [48]. Few have investigated the impact of laparoscopic colectomy or proctectomy on maternal and fetal morbidity. A systemic review of all publications on the surgical management of inflammatory bowel disease during pregnancy reported four cases of attempted laparoscopy [52]. Only two were completed laparoscopically, and one experienced preterm labor at 28 weeks of gestation [53]. To date, insufficient evidence supports the use of laparoscopy in the operative management CRC in pregnancy.

Debate exists on whether bilateral salpingo-oophorectomy at the time of resection should be performed given the described risk of metastasis. Ovarian metastasis occurs in 24% of patients with CRC during pregnancy [54–57]. If they are frankly involved, they should be removed at the time of surgery; otherwise, wedge biopsies with frozen sections can be performed to establish diagnosis. Prophylactic removal of bilateral

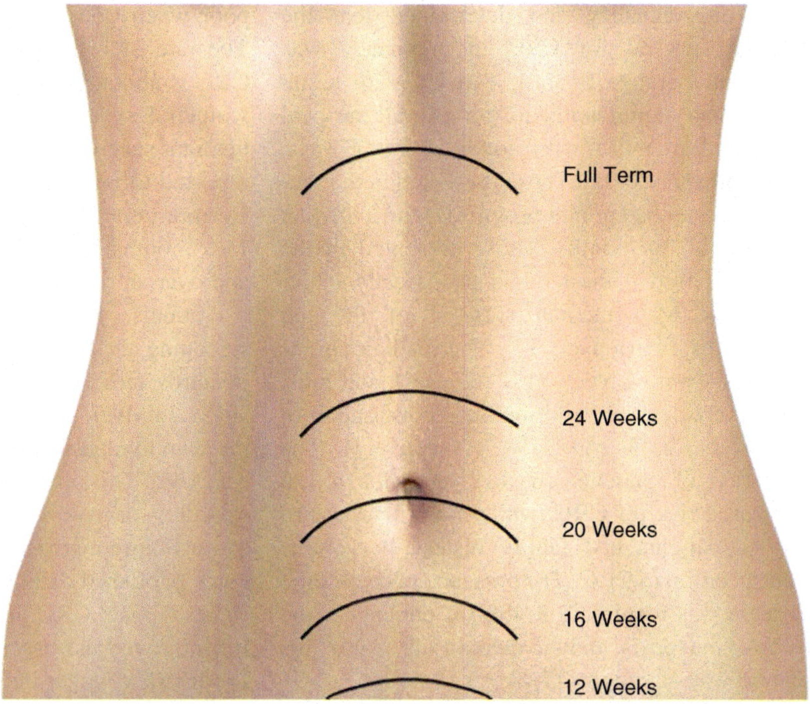

Fig. 15.3 Uterine size based on weeks of gestation

ovaries is not recommended because of the risk of spontaneous abortion, even if hormonal replacement is administered [55].

Surgical Emergency

Tumor complications such as perforation, obstruction, or hemorrhage further complicate the management algorithm for CRC in pregnancy. Colonic perforation and resultant fecal peritonitis carry devastating maternal and fetal outcomes. Intestinal perforation due to CRC is rare and only constitutes 2.4% of initial presentations [7]. Published data on maternal and fetal morbidity and mortality are largely based on appendiceal perforation in pregnancy, which is associated with a 20–35% fetal loss rate and a 4% rate of maternal mortality [58, 59]. The incidence of intestinal obstruction is estimated to be between 1 in 1500 and 1 in 66,000 pregnancies and was the presenting symptom in 9.4% of pregnant patients with CRC [7, 60, 61]. A midline laparotomy provides the best operative exposure, and definitive operative treatment with colonic resection and/or diverting stoma should be performed. In a literature review by Perdue, 23% of pregnant patients with intestinal obstruction required bowel resection, pregnancy was completed to term in only 38%, maternal mortality rate was 6%, and fetal mortality rate was 26% [61]. Rectal bleeding is the most common presenting symptom and rarely leads to operative intervention alone. However, when gastrointestinal hemorrhage is rapid or requiring prolonged resuscitation, definitive surgical resection should be considered.

Prognosis

Patients with CRC during pregnancy have a poor prognosis. This apparent predisposition has been attributed to a variety of factors including age at diagnosis, aggressive histology, delayed diagnosis, and advanced pathologic stage [2, 62, 63]. The 5-year disease-free survival was found to be 42% in a study of 26 pregnant patients with rectal cancer and 38% with colon cancer [2]. Pellino et al. conducted a review of all published cases of

CRC in pregnancy and determined that the median survival for CRC in pregnancy was 36 months (range 0–360). Patients with rectal cancer had significantly longer overall survival compared to those with colon cancer (73 vs. 26 months, $P < 0.01$). Those presented in the second trimester had poorer prognosis with a median survival of 30 months. Those presented in the first and third trimester had statistically better prognosis with median survival of 36 and 73 months, respectively [7]. The median age of diagnosis was 32 years (17–46 years), and most cases were diagnosed during the second and third trimesters (41% and 47%, respectively). The majority of patients (65%) were not at an increased risk for CRC, while more than a third of the patients had family history or genetic redisposition to CRC. The presence of metastatic disease was identified in 48% of patients at the time of diagnosis, and the median survival in this cohort was 42 months [7].

Age

The poor prognosis of pregnant women with CRC may, in part, be a reflection of the patient age [2]. With improved accessibility to screening and improved treatment armamentarium, mortality has decreased (by 2–3% annually between 1992 and 2009) for CRC patients in all age groups except for younger patients, whose mortality rate has been rising in the last few years. Colorectal cancer incidence rates have been increasing by 2.4% per year in adults age 20–29 and by 1.0% per year in adults age 30–39 [62]. Currently, nearly one-third of rectal cancer patients are younger than 55 years of age.

Whether this increase in incidence of CRC in young patients affects disease-specific survival is yet to be elucidated. A recent epidemiological investigation of 258,024 patients of the Surveillance, Epidemiology, and End Result (SEER) database of the National Cancer Institute (NCI) demonstrated that young patients were more likely to present with regional (relative risk ratio, 1.3; $P < 0.001$) or distant (relative risk ratio, 1.5; $P < 0.001$) disease. Prognosis is particularly poor when CRC is metastasized to the ovaries. The rate of ovarian metastases in women with CRC is about 3–8% [56, 57] but rises to 31% in women less than 40 years old [54, 64]. The median survival for this population has been reported to be between 3 months to 1 year [56]. Herrera-Ornelas reported the median survival of 16.5 months in 54 pregnant patients with CRC and ovarian metastasis [65].

Patients younger than the recommended screening age have better overall disease-specific (hazards ratio, 0.77; $P < 0.001$) and stage-for-stage survival, despite a larger percentage of these individuals presenting with advanced disease [66]. This apparent improvement in disease-specific survival is likely due to a tendency toward more aggressive treatment. As more and more published data began to elucidate the trend of early onset CRC, multiple groups have called for improved risk assessment and early screening for at-risk younger individuals [62, 66–69].

Tumor Histology

Younger patients, specifically patients under the age of 40, with CRC often exhibit signet cell tumor morphology and are associated with a higher incidence of lymphovascular invasion; are frequently diagnosed in an advanced stage of disease; and carry a worse prognosis [63, 70, 71]. Signet cell histology is defined by greater than 50% presence of tumor cells possessing prominent intracytoplasmic mucin and lack of cell-to-cell adhesion molecules. Its aggressive potential is secondary to the deregulation of cell-to-cell adhesion molecule E-cadherin, which, in turn, enhances its tendency to spread. Carriers of CDH-1 germline mutation leading to E-cadherin deficiency are predisposed to early onset hereditary diffuse gastric cancer with a 70% lifetime risk and median age of diagnosis at 33 [72, 73]. Although largely studied in patients with hereditary diffuse gastric adenocarcinoma, a subset of these patients also has increased risk of developing colorectal cancer in the third decade of life [74].

Recently, Tawadros et al. demonstrated a 3.6-fold increase risk of signet cell histology in the cohort under 40 years of age in a review of more than 38,000 patients diagnosed with rectal cancer from the SEER database [63]. This increased prevalence of signet cell adenocarcinoma histology was significantly associated with advanced stage, poorly differentiated tumor grade, and worse prognosis than its mucinous and non-mucinous counterparts. Adenocarcinoma of signet cell histology was found to impact survival by nearly twofold. The median survival for signet cell type is 14 months compared to 27 months ($P < 0.001$) in mucinous-type [63].

Hormonal Effects of Pregnancy

With respect to the hormonal influence on CRC during pregnancy, earlier investigators suggested that the increase circulation of estrogen and progesterone may stimulate rapid growth by activating estrogen and progesterone receptor-binding capacity of the tumor cells. This hypothesis was supported by several small reports demonstrating high levels of estrogen and progesterone receptor positivity in CRC tumor cells [75, 76]. However, recent experience with larger cohorts (n = 29–156) demonstrated low detection of estrogen or progesterone receptor expressivity on CRC tumor cells via immunohistochemical staining [77, 78]. Furthermore, a growing body of evidence from preclinical studies indicate that expression of the estrogen receptor beta (ERβ) demonstrates an inverse relationship with the presence of colorectal polyps and stage of tumors and can mediate a protective response [79, 80].

In two large trials launched by the Women's Health Initiative (WHI), combination estrogen plus progestin therapy was associated with 40% reduction in incidence of colorectal cancer [81, 82]. This conclusion was later refuted in several large-scale follow-up studies that demonstrated combination estrogen and progestin therapy had no clinically significant influence on CRC mortality [83–85]. In 2014, the WHI published its 11.6-year follow-up data of the initial randomized controlled study and concluded that combination hormonal therapy was not compatible with clinically meaningful reduction in colorectal cancer [84]. Despite enormous scale and effort of these trials, it is difficult to extrapolate discernable insight in regard to CRC patients during pregnancy. To date, no dedicated studies have investigated the influence of estrogen and progestin during pregnancy with respect to the development and progression of colorectal cancer.

Another unique challenge to the treatment of CRC is the complex interactions between growth factors, immune system, and environmental factors underlying pregnancy. The state of pregnancy promotes a myriad of physiologic changes on the molecular level. Current research is beginning to elucidate the overexpression of growth factors such as cyclooxygenase-2 (COX-2) enzymes, insulin-like growth factor 1 (IGF-1), and placental growth factor (PGF) and its impact on cancer biology [86–88]. However, sufficient evidence has not yet revealed a direct link between physiologic changes of pregnancy and the apparent rapid growth and spread of colorectal cancer in this cohort.

Advanced Stage of Presentation

Another factor likely to contribute to the aggressive nature of CRC in pregnancy is the advanced stage of disease at presentation. Unfortunately, metastatic disease at the time of diagnosis is found in 48% of patients in a review of 119 published cases of CRC during pregnancy. Only 12% of patients were diagnosed during the first trimester of gestation, 41% and 47% during the second and third trimester, respectively. Those 87 who presented in the third trimester had significantly advanced disease, and over 25% of patients presented in an emergent setting requiring hospitalization and intervention [7]. The cause for the apparent delay in diagnosis is multifaceted. Factors including low threshold for suspicion, confounding clinical features of early pregnancy, and reluctance for invasive examination all hinder early identification and treatment.

In addition to a low incidence of CRC in this age cohort, the majority of patients were not at an increased risk of CRC based on personal and family history [7]. This finding is confounded as patients with a known genetic disposition for CRC are likely to be screened early in life and excluded from these studies. Regardless, this further lowers the suspicion of CRC in pregnant patients on the list of differential diagnosis. Its rarity along with a seemingly insignificant group of presenting symptoms compounds the difficulty of diagnosing of CRC in pregnancy.

The most commonly presenting complaints for pregnant patients with CRC are rectal bleeding, abdominal pain, and constipation [8, 63, 89, 90]. These symptoms are routinely attributed to the natural physiological changes during early gestation and often overlooked without additional investigation. Rectal bleeding, the most common initial symptom and found in almost half of the patients with CRC in pregnancy, is frequently accredited to hemorrhoidal disease pervasive in the population in question [2, 7].

Diagnosis of CRC in pregnancy at its earliest symptomatic presentation is a challenging task faced by many obstetricians and primary care physicians. Although the incidence of CRC remains low during pregnancy, a high index of suspicion is important for the early diagnosis and treatment of this devastating disease. With rising occurrence of CRC in women of childbearing age, patients with rectal bleeding, constipation, persistent nausea, and vomiting should be offered the same consideration and investigation as their nonpregnant counterparts.

Another factor contributing to the overall poor prognosis of CRC in pregnancy is the complicated decision-making process related to disease management. Often riddled with emotional, religious, and ethical convictions, patients are frequently faced with choice between optimal cancer treatment and the welfare of the fetus. Under these difficult prevailing circumstances, therapeutic options should be individualized, and a multidisciplinary team consisting of the surgeon, obstetrician, oncologist, maternal-fetal medicine specialist, and social worker should collaborate in the care of the patient.

Conclusion

Colorectal cancer during pregnancy presents a variety of challenges to a clinician. Frequently disguised as common ailments of pregnancy, CRC is difficult to diagnose and even more bewildering to treat. A high index of suspicion, a proficient knowledge of the available diagnostic tools, and a full understanding of treatment options can provide valuable guidance to the complex and delicate therapeutic decision-making process.

References

1. Cruveilhier J. Anatomie pathologique du corps humaine. Livre Maison. 1842;2:7–10.
2. Bernstein MA, Madoff RD, Caushaj PF. Colon and rectal cancer in pregnancy. Dis Colon Rectum. 1993;36(2):172–8.
3. Donegan WL. Cancer and pregnancy. Cancer J Clin. 1983;33(4):194–214.
4. Minter A, Malik R, Ledbetter L, Winokur TS, Hawn MT, Saif MW. Colon cancer in pregnancy. Cancer Control. 2005;12(3):196–202.
5. Girard RM, Lamarche J, Baillot R. Carcinoma of the colon associated. Dis Colon Rectum. 1981;24:473–5.
6. Woods JB, Martin JN, Ingram FH, Odom CD, Scott-Conner C, Rhodes RS. Pregnancy complicated by carcinoma of the colon above the rectum. Am J Perinatol. 1992;9(2):102–10.
7. Pellino G, Simillis C, Kontovounisios C, Baird DL, Nikolaou S, Warren O, et al. Colorectal cancer diagnosed during pregnancy. Eur J Gastroenterol Hepatol. 2017;29(7):743–53.
8. Yaghoobi M, Koren G, Nulman I. Challenges to diagnosing colorectal cancer during pregnancy. Can Fam Physician. 2009;55:881–5.
9. Cappell MS, Colon VJ, Sidhom OA. A study at 10 medical Centers of the safety and efficacy of 48 flexible Sigmoidoscopies and 8 colonoscopies during pregnancy with follow-up of Fetal outcome and with comparison to control groups. Dig Dis Sci. 1996;41(12):2353–61.
10. Savas N. Gastrointestinal endoscopy in pregnancy. World J Gastroenterol. 2014;20(41):15241–13.
11. Gilinsky NH, Muthunayagam N. Gastrointestinal endoscopy in pregnant and lactating women: emerging standard of care to guide decision-making. Obstet Gynecol Surv. 2006;61(12):791–9.
12. Cappell MS, Fox SR, Gorrepati N. Safety and efficacy of colonoscopy during pregnancy. J Reprod Med. 2010;55(3–4):115–23.
13. Cappell MS. Colon cancer during pregnancy. Gastroenterol Clin N Am. 2003;32:341–83.
14. Vinod J, Bonheur J, Korelitz B, Panagopoulos G. Choice of laxatives and colonoscopic preparation in pregnant patients from the viewpoint of obstetricians and gastroenterologists. World J Gastroenterol. 2007;13(48):6549–52.

15. Sultana F, Al-Azad S, Sattar A, Hossain MZ, Deepa ZS, Chatterjee S. Ultrasonographic evaluation of hepatic metastases of malignant diseases with cytopathological correlation. J Dhaka Med Coll. 2014;23(2):239–44.
16. Türkay C, Elagöz S, Yüksel I, Yönem O, Murat I. The diagnostic value of ultrasonography-guided fine needle aspiration biopsy from liver and pancreas. Turk J Gastroenterol. 2002;13(1):53–5.
17. Dick R, Watkinson A. The liver and spleen. In: Sutton D, editor. Textbook of Radiology and Imaging. 7th ed. London: Churchill Livingstone; 2003. p. 737–8. 772–773.
18. Marone P, de BM, D'Angelo V, Delrio P, Passananti V, Girolamo ED, et al. Role of endoscopic ultrasonography in the loco-regional staging of patients with rectal cancer. World J Gastrointest Endosc. 2015;7(7):688–15.
19. Serra-Aracil X, Galvez A, Mora-López L, Rebasa P, Serra-Pla S, Pallisera-Lloveras A, et al. Endorectal ultrasound in the identification of rectal tumors for transanal endoscopic surgery: factors influencing its accuracy. Surg Endosc. 2017. https://doi.org/10.1007/s00464-017-5988-9.
20. Liu Z-L, Zhou T, Liang X-B, Ma J-J, Zhang G-J. Learning curve of endorectal ultrasonography in preoperative staging of rectal carcinoma. Mol Clin Oncol. 2014;2(6):1085–90.
21. Garcia-Aguilar J, Pollack J, Lee S-H, Hernandez de Anda E, Mellgren A, Wong WD, et al. Accuracy of endorectal ultrasonography in preoperative staging of rectal tumors. Dis Colon Rectum. 2002;45(1):10–5.
22. Nesbakken A, Lovig T, Lunde OC, Nygaard K. Staging of rectal carcinoma with Transrectal ultrasonography. Scand J Surg. 2013;92:125–9.
23. Mackay SG, Pager CK, Joseph D, Stewart PJ, Solomon MJ. Assessment of the accuracy of transrectal ultrasonography in anorectal neoplasia. Br J Surg. 2003;90:346–50.
24. Koren G, Weiner L, Lishner M, Zemlickes D, Finegen J. Cancer in pregnancy: identification of unanswered questions on maternal and Fetal risks. Obstet Gynecol Surv. 1990;45(8):509–14.
25. Streffer C, Shore R, Konermann G, Meadows A, Uma Devi P, Preston Withers J, et al. Biological effects after prenatal irradiation (embryo and fetus). A report of the international commission on radiological protection. Ann ICRP. 2003;33(1–2):5–206.
26. Klessen C, Rogalla P, Taupitz M. Local staging of rectal cancer: the current role of MRI. Eur Radiol. 2006;17(2):379–89.
27. Botterill ID, Blunt DM, Quirke P, Sebag-Montefiore D, Sagar PM, Finan PJ, et al. Evaluation of the role of pre-operative magnetic resonance imaging in the management of rectal cancer. Color Dis. 2001;3:295–303.
28. Mathur P, Smith JJ, Ramsey C, Owen M, Thorpe A, Karim S, et al. Comparison of CT and MRI in the pre-operative staging of rectal adenocarcinoma and prediction of circumferential resection margin involvement by MRI. Color Dis. 2003;5:396–401.
29. Purkayastha S, Tekkis PP, Athanasiou T, Tilney HS, Darzi AW, Heriot AG. Diagnostic precision of magnetic resonance imaging for preoperative prediction of the circumferential margin involvement in patients with rectal cancer. Color Dis. 2006;9(5):402–11.
30. Brown MA, Birchard KR, Semelka RC. Magnetic resonance evaluation of pregnant patients with acute abdominal pain. Semin Ultrasound CT MR. 2005;26(4):206–11.
31. Oto A, Ernst R, Jesse M, Chaljub G, Saade G. Magnetic resonance imaging of the chest, abdomen, and pelvis in the evaluation of pregnant patients with neoplasms. Am J Perinatol. 2007;24(4):243–50.
32. De Santis M, Straface G, Cavaliere AF, Carducci B, Caruso A. Gadolinium periconceptional exposure: pregnancy and neonatal outcome. Acta Obstet Gynecol Scand. 2007;86(1):99–101.
33. Marcos HB, Semelka RC, Worawattanakul S. Normal Placenta: Gadolinium-enhanced, dynamic MR imaging. Radiology. 1997;205(2):493–6.
34. Tanaka YO, Sohda S, Shigemitsu S, Niitsu M, Itai Y. High temporal resolution dynamic contrast MRI in a high risk group for placenta accreta. Magn Reson Imaging. 2001;19:635–42.
35. Bouyou J, Gaujoux S, Marcellin L, Leconte M, Goffinet F, Chapron C, et al. Abdominal emergencies during pregnancy. J Visc Surg. 2015;152(6):S105–15.
36. Van Calsteren K. Chemotherapy during pregnancy: pharmacokinetics and impact on foetal neurological development. Facts Views Vis Obgyn. 2010;2(4):278–86.
37. Zemlickes D, Lishner M, Degendorfer P, Panzarella T, Sutcliffe SB, Koren G. Fetal outcome after in utero exposure to cancer chemotherapy. Arch Intern Med. 1992;152:573–6.
38. Buekers TE, Lallas TA. Chemotherapy in pregnancy. Obstet Gynecol Clin N Am. 1998;25(2):323–9.
39. Kozlowski RD, Steinbrunner JV, MacKenzie AH, Clough JD, Wilke WS, Segal AM. Outcome of first-trimester exposure to low-dose methotrexate in eight patients with rheumatic disease. Am J Med. 1990;88(6):589–92.
40. Garofalo S, Degennaro VA, Salvi S, De Carolis MP, Capelli G, Ferrazzani S, et al. Perinatal outcome in pregnant women with cancer: are there any effects of chemotherapy? Eur J Cancer Care. 2016;26(6):e12564–7.
41. Jeppesen JB, Østerlind K. Successful twin pregnancy outcome after in utero exposure to FOLFOX for metastatic colon cancer: a case report and review of the literature. Clin Colorectal Cancer. 2011;10(4):348–52.
42. Shuey DL, Buckalew AR, Wilke TS, Rogers JM, Abbott BD. Early events following maternal exposure to 5-fluorouracil lead to dysmorphology. Teratology. 1994;50:379–86.
43. Taylor J, Amanze A, Di Federico E, Verschraegen C. Irinotecan use during pregnancy. Obstet Gynecol. 2009;114:451–2.
44. Bamdad S, Bamdad M, Khanlari M, Daneshbod Y, Khademi B. Teratogenic effects of Intravitreal

injection of Bevacizumab in a pregnant rat model. Iran J Pharm Res. 2017;16(2):670–6.
45. FDA. XELODA (capecitabine) tablets, for oral use. 2015 24:1–46. https://www.accessdata.fda.gov/drugsatfda_docs/label/2015/020896s037lbl.pdf.
46. Avilés A, Neri N. Hematological malignancies and pregnancy: a final report of 84 children who received chemotherapy in utero. Clin Lymphoma. 2011;2(3):173–7.
47. Cardonick E, Usmani A, Ghaffar S. Perinatal outcomes of a pregnancy complicated by cancer, including neonatal follow-up after in utero exposure to chemotherapy. Am J Clin Oncol. 2009;33(3):221–8.
48. Cohen-Kerem R, Railton C, Oren D, Lishner M, Koren G. Pregnancy outcome following non-obstetric surgical intervention. Am J Surg. 2005;190(3):467–73.
49. Quddus A, Martin-Perez B, Schoonyoung H, Albert M, Atallah S. Toxic megacolon during pregnancy in ulcerative colitis: a case report. Int J Surg Case Rep. 2015;11:83–6.
50. Parker AR, Baker N, Maxwell D. A modification of the surgical indications for the treatment of ulcerative colitis during pregnancy. Am Surg. 2011;77(12):281–3.
51. Toiyama Y, Araki T, Yoshiyama S, Sakamoto N, Miki C, Kusunoki M. Fulminant ulcerative colitis during pregnancy successfully treated by three-stage operation. J Gastroenterol. 2004;39(3):300–1.
52. Killeen S, Gunn J, Hartley J. Surgical management of complicated and medically refractory inflammatory bowel disease during pregnancy. Color Dis. 2017;19(2):123–38.
53. Czymek R, Limmer S, Kleemann M, Hildebrand P, Schmidt A, Jungbluth T, et al. Crohn's disease—a chameleon during pregnancy. Langenbeck's Arch Surg. 2008;394(3):517–27.
54. Tsukamoto N, Uchino H, Matsukuma K, Kamura T. Carcinoma of the colon presenting as bilateral ovarian Tumors during pregnancy. Gynecol Oncol. 1986;24:386–91.
55. Nesbitt JC, Moise KJ, Sawyers JL. Colorectal Carcinoma in Pregnancy. Arch Surg. 1985;120:636–40.
56. Mason M, Kovalcik P. Ovarian metastases from colon carcinoma. Eur J Surg Oncol. 1981;17:33–8.
57. Knoepp LF, Ray JE, Overby I. Ovarian metastases from colorectal carcinoma. Dis Colon Rectum. 1973;16(4):305–11.
58. Firstenberg MS, Malangoni MA. Gastrointestinal surgery during pregnancy. Gastroenterol Clin N Am. 1998;27(1):73–88.
59. Alkis I, Kurdoglu M, Kurdoglu Z. Nonobstetric surgical intervention in pregnancy. East J Med. 2010;15:1–6.
60. Ballantyne GH. Review of sigmoid volvulus. Dis Colon Rectum. 1982;25:823–30.
61. Perdue PW, Johnson HW, Stafford PW. Intestinal obstruction complicating pregnancy. Am J Surg. 1992;164:384–8.
62. Siegel RL, Fedewa SA, Anderson WF, Miller KD, Ma J, Rosenberg PS, et al. Colorectal cancer incidence patterns in the United States, 1974–2013. J Natl Cancer Inst. 2017;109(8):1–6.
63. Tawadros PS, Paquette IM, Hanly AM, Mellgren AF, Rothenberger DA, Madoff RD. Adenocarcinoma of the rectum in patients under age 40 is increasing. Dis Colon Rectum. 2015;58(5):474–8.
64. Pitt J, Dawson PM. Oophorectomy in women with colorectal cancer. Eur J Surg Oncol. 1999;25:432–8.
65. Herrera-Ornelas I, Natarajan N, Tsukada Y, Prado-Alcala F, Gutierrez-Garcia CJ, Piver S, et al. Adenocarcinoma of the colon masquerading as primary ovarian Neoplasia. Dis Colon Rectum. 1983;26:377–80.
66. Abdelsattar ZM, Wong SL, Regenbogen SE, Jomaa DM, Hardiman KM, Hendren S. Colorectal cancer outcomes and treatment patterns in patients too young for average-risk screening. Cancer. 2016;122(6):929–34.
67. Bailey CE, Hu C-Y, You YN, Bednarski BK, Rodriguez-Bigas MA, Skibber JM, et al. Increasing disparities in the age-related incidences of colon and rectal cancers in the United States, 1975-2010. JAMA Surg. 2015;150(1):17–4.
68. Tsai M-H, Xirasagar S, Li Y-J, de Groen PC. Colonoscopy screening among US adults aged 40 or older with a family history of colorectal cancer. Prev Chronic Dis. 2015;12(E80):140533–9.
69. Ahnen DJ, Wade SW, Jones WF, Sifri R, Mendoza Silveiras J, Greenamyer J, et al. The increasing incidence of young-onset colorectal cancer: a call to action. Mayo Clin Proc. 2014;89(2):216–24.
70. Goldvaser H, Purim O, Kundel Y, Shepshelovich D, Shochat T, Shemesh-Bar L, et al. Colorectal cancer in young patients: is it a distinct clinical entity? Int J Clin Oncol. 2016;21(6):684–95.
71. Psathakis D, Schiedeck THK, Krug F, Oevermann E, Kujath P, Bruch H-P. Ordinary Colorectal Adenocarcinoma. Dis Colon Rectum. 1999;42(12):1618–25.
72. Melo S, Figueiredo J, Fernandes M, Gonçalves M, Morais-de-Sá E, Sanches J, et al. Predicting the functional impact of CDH1 missense mutations in hereditary diffuse gastric cancer. Int J Mol Sci. 2017;18(12):2687–19.
73. Blair V, Martin I, Shaw D, Winship I, Kerr D, Arnold J, et al. Hereditary diffuse gastric cancer: diagnosis and management. Clin Gastroenterol Hepatol. 2006;4(3):262–75.
74. Richards FM, Mckee SA, Rajpar MH, Cole TRP, Evans DG, Jankowski JA, et al. Germline E-cadherin gene (CDH1) mutations predispose to familial gastric cancer and colorectal cancer. Hum Mol Genet H. 1999;8(4):607–10.
75. Alford TC, Do HM, Geelhoed GW, Tsangaris NT, Lippman ME. Steroid receptors in human colon cancers. Cancer. 1979;43:980–4.
76. Stedman KE, Moore GE, Morgan RT. Estrogen receptor proteins in diverse human tumors. Arch Surg. 2017;115:244–8.
77. Slattery ML, Samowitz WS, Holden JA. Estrogen and progesterone receptors in colon Tumors. Am J Clin Pathol. 2000;113:364–8.

78. Dawson PM, Shousha S, Blair SD, Carter GD, Jones J, Alaghband-Zadeh J, et al. Oestrogen receptors in colorectal carcinoma. J Clin Pathol. 1990;43:149–51.
79. Niv Y. Estrogen receptor β expression and colorectal cancer. Eur J Gastroenterol Hepatol. 2015;27(12):1438–42.
80. Williams C, DiLeo A, Niv Y, Gustafsson J-Å. Estrogen receptor beta as target for colorectal cancer prevention. Cancer Lett. 2016;372(1):48–56.
81. Chlebowski RT, Ritenbaugh C, Ascensao J, Rosenberg CA, Harris R, White E. Estrogen plus progestin and colorectal cancer in postmenopausal women. N Engl J Med. 2004;350(10):991–1004.
82. Anderson GL, Chlebowski RT, Aragaki AK, Kuller LH, Manson JE, Gass M, et al. Conjugated equine oestrogen and breast cancer incidence and mortality in postmenopausal women with hysterectomy: extended follow-up of the Women's Health Initiative randomised placebo-controlled trial. Lancet Oncol. 2012;13(5):476–86.
83. Simon MS, Chlebowski RT, Wactawski-Wende J, Johnson KC, Muskovitz A, Kato I, et al. Estrogen plus progestin and colorectal cancer incidence and mortality. J Clin Oncol. 2012;30(32):3983–90.
84. Chlebowski RT, Anderson GL. Menopausal hormone therapy and cancer: changing clinical observations of target site specificity. Steroids. 2014;90:53–9.
85. Prentice RL, Pettinger M, Beresford SAA, Wactawski-Wende J, Hubbell FA, Stefanick ML, et al. Colorectal cancer in relation to postmenopausal Estrogen and Estrogen plus progestin in the Women's Health Initiative clinical trial and observational study. Cancer Epidemiol Biomark Prev. 2009;18(5):1531–7.
86. Ho MY, Cassano-Bailey A, Czaykowski P. Colorectal cancer in pregnancy: driven by pregnancy-associated growth factors? J Gastrointest Cancer. 2012;43(S1):239–42.
87. Eberhart CE, Coffey RJ, Radhika A, Giardiello FM, Ferrenbach S, Dubois RN. Up-regulation of cyclooxygenase 2 gene expression in human colorectal adenomas and adenocarcinomas. Gastroenterology. 1994;107:1183–8.
88. Giovannucci E. Insulin, insulin-like growth factors and colon cancer: a review of the evidence. J Nutr. 2001;131(11 Suppl):3109S–20S.
89. Salani R, Billingsley CC, Crafton SM. Cancer and pregnancy: an overview for obstetricians and gynecologists. Am J Obstet Gynecol. 2014;211(1):7–14.
90. Aytac E, Ozuner G, Isik O, Gorgun E, Stocchi L. Management of colorectal neoplasia during pregnancy and in the postpartum period. World J Gastrointest Oncol. 2016;8(7):550–6.

Hernia Complications During Pregnancy

16

Ivy N. Haskins and Michael J. Rosen

Introduction

Approximately four million live births occur annually in the United States, with the risk of acute abdomen requiring surgical intervention occurring in up to 1 in 500 pregnancies [1, 2]. While many of the causes of acute abdomen are related to the pregnancy itself, general surgery disease processes must be considered in the differential diagnosis. Within this chapter, we will detail the evaluation and management of pregnant patients who present with a symptomatic abdominal wall hernia.

Incidence of Abdominal Wall Hernias in Pregnancy

To date, no randomized controlled trial or prospective analysis has detailed the incidence or management of abdominal wall hernias during pregnancy [3]. Therefore, the true incidence of abdominal wall hernias in pregnant patients remains unknown. Nevertheless, in a large, registry-based trial, Oma et al. found that the incidence of umbilical hernias in pregnant patients was 0.08% and that the incidence of inguinal and femoral hernias was 0.12% [4]. While the overall percentage of abdominal wall hernias in pregnant patients is less than 1%, when considered in the context of four million live births, upward of 3200 pregnant women will have a concomitant umbilical hernia and nearly 4800 pregnant women will have a concomitant groin hernia annually. Therefore, both obstetricians and general surgeons must be equipped to evaluate and manage pregnant patients with abdominal wall hernias.

Etiology of Abdominal Wall Hernias in Pregnancy

The incidence of abdominal wall hernias rises dramatically in women, starting at 20 years of age and plateauing at approximately 40 years of age [5, 6]. Because of this pattern, it has been postulated that pregnancy is a risk factor for abdominal wall hernia formation [5]. Furthermore, additional studies have found that pregnancy is associated with an increased risk of abdominal wall hernia recurrence [4]. While the association between pregnancy and abdominal wall hernia formation and recurrence is not completely understood, it is believed that the increased intra-abdominal pressure and hormonal changes associated with pregnancy leads to increased abdominal wall compliance and elasticity, facilitating abdominal wall hernia formation [4, 5].

I. N. Haskins · M. J. Rosen (✉)
Department of Digestive Disease and Surgical Institute, Cleveland Clinic Foundation, Cleveland, OH, USA
e-mail: ihaskins@gwu.edu; rosenm@ccf.org

C. H. Nezhat (ed.), *Non-Obstetric Surgery During Pregnancy*,
https://doi.org/10.1007/978-3-319-90752-9_16

Evaluation of Abdominal Wall Hernias in Pregnancy

In their most severe form, abdominal wall hernias can progress to symptoms of incarceration or strangulation. While pain, nausea, and emesis often accompany symptomatic abdominal wall hernias, these are also common symptoms of pregnancy, which can make the diagnosis of an abdominal wall hernia challenging [3, 7]. Therefore, a thorough history and physical examination is an important first step in evaluating a pregnant patient with a suspected abdominal wall hernia. Specifically, these patients should be asked if they have ever been diagnosed with an abdominal wall hernia, if they have noticed a new bulge in their abdominal wall or in their groin independent from their pregnancy, and about their surgical history. Next, in addition to a routine obstetric examination, the abdominal wall and inguinal regions should be inspected and palpated to rule out a hernia.

When there is a high suspicion for an abdominal wall hernia in a pregnant patient that cannot be identified on physical examination, imaging may be necessary. Due to the risk of radiation exposure to the fetus, ultrasound, rather than computed tomography or x-ray, is the preferred imaging modality [3, 8]. The use of ultrasound is advantageous as it can simultaneously rule out an obstetric cause of the patient's symptoms in addition to other general surgery considerations, including appendicitis and cholecystitis [9]. Furthermore, in addition to the diagnosis of abdominal wall hernias, ultrasound can help to rule out varicose veins around the round ligament, which is a potential alternative source of groin swelling [4, 10].

Management of Abdominal Wall Hernias in Pregnancy

Pregnant women present unique challenges to the general surgeon regardless of operative or nonoperative treatment. Nonoperative management can increase the risk of progression to bowel incarceration and strangulation, while operative intervention exposes the mother and fetus to increased physiologic stress and potentially teratogenic medications [11]. As previously discussed, there is a paucity of literature directing the management of pregnant patients with abdominal wall hernias. Herein, we will detail the most recent case series and attempt to make recommendations for these patients.

In a small study by Buch et al., 12 female patients with a known umbilical or groin hernia were followed through the course of their pregnancies [9]. No patient developed hernia incarceration or strangulation, and no patient required emergency hernia repair during pregnancy [9]. All patients underwent hernia repair postpartum. Based on their observations, the authors concluded that umbilical and groin hernias in pregnant patients should be managed with watchful waiting during pregnancy with planned surgical intervention postpartum [9].

A recent study by Oma et al. followed 224 female patients who went on to become pregnant following primary umbilical hernia repair. Although previous studies have shown a lower recurrence rate with mesh versus primary repair in nonpregnant patients, this study found no difference in hernia recurrence rate at an average follow-up time of 3.8 years in female patients who went on to become pregnant regardless of surgical approach or mesh utilization [5, 12, 13].

A systematic review of abdominal wall hernias and pregnancy was performed by Jensen et al. in 2015. In this review, the terms "abdominal wall hernias" and "pregnancy" were searched with PubMED and Embase [3]. Thirty-one studies were reviewed; 4 detailed the outcomes of abdominal wall hernia repair prior to pregnancy, 12 detailed the results of abdominal wall hernia repair at the time of pregnancy, and 15 detailed the results of abdominal wall hernia at the time of cesarean section [3]. A total of 40 patients were described in the case series detailing abdominal wall hernia repair prior to pregnancy. Interestingly, 12 patients had pain during pregnancy related to hernia repair with mesh, and 2 of these patients experienced a hernia recurrence [3, 14, 15]. Of the 12 articles that detailed abdominal wall hernia repair during pregnancy, all studies were case reports and all patients underwent emergency surgical intervention for hernia incarceration or strangulation, with one patient spontaneously aborting 4 weeks postoperatively [3]. With respect to abdominal wall hernia repair at the time of cesarean section, patients had a higher analgesic requirement and a higher wound infection rate, and short-term recurrence was as high as 29% [3, 16].

Finally, in a large, retrospective database study examining 20,714 women in Denmark, Oma et al. attempted to determine the incidence of umbilical and groin hernias in women of reproductive age [3]. They found that the incidence of umbilical hernias during pregnancy was 0.08% and that no patient with an umbilical hernia required surgical intervention during pregnancy [3]. They also found that the incidence of groin hernias during pregnancy was 0.12% and that no patient with a groin hernia required surgical intervention during pregnancy [3]. Interestingly, 40% of the women who were diagnosed with a groin hernia during pregnancy had spontaneous resolution postpartum, which may be related to round ligament varicosities [3].

Recently accepted for publication in *Hernia* is a study from our institution which uses the American College of Surgeons National Surgical Quality Improvement Program (ACS-NSQIP) database to detail the incidence and management of umbilical hernias during pregnancy. A total of 126 pregnant patients underwent umbilical hernia repair from 2005 through 2014. A majority of these patients (58%) had incarceration or strangulation at the time of surgical intervention, and almost all patients (95%) underwent open, primary tissue repair of their umbilical hernia. While umbilical hernia repair during pregnancy was associated with minimal maternal morbidity, the risk to the fetus cannot be elucidated from the ACS-NSQIP database.

Unfortunately, it is not known how often abdominal wall hernias become symptomatic during pregnancy [3]. Nevertheless, there are some general conclusions that can be made from the aforementioned studies. First and foremost, approximately 8000 pregnant women in the United States will have a concomitant abdominal wall hernia annually. Therefore, the likelihood of a general surgeon having to evaluate or operate on a pregnant patient during their career is almost inevitable. Second, pregnancy is associated with an increased risk of abdominal wall hernia formation and recurrence. Therefore, ideally, these hernias should be managed nonoperatively until a patient has completed childbearing. Furthermore, because of the higher rate of wound events and hernia recurrence at the time of cesarean section compared to routine abdominal wall hernia repair, pregnant patients with abdominal wall hernias should not undergo routine simultaneous abdominal wall hernia repair at the time of cesarean section. Finally, general surgeons should be reassured that patients who progress to hernia incarceration or strangulation during pregnancy can undergo primary tissue repair with minimal associated maternal morbidity. What remains to be determined is the ideal surgical approach and need for mesh utilization at the time of definitive abdominal wall hernia repair and the effect of general anesthesia and symptomatic abdominal wall hernias on the health of the fetus.

Conclusion

Abdominal wall hernias can be a source of acute abdomen in the pregnant patient. Unless symptoms of incarceration or strangulation are present, abdominal wall hernias should be managed nonoperatively until the postpartum period. Additional research in this area is needed to determine the true incidence and ideal management of abdominal wall hernias in pregnant patients.

References

1. Augustin G, Majerovic M. Non-obstetrical acute abdomen during pregnancy. Eur J Obstet Gynecol Reprod Biol. 2007;131(1):4–12.
2. 4 Pregnancy Statistics. http://www.statisticbrain.com/pregnancy-statistics/. Accessed 30 May 2017.
3. Jensen KK, Henriksen NA, Jorgensen LN. Abdominal wall hernia and pregnancy: a systematic review. Hernia. 2015;19:689–96.
4. Oma E, Bay-Nielsen M, Jensen KK, Jorgensen LN, Pinborg A, Bisgaard T. Primary ventral or groin hernia in pregnancy: a cohort study of 20,714 women. Hernia. 2017;21:335–9.

5. Oma E, Jensen KK, Jorgensen LN. Recurrent umbilical or epigastric hernia during and after pregnancy: a nationwide cohort study. Surgery. 2016;159(6):1677–83.
6. Burcharth J, Pedersen MS, Pommergaard HC, Bisgaard T, Pedersen CB, Rosenberg J. The prevalence of umbilical and epigastric hernia repair: a nationwide epidemiologic study. Hernia. 2015;19(5):815–9.
7. Vikanes AV, Stoer NC, Magnus P, Grjibovski AM. Hyperemesis gravidarum and pregnancy outcomes in the Norwegian mother and child cohort- a cohort study. BMC Pregnancy Childbirth. 2013;13:169.
8. Shetty MK. Abdominal computed tomography during pregnancy: a review of indications and fetal radiation exposure issues. Semin Ultrasound CT MR. 2010;31(1):3–7.
9. Cox TC, Huntington CR, Blair LJ, Prasad T, Lincourt AE, Augenstein VA, et al. Laparoscopic appendectomy and cholecystectomy versus open: a study in 1999 pregnant patients. Surg Endosc. 2016;30:593–602.
10. Lechner M, Fortlenly R, Ofner D, Mayer F. Suspected inguinal hernias in pregnancy—handle with care! Hernia. 2014;18(3):375–9.
11. Buch KE, Tabrizian P, Divino CM. Management of hernias in pregnancy. J Am Coll Surg. 2008;207(4):539–42.
12. Arroya A, Garcia P, Perez F, Andreu J, Andreu J, Candela F, Calpena R. Randomized clinical trial comparing suture and mesh repair of umbilical hernia in adults. Br J Surg. 2001;88(10):1321–3.
13. Sanjay P, Reid TD, Davies EL, Arumugam PJ, Arumugam PJ, Woodward A. Retrospective comparison of mesh and sutured repair for adult umbilical hernias. Hernia. 2005;9(3):248–51.
14. Aean V, Cown L, Sakala PP, Small ML. Prolonged parenteral meperidine analgesia during pregnancy for pain from an abdominal wall mesh graft. Obstet Gynecol. 1993;82:721–2.
15. Schoenmaeckers E, Stirler V, Raymakers J, Rakic S. Pregnancy following laparoscopic mesh repair of ventral abdominal wall hernia. JSLS. 2012;16(1):85–8.
16. Steinemann DC, Limani P, Ochsenbein N, Krähenmann F, Clavien PA, Zimmermann R, et al. Suture repair of umbilical hernia during caeserean section: a case-control study. Hernia. 2013;17(4):521–6.

Breast Surgery in the Pregnant Patient

17

Meredith Redden, Natalie Kessler, and Amelia Donlan

Introduction

The breast undergoes significant transformation during pregnancy making surveillance and identification of changes challenging. The physiologic changes of pregnancy include breast growth and enlargement, tenderness and hypersensitivity, darkened nipples and areolas, darkened veins along breasts, nipple enlargement and projection, and raised Montgomery tubercles. Estrogen and progesterone production stimulates ductal and lobule development and proliferation, adipose tissue involution, and increased vascularization. These hormonal changes of pregnancy can produce palpable nodularity, firmness, and increased parenchymal density secondary to an increase in breast volume and water content, making clinical and radiologic evaluation challenging. Most women presenting with breast changes during pregnancy will not require surgical intervention. We will review both malignant and benign breast diseases that can affect women during their pregnancy and the management for their disease during pregnancy.

M. Redden (✉)
Northside Hospital, Atlanta, GA, USA
e-mail: mredden@breastcareatlanta.com

N. Kessler
Sandy Springs, GA, USA
e-mail: npk5ns@virginia.edu

A. Donlan
Athens, GA, USA

Evaluation and Diagnosis

Initial evaluation of breast changes noted during pregnancy begins with a thorough history and clinical examination. A palpable breast mass that persists for greater than 2 weeks mandates further evaluation with a clinical breast examination and ultrasonography [1]. The common differential diagnosis of a palpable breast mass during pregnancy includes gestational breast cancer, fibroadenoma, lactating adenoma, fibrocystic changes, or cyst. Breast ultrasound has demonstrated an excellent degree of accuracy in the evaluation of both benign and malignant pregnancy-associated breast masses, and it can accurately and safely differentiate between cystic and solid lesions. Ultrasound is particularly accurate in the evaluation of breast cancers in pregnancy, with studies demonstrating 100% sensitivity and 100% negative predictive value for pregnancy-associated breast cancers [2–5].

Ultrasound-guided incisional breast biopsy has been demonstrated to be safe during pregnancy and allows for pathologic evaluation of new or enlarging solid nodules [6]. If core needle biopsy yields malignant pathology, bilateral whole-breast ultrasound and ipsilateral axillary

C. H. Nezhat (ed.), *Non-Obstetric Surgery During Pregnancy*,
https://doi.org/10.1007/978-3-319-90752-9_17

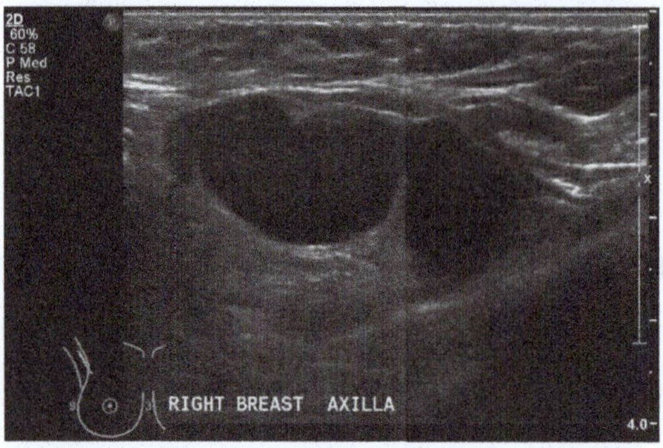

Fig. 17.1 Abnormal axillary lymph node in pregnant patient. Ipsilateral abnormal appearing axillary lymph node in patient with newly palpable breast cancer. Pathology from USIBB demonstrated metastatic carcinoma

ultrasound are necessary to evaluate for the extent of disease, including multifocal or multicentric disease and metastatic disease in the axillary lymph node basin (Fig. 17.1). An ultrasound-guided axillary core needle biopsy can pathologically evaluate suspicious lymph nodes for metastatic disease.

Further imaging evaluation with mammography is necessary in the setting of a gestational breast cancer or a clinically suspicious presentation for a breast malignancy. Routine mammographic screening is not recommended during the gestational period because of concern for radiation exposure to the developing fetus and the potentially teratogenic consequences. However, mammography has been shown to be safe during pregnancy with fetal shielding, with minimal radiation exposure to the fetus. A bilateral mammogram during pregnancy is limited to patients diagnosed with breast cancer and can be indispensable in evaluating for microcalcifications not detected by ultrasound and in determining the full extent of disease prior to treatment initiation [5].

Contrast-enhanced MRI has not been demonstrated to be safe during pregnancy because of the concern regarding gadolinium-based contrast agents crossing the placenta. Therefore, breast MRI is not recommended in the imaging evaluation of a newly diagnosed gestational breast cancer.

Malignant Breast Disease in Pregnancy

Gestational Breast Cancer

Pregnancy-associated breast cancer accounts for 3% of all newly diagnosed breast cancers and presents in 1 in 3000 to 1 in 10,000 pregnancies [7]. It is defined as a breast cancer presenting during pregnancy, the first postpartum year, or anytime during lactation. We will focus specifically on gestational breast cancers and their unique management considerations. The majority of all gestational breast cancers are diagnosed in young women, with a mean age of 32–34 years old [6]. Some studies indicate that the incidence of gestational pregnancy is increasing as women delay childbearing [8, 9]. It can present a challenging clinical dilemma because treatment plans must maximize treatment of the known malignancy while minimizing risk to the fetus. Pregnancy termination has not been demonstrated to improve outcomes in gestational breast cancer [10]. A multidisciplinary team approach to treatment, incorporating medical oncology, breast surgical oncology, radiation oncology, and maternal-fetal medicine, is essential to achieving the best clinical outcome oncologically and maternally.

One of the greatest challenges in evaluating a newly diagnosed gestational breast cancer is managing the need for a thorough evaluation of the extent of disease, to ensure that all disease is clearly noted, against potential radiologic side effects to the fetus. Many breast cancers presenting in this patient population present in a delayed fashion because of the challenges of clinical examination, as natural breast changes of pregnancy may obscure new breast masses, and because pregnant women are not undergoing surveillance with screening mammography (Fig. 17.2a, b). Regardless, a complete imaging evaluation is necessary, particularly if breast-conserving surgery is being considered or if neoadjuvant chemotherapy is planned. Documenting the full extent of disease is essential for oncologically safe and successful surgery.

For women with advanced-stage breast cancer or symptoms suspicious for metastatic disease,

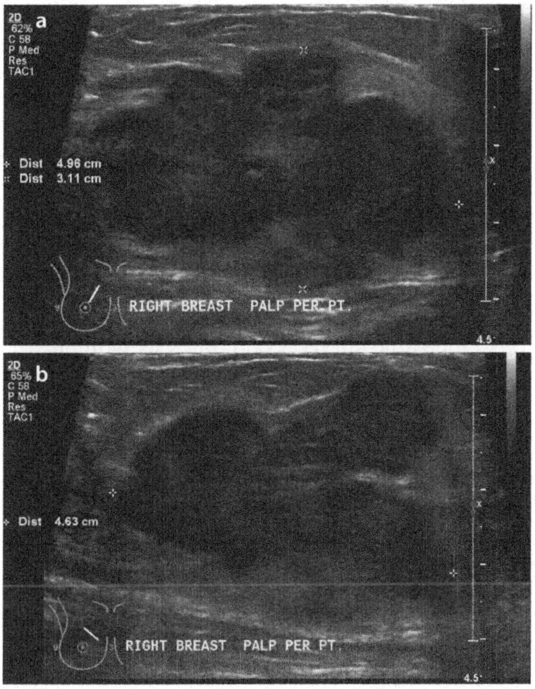

Fig. 17.2 (**a**, **b**) Palpable breast cancer in pregnant patient. 32yo female with newly palpable mass on self breast examination and clinical breast examination. Pathology from USIBB demonstrated poorly differentiated invasive ductal carcinoma

additional evaluation for metastatic disease prior to the initiation of treatment is required. This can be safely accomplished with a chest radiograph with fetal shielding, a liver US, and a spine MRI without contrast. This is of utmost importance because it impacts treatment recommendations and treatment goals.

Surgical Treatment

The management of gestational breast cancer is influenced both by the trimester at diagnosis and the stage of disease. NCCN guidelines for the management of gestational breast cancer are organized based on trimester of presentation:

First Trimester

NCCN guidelines recommend mastectomy with sentinel lymph node biopsy (SLNB) versus axillary lymph node dissection (ALND) for breast cancers diagnosed during the first trimester of pregnancy. Following mastectomy and axillary surgery, adjuvant chemotherapy can be started in the second trimester, as it is ideally avoided during the organogenesis period of the first trimester. Adjuvant radiation treatment and endocrine therapy are delayed until after the baby is born, as both pose significant fetal risks.

Second Trimester

Breast cancer diagnosed in the second trimester or early third trimester can be treated first with neoadjuvant chemotherapy with delay in surgical treatment until after delivery or with upfront surgery with either mastectomy or partial mastectomy with SLNB or ALND. If breast-conserving surgery is chosen, whole-breast radiation treatment is delayed until after delivery, typically after the completion of adjuvant chemotherapy through the third trimester. Adjuvant endocrine therapy follows postpartum radiation therapy, when biologically indicated.

Third Trimester

Breast cancer diagnosed late in the third trimester can be treated with mastectomy or partial mastectomy and SLNB or ALND. Adjuvant chemotherapy, radiation treatment, and endocrine therapy, if indicated, can be safely delivered in the postpartum setting.

The treatment for gestational breast cancer follows the same NCCN guidelines established for nonpregnant breast cancer, with modifications to protect the developing fetus. Breast and axillary lymph node surgery has been shown to be associated with minimal fetal risk during any trimester [1, 11–15]. However, it is ideally positioned between the beginning of second trimester and 34–37 weeks' gestation. Avoiding surgery during the first trimester allows the initial phase of organogenesis to be completed. Additionally, surgery can increase the risk of preterm labor at the end of the third trimester; obstetricians can deliver a full-term infant at 37 weeks, to be followed by either continued medical treatment or surgical intervention. Ideally delivery is positioned 3–4 weeks following the last chemotherapy cycle to allow for hematopoietic recovery for the mother and fetus prior to delivery.

Historically, the only surgical option for gestational breast cancer was a modified radical mastectomy. Recently, studies have demonstrated the safety and feasibility of breast-conserving surgery in gestational breast cancer [16, 17]. The exception is for breast-conserving surgery patients who would not be able to receive radiation treatment within the standard time period following surgical excision with or without adjuvant chemotherapy. Whole-breast radiation has not been demonstrated to be safe to administer during pregnancy as it would expose the fetus to teratogenic doses of radiation.

Immediate breast reconstruction has been safely performed in small series [18]. However, delayed reconstruction has traditionally been preferred to minimize operative time and potential complications from placement of a foreign body.

In clinically lymph node-negative patients, sentinel lymph node biopsy with the use of technetium-99m or methylene blue has been demonstrated to be safe and effective in pregnant patients in small studies [17, 19–23]. Isosulfan blue dye should not be used for sentinel lymph node biopsy because of the small but catastrophic risk of anaphylaxis associated with administration of the dye. Many patients present with locally advanced disease, mandating an axillary dissection at the time of surgical intervention.

Neoadjuvant and Adjuvant Chemotherapy Treatment

Recommendations for utilization of chemotherapy treatment are the same for the gestational breast cancer patient as for the nonpregnant, stage-matched patient. Gestational timing of diagnosis in light of the clinical stage influences the decision for neoadjuvant versus adjuvant chemotherapy. Chemotherapy is avoided during the first trimester when possible to avoid potentially teratogenic treatment during critical fetal organogenesis. The typical treatment regimen includes adriamycin with cyclophosphamide and fluorouracil. Endocrine therapy is withheld until after delivery because of the potential risk for birth defects [24].

Prognosis

Outcomes data suggests that stage-matched women diagnosed with gestational breast cancer have the same survival outcomes as women who are not pregnant.

Benign Breast Disease in Pregnancy

Gestational Gigantomastia

Gestational gigantomastia is defined as the enormously exaggerated increase in the size and weight of the breasts during pregnancy. Breast weights of 4000–7000 g per breast have been reported with this condition. While very rare, affecting about 1 in 100,000 pregnancies, the rapid physiologic changes in the breast are both grossly deforming and can result in significant complications, including skin ulceration, infection, and massive bleeding from vascular wall compromise of massively dilated subcutaneous veins [25]. At times, these secondary complications can become life threatening if not rapidly addressed.

The etiology of this disease process remains unknown. It is hypothesized to be secondary to an abnormal breast tissue response to the normal increases in progesterone level during pregnancy. The exaggerated breast tissue hypertrophy does not always present during a woman's first pregnancy; however, once the condition has developed during a pregnancy, it is highly likely to recur with each subsequent pregnancy.

Ultrasound evaluation will demonstrate primarily normal breast hypertrophy. Biopsies of breast tissue changes are imprudent because of the increased risk for bleeding and infection. However, if the diagnosis is unclear, ultrasound-guided incisional breast biopsy can be used to exclude a malignant process, most commonly a lymphoma.

Treatment is initially limited to medical. Bromocriptine has been demonstrated to halt the growth of breasts and has demonstrated the greatest medical success in management [26]. Surgical intervention, primarily bilateral mastectomies with delayed breast reconstruction, becomes necessary when life-threatening complications develop, primarily uncontrolled bleeding. Some case reports describe preterm delivery followed by urgent breast reduction surgery.

Following delivery, most breasts do not revert to normal size, requiring breast reduction surgery to prevent complications of macromastia. Breastfeeding is not recommended because breasts may continue to hypertrophy, resulting in continued risk for serious complications. Recurrence can develop in subsequent pregnancies following breast reduction. Therefore, all patients considering future pregnancies should be offered mastectomies.

Lactating Adenomas

Lactating adenomas are benign breast lesions most commonly presenting during the third trimester of pregnancy, rather than during lactation. Because they can be sizeable, patients typically present with a new palpable breast mass on self-breast examination most commonly in the upper outer quadrant. Evaluation by ultrasound will demonstrate an oval or round, hypoechoic, homogenous, well-circumscribed lobulated nodule, potentially with large cystic areas of infarction and necrosis [27]. As malignancy must be excluded, an ultrasound-guided incisional breast biopsy can be safely performed for pathologic evaluation. The histologic presentation of lactating adenomas is characteristic, demonstrating lobulated masses of acini or lobules densely packed together with little intervening stroma and an intact basement membrane. Surveillance with clinical examination and ultrasound through pregnancy and lactation can monitor for stability and then involution.

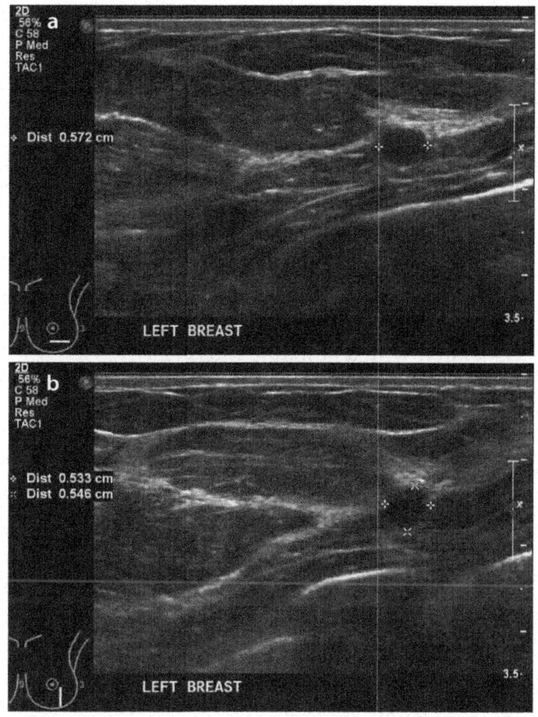

Fig. 17.3 (**a**, **b**) Lactating Adenoma in pregnant patient. 38yo female with new oval hypoechoic nodule on US imaging. Pathology from USIBB demonstrated lactating adenoma

Lactating adenomas can recur with subsequent pregnancies (Fig. 17.3a, b).

Breast Infarcts

Vascular insufficiency secondary to increased metabolic demands may cause infarction in fibroadenomas, hamartomas, lactating adenomas, and hypertrophic breast tissue (Figs. 17.4a, b and 17.5a, b). Clinically, focal tenderness, skin fixation, and a palpable, ill-defined, tethered mass may be associated with the presentation of an area of infarct. An ultrasound-guided incisional breast biopsy is required for definitive diagnosis. Histologically, extensive necrosis may distort the normal architecture of the underlying benign breast lesion. Treatment is conservative until the postpartum period when the necrotic area can safely undergo wide local excision [28].

Bloody Nipple Discharge

In the third trimester of pregnancy, ductal proliferative changes can result in bloody nipple discharge from ductal epithelial trauma. Bleeding often ceases with the onset of nursing. Further evaluation with mammogram and ductogram or breast biopsy is only indicated if the bloody nipple discharge persists more than 2 months following delivery, is from a single duct, or is associated with a palpable mass [29].

Fibroadenoma, Breast Hamartoma, and Axillary Breast Tissue

Benign breast lesions present prior to pregnancy may proliferate during pregnancy secondary to hormonal stimulation. These benign breast lesions do not require surgical intervention during pregnancy but should be followed during and after pregnancy with imaging and clinical surveillance to ensure return to prepregnancy size with the completion of breastfeeding. Failure of a fibroadenoma to return to its prepregnancy dimensions should prompt either close surveillance with ultrasound and clinical examination at 6-month intervals for 2 years to ensure stability or surgical excision.

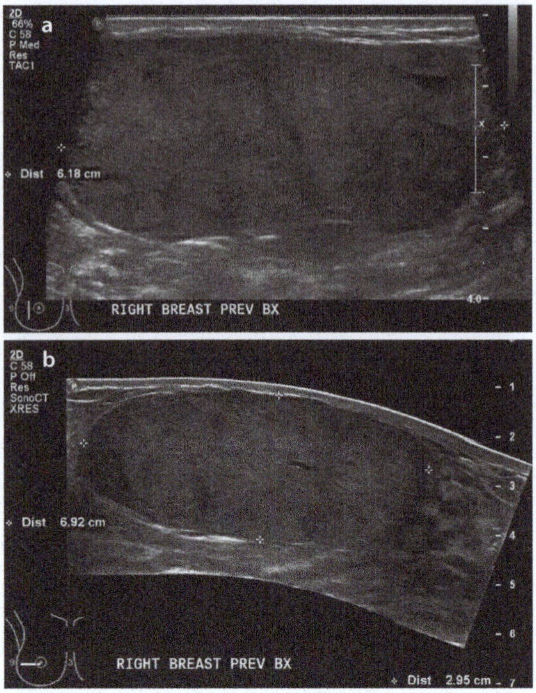

Fig. 17.5 (**a**, **b**) Fibroadenoma increased in size during pregnancy to 6.18 cm x2.95 cm x6.92 cm. Fibroadenoma regressed to pre-pregnancy size following breastfeeding

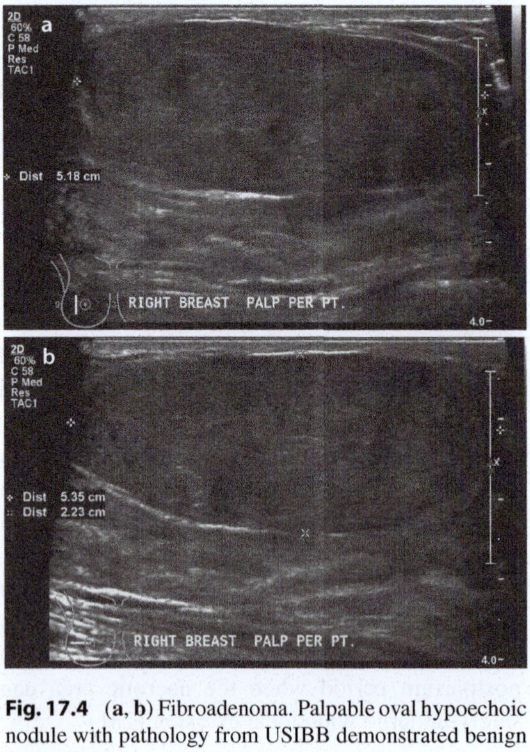

Fig. 17.4 (**a**, **b**) Fibroadenoma. Palpable oval hypoechoic nodule with pathology from USIBB demonstrated benign fibroadenoma

> **Conclusion**
>
> The majority of breast changes noted during pregnancy are benign and attributable to normal breast tissue responses to increased estrogen and progesterone levels. Ultrasound is a safe and accurate method for evaluating these changes and can guide core needle biopsy if pathologic evaluation is warranted to exclude malignancy. When gestational breast cancer or gestational gigantomastia require surgical intervention, surgical timing is important to minimize risk to the developing fetus. These are challenging clinical scenarios in which the welfare of both mother and baby must be prioritized. For benign disease, clinical and imaging

surveillance is sufficient through pregnancy and in the postpartum period. Most gestational changes will involute or return to pre-pregnancy size, not requiring additional intervention.

References

1. Woo JC, Yu T, Hurd TC. Breast cancer in pregnancy: a literature review. Breast cancer in pregnancy: a literature review. Arch Surg. 2003;138:91–8.
2. Ahn BY, Kim HH, Moon WK, Pisano ED, Kim HS, Cha ES, et al. Pregnancy-and lactation-associated breast cancer: mammographic and sonographic findings. J Ultrasound Med. 2003;22:491–7.
3. Robbins J, Jefferies D, Roubidoux M, Helvie M. Accuracy of diagnostic mammography and breast ultrasound during pregnancy and lactation. AJR. 2011;196:716–22.
4. Liberman L, Giess CS, Dershaw DD, Deutch BM, Petrek JA. Imaging of pregnancy-associated breast cancer. Radiology. 1994;191:245–8.
5. Yang WT, Dryden MJ, Gwyn K, Whitman GJ, Theriault R. Imaging of breast cancer diagnosed and treated with chemotherapy during pregnancy. Radiology. 2006;239:52–60.
6. Vashi R, Hooley R, Bulter R, Geisel J, Philpotts L. Breast imaging of the pregnant and lactating patient: imaging modalities and pregnancy-associated breast cancer. AJR. 2013;200:321–8.
7. Anderson JM. Mammary cancers and pregnancy. Br Med J. 1979;1:1124–7.
8. Stensheim H, Moller B, van Dikj T, Fossa SD. Cause-specific survival for women diagnosed with cancer during pregnancy or lactation: a registry-based cohort study. J Clin Oncol. 2009;27:45.
9. Ventura SJ. First births to older mothers, 1970-86. 1989 йил. Am J Public Health. 1989;79:1675.
10. Nugent P, O'Connell TX. Breast cancer and pregnancy. Arch Surg. 1985;120:1221.
11. Byrd BF Jr, Bayer DS, Robertson JC, Stephenson SE Jr. Treatment of breast tumors associated with pregnancy and lactation. Ann Surg. 1962;155:940.
12. Mazze RI, Kallen B. Reproductive outcome after anesthesia and operation during pregnancy: a registry study of 5405 cases. Am J Obstet Gynecol. 1989;161:1178.
13. Gianopoulos JG. Establishing the criteria for anesthesia and other precautions for surgery during pregnancy. Surg Clin North Am. 1995;75:33.
14. Duncan PG, Pope WD, Cohen MM, Greer N. Fetal risk of anesthesia and surgery during pregnancy. Anesthesiology. 1986;64:790.
15. Barron WM. The pregnant surgical patient: medical evaluation and management. Ann Intern Med. 1984;101:683.
16. Petrek JA, Dukoff R, Rogatko A. Prognosis of pregnancy-associated breast cancer. Cancer. 1991;67:869–72.
17. Berry DL, Theriault RL, Holmes FA, Parisi VM, Booser DJ, Singletary SE, et al. Management of breast cancer during pregnancy using a standardized protocol. J Clin Oncol. 1999;17:855–561.
18. Meisel JL, Economy KE, Calvillo KZ, Schapira L, Tung NM, Gelber S, et al. Contemporary multidisciplinary treatment of pregnancy-associated breast cancer. Springerplus. 2013;2:297.
19. Mondi MM, Cuenca RE, Ollila DW, Stewart JH 4th, Levine EA. Sentinel lymph node biopsy during pregnancy: initial clinical experience. Ann Surg Oncol. 2007;14:218.
20. Khera SY, Kiluk JV, Hasson DM, Meade TL, Meyers MP, Dupont EL, et al. Pregnancy-associated breast cancer patients can safely undergo lymphatic mapping. Breast J. 2008;14:250.
21. Gropper AB, Calvillo KZ, Dominici L, Troyan S, Rhei E, Economy KE, et al. Sentinel lymph node biopsy in pregnant women with breast cancer. Ann Surg Oncol. 2014;21(8):2506–11.
22. Gentilini O, Cremonesi M, Toesca A, Colombo N, Peccatori F, Sironi R, et al. Sentinel lymph node biopsy in pregnant patients with breast cancer. Eur J Nucl Med Mol Imaging. 2010;37:78–83.
23. Keleher A, Wendt R 3rd, Delpassand E, Stachowiak AM, Kuerer HM. The safety of lymphatic mapping in pregnant breast cancer patients using Tc-99m sulfur colloid. Breast J. 2004;10:492–5.
24. Cullins SL, Pridjian G, Sutherland CM. Goldenhar's syndrome associated with tamoxifen given to the mother during gestation. JAMA. 1994;271:1905–6.
25. Agrawal N, Kriplani A, Gupta A, Bhatla N. Management of gigantomastia complicating pregnancy. A case report. J Reprod Med. 2002;47:871–4.
26. Rezai S, Nakagawa JT, Tedesco J, Chadee A, Gottimukkala S, Mercado R, et al. Gestational gigantomastia complicating pregnancy: a case report and review of the literature. Case Rep Obstet Gynecol. 2015;2015:892369.
27. Sumkin JH, Perrone AM, Harris KM, Nath ME, Amortegui AJ, Weinstein BJ. Lactating adenoma: US features and literature review. Radiology. 1998;206:271–4.
28. Behrndt VS, Barbakoff D, Askin FB, Brem RF. Infarcted lactating adenoma presenting as a rapidly enlarging breast mass. Am J Roentgenol. 1999;173:933–5.
29. Lafreniere R. Bloody nipple discharge during pregnancy: a rationale for conservative treatment. J Surg Oncol. 1990;43(4):226–30.

Part III

Subspecialty Surgery During Pregnancy

18 Neurosurgery During Pregnancy

Nicholas S. Szuflita, Jason H. Boulter,
Jonathan E. Gilhooly, and Chris J. Neal

Introduction

The indications for neurosurgical intervention in the pregnant patient often include mitigation of serious injury or pathology for the purposes of preventing a neurological deficit, preserving life, or treating pain. In general, elective procedures are often delayed until after delivery to prevent complicating factors for the fetus. However, there are times when neurosurgical intervention is required to save the life of the mother and fetus or to prevent debilitating neurological deficit. The goal of this chapter is to provide the non-neurosurgeon with information on common intracranial and spinal pathology, as well as aspects of neurocritical care that can be applied to the gravid patient.

N. S. Szuflita · J. H. Boulter · J. E. Gilhooly
Department of Neurosurgery, Walter Reed National Military Medical Center-Bethesda, Bethesda, MD, USA
e-mail: jonathan.e.gilhooly.mil@mail.mil

C. J. Neal (✉)
Department of Neurosurgery, Walter Reed National Military Medical Center-Bethesda, Bethesda, MD, USA

Uniformed Services University of the Health Sciences, Bethesda, MD, USA
e-mail: christopher.j.neal3.mil@mail.mil

General Considerations

Initial management of neurosurgical patients depends on the clinical presentation, underlying etiology, comorbidities, disease severity, and other ongoing clinical considerations including pregnancy or parturition. Specific management decisions should be made in a multidisciplinary manner balancing the unique considerations of each patient. The presenting history and neurologic examination are of the utmost importance in determining the nature and acuity of a patient's pathology or injuries. Important factors for consideration include the patient's vital signs, level of alertness, cranial nerve exam, and strength in all four limbs. In the setting of trauma, a pupillary exam and enough information to calculate a Glasgow Coma Score (GCS) should be ascertained whenever possible. However, if a provider is sufficiently concerned about a patient to consider neurosurgical consultation, doing so should not be delayed—especially in acutely ill or unstable patients.

Imaging

The correct interpretation of appropriate imaging is a crucial aspect of neurosurgical decision-making for both cranial and spinal pathologies. For most neurosurgical emergencies, the initial imaging modality of choice is computed

C. H. Nezhat (ed.), *Non-Obstetric Surgery During Pregnancy*,
https://doi.org/10.1007/978-3-319-90752-9_18

tomography (CT) because of the speed with which it can be completed as well as its ability to discriminate a wide variety of pathologies. Moreover, CT is often requisite to identify whether a given clinical presentation even represents a neurologic problem for which surgery is indicated or one that can be safely managed without operative intervention. The use of ionizing radiation and IV contrast, however, is not benign for mothers or fetuses and should therefore be used judiciously and only when the results of a study have the potential to change management. Magnetic resonance imaging (MRI) may be preferable in some circumstances (e.g., concern for acute radiculopathy or stroke) due to the lack of ionizing radiation but can be unsafe for patients who are unable to safely remain supine for the duration of the study.

Radiation Exposure

The effects of radiation on developing fetuses are dose-dependent. Lower doses (10–100 mGy) can increase the risk for developing certain childhood cancers. Larger doses are associated with an increased risk of intellectual consequences (>100 mGy at an estimated rate of 30 IQ points/Gy), microcephaly, and loss of pregnancy (500–1000 mGy) [1, 2]. The threshold for development of fetal malformations attributable to exposure to ionizing radiation is approximately 100 mGy, with the period of highest risk during gestational weeks 8–25 [1, 2].

For the majority of pregnant patients, the important threshold of 10 mGy exposure to the fetus will never be reached. Conventional X-ray studies of the lumbar spine expose the fetus to 1.7 mGy on average, and CT of the lumbar spine typically delivers 2.4 mGy [3].

IV Contrast

The use of IV contrast is critical to the ability to diagnose multiple pathologies and safely prepare for a neurosurgical intervention. The existing literature acknowledges that available data is scarce but suggests that gadolinium transmission across the placenta is limited resulting in decreased gadolinium concentrations for the fetus (up to 170 times less than in maternal serum in some animal models). Additionally, in vitro studies, animal model testing, and several case reports of gadolinium administration to pregnant women have demonstrated no mutagenic or teratogenic potential [4]. Similarly, placental transmission of iodinated contrast is limited with animal studies demonstrating a 0.003% transmission rate, and in vitro studies and animal models have demonstrated no mutagenic or teratogenic properties. There is, however, the potential for iodine exposure to depress neonatal thyroid function. Infants exposed to iodinated contrast during development should be screened for hypothyroidism within 1 week of delivery [4].

Antiepileptics

Antiepileptic drugs (AEDs) represent an important adjunct to the neurosurgical care of supratentorial pathology (e.g., hemorrhage, tumor, trauma) or the control of a known seizure disorder. Older-generation AEDs have been associated with higher rates of teratogenicity and congenital malformations including heart defects, cleft lip/palate, neural tube defects, and dysmorphic syndromes. Valproic acid and phenobarbital have been associated with rates of major structural malformation as high as 9.3% and 5.5%, respectively [5]. By comparison, newer AEDs have improved safety profiles in pregnant patients. Lamotrigine, for example, has been associated with structural malformation at rates of 2.0%, and levetiracetam, perhaps the most commonly used AED in neurosurgery patients, demonstrates rates of malformation ranging from 0.7% to 2.4% [5, 6]. Whenever possible, AEDs should be used for the shortest length of time in the pregnant patient and at the minimum effective dose to achieve proper seizure control.

Cranial Pathology

Intracranial pathologies are potentially among the most emergent and devastating of neurosurgical disorders. When suspected, any of the pathologies discussed below—cerebrovascular disease and subarachnoid hemorrhage, cerebral venous sinus thrombosis, tumor, ventriculoperitoneal shunt malfunction, and traumatic brain injury—warrant urgent or emergent neurosurgical consultation. Initial workup often includes noncontrast head CT; cerebrovascular pathologies may warrant urgent or emergent CT angiography.

Subarachnoid Hemorrhage

Subarachnoid hemorrhage (SAH) is one form of intracranial hemorrhage and can be seen in isolation or in conjunction with intraparenchymal or intraventricular hemorrhage (Fig. 18.1). SAH in pregnancy is rare, affecting up to 5.8 to 15 per 100,000 pregnancies [7, 8], but represents a true neurosurgical emergency and is responsible for 4.1–12% of total mortality during pregnancy [7–9]. In the general population, ruptured cerebral aneurysms comprise the most common etiology other than trauma underlying SAH. A lower mortality is observed in pregnancy-associated SAH (10.3%) as compared to non-pregnancy-associated SAH (18.3%) and may be due in part to the relative predominance of nonaneurysmal SAH observed among pregnant women.

Risk factors for peripartum subarachnoid hemorrhage include African-American or Hispanic racial background, hypertension, coagulopathy, drug, alcohol or tobacco abuse, sickle cell disease, hypercoagulability, and cerebral venous sinus thrombosis [7]. Other etiologies underlying SAH or frank intraparenchymal hemorrhage during pregnancy include ruptured arteriovenous malformations (AVM), cerebral venous thrombosis with venous hypertension and hemorrhage, moyamoya disease, and angiopathy in the postpartum period. The hypertensive rupture of pial vessels can be seen in the setting of eclampsia and stresses the need for appropriate blood pressure control and management.

The most common presenting symptom of pregnancy-associated intracranial hemorrhage or SAH is sudden-onset headache, which is often associated with nausea and vomiting. Other features include focal neurologic deficits, syncope at onset of symptoms, or seizure. The severity of symptoms and rapidity of onset help differentiate SAH from more benign causes of headache (e.g., tension headache, migraine) or the gradual-onset positional headaches associated with persistent spinal fluid leaks caused by administration of epidural analgesia. Initial management includes immediate noncontrast head CT as well as possible CT angiogram if SAH is detected or clinical suspicion for cerebrovascular pathology is high.

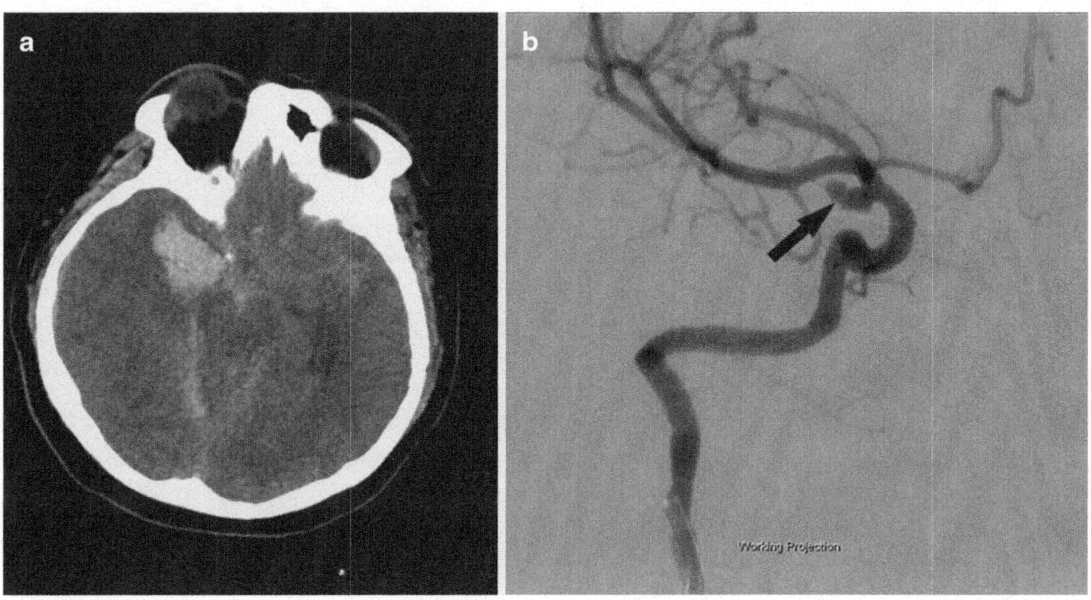

Fig. 18.1 (**a**) Noncontrast CT scan of the head showing a subarachnoid hemorrhage and right temporal hematoma. (**b**) An angiogram shows an aneurysm (*black arrow*) of the posterior communicating artery

Further recommendations will depend upon the results of the initial CT and may include a consultation to neurosurgery or neurology, especially in the setting of new focal neurologic deficits or decreased level of consciousness.

Given the distribution of etiologies underlying SAH in pregnancy relative to the nonpregnant state, there is conflicting evidence about the contribution of pregnancy and labor to the risk of SAH. However, the majority of hemorrhages appear to occur around delivery and the initial postpartum period. Following a hemorrhage, the highest risk of rebleeding from unsecured aneurysms is within the first 2–12 h and occurs in 4–14% within the first day. Ultimately, 10–50% of cases will demonstrate rehemorrhage within the first month. Mortality rates for recurrent bleeds can be as high as 50–68% in both pregnant and nonpregnant patients [8, 9].

Arteriovenous Malformations

Arteriovenous malformations (AVMs) are abnormal, congenital connections between cerebral arteries and veins (Fig. 18.2). The associated brain parenchyma is nonfunctional, gliotic tissue. Whether pregnancy increases the risk of hemorrhage from AVMs is controversial. Recently published series by Gross and Du and Porras et al. specifically designed to mitigate biases in incidence rate calculations indicate that pregnant women may in fact have elevated risks of hemorrhage [10, 11]. Gross and Du observed an 8.1% risk of hemorrhage per pregnancy (10.8% annual risk) as compared to a cumulative annual incidence of 1.1% among these same patients while not pregnant [10]. Similarly, Porras et al. observed an annual incidence of AVM hemorrhage of 1.3% in nonpregnant women versus a risk of 5.7% during pregnancy and the puerperium. In the cohort studied by Porras, all AVM ruptures occurred in the second (62.7%) or third trimester (37.5%). Two of these patients had a recurrent hemorrhage during the same pregnancy or during the puerperium, and all of these patients delivered via cesarean section. There were no maternal or fetal deaths [11].

Cerebral Venous Sinus Thrombosis

Cerebral venous sinus thrombosis (CVST) is a rare disease with an incidence of approximately 10–12 per million women per year that affects 0.004–0.01% of all pregnancies [12]. However,

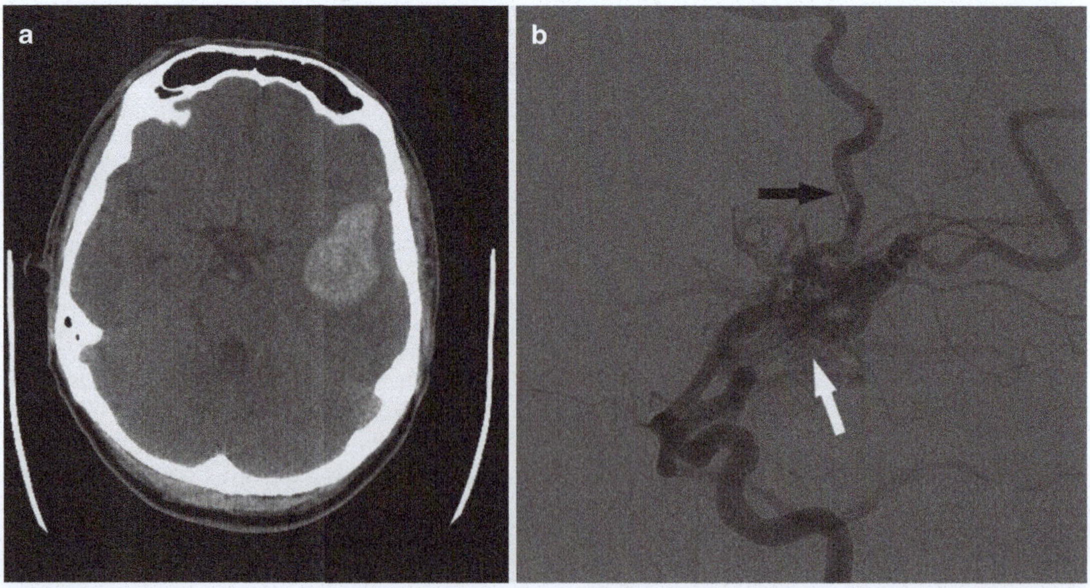

Fig. 18.2 (**a**) Noncontrast CT scan showing an acute left temporal lobe hematoma. (**b**) Underlying the hematoma is an arteriovenous malformation. Notice the abnormal tangle of blood vessels (*white arrow*) that comprise the nidus of the AVM and the early venous drainage (*black arrow*)

approximately 59% of all CVST occur during pregnancy or the puerperium [13]. Pregnancy itself comprises an independent risk factor for CVST. In hospital mortality rates from CVST are approximately 6%, and 30-day mortality rates are approximately 4% [12].

The majority of patients present with headache (74%), followed by seizure (50%), motor weakness (38%), severe alteration in mental status including coma or obtundation (45%), or visual disturbance (24%). Initial management includes control of intracranial hypertension to prevent additional brain injury. Special attention is paid to optimizing blood rheology by keeping patients on generous IV fluids (e.g., 1.5 times maintenance rates with 0.9% normal saline) and keeping the head of bed elevated to maximize venous outflow. It is important to differentiate CVST from idiopathic intracranial hypertension (IIH or pseudotumor cerebri), as treatment strategies vary. Diagnostic imaging studies include magnetic resonance imaging (MRI) and magnetic resonance venogram (MRV), although occasionally computed tomography venogram (CTV) is utilized.

Neurosurgeons are frequently consulted early in the assessment of suspected CVST, especially in the setting of venous hypertension, infarction, and intracranial hemorrhage. However, this is generally not a diagnosis that requires surgical intervention and is the rare case when anticoagulation is used even with existing intracranial hemorrhage. A pooled meta-analysis revealed 91% of patients were started on anticoagulation, 26% received intra-arterial thrombolysis alone, and 5% necessitated endovascular thrombectomy. While cerebral venous hypertension and infarction is potentially catastrophic, this outcome is a rarity, and the majority of patients have good to excellent clinical outcomes.

Intracranial Tumors

The incidence of brain tumors in pregnant women is an exceedingly rare phenomenon, but one that presents potential management dilemmas as well as possible obstetric and neurosurgical emergencies. Gliomas are the most frequently diagnosed histopathologic type (34%), although pituitary tumors (27%) and meningiomas (14%) are also common [14]. Some tumor types, most notably meningiomas (Fig. 18.3) and astrocytomas (Fig. 18.4), have been noted to become more clinically apparent during pregnancy. Meningiomas may be affected by the trophic effects of increased levels of circulating steroid hormones, while astrocytomas have been posited to become more symptomatic due to the relatively immunologically permissive environment. This can lead to vascular engorgement and subsequent peritumoral edema, particularly during the late second and third trimesters. Indications for surgical management (resection or debulking) of intracranial tumors during pregnancy depend on the anatomic location, biology, patient symptoms, and aggressiveness of the tumor. If possible, surgical intervention is delayed until after delivery of the fetus since many treatment strategies for the tumor may be contraindicated during pregnancy.

In a large population-based epidemiologic study of brain tumors in pregnancy, Isla et al. [15] analyzed a population of over 1.4 million individuals in which 126,413 births occurred between 1983 and 1995. There was a cumulative incidence of seven intracranial tumors among pregnant women (two meningiomas, two ependymomas, two other gliomas, and one tumor of uncertain histopathology). Three of the seven patients presented with new onset seizures. One other patient experienced tumor hemorrhage during labor and expired despite an emergency craniotomy. Another patient presented with diplopia and multiple cranial nerve deficits but was able to deliver at 33 weeks' gestation. She subsequently underwent radiotherapy and passed away 3 months later (histopathology unknown). Three of the patients had craniotomies while pregnant, and one experienced fetal loss due to a spontaneous abortion 10 weeks after her craniotomy at an estimated gestational age of 20 weeks.

A recent retrospective review by Laviv et al. [16] identified 104 published cases of meningiomas managed surgically, with 86 of these reports having sufficient data to form the basis for potential recommendations. In their series, 40% of patients had craniotomies for resection during pregnancy, and 60% underwent resection postpartum. A greater proportion of those who had craniotomies during pregnancy were emergent craniotomies (40% vs. 19.6%). This same group also had a higher proportion of

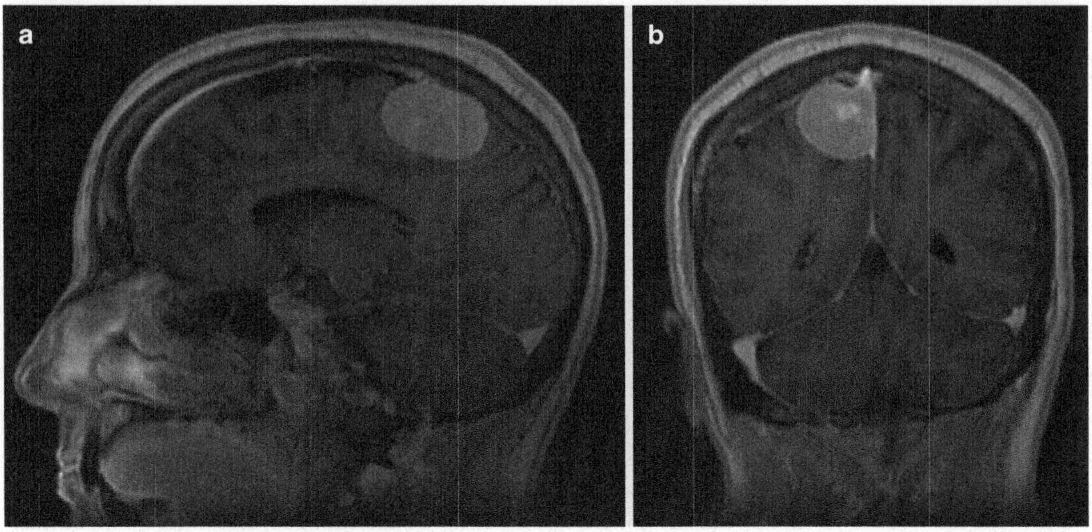

Fig. 18.3 (**a**) Sagittal and (**b**) coronal post-contrast T1-weighted MR images showing a convexity meningioma involving the falx and the superior sagittal sinus

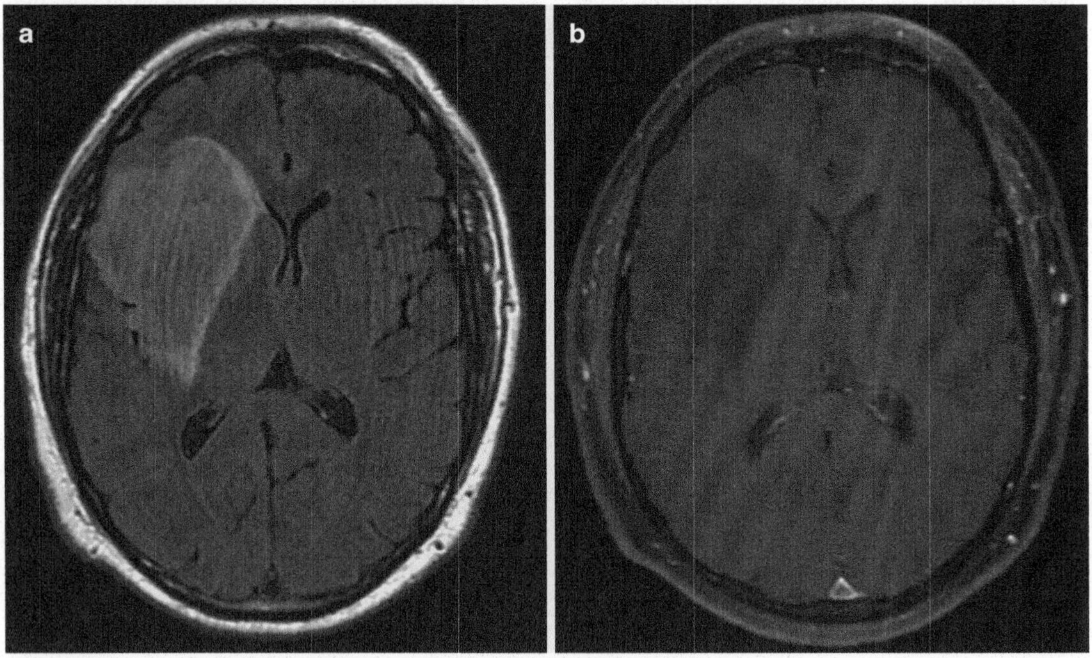

Fig. 18.4 (**a**) T2 flair and (**b**) post-contrast T1 axial MR images showing an example of a right insular, low-grade astrocytoma, also known as a glioma

emergent C-sections (47% vs. 17.8%). The risk of maternal or fetal mortality was higher with the earlier craniotomy group, but this was not statistically significant. For these reasons, the authors recommended term deliveries whenever possible.

Brain Tumor Outcomes

Terry et al. [14] utilized the Nationwide Inpatient Sample, an epidemiologically representative sample of all non-federal US hospitalizations, to perform a retrospective cohort study of pregnancy-related hospitalizations among women with malignant and benign brain tumors as well as spine tumors from 1988 to 2009. From among the more than 19.75 million pregnancy-associated admissions in this time period, 397 were associated with malignant brain tumors, including 165 (44%) for deliveries. Four hundred and-thirty-seven admissions were associated with benign brain tumors, 265 (61%) of which were deliveries. Among the pregnant population without brain tumors, approximately 90% of admissions were for delivery.

Hospitalizations for reasons other than delivery were significantly more likely in pregnant patients with malignant or benign brain tumors. Pregnancy complications including preterm labor, intrauterine growth restriction, and stillbirth were more common among patients with malignant tumors. Benign tumors were associated with preterm labor as well as gestational diabetes and gestational and chronic hypertension. Notably while 48% of patients with malignant tumors and 19% of those with benign tumors underwent some type of neurosurgical procedure, these adverse outcomes were not associated with neurosurgical intervention itself. The authors posited that these complications were secondary to the underlying tumor as opposed to neurosurgical intervention since the clinical sequelae of intracranial neoplasia such as hydrocephalus, seizures, hyperemesis, etc. can have detrimental effects on a pregnancy. The most commonly performed neurosurgical procedures were craniotomies in both the malignant (31.4%) and benign (16%) cases, followed by biopsy (9%) among those patients with malignant tumors. Rates of biopsy, ventriculostomy, and shunt implantation were too low among women with benign tumors to be reported.

Cesarean section was much more common among women with malignant (odds ratio 3.3, 95% confidence interval 1.2–9.2) and benign (OR 2.8, 95% CI 2.1–3.6) tumors than the general population. Spine tumors were also associated with increased rates of cesarean section (OR 3.9, 95% CI 1.8–8.2), which may indicate that, overall, pregnancies with comorbid CNS tumors are viewed as higher risk, thus lowering the threshold for elective cesarean section.

Shunts and Hydrocephalus

Ventriculoperitoneal shunts (VPS) are devices designed to treat hydrocephalus by diverting cerebrospinal fluid (CSF) into the peritoneal space. CSF diversion into other locations including the pleural space (ventriculopleural) or right atrium (ventriculoatrial) is much less common but represents viable alternatives when the abdominal compartment cannot be utilized. Despite technological advancements, the function of shunts depends fundamentally on a pressure gradient or differential between the intracranial/intraventricular compartment and that of the body cavity into which CSF is being diverted. Thus, intuitively, the elevated intraabdominal pressure associated with pregnancy may predispose a VPS to failure, with resultant worsening of hydrocephalus and intracranial hypertension.

In a retrospective series of 77 pregnancies among 37 women (with 38 shunts) [17], shunts were revised ten total times either during pregnancy or the subsequent 6 months. Eighty-four percent of all pregnancies were unassociated with shunt malfunctions or failures. Of the three revisions that were done during pregnancy, two were in the same patient who also required a third revision 2 days postpartum. More than 60% of deliveries were vaginal. Three C-sections were done because of the presence of a shunt, two in mothers known to be in shunt failure and the third because the attending physicians deemed the presence of a shunt to be sufficient to require a cesarean. Of note, the distal shunt catheters of two other patients with a VPS were found to have disconnected and become entangled with reproductive organs. Neither of these instances occurred while the patient was pregnant.

More recently, Rajagopalan et al. conducted a literature review and noted a cumulative shunt malfunction rate of 29% with 71% of these women requiring shunt revision antenatally (4/28), during delivery (2/28), or within 6 months of delivery (14/28). In this series, 14 women (24%) had a C-section performed because of concerns for elevated ICP [18].

Cusimano and others have suggested that given the high shunt failure rates associated with VPS in pregnancy, revision to ventriculoatrial

(VA) systems may be indicated for pregnant women [19]. However, VA shunts carry other significant attendant risks, including development of arrhythmias, infection, and valvular dysfunction. Thus, the risk-benefit ratio does not seem to justify revision to VA systems for pregnant women in all cases. Rather, the preponderance of available evidence supports allowing pregnancies to progress naturally with close attention paid to signs and symptoms of shunt failure. Managing physicians should maintain a high suspicion for shunt malfunction antenatally and during parturition as well as for infection [20] in the postpartum period.

Traumatic Brain Injury (TBI)

Mild and moderate traumatic brain injury, usually resulting from a fall or motor vehicle accident, is usually managed with standard conservative and nonsurgical measures. Previous studies hinted at the possibility that the increased levels of estrogen and progesterone in pregnancy might have neuroprotective effects in pregnant women. Unfortunately, clinical trial [21] and population-based studies [22] failed to corroborate this data and even showed trends toward worsened outcomes in pregnant women.

Management of severe traumatic brain injury (sTBI) in pregnant women is fraught with ethical dilemmas. While case reports establish that maintenance of viable pregnancies among neurologically devastated patients is possible, many of the interventions required in such circumstances may present significant risk to developing fetuses. Careful consideration should be given to the risk-benefit analysis of extraordinary interventions in a neurocritical care setting. Concomitant injuries and fetal gestational age may allow for more accurate recommendations about the aggression of intervention. The ethical justifiability of such invasive surgical measures as decompressive hemicraniectomy must be determined on a case-by-case basis in close consultation with patients' families after they have been well informed about the prognosis of both an expectant mother and the fetus.

Fundamental Tenets of Neurocritical Care

When a pregnant patient presents with depressed mental status from a neurological condition, immediate interventions should focus on maintaining a patient's airway and appropriate oxygenation. Rapid sequence intubation should be considered in patients with an initial post-resuscitation GCS of eight or less. Short-acting agents are preferred to enable an examining neurosurgeon to obtain an accurate exam. Even if concern exists about increased intracranial pressure, there is rarely an indication for prolonged hyperventilation as excessive vasoconstriction can precipitate further neurologic injury [23]. A possible exception would be a unilaterally dilated pupil in a patient with a known mass lesion or increased intracranial pressure as a short-term emergent treatment. Intubated patients should be maintained at the lowest positive end-expiratory pressure deemed safe by the primary treatment team.

Blood pressure should be controlled with short-acting agents with the goal of modest reduction while avoiding hypotension. Initial blood pressure goals should be systolic blood pressure <160 mmHg and mean arterial pressure (MAP < 90). The classic "Cushing's triad" of hypertension, bradycardia, and disordered breathing is often a late finding and portends a poor prognosis.

When intracranial hypertension is suspected, initial interventions include head of bed elevation, correction of hypercarbia, and administration of hypertonic saline or mannitol. In most scenarios, hypertonic saline (e.g., 3%, 7%, or 23.4%) is the preferred first-line agent. Mannitol is another commonly used osmotic agent but has been tested in pregnant rabbits and found to cross the placenta, increasing fetal osmotic pressure and precipitating both intravascular and extravascular fluid losses [24]. In the setting of hypovolemia, this may exacerbate hemodynamic instability and/or worsen renal function. Uterine hypoperfusion and accumulation of osmotic agents in the fetus should be considered prior to their administration to pregnant patients [25]. Neurosurgical consultation is warranted prior to administration of hypertonic agents as intracranial pressure monitoring may be recommended to help guide therapy. Similarly, in the third trimester, the use of corticosteroids to manage cerebral edema may cause fetal adrenal suppression, and their use should be weighed carefully against the risks of urgent/emergent delivery [25].

Spinal Pathology

Surgical Timing Considerations

Spinal pathology often presents with symptoms that can be used clinically to estimate both the anatomic location and the nature of the pathology (e.g., radiculopathy vs. myelopathy). A careful history and physical examination can be tremendously useful in elucidating whether a patient's symptoms are pregnancy-associated or due to neural injury. This in turn helps guide decision-making about timing of potential neurosurgical interventions. With few exceptions, surgical interventions are not undertaken unless the patient is experiencing a neurological deficit and the procedure can be performed without harm to the fetus. Many spinal conditions, including radiculopathy, may appear or worsen during pregnancy but then spontaneously improve following delivery eliminating the need for surgical intervention.

Back Pain

Back pain in pregnancy is a common complaint affecting over 50% of patients, with some studies suggesting up to 90% incidence [26]. The majority of these patients present with pelvic girdle pain or pregnancy-related lower back pain that can be treated by a nonelastic pelvic belt and/or exercise regimens [26]. Typically, axial and paraxial back pain without radiation into the extremities or focal muscle weakness does not require neurosurgical consultation in the absence of known trauma or a history of cancer. Conservative measures including rest, physical therapy, and judicious use of appropriate pain medications constitute the mainstay of treatment. A low threshold for neurosurgical consultation should prevail in the setting of progressing deficit, urinary retention, or intractable symptoms.

Disc Herniation

Herniated discs represent the most common spinal pathology causing pain in the pregnant population but overall remain rare [26]. Symptoms related to herniated vertebral discs (and any other compressive lesion) can be grossly divided into two categories by what structure is being compressed: radiculopathy and myelopathy. Radiculopathy is caused by compression of nerve roots emanating from the spinal cord (Fig. 18.5). This is a lower motor neuron lesion and stereotypically manifests as shooting pain, numbness, or paresthesias in a dermatomal distribution. There may also be weakness in the corresponding myotome. It is important to note that more than one dermatome or myotome may be involved depending on the exact nature and location of the compressive lesion. In myelopathy, the spinal cord itself is being compressed leading to an upper motor neuron lesion. This can result in numbness, dyscoordination, weakness, and spasticity or hyperreflexia, which often manifest as difficulty with coordination or gait instability.

Diagnosis of a disc herniation is made with a MRI (without contrast) of the suspected spinal segment. In the absence of frank muscle weakness, the vast majority of vertebral disc herniations do not require emergent surgical intervention. Moreover, most patients with disc herniations will experience symptomatic improvement with the existing data suggesting that 50% will experience major improvement within 3 months [27]. First-line management in patients with isolated radiculopathy without acute weakness therefore is founded on multimodal pain control, physical therapy, and close observation.

Cauda Equina Syndrome

Cauda equina syndrome represents a rare but important entity with an estimated incidence of approximately 2 per million. Due to its severity and potential for permanent morbidity [28], concern for cauda equina syndrome is an indication for urgent neurosurgical consultation. This syndrome, which can present acutely or chronically,

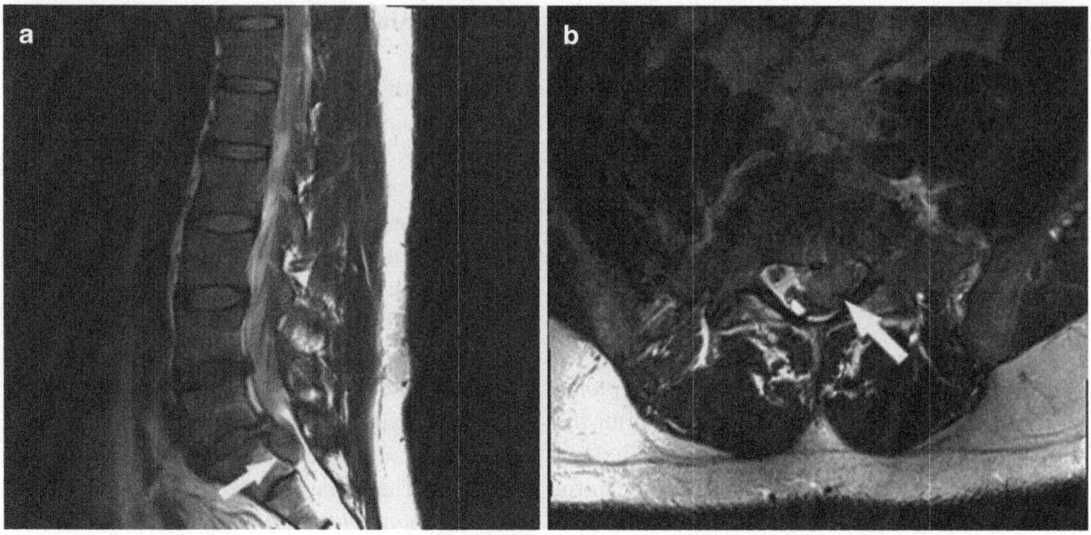

Fig. 18.5 (**a**) T2 sagittal and (**b**) T2 axial MR images of the lumbar spine showing a herniated L5–S1 disc (*white arrow*) to the left causing significant nerve compression

is usually due to the herniation of a large amount of disc material into the spinal canal, causing compression of multiple nerve roots comprising the cauda equine [29].

Lower extremity symptoms include radiculopathy (i.e., sensory deficits, paresthesias, and weakness). Sacral root compression produces the hallmark symptoms of saddle anesthesia, urinary retention, and decreased or absent rectal tone that may result in bowel incontinence. When cauda equina syndrome is suspected, a detailed lower-extremity neurological exam and rectal exam must be performed to document the presence or absence of these findings. Bladder scans and urinary post-void residuals are also of great diagnostic value. If the physical exam corroborates concerns for cauda equina syndrome, MRI of the lumbar spine should be performed emergently to evaluate for a causative lesion, and neurosurgical consultation should be made.

Treatment of cauda equina syndrome is emergent surgical decompression. Delay can lead to the associated deficits, including bowel and bladder dysfunction, becoming permanent [28, 30]. Despite the possibility for poor outcomes, surgical decompression is very effective in correcting the symptoms associated with cauda equina syndrome [28, 30, 31].

Compression Fracture

Calcium homeostasis during pregnancy is altered to provide the developing fetus with enough calcium to mineralize the skeleton. Parathyroid hormone-related protein (PTHrP) leads to increased calcium through multiple mechanisms including increased resorption from the maternal skeleton [32]. Most patients tolerate this increased resorption without issue, but in some patients this can lead to pregnancy-associated osteoporosis and vertebral compression fracture. Patients with a family history of early osteoporotic fractures may be at increased risk [33].

These fractures most commonly occur during the third trimester when mineralization of the fetal skeleton is at its peak and the gravid uterus adds an extra 12 kg on average to the axial load placed on the spine [34]. Patients predominantly present with complaints of acute-onset axial and paraxial back pain at the affected levels, and physical examination may demonstrate point tenderness over the spinous processes [35]. Fractures are typically diagnosed with plain films or CT, but some providers opt for MRI to decrease maternal and fetal radiation exposure. Additionally, MRI can provide information on the chronicity of the fracture with marrow edema being a marker of an acute fracture.

The majority of compression fractures are not associated with neurological deficit, and treatment of these fractures centers on pain control. Adjunctive measures include thoracolumbar orthotics with the specific brace used dependent on the levels injured. Other treatments include a bone density-increasing regimen with vitamin D and calcium supplementation, weight-bearing exercises, and possibly the use of anti-resorptive medications [34, 36, 37]. Endocrinological consultation may be indicated for patients thought to require pharmacologic management of their osteoporosis.

For patients whose pain is not controlled with conservative management, percutaneous vertebroplasty or kyphoplasty can be considered. Recent randomized controlled trials have called into question the benefit of vertebroplasty for compression fractures after failing to demonstrate an improvement in pain or functional status over sham surgery [38, 39]. However, the patient populations in these studies were significantly older than the patient population addressed in this review, and there have been multiple case reports reflecting successful treatment of acute pain with vertebroplasty [35, 36, 40]. For the rare patient who presents with pain and neural element compression, vertebroplasty is not sufficient as no decompression can be obtained. These patients may require an open procedure to relieve the compression on the spinal cord and/or nerve roots.

Vertebral Hemangiomas

Vertebral hemangiomas are common, asymptomatic tumors found in approximately 10% of the population, with symptoms arising in only 1% (Fig. 18.6). Published data about vertebral hemangiomas in pregnancy consists primarily of case reports, but the majority of patients who present with this pathology do so in the third trimester. This is likely the consequence of the increased blood volume and inferior vena cava compression causing expansion of the hemangioma [41, 42]. Generally, patients with vertebral hemangiomas present with pain from mass effect causing subperiosteal expansion or from compression fractures as the vertebral body is replaced by tumor causing structural weakness. Less commonly, patients may present with a neurological deficit due to compression caused directly by hemangioma expansion or tissue ischemia due to vascular steal [43]. Diagnosis of

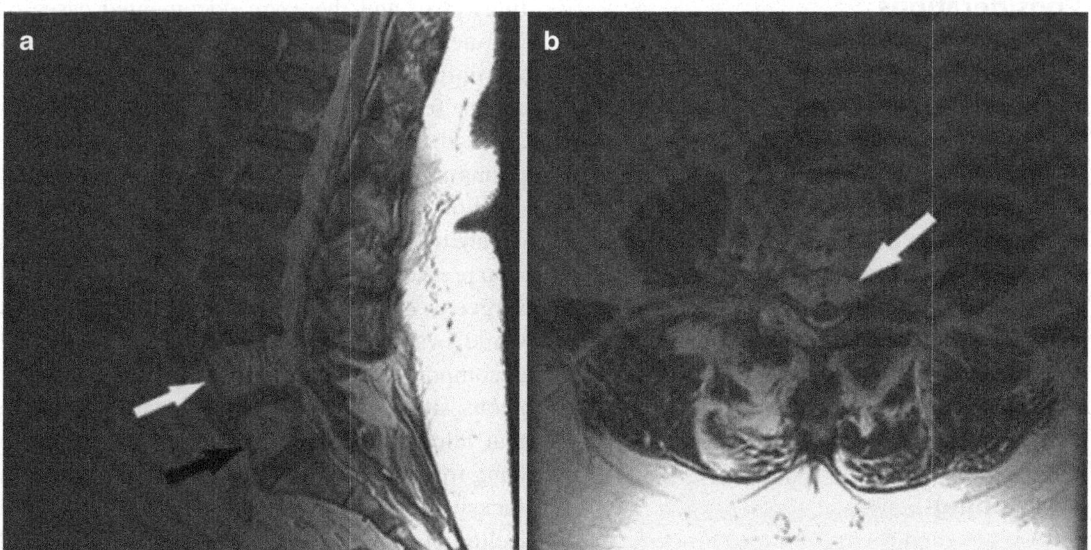

Fig. 18.6 (**a**) T2 sagittal and (**b**) T2 axial MR image of the lumbar spine showing a typical (*black arrow*) and atypical (*white arrow*) hemangioma. Notice how the atypical hemangioma violates the posterior cortex of the vertebral body, causing stenosis

a vertebral hemangioma is made primarily by MRI with gadolinium. The lesion will appear hyperdense on T1 and T2 sequences and enhance with contrast [41, 43].

Treatment of vertebral hemangiomas depends on the presence or absence of neurologic deficit. For patients who present solely with pain but who desire intervention during pregnancy, endovascular embolization or vertebroplasty can be offered [44]. For patients with neurological compromise, more invasive surgical measures ranging from laminectomy to corpectomy may be required to provide the necessary decompression [41, 44]. As surgical intervention increases in scope and complexity, the associated blood loss, potential for complications, and risk to both the mother and fetus concomitantly increase. Thus, many providers will prefer minimal safe and effective intervention until the postpartum period at which point a larger, more definitive surgery can be performed with less risk to the fetus [41, 44]. Of note, spontaneous improvement following delivery has been seen in some patients and may obviate the need for more aggressive intervention [44].

General Perioperative Considerations

The gravid patient presents some unique challenges in the perioperative and intraoperative setting. While most of these will not preclude neurosurgical intervention, providers are again strongly encouraged to take a multidisciplinary approach to the pregnant neurosurgery patient, by discussing considerations with the operating neurosurgeon, obstetrician, and anesthesiologist, as well as perioperative and surgical nurses. The following are select aspects of operative management of pregnant neurosurgery patients.

Positioning

Careful positioning of neurosurgical patients is of the utmost importance. For cranial neurosurgery, the orientation of the skull—and therefore intracranial contents—enables not only access to a surgical target in a complicated three-dimensional space but is also used to manipulate blood and CSF flow and drainage, to use gravity to assist with retraction of neural structures so that operative corridors can be established and maintained with minimal direct retraction on the brain or its vasculature, and to prevent intraoperative and postoperative complications such as venous air emboli. Similarly, successful spine surgery requires appropriate positioning to maintain cord perfusion, minimize venous congestion in Batson's plexus, and foster proper vertebral alignment for cases of decompression and fusion.

Unfortunately, having patients in ideal neurosurgical positions may sometimes present risks by placing unacceptable pressure on the gravid pelvis or by causing aortocaval compression. As a corollary, sacrificing sound neurosurgical positioning because of a patient's pregnancy may make a surgery technically more challenging and thereby place both the mother and fetus at increased risk indirectly, by prolonging the operation, or by increasing the risk of hemorrhage, or neurologic compromise [45].

Neurosurgical interventions on pregnant patients have been carried out successfully in multiple positions (e.g., lateral, prone, and sitting) [46], and there are documented cases of non-neurosurgical procedures being performed in similar positions that did not cause adverse events for fetuses [47]. Surgeons are encouraged to take great care to ensure all pressure points are padded adequately. Furthermore, all position changes should be made slowly to ensure there are no deleterious changes in perfusion pressures to either mother or fetus [46], and surgeons should consider positioning patients while awake whenever possible [48]. For spinal decompression and/or fusion surgeries, surgeons should consider using a table or frame that allows the gravid abdomen and pelvis to hang free without compression, such as an open Jackson frame, a four-post frame such as a Relton-Hall frame, or laminectomy rolls placed to accomplish the same effect [48]. If fluoroscopy is required for the surgery, every attempt should be made to provide extra shielding for the fetus.

Intraoperative Fetal Monitoring

Intraoperative fetal heart rate monitoring should be considered. In general most authors believe that fetal heart rate monitoring is not indicated before 20 weeks' gestation, may have value between 20 and 23 weeks, and is indicated after 23 weeks [49]. In situations where the operating neurosurgeon expects substantial fluid shifts, blood pressure swings, or possible compromise of the fetal circulation secondary to maternal positioning, fetal heart rate monitoring may be of particular utility. Decisions about this monitoring and interpretation of data obtained should be done in close consultation with a qualified obstetrician.

Conclusion

Neurosurgical emergencies in the pregnant patient will continue to present a diagnostic and treatment challenge to physicians. Although the deferral of treatment until after delivery is preferred when appropriate, many neurosurgical disorders may present an urgent threat to the mother and fetus and necessitate intervention. New and different neurologic complaints or mental status change may be a harbinger of serious pathology that can result in loss of function, paralysis, and death if not treated appropriately. In many instances, available data and treatment guidelines for neurosurgical emergencies during pregnancy are scarce, and decisions will have to be made on a case-by-case basis in the best interest of the mother and fetus. Early consultation and close coordination between obstetricians and neurosurgeons will help to minimize the impact of neurosurgical pathology and maximize outcomes for the pregnant patient, baby, and family.

References

1. ICRP. Pregnancy and medical radiation. ICRP Publication 84 An ICRP. 2000;30(1).
2. Shaw P, Duncan A, Vouyouka A, Ozsvath K. Radiation exposure and pregnancy. J Vasc Surg. 2011;53(1):28S–34S.
3. Nikolaos K, Dimitrios M, Nikolaos T, Alexandros R. Exposure to ionizing radiation and pregnancy. HJOG. 2015;14(2).
4. Webb J, Thomsen H, Morcos S. The use of iodinated and gadolinium contrast media during pregnancy and lactation. Eur Radiol. 2005;15(6):1234–40.
5. Hernandez-Diaz S, Smith C, Shen A, Mittendorf R, Hauser W, Yerby M, et al. Comparative safety of antiepileptic drugs during pregnancy. Neurology. 2012;78:1692–9.
6. Mawhinney E, Craig J, Morrow J, Russell A, Smithson W, Parsons L, et al. Levetiracetam in pregnancy: results from the UK and Ireland epilepsy in pregnancy registers. Neurology. 2013;80(4):400–5.
7. Bateman BT, Olbrecht VA, Berman M, Minehart RD, Schwamm LH, Leffertr LR. Peripartum subarachnoid Hemorrhage, Nationwide Data and Institutional Experience. Anesthesiology. 2012;116(2):524–33.
8. Tarnaris A, Haliasos N, Watkins LD. Endovascular treatment of ruptured intracranial aneurysms during pregnancy: is this the best way forward? Case report and review of the literature. Clin Neurol Neurosurg. 2012;114(6):703–6.
9. Robba C, Bacigaluppi S, Bragazzi NL, Bilotta F, Sekhon MS, Bertuetti R, et al. Aneurysmal subarachnoid Hemorrhage in pregnancy-case series, review, and pooled data analysis. World Neurosurg. 2016;88:383–98.
10. Gross BA, Du R. Hemorrhage from arteriovenous malformations during pregnancy. Neurosurgery. 2012;71(2):349–55; discussion 55–6.
11. Porras JL, Yang W, Philadelphia E, Law J, Garzon-Muvdi T, Caplan JM, et al. Hemorrhage risk of brain Arteriovenous malformations during pregnancy and Puerperium in a north American cohort. Stroke. 2017;48(6):1507–13.
12. Kashkoush AI, Ma H, Agarwal N, Panczykowski D, Tonetti D, Weiner GM, et al. Cerebral venous sinus thrombosis in pregnancy and puerperium: a pooled, systematic review. J Clin Neurosci. 2017;39:9–15.
13. Coutinho JM, Ferro JM, Canhao P, Barinagarrementeria F, Cantu C, Bousser MG, et al. Cerebral venous and sinus thrombosis in women. Stroke. 2009;40(7):2356–61.
14. Terry AR, Barker FG 2nd, Leffert L, Bateman BT, Souter I, Plotkin SR. Outcomes of hospitalization in pregnant women with CNS neoplasms: a population-based study. Neuro-Oncology. 2012;14(6):768–76.
15. Isla A, Alvarez F, Gonzalez A, Garcia-Grande A, Perez-Alvarez M, Garcia-Blazquez M. Brain tumor and pregnancy. Obstet Gynecol. 1997;89(1):19–23.
16. Laviv Y, Bayoumi A, Mahadevan A, Young B, Boone M, Kasper EM. Meningiomas in pregnancy: timing of surgery and clinical outcomes as observed in 104 cases and establishment of a best management strategy. Acta Neurochir. 2017. https://doi.org/10.1007/s00701-017-3146-8.
17. Bradley NK, Liakos AM, McAllister JPI, Magram G, Kinsman S, Bradley MK. Maternal shunt dependency: implications for obstetric care, neurosurgical management, and Pregnancy Outcomes and a review of selected literature. Neurosurgery. 1998;43(3):448–60.

18. Rajagopalan S, Gopinath S, Trinh VT, Chandrasekhar S. Anesthetic considerations for labor and delivery in women with cerebrospinal fluid shunts. Int J Obstet Anesth. 2017;30:23–9.
19. Cusimano MD, Meffe FM, Gentili F, Sermer M. Management of pregnant women with cerebrospinal fluid shunts. Pediatr Neurosurg. 1991;17(1): 10–3.
20. Kane JM, Jackson K, Conway JH. Maternal postpartum group B beta-hemolytic streptococcus ventriculoperitoneal shunt infection. Arch Gynecol Obstet. 2004;269(2):139–41.
21. Skolnick BE, Maas AI, Narayan RK, van der Hoop RG, MacAllister T, Ward JD, et al. A clinical trial of progesterone for severe traumatic brain injury. N Engl J Med. 2014;371(26):2467–76.
22. Berry C, Ley EJ, Mirocha J, Margulies DR, Tillou A, Salim A. Do pregnant women have improved outcomes after traumatic brain injury? Am J Surg. 2011;201(4):429–32.
23. Carney N, Totten AM, O'Reilly C, Ullman JS, Hawryluk GW, Bell M, et al. Guidelines for the management of severe traumatic brain injury. Neurosurgery. 2017;80(1):6–15.
24. Bruns P, Linder R, Drose V, Battaglia F. The placental transfer of water from fetus to mother following the intravenous infusion of hypertonic mannitol to the maternal rabbit. Am J Obstet Gynecol. 1963;86(2):160–7.
25. Cohen-Gadol AA, Friedman JA, Friedman JD, Tubbs RS, Munis JR, Meyer FB. Neurosurgical management of intracranial lesions in the pregnant patient: a 36-year institutional experience and review of the literature. J Neurosurg. 2009;111(6):1150–7.
26. Han I. Pregnancy and spinal problems. Curr Opin Obstet Gynecol. 2010;22:477–81.
27. Weinstein J, Lurie J, Tosteson T, Skinner J, Hanscom B, Tosteson A, et al. Surgical vs nonoperative treatment for lumbar disk herniation: the spine patient outcomes research trial (SPORT) observational cohort. JAMA. 2006;296(20):2451–9.
28. Kim H, Kim S, Lee S, Shin H. Endoscopic discectomy for the cauda equina syndrome during third trimester of pregnancy. J Korean Neurosurg Soc. 2007;42(5):419–20.
29. Lavy C, James A, Wilson-MacDonald J, Fairbank J. Cauda Equina Syndrome. Obstet Anesth Dig. 2010;30(1):16–7.
30. Brown M, Levi A. Surgery for lumbar disc herniation in pregnancy. Spine. 2001;26(4):440–3.
31. Hakan T. Lumbar disk herniation presented with cauda equina syndrome in a pregnant woman. J Neurosci Rural Pract. 2012;2012(3):2.
32. Raffaeta G, Mazzantini M, Menconi A, Bottai V, Falossi F, Celauro I, et al. Osteoporosis with vertebral fractures associated with pregnancy: two cases reports. Clin Case Min Bone Metab. 2014;11(2):136–8.
33. Dunne F, Walters B, Marshall T, Heath D. Pregnancy associated osteoporosis. Clin Endocrinol. 1993;39(4): 487–90.
34. Kovacs C, Ralston S. Presentation and management of osteoporosis presenting in association with pregnancy or lactation. Osteoporos Int. 2015;26:2223–41.
35. Bonacker J, Janousek M, Krober M. Pregnancy-associated osteoporosis with eight fractures in the vertebral column treated with kyphoplasty and bracing: a case report. Arch Orthop Trauma Surg. 2014;134(2):173–9.
36. Kim H, Song J, Kwon A, Kim H. Percutaneous vertebroplasty for pregnancy-associated osteoporotic vertebral compression fractures. J Korean Neurosurg Soc. 2010;47(5):99–102.
37. Iwamoto J, Sato Y, Wzawa M, Matsumoto H. Five year follow up of a woman with pregnancy and lactation-associated osteoporosis and vertebral fractures. Ther Clin Risk Manag. 2012;8:195–9.
38. Buchbinder R, Osborne R, Ebeling P, Wark J, Mitchell P, Wriedt C, et al. A randomized trial of vertebroplasty for painful osteoporotic vertebral fractures. N Engl J Med. 2009;361(6):557–68.
39. Kallmes D, Comstock B, Heagerty P, Turner J, Wilson D, Diamond T, et al. A randomized trial of vertebroplasty for osteoporotic spinal fractures. N Engl J Med. 2009;361:569–79.
40. Bayram S, Ozturk C, Sivrioglu K, Aydinli U, Kucukoglu S. Kyphoplasty for pregnancy-associated osteoporotic vertebral fractures. Joint Bone Spine. 2006;73(5):564–6.
41. Moles A, Hamel O, Perret C, Bord E, Robert R, Buffenoir K. Symptomatic vertebral hemangiomas during pregnancy. J Neurosurg. 2014;20:585–91.
42. Newman M. Spinal angioma with symptoms in pregnancy. J Neurol Neurosurg Psychiatry. 1958;21:38–41.
43. Chi J, Manley G, Chou D. Pregnancy-related vertebral hemangioma: case report, review of the literature, and management algorithm. Neurosurg Focus. 2005;19(3):E7–E13.
44. Kiroglu Y, Benek B, Yagci B, Cirak B, Thata K. Spinal cord compression caused by vertebral hemangioma being symptomatic during pregnancy. Surg Neurol. 2009;71:487–92.
45. Samali M, Elkoundi A, Tahri A, Bensghir M, Haimeur C. Anesthetic management of spontaneous cervical epidural hematoma during pregnancy: a case report. J Med Case Rep. 2017;11(1):171.
46. Chowdhury T, Chowdhury M, Schaller B, Cappellani RB, Daya J. Perioperative considerations for neurosurgical procedures in the gravid patient: continuing professional development. Can J Anaesth. 2013;60(11):1139–55.
47. Julien F, Drolet S, Levesque I, Bouchard A. The right lateral position for laparoscopic diaphragmatic hernia repair in pregnancy: technique and review of the literature. J Laparoendosc Adv Surg Tech A. 2011;21(1):67–70.
48. Brown MD, Levi AD. Surgery for lumbar disc herniation during pregnancy. Spine (Phila Pa 1976). 2001;26(4):440–3.
49. Katz JD, Hook R, Barash PG. Fetal heart rate monitoring in pregnant patients undergoing surgery. Am J Obstet Gynecol. 1976;125(2):267–9.

Ophthalmology Surgery During Pregnancy

19

Michael S. Jacobson

Who Is Pregnant?

One issue ophthalmologists often forget to address is the absolute requirement for pregnancy tests on all women of childbearing age whose ocular condition may worsen during pregnancy, require medications, or require eye surgery. Without that knowledge, ophthalmologists may accidentally operate on a pregnant patient, and all the information/precautions presented in this chapter may go unutilized, thereby unknowingly exposing the fetus to teratogens or other dangers and endangering the pregnancy. Interestingly, this lack of pregnancy testing on pregnant patients unintentionally provides the data found in case reports. Verbal confirmation of pregnancy status is not sufficient, and patients should all be tested prior to all planned ophthalmology surgery. This needs to be well notated in the medical record, and it needs to state explicitly that the patient was counseled about not getting pregnant while under treatment, and if there is any ambiguity, the patient should be retested.

The Exam of the Pregnant Patient

Is it safe for the ophthalmologist to do a conventional dilated exam on a pregnant patient? **It is not thought that standard dilating drops pose any risks for the mother or fetus** [1, 2]. However, intravenous injection of phenylephrine would pose a potential risk, and intravenous atropine, homatropine, and epinephrine early in pregnancy have been associated with minor fetal malformations, so obviously excessive dilating drops should be avoided. It is thought that the stimulation of bright lights can dispose susceptible woman to seizures, but there is no question that the additional information gained in the ophthalmic exam outweighs the risk when such an examination is necessary. Unfortunately, some patients may feel uncomfortable undergoing dilation and having ophthalmologic examinations or may not trust the safety of some of the noninvasive testing. For those patients with reduced vision or ocular symptoms who are too anxious or cannot be educated and persuaded that there is no risk to exam, there will be an inadequate assessment of their ocular pathology. This could be particularly dangerous for them and increases the risk of permanent vision loss.

M. S. Jacobson
Georgia Retina, Tucker, GA, USA

Northside Hospital, Atlanta, GA, USA

Georgia Retina Surgery Center, LLC, Atlanta, GA, USA

Dekalb Medical Center, Decatur, GA, USA
e-mail: mjacobson@garetina.com

C. H. Nezhat (ed.), *Non-Obstetric Surgery During Pregnancy*,
https://doi.org/10.1007/978-3-319-90752-9_19

What Ophthalmological Testing or Imaging Is Safe to Do?

There have been significant improvements in noninvasive methods to evaluate ocular pathology [3]. Up until just 20 years ago, the only way to properly evaluate retinal and choroidal circulation was fluorescein angiography (FA) [4]. Fluorescein dye, a vegetable-based dye injected intravenously, is considered FDA risk category B, but most retinologists choose to avoid it in the pregnant patient as its true teratogenicity is unknown. The fluorescein dye toxicity is also unknown for newborns, so its use should probably be avoided in a lactating mother, or the mother should breast pump and dispose of any milk that has an orange dye color to it, which would suggest residual fluorescein dye that has not yet been fully excreted by the kidneys.

Optical coherence tomography (OCT) was developed in the late 1990s. Using this scanning laser device, the ophthalmologist can see cross sections revealing each of the retina's distinctive layers, often without dilation. This retinal mapping and thickness measurements are fundamental to guide treatment for glaucoma and diseases of the retina. While not as useful as FA, it is still quite excellent and there are no safety concerns (Fig. 19.1) [4].

In the past 5 years, optical coherence tomography angiography (OCTA) has been developed. It is the next evolution of OCT. It is a new, noninvasive imaging technique (dye-free) that quickly generates volumetric angiography images, and it has some clinical capability of evaluating pathology of the retinal and choroidal vasculature. Its value and limitations are still being defined. It is safe but still less useful than FA (Fig. 19.2a, b).

Historically, ocular photography necessitated a dilated exam, but now there are cameras that can take fundus photos without dilation (nonmydriatic) and ones that can even provide a panoramic view (Optos and Zeiss Clarus). So instead of having a conventional 45° view, one can obtain a much more extensive view up to 200° which increases the chance of capturing peripheral retinal pathology. These tests provide very quick screening (Fig. 19.3a, b).

As described, we now have many other excellent noninvasive methods to evaluate retinal and choroidal pathology. Employing these newer noninvasive techniques, it is less frequent that a diagnosis remains elusive. So, while some tests cannot be undertaken in the pregnant patient, these alternate tests are often good enough to allow us to reach a diagnosis or in other cases at least postpone riskier, more informative diagnostic testing until the postpartum period.

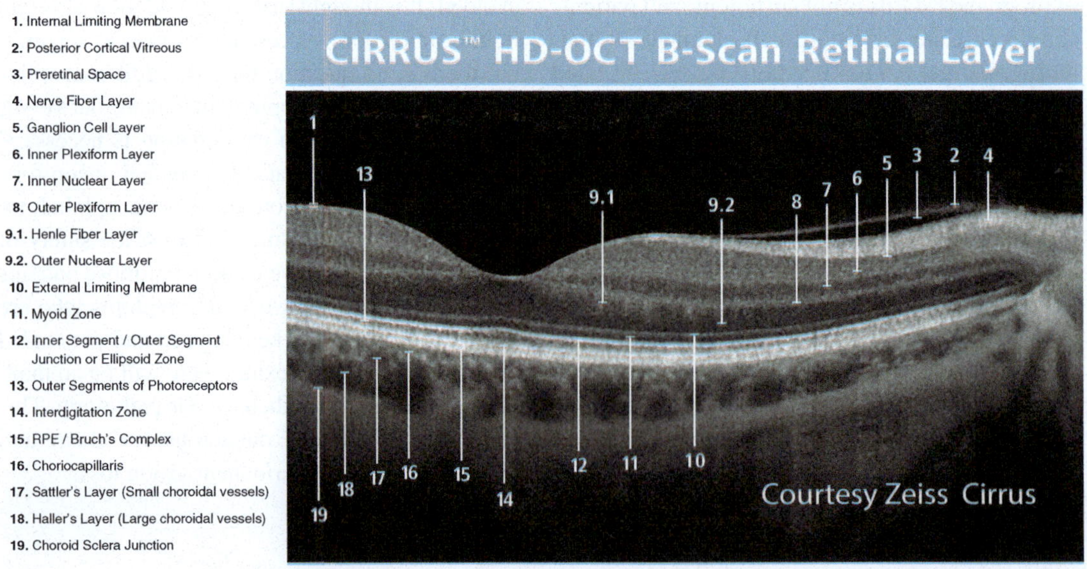

Fig. 19.1 OCT revealing the various layers of the retina. Photo: Courtesy of ZEISS

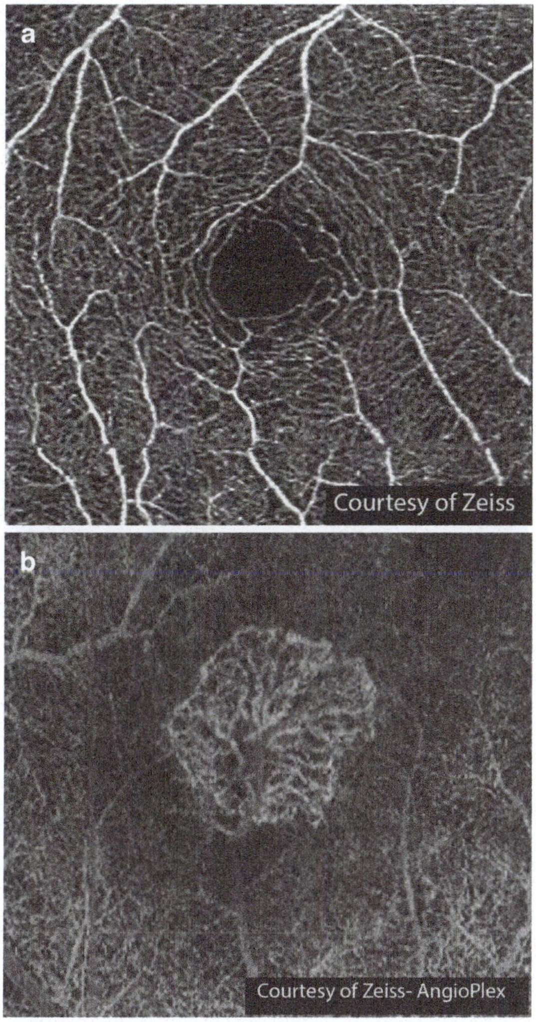

Fig. 19.2 (**a**) OCTA revealing normal vascular pattern of the fovea. (**b**) OCTA revealing abnormal choroidal neovascularization in the fovea. Photos: Courtesy of ZEISS

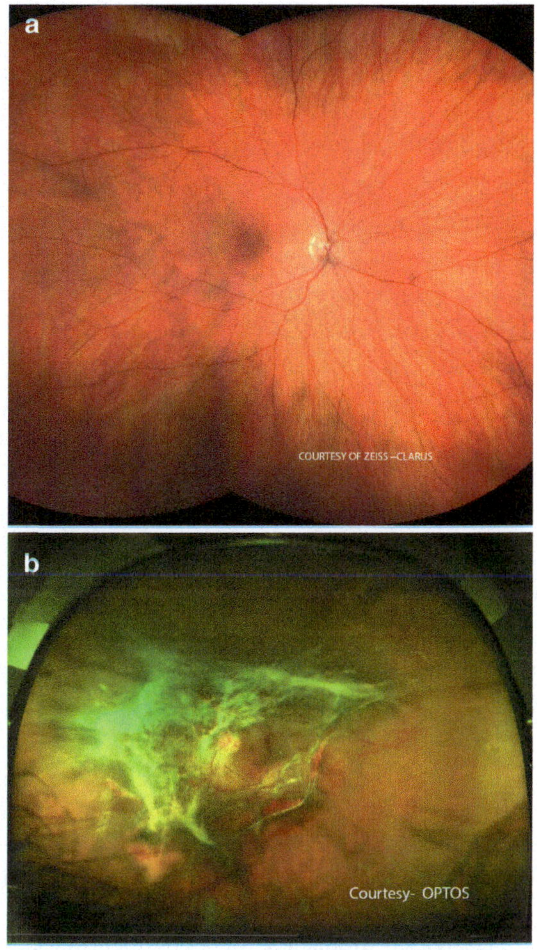

Fig. 19.3 (**a**) A 200-degree ultra-field view of a normal fundus. Photo: Courtesy of ZEISS. (**b**) Optos wide-field angle view of the retina revealing an extensive traction diabetic retinal detachment. Courtesy of Optos

The Impact of Pregnancy on Preexisting Disease

The impact of pregnancy on preexisting disease is well known, and this manifests itself in both good and pathological ways [2–11]. Pregnant women are known to have increasing episodes of central serous retinopathy (CSR). CSR is an episodic condition in which fluid blisters form under the retina, diminishing central vision and resulting in significant distortion (Fig. 19.4). Higher steroid levels present in pregnant women are the cause. These CSR episodes are more frequent among pregnant patients. Laser surgery treatment of this condition works well and is safe but may be worth postponing since the condition will often go away spontaneously after delivery. There are documented increased episodes of retinal vein and artery occlusions [8]. These occlusive vascular disorders are known to be more common in pregnancy because of the hypercoagulable state. Thrombotic thrombocytopenic purpura (TTP) is rare, but is more likely to occur during pregnancy. If these conditions occur, laser surgery or medications would be utilized and can deal with most of the consequences. Nonetheless, these occlusions do lead to varying degrees of irreversible vision loss.

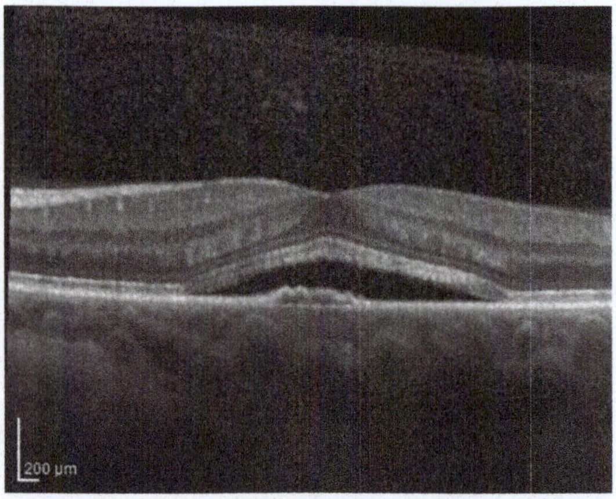

Fig. 19.4 OCT showing the blister from CSR

Conventional treatments using anti-VEGF drugs would be avoided as detailed earlier in this chapter. Acceleration of diabetic retinopathy (DR) often occurs (Fig. 19.5a, b) [11, 12]. The acute onset of hypertensive retinopathy related to preeclampsia or eclampsia is well documented.

As noted, some conditions benefit from the gravid state. Specifically, decreased frequency of uveitis episodes has been observed [3]. Diminished intraocular pressure in patients with glaucoma is well known as well [9].

Decreased frequency of optic neuritis has been observed and likely is related to immunosuppressive effects seen in pregnancy. Unfortunately, most of these beneficial effects disappear in the early postpartum period [2].

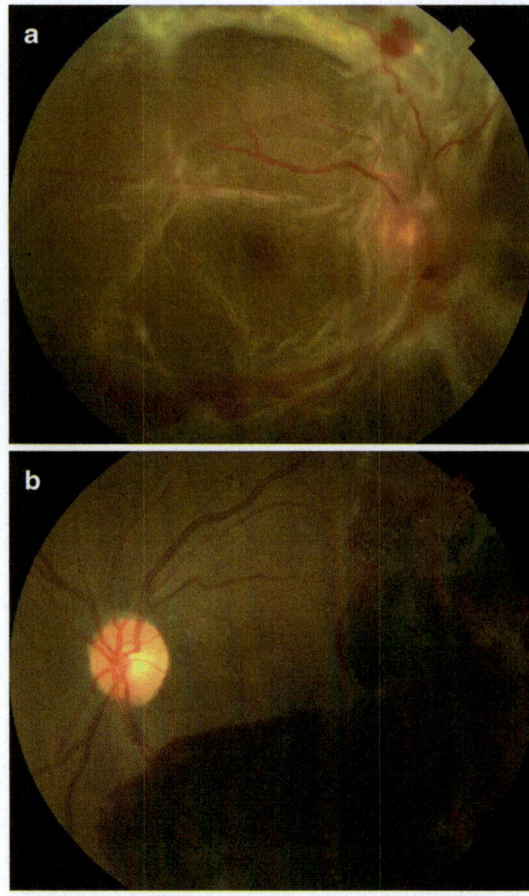

Fig. 19.5 (**a**) Fundus photograph of pregnant diabetic patient whose right eye suddenly developed severe vision loss from rapidly evolving proliferative DR with its associated traction retinal detachment and vitreous hemorrhage. (**b**) Fundus photograph of the left eye of a pregnant diabetic patient complaining of loss of their superonasal visual field after they developed a sudden subhyaloid hemorrhage (bleeding between the retina and posterior hyaloid face of the vitreous) after the eye transitioned to proliferative disease

New Eye Surgery Breakthroughs

The surgical management of pregnant eye patients is radically different today than 20 years ago, not so much because of enhancement of obstetrical management or maternal-fetal subspecialist care, but mostly due to significant strides in ocular surgery. Improvements in equipment, techniques, pharmacology, and other technologies are what have contributed to these substantial improvements. Of course, these breakthroughs make it safer for the mother and the fetus since the newer surgery can usually be accomplished with monitored anesthesia care (twilight anesthesia) and seldom requires general anesthesia. Twenty-five years ago, general anesthesia was much more common, especially for retinal surgery. Regarding cataract and retinal surgery, the duration of the cases is much shorter as well and in many cases 50–75% shorter operative time. The advent of small-incision surgery and *sutureless* surgery has been accomplished today because of improvements in newer techniques, surgical instruments, phacoemulsification (ultrasonic handpieces that dissolve/vacuum cataracts), and cutting handpieces with

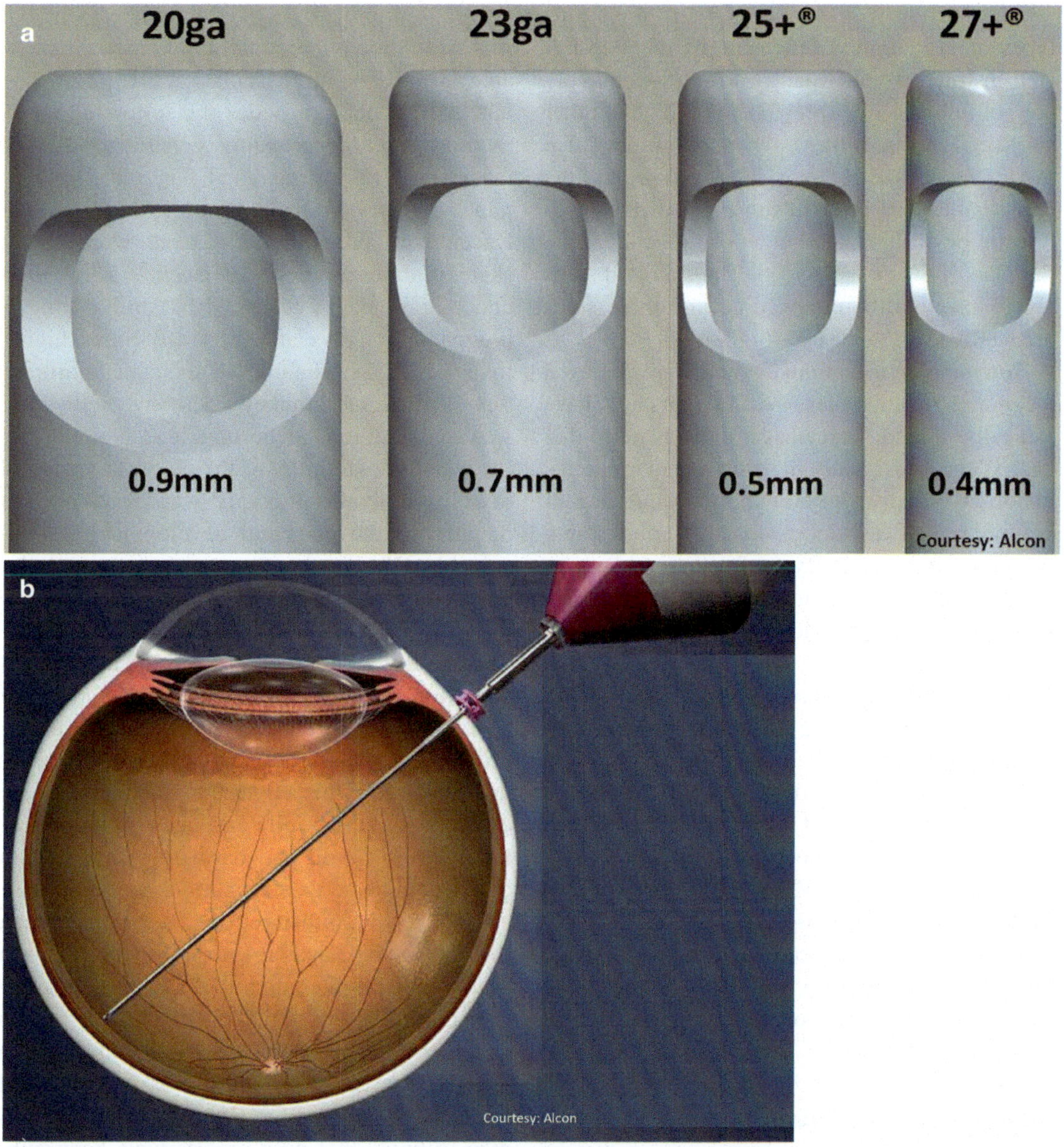

Fig. 19.6 (**a**) Various gauges of vitrectomy handpieces ranging from 20 gauge to 27 gauge and the diameter of the cutting aperture. (**b**) Vitreous cutter in the eye. Photos: courtesy of Alcon

higher-speed cutters and smaller-gauge instruments (less invasive) (Fig. 19.6a, b). In fact, the magnitude of improvements in ocular surgery technique routinely using 25-gauge instrument where surgery is all performed through these tiny 25-gauge perforations is not so different from how video-assisted laparoscopic surgery (VALS) small incisions started with gynecology and eventually revolutionized MIS in all surgical disciplines.

What Do They Mean by Eye Surgery?

Eye surgery is likely different than the general conception that most doctors may have regarding eye surgery. To the ophthalmologist, it ranges from pharmaceutical injections into the eye to in-office laser photocoagulation to more conventional incisional surgery employed for glaucoma, cataracts, plastics, and retina.

This section is broken down into the various types of eye surgery. Interestingly, the step-by-step instructions on what to do intraoperatively are not influenced by pregnancy unlike the other surgical subspecialties where intraoperative modifications are common. For eye surgery, the *game plan* is set prior to surgery on whether to operate or postpone. If surgery is pursued, then the plan of attack is decided. The standard steps are followed without deviation, and these steps are well known to the eye surgeon.

Intraocular injections, which were not even a common treatment less than 10 years ago, have radically altered the management of many disease states, specifically diabetic macular edema, abnormal blood vessel growth in macular degeneration, retinal vascular occlusions (arteries and/or veins), and uveitis. Typically, patients receive intravitreal injections monthly which stabilize their condition, and vision improvement is often achieved (Fig. 19.7).

The anti-VEGF (anti-vascular endothelial growth factor) drugs are Avastin (bevacizumab), Lucentis (ranibizumab), and Eylea (aflibercept) [13, 14]. These three drugs have revolutionized retina care and are used routinely with excellent success. They are bioengineered drugs that work by scavenging VEGF, and this inhibits both normal and pathologic blood vessel growth. This reduction of abnormal growth and leakage helps to stabilize vision loss and, in some cases, improves sight. Injection directly into the eye (vitreous) minimizes systemic side effects, but it is well known that small amounts are detectable in the systemic circulation [10]. The drug label of Lucentis provides the following information, and this probably generalizes for all these anti-VEGF drugs [15]. There are no adequate or well-controlled clinical studies of Lucentis in pregnant or nursing women, but skeletal abnormalities were seen at a low incidence in monkey fetuses, when administered to pregnant monkeys at a dose 13 times higher than normal for humans. No skeletal abnormalities were seen in monkey fetuses when the drug was administered at a normal dose. No effect on the weight or structure of the placenta, maternal toxicity, or embryotoxicity was observed, but damage to the placental development is conceivable. Whether it can cross the maternal placental barrier is not clear. There is no question that fetal blood vessel development might be affected if it gained access due to its mechanism of action. It may pose a risk to embryo-fetal development and reproductive capacity risking birth defects or stillborn, even if animal studies do not reveal this. Because many drugs are excreted in human milk and because the potential for absorption and harm to infant growth and development exists, caution should be exercised when administered to a nursing woman there are no data available to assess the presence or absence in human milk nor to assess the effects on the breastfed child and no data to assess the effects on milk production/excretion [15]. As an aside, if a woman is pregnant and does not know it and receives these drugs, it is nice to know that case reports have been published in women who received Lucentis during pregnancy or during lactation and that no fetal deformations or impacts on the newborn were reported, but these reports are very few. Based on all this data, most ophthalmologists suspend these treatments when the patient is in the pregnant state or puerperium or if the mother is breastfeeding. The consequence of stopping these treatments in patients with preexisting disease poses a therapeutic dilemma. If the need arises in pregnancy to address one of these diseases, then alternate less effective treatments

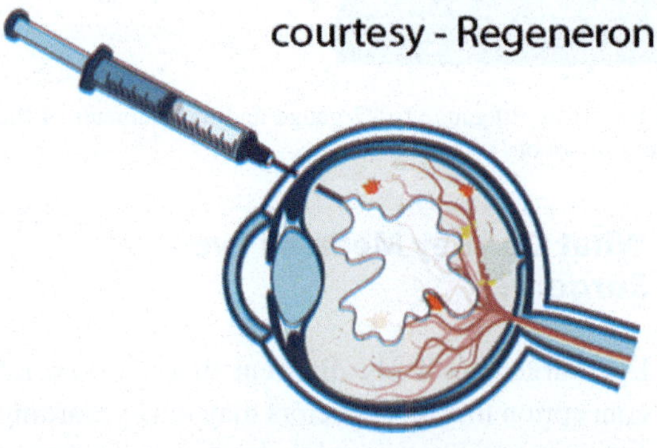

Fig. 19.7 Intravitreal injection illustrating injection of a drug with a 30-gauge needle through the pars plana. Copyright Regeneron Pharmaceuticals, Inc., 2017. All rights reserved. Used with permission

such as steroids (intravitreal or systemic) and/or laser photocoagulation may need to be substituted. Utilization of these drugs is worthy of consideration if there is a risk of permanent loss of vision or eye, but a very comprehensive informed consent is mandatory [4].

Regarding **laser photocoagulation** (laser surgery), there is no contraindication for these treatments when they are medically necessary [4]. Fitting the pregnant woman with her distended abdomen into the conventional slit-lamp apparatus to do the laser can be challenging, but now alternatively, some laser treatments can be performed where the surgeon employs a headlamp-mounted laser and the patient can be reclined into a more comfortable supine position. Laser treatments are extremely valuable in treating retinal tears, small retinal detachments, retinal vascular occlusions, glaucoma (open or closed), as well as diabetic retinopathy. Keep in mind that a laser treatment can also sometimes stabilize the condition enough so that the completion of a more extensive incisional procedure can be postponed until after the baby is delivered and then incisional surgery can be accomplished without limitations. Generally, the success of these lasers is not influenced by the patient's pregnancy. However, diabetic retinopathy laser treatments certainly may not be as effective due to sometimes rapid acceleration of diabetic eye disease (Fig. 19.8a, b) [11].

Regarding **incisional surgery**, only necessary eye surgery should be performed during pregnancy. Elective surgery, such as cosmetic, refractive, or cataract surgery, is best postponed. There is no reason to expose the mother or fetus to any additional stress or medications. In fact, there are specific reasons to avoid these types of surgeries [2]. Regarding oculoplastic surgery, ptosis is known to increase in the pregnant patient (either due to retained fluid or weight gain), so a cosmetic blepharoplasty ("lid job") would obtain less predictable results and potentially even overcorrect the lid position. Refractive surgery during pregnancy should be avoided, since myopia (nearsightedness) increases in pregnancy resulting from both increased corneal thickness and curvature of the crystalline lens [1, 2, 9, 11].

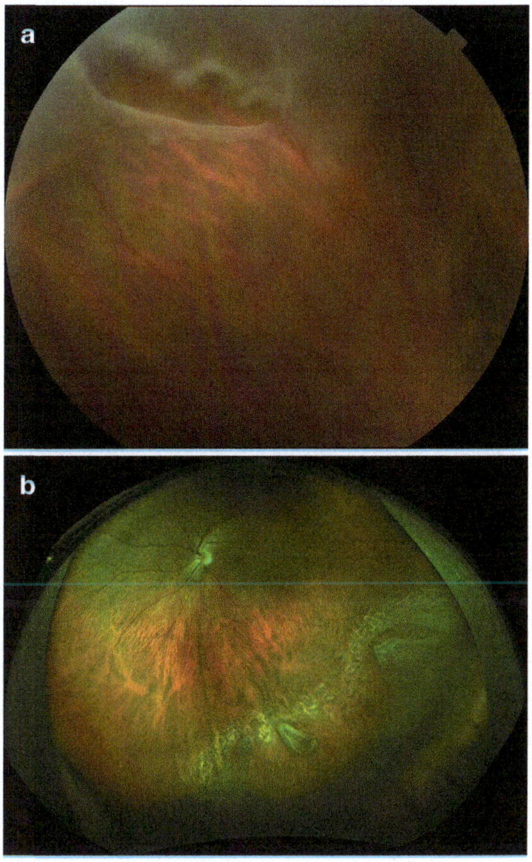

Fig. 19.8 (**a**) Fundus photograph of a retinal tear. (**b**) Fundus photograph of a cluster of treated retinal tears of the inferotemporal retina

Other issues can arise from decreased corneal sensitivity and decreased tear production (80% of women) and/or transient loss of accommodation (difficulty focusing up close).

LASIK (*laser-assisted* in situ *keratomileusis)* and photorefractive keratectomy (PRK), which are based on biometric calculations, would likely not achieve the desired refractive outcome. The same biometric measurements would be influenced in cataract surgery. Likewise, changing glasses during pregnancy should be avoided because there is temporary increased myopia and there is transient loss of accommodation (focusing up close). As mentioned, all surgery that is not obligatory should be postponed. However, if a pregnant woman is involved in an accident or sustains trauma and ends up with a lid laceration, globe perforation, or a traumatic cataract, then – of course – surgery must be undertaken for this compelling surgical need.

Regarding glaucoma surgery, glaucoma surgeons try to postpone surgery until the completion of the pregnancy because the intraocular pressure is known to become lower during pregnancy [16]. Consequently, pregnancy may make a patient who needs surgery seem like she does not need surgery, and in a patient who undergoes surgery to achieve a specific intraocular pressure target, the effect may be excessive. Furthermore, the immunosuppressive drugs, mitomycin C and 5-FU (Fluorouracil), are often topically applied during trabeculoplasties (a type of glaucoma surgery where a filtering bleb is created on the eye to reduce the pressure) to enhance their success, but these teratogenic drugs (category X) should be avoided, even though the amount of systemic absorption is minimal. Mitomycin has not been formally assigned to a pregnancy category by the FDA, but animal studies have revealed evidence of teratogenicity. 5-FU is classified as US FDA pregnancy category D. Acute-angle-closure glaucoma (narrow angles) occurring during delivery has been described, and laser peripheral iridotomy may be required to open alternate pathways for the fluid egress [17].

Regarding retinal surgery, if the retinal specialist cannot temporize with steroid injections and/or laser and there is a true risk of blindness, then incisional surgery will be obligatory. For retinal detachment, the common procedures of vitrectomy surgery and/or scleral buckling are quite effective (Fig. 19.9). In choosing one procedure over the other in the pregnant patient, they both have their advantages and disadvantages, mostly in terms of the postoperative positioning which may or may not be required. Some unique retinal detachments can be fixed in the office with a procedure called pneumatic retinopexy, and this avoids a trip to the operating room. Many of these retinal reattachment procedures involve gas tamponade. The gas is injected directly into the eye, and it not only inflates the globe but most importantly serves to "splint" the retina in the correct position as the welding that was accomplished by cryopexy and/or laser photocoagulation has the necessary time to strengthen. After a procedure

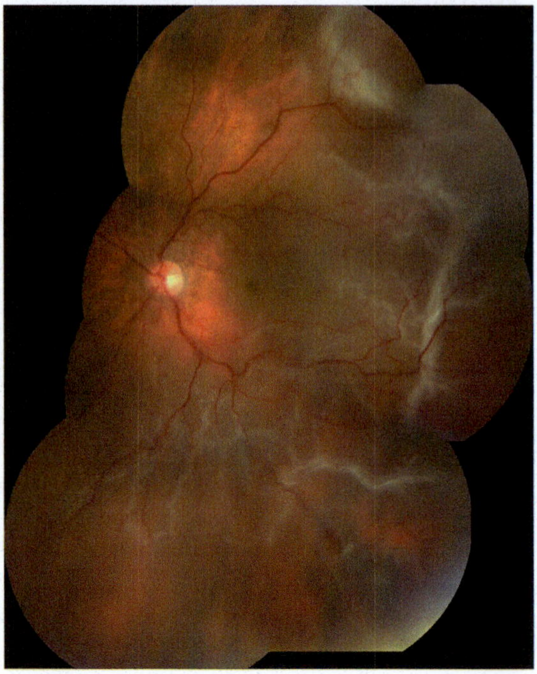

Fig. 19.9 Fundus photograph of a young woman with a macula involved retinal detachment of the left eye; a small tear is seen in the inferotemporal periphery

with gas, the patient must stay in a very specific position which depends on the location of the tears. It varies from right or left side down, face down, or head of bed elevated with head forward. This requirement is usually for an entire week, both day and night, with only 10- to 15-min breaks per hour. The decision of which is the best retinal reattachment procedure needs to take into account the size of the pregnant patient and whether such postoperative positioning is even feasible. For example, the gravid patient with profound abdominal enlargement may find it impossible to face-down position, so a scleral buckle is probably the best choice as it usually requires no positioning. For those that cannot comply with the position, tamponade with silicone oil liquid may be the best management strategy, as that gives the patient the greatest flexibility of position. However, using ingenuity, the retinal surgeon can often devise a successful plan. These position requirements cannot be simply treated in a casual manner, or the surgery will fail or lead to the predictable complications of accelerated cataract

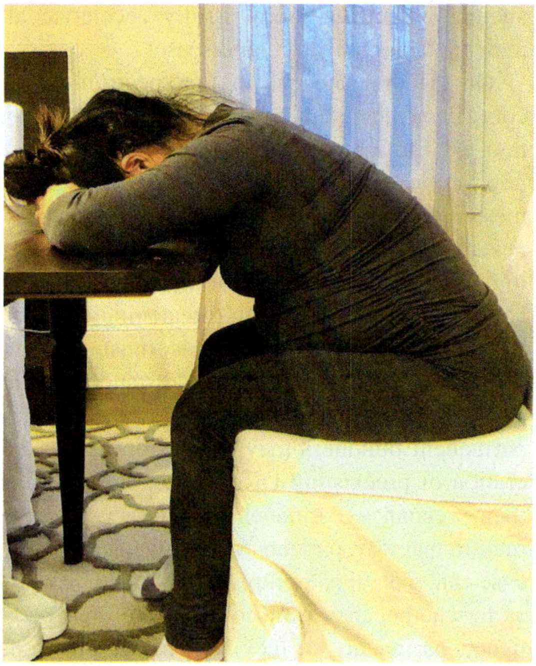

Fig. 19.10 Photograph of a 36-week pregnant woman trying to comply with her face-down positioning requirement

and/or glaucoma so the patient should practice positioning prior to the procedure and to determine what is feasible. This will assure appropriate decisions are made at surgery (Fig. 19.10). Remember, if a patient with eclampsia develops an exudative retinal detachment, these retinal detachments spontaneously reattach in the postpartum period, so no surgical intervention is necessary. But even with reattachment, modest permanent vision reduction may occur, and retinal pigmentary alterations are common [11].

Anesthesia

Since the majority of eye cases are short and done without general anesthesia, we may assume that it is safer for the mother and fetus, but given that narcotics can be considered unsafe for the fetus, no anesthesia exposure is without risk [18]. Fortunately, the American College of Obstetricians and Gynecologists' (ACOG) Committee on Obstetric Practice jointly with the American Society of Anesthesiologists issued a committee opinion on April 2017 giving some guidelines regarding nonobstetric surgery during pregnancy [19]. They acknowledged that the issue of nonobstetric surgery during pregnancy is an important concern for physicians who care for women, and they advised that a physician obtain an obstetric consultation before performing nonobstetric surgery as well as some other invasive procedures because obstetricians are uniquely qualified to discuss aspects of maternal physiology and anatomy that may affect intraoperative maternal-fetal well-being. Ultimately, each case warrants a team approach (anesthesia and obstetric care providers and eye surgeons) for optimal safety of the woman and the fetus. Because of the difficulty of conducting large-scale randomized clinical trials in this population as in ophthalmology, there are no data to allow for specific recommendations. The following generalizations may be helpful to guide decision-making:

- No currently used anesthetic agents have been shown to have any teratogenic effects in humans when using standard concentrations at any gestational age. However, the FDA, in 2016, released some conflicting guidance in a practice advisory without feedback from ACOG which was not based on pregnant women and has not gained much traction even though it has muddied the water.
- A pregnant woman should never be denied indicated surgery, regardless of trimester, but as we noted, elective surgery should be postponed until after delivery. If possible, nonurgent surgery should be performed in the second trimester when preterm contractions and spontaneous abortion are least likely.
- The decision to use fetal monitoring should be individualized and, if used, should be based on gestational age, type of surgery, and facilities available. This will be more completely addressed in the chapter on anesthesia as there are a lot of concurrent recommendations that fetal monitoring necessitates.

Today's improvements in anesthesia and intraoperative monitoring will diminish the risk to the mother and fetus and still allow the mother to have surgery when it is necessary and not choose an inferior solution. Today's guidelines provide a more affirmative pathway for anesthesiologists and ophthalmologists. So together with the obstetrician feedback, they as a team can collectively navigate the route to successful surgery and minimize the risk to the pregnant patient and her fetus. All of this is much more extensively detailed in its own dedicated chapter (e.g., see Chap. 7 "Anesthetic Considerations for the Gravid Patient for Non-obstetric Surgery").

Planning Ahead

An underestimated strategy in a planned pregnancy is for the team of physicians to plan ahead. If a patient has known eye issues, then an eye consult prior to pregnancy is essential. That type of coordinated care allows the ophthalmologist to address issues that may worsen during pregnancy. In that way, those problems can be addressed beforehand. In some cases, pretreatment prior to pregnancy can be accomplished to put the patient in a better position [2]. This is probably most important in diabetic patients, particularly one-eyed patients. This allows the doctor team to decide whether to elect or postpone a pregnancy and address in detail the effect of pregnancy on patients with diabetic retinopathy and how blindness is a risk. As we are all too familiar, many people are unaware that they have diabetes, and even if they have it, they may be unaware that they have diabetic retinopathy. Fifty percent of pregnant patients with nonproliferative diabetic retinopathy (DR) show worsening, but it might improve by the third trimester. Five to ten percent of women convert to proliferative DR, the form that carries the highest risk of blindness [1, 8]. Discussion on whether the baby would need to be delivered preterm if the mother is headed towards permanent blindness is necessary even prior to conception. Obstetricians know better than ophthalmologists that in a poor controlled diabetic patient, the fetus has a high risk of prematurity and/or morbidity. To make matters even more severe, superimposed vascular-related conditions, such as sickle cell trait and/or sickle cell anemia, will even more rapidly accelerate all underlying retinal vascular diseases.

On the opposite end of the spectrum is the completely unplanned pregnancy. It is not unusual for a retina specialist to be referred a poorly controlled diabetic patient in her first trimester excited about her pregnancy, and who had never had recommended annual eye exams, only to be informed during their consult that they now have very advanced, vision-threatening DR. The discussions with these patients must be very frank, and the patient must understand, particularly if they are in the early first trimester, that permanent blindness may result from the acceleration of preexisting DR that can occur during their pregnancy. Permanent blindness is rare, but real. In that way, patients with very advanced disease can make the appropriate informed decision as to whether they want to terminate their pregnancy, particularly if they have already lost one eye from advanced DR and the other eye is at high risk [20]. In fact, this patient may be best served by never becoming pregnant or becoming pregnant in the future after there is an opportunity to intercede and stabilize their retinal condition so that it does not catapult out of control. In that way, the prospect of a blind mother trying to raise her newborn and/or other children is often avoidable.

How to Manage Medications and Postoperative Medications

First of all, use of punctal occlusion in patients taking therapeutic eye drops will lessen their systemic absorption and will minimize any unknown toxicity. Punctal occlusion involves blocking the tear duct with finger pressure for 2–3 min after eyedrop instillation. Do not blink prior to this step as this will pump the medicine into the puncta (Fig. 19.11). Regarding glaucoma medications, be careful with use of the commonly used beta blockers (i.e., timolol) or prostaglandin (PG) analogs [1, 10]. Topical beta blockers are considered category C in the first trimester and category D in the second and third trimesters as they might cause intrauterine

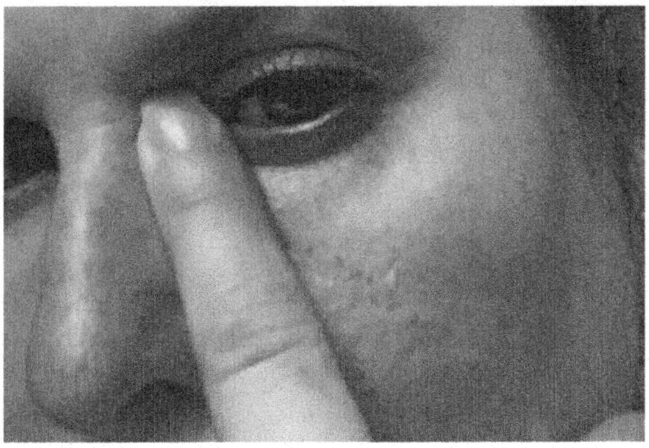

Fig. 19.11 Photo of model demonstrating punctal occlusion pressing just medial to the medial canthus

growth retardation and persistent neonatal blockade if used near delivery. Avoid prostaglandin analogs because they are considered category C and they have not been well studied and safety reports are conflicting. The potent oral glaucoma drug Diamox, a carbonic anhydrase inhibitor, is contraindicated because of potential teratogenic effects [11].

Regarding other topical agents, steroid drops are considered safe when used with care, but systemic prednisone would need to be approved by the OB/GYN doctor. Antihistamine eye drops should be avoided, but those are seldom used. Most of the topical antibiotics are considered category C, including commonly used ones such as aminoglycosides and/or fluoroquinolones. New data implicating fluoroquinolone with arthropathy has made it an even less attractive choice. Tetracycline eye ointment is considered category D. The use of systemic antibiotics would be chosen in consult with the OB/GYN colleague, but clearly intravenous aminoglycosides and fluoroquinolones should be avoided. Antiviral eye medications, such as acyclovir, are considered category B and are generally considered safe. The safety of systemic acyclovir is less well known. Be aware that this FDA letter classification system is soon to be replaced with a more comprehensive, individualized system that even addresses safety through the various trimesters, so the categories provided here should be seen as a rough guideline.

Odds and Ends

While outside the scope of this ophthalmic surgery discussion, pituitary adenomas are known to grow rapidly, as well as meningiomas, but the management of those conditions, which are often discovered by ophthalmologists because they manifest with visual symptoms, is more appropriately addressed by neurology and a neurosurgeon (e.g., see Chap. 18 "Neurosurgery During Pregnancy") [2].

References

1. Bhatia J, Sadiq MN, Chaudhary TA, Bhatia A. Eye changes and the risk of ocular medications during pregnancy and their management. Pak J Ophthalmol. 2007;23(1):1–5.
2. Sharma S, Wuntakal R, Anand A, Sharma TK, Downey G. Pregnancy and the eye. Obstet Gynaecol. 2006;8:141–6.
3. Guidelines for diagnostic imaging during pregnancy and lactation. Committee Opinion No. 723. American College of Obstetricians and Gynecologists. Obstet Gynecol. 2017;130:e210–6.
4. Park YJ, Park KH, Woo SJ. Clinical features of pregnancy-associated retinal and Choroidal diseases causing acute visual disturbance. Korean J Ophthalmol. 2017;31(4):320–7.
5. Garg P, Aggarwal P. Ocular changes in pregnancy. Nepal J Ophthalmol. 2012;4(1):150–61.
6. Gotovac M, Kastelan S, Lukenda A. Eye and pregnancy. Coll Antropol. 2013;37(Suppl 1):189–93.
7. Omoti AE, Waziri-Erameh JM, Okeigbemen VW. A review of the changes in the ophthalmic and visual system in pregnancy. Afr J Reprod Health. 2008;12(3):185–96.
8. Errera MH, Kohly RP, da Cruz L. Pregnancy-associated retinal diseases and their management. Surv Ophthalmol. 2013;58(2):127–42.
9. Efe YK, Ugurbas SC, Alpay A, Ugurbas SH. The course of corneal and intraocular pressure changes during pregnancy. Can J Ophthalmol. 2012;47(2):150–4.
10. Yenerel NM, Küçümen RB. Pregnancy and the eye. Turk J Ophthalmol. 2015;45(5):213–9.
11. Dinn RB, Harris A, Marcus PS. Ocular changes in pregnancy. Obstet Gynecol Surv. 2003;58(2):137–44.
12. Sheth BP. Does pregnancy accelerate the rate of progression of diabetic retinopathy? An update. Curr Diab Rep. 2008;8(4):270–3.
13. Polizzi S, Mahajan VB. Intravitreal anti-VEGF injections in pregnancy: case series and review of literature. J Ocul Pharmacol Ther. 2015;31(10):605–10.

14. The IVAN Study Investigators. Ranibizumab versus bevacizumab to treat neovascular age-related macular degeneration: one-year findings from the IVAN randomized trial [published correction appears in Ophthalmology 2012;119;1508]. Ophthalmology. 2012;119:1399–411.
15. Lucentis® [package insert]. Genentech, South San Francisco, CA.
16. Sunness JS. The pregnant woman's eye. Surv Ophthalmol. 1988;32:219–38.
17. Razeghinejad MR, Masoumpour M, Eghbal MH, Myers JS, Moster MR. Glaucoma surgery in pregnancy: a case series and literature review. Iran J Med Sci. 2016;41(5):437–45.
18. Cheek TG, Baird E. Anesthesia for nonobstetric surgery: maternal and fetal considerations. Clin Obstet Gynecol. 2009;52(4):535–45.
19. American College of Obstetricians and Gynecologists. Committee Opinion No. 696: Nonobstetric surgery during pregnancy. Obstet Gynecol. 2017;129:777–8.
20. Mohammadi SF, Letafat-Nejad M, Ashrafi E, Delshad-Aghdam H. A survey of ophthalmologists and gynecologists regarding termination of pregnancy and choice of delivery mode in the presence of eye diseases. J Curr Ophthalmol. 2017;29(2):126–32.

Oral and Maxillofacial Surgery for the Pregnant Patient

20

Pooyan Sadr-Eshkevari, Roger A. Meyer, Behnam Bohluli, and Shahrokh C. Bagheri

Introduction

The primary concerns of the obstetrician during pregnancy are for the health and well-being of the mother and the protection of the developing fetus from factors which might impair or obstruct normal development before birth. However, the pregnant female is at risk of developing dental caries (decayed teeth), gum disease (periodontitis), abscessed teeth, or other diseases, injuries, or conditions of the oral cavity and jaws, just as in other patients [1]. Such adverse events require timely treatment in order to prevent the development of more serious conditions which might compromise the mother's health and/or adversely affect the developing fetus. Indeed, the hormonal, vascular, and other anatomic changes (e.g., enlargement of the uterus and its effect on adjacent arteries and veins), as well as the preoccupation of the mother with her pregnancy which may cause her to ignore good oral hygiene practices or avoid dental care, make the pregnant female *more likely* to develop an abscessed tooth or gum infection [2]. Such situations require the prompt attention of an oral and maxillofacial surgeon (OMFS) to prevent the development of regional or systemic complications that put the pregnancy at serious risk [3]. The pregnant female often considers her obstetrician (OB-GYN) to be her "primary health care provider." In this situation, the OB-GYN should consider the OMFS to be a "friend in need" or consultant for pregnant women in matters of oral health. In this chapter, the authors give an overview of oral and maxillofacial surgery (OMS) for the female patient who might require this specialty care during pregnancy. Close cooperation between the OMFS and the OB-GYN and an understanding of each other's role in the care of the pregnant female are essential to the best outcome for the patient and the fetus.

P. Sadr-Eshkevari (✉)
Department of Oral and Maxillofacial Surgery, University of Louisville, Louisville, KY, USA

R. A. Meyer
Northside Hospital, Atlanta, GA, USA

B. Bohluli
Deaprtment of Oral and Maxillofacial Surgery, University of Toronto, Toronto, ON, Canada

S. C. Bagheri
Department of Surgery, Northside Hospital, Georgia Oral and Facial Surgery, Atlanta, GA, USA

Definition and Scope of Practice

Oral and maxillofacial surgery (OMS) is defined as "that specialty of dentistry which includes the diagnosis, surgical and adjunctive treatment of diseases, injuries and defects involving both the functional and esthetic aspects of the hard and soft tissues of the oral and maxillofacial and contiguous head and neck regions" [4]. OMFSs are

C. H. Nezhat (ed.), *Non-Obstetric Surgery During Pregnancy*,
https://doi.org/10.1007/978-3-319-90752-9_20

graduates of dental school (Doctor of Dental Medicine, DMD, or Doctor of Dental Surgery, DDS). In the 1970s, it became recognized that OMFSs could benefit from basic medical education and general surgery training as the foundation of postgraduate training in OMS [5]. OMS trainees complete a residency of 4–7 years' duration in an accredited JCAHO hospital program [2]. The longer training period includes qualification for a medical degree (MD) and one or more years of general surgery, in addition to training specific to OMS. Such programs have been developed in the succeeding years to the point where currently nearly 50% of OMS residency programs offer the "double-degree" training track. OMFSs have been recognized by the American College of Surgeons (with or without MD degrees) and can qualify for Fellowship (FACS), if all other requirements are met [6]. OMFSs can become "board-certified," similar to that of other surgical specialists, upon successful completion of the oral and written examinations of the American Board of Oral and Maxillofacial Surgery. Post-residency fellowships are now available for additional subspecialty training in pediatric craniomaxillofacial surgery, head and neck oncologic surgery and microsurgery, and facial esthetic surgery [7].

The modern practice of OMS includes much more than just "pulling teeth" which was the original impetus for dental specialization during after World War I [8]. That practice, which has continuously broadened as training opportunities expanded in the past 50 years [9, 10] includes, but is not limited to, the following:

1. Removal of nonrestorable, malposed, or impacted teeth and other dentoalveolar operations.
2. Placement of dental implants.
3. Treatment of acute and chronic oral or facial infections.
4. Removal of cysts and tumors (benign and malignant), ablative and reconstructive.
5. Treatment of salivary gland diseases.
6. Maxillofacial trauma (bone and soft tissue).
7. Congenital, developmental, and acquired deformities of the jaws and other facial bones.
8. Microsurgical repair of peripheral nerve injuries (esp. trigeminal and facial nerves).
9. Paranasal sinus disease secondary to oral or dental conditions or injuries.
10. Temporomandibular joint and associated musculoskeletal disorders.
11. Facial esthetic surgery.
12. By virtue of additional training and experience, additional expertise may exist in any given OMS practice.

The pregnant patient requiring the services of the OMFS often presents with complex and precarious medical and surgical considerations. The surgeon should be cognizant of the hormonal, anatomic, physiologic, and vascular changes that occur during pregnancy and how these changes might require modification of treatment to minimize risk to both the mother and the fetus. As in many aspects of surgery, the risk and extent of the intervention have to be weighed against the benefits to both patients (mother and fetus). Consultation between the OMFS and the OB-GYN opens the door to communication, shared risks, and a mutually satisfactory treatment plan [2].

Prevention

Being proactive in the care of the obstetric patient can prevent development of dental or oral disease and the attendant risks to mother and fetus. At the initial visit with the OB-GYN, the pregnant female should be questioned about her dental status: When was your last dental check-up? Do you have any decayed teeth, painful teeth, or defective fillings that need attention? Do you brush your teeth twice daily? Do you have an ulcer or sore spot in your mouth that has failed to heal in a reasonable period of time (e.g., 2 weeks)? Do you have any food cravings?

Although the OB-GYN is not expected to be an expert in dentistry, at least a cursory examination of the oral cavity should be done to determine if there are obvious grossly decayed teeth, red or swollen gingiva, heavy deposits of food or calculus about the teeth, bad breath, or suspicious changes in appearance or ulceration of the tongue, palate, buccal mucosa, or floor of the mouth. Any such findings should prompt a referral to a dentist without delay. In the absence of such findings, the patient is encouraged to see her family dentist for a regular check-up and cleaning before the end of the first trimester. Then, if any elective dental care is necessary during the pregnancy, it can be scheduled for the middle trimester when it will be well-tolerated and pose less risk to the development of the fetus than during the first trimester or to maternal and fetal circulation during the third trimester. Pregnant females often have food cravings, many of which contain large amounts of sugar which can lead to dental decay. Dietary counseling from her dentist would be helpful. Due to hormonal and vascular changes resulting from pregnancy, the gingiva becomes engorged, tender, and likely to bleed easily with toothbrushing. A dental hygienist can give the patient good suggestions for maintaining appropriate oral hygiene despite the increased susceptibility of the gingiva to the development of gingivitis during pregnancy. A tooth with decay or a broken or otherwise defective filling should be restored by the dentist; otherwise it might become infected. The resulting pain and infection of an abscessed tooth are better avoided by proactive dental treatment, rather than wait until a dental infection requires control with pain medications and antibiotics and perhaps removal of a tooth or teeth, which might have adverse effects on the developing fetus. It is always best to avoid these situations, if possible, by regular dental care.

Preoperative Assessment

There are a number of considerations regarding management of the pregnant patient in the OMS setting. The first and foremost is the OMFS's assessment of the patient's situation to determine if the nature of her condition is routine/elective, urgent, or life-threatening (Table 20.1). *Elective* or routine oral and maxillofacial surgical procedures are considered as "relative contraindications" in the pregnant female, and they should be delayed until after delivery [11]. Common elective procedures include extraction of *asymptomatic* third molars and other impacted (or erupted) teeth, surgeries to modify the oral anatomy in preparation for future dentures or for the placement of dental implants, removal of benign lesions of the jaws (a biopsy may be needed to confirm that a suspicious lesion is, indeed, benign), cleft repairs, microneurosurgery for repair of peripheral trigeminal nerve injury in absence of pain, temporomandibular joint surgeries (except for fractures, dislocations, and closed locks), orthognathic surgery to correct jaw deformities or obstructive sleep apnea, and facial esthetic surgeries.

Urgent conditions are those which, if left untreated, could pose a risk for development of more serious local, regional, or systemic complications. Examples include decayed, painful teeth, localized dental infections or abscesses, minor lacerations or loosened or avulsed teeth due to trauma, and suspicious soft tissue lesions. Prompt surgical treatment can usually be done under local anesthesia with minimal risk [12].

The standard approach to a gravid female who presents to an OMS office with an urgent condition includes the taking the patient's history (chief complaint, history of present illness, review of the medical history with emphasis on the duration and progress of the pregnancy), vital signs, and body mass index; oral, head, and neck clinical examination; imaging studies (with protective lead shield: periapical, panoramic, or cone-beam computed tomography, none of which expose the fetus to harmful radiation) to determine the status of the offending tooth and any associated pathology; and consultation with the patient's OB-GYN to discuss the best possible treatment options for the patient's present condition. If local anesthesia, antibiotics, or pain medications are indicated, the decision about the best choices will be a mutually agreed-upon regimen. For instance, local anesthetics are safe for most pregnant women with the exception of bupivacaine. Penicillin and clindamycin are antibiotics which are effective against most oral pathogens, and hydrocodone and acetaminophen or tramadol are effective and safe analgesics for most pregnant

Table 20.1 Classification of oral and maxillofacial surgery operations in relation to the pregnant patient

Classification	Operation	Must be done during pregnancy
Elective	Removal of asymptomatic tooth/teeth	No; defer until after delivery
	Dental implant placement	
	Correction of jaw deformity	
	Facial cosmetic operations	
	Removal of painful, infected tooth/teeth	
Urgent	Incision/drainage of localized oral abscess	Yes; ASAP[a]
	Biopsy of suspicious lesion	
	Localized trauma to soft tissue and teeth	
	Repair of painful nerve injury[b]	
	Closed lock of TMJ[c]	
	Treatment for malignancy	
	Maxillofacial trauma	
	Fascial space infection of head/neck	
Emergency		Yes; immediate hospitalization

[a]Provide immediate treatment in either the office or hospital, depending on severity of condition and patient's overall status

[b]Injury to peripheral branch of trigeminal nerve secondary to trauma or dental treatment may be necessary to relieve unremitting neuropathic pain that cannot be controlled with acceptable medications for the remaining duration of the pregnancy

[c]TMJ closed lock causes severe pain, inability to open the mouth, and limitation of oral intake

women and their fetuses. Aspirin and other non-steroidal anti-inflammatory medications are eschewed in order to avoid enhancing the risk of intrauterine bleeding or bleeding in the fetus.

The patient will have decreased urinary bladder capacity due to pressure from the gravid uterus during the last trimester of pregnancy. She should be asked to visit the restroom and empty her bladder before being seated in the surgical chair. As the gravid uterus expands, it progressively increases the pressure on the underlying vena cava and the abdominal aorta. When seated in a reclined or supine position, the patient may experience the "supine hypotension syndrome." Therefore, the patient should be positioned in a 15° left lateral tilted position for treatment in a dental chair [2].

More serious or *life-threatening* conditions require prompt diagnosis and treatment. These include fascial space infections which have spread from the alveolar processes of the jaws to involve the paranasal sinuses, neck, or pharynx [12]. Airway involvement can rapidly cause hypoxia and an acute need for airway management (endotracheal intubation or tracheostomy). Infection may spread via the angular facial veins to the cavernous sinus with life-threatening consequences (cavernous sinus thrombosis). Such situations must be managed without delay, and both the OMFS and the obstetrician should manage the patient simultaneously in the hospital setting. Consultation with other specialists may be indicated as well (infectious disease, otolaryngology, pulmonology, etc.).

Anesthesia

Local Anesthesia

Sensation to the teeth, jaws, and facial regions is supplied by the peripheral branches of the fifth cranial (trigeminal) nerve (V), which has three major divisions (Table 20.2). The ophthalmic division of V (V-1) carries sensory input from the corneas of the eyes, the upper eyelids, portions of the nose, and forehead. The midfacial area including the nose, infraorbital area, upper lip, paranasal sinuses, portions of the nose, maxilla, upper teeth, gingiva and proximate buccal mucosa, and palate receive their sensation from branches of the maxillary division (V-2). The mandibular division (V-3) supplies sensation to the lower lip, chin, lower teeth, gingiva and

Table 20.2 The divisions of the trigeminal (fifth cranial) nerve (N5) and the areas supplied by its sensory branches in the mouth and face

Division	Anatomic areas supplied
Ophthalmic (V-1)	Forehead
	Upper eyelids
	Cornea of eye
	Portions of the nose, external and internal
Maxillary (V-2)	Midface
	Lower eyelids
	Paranasal sinuses
	Upper lip
	Portions of the nose, external and internal
	Maxillary teeth and gingiva
	Hard and soft palate
	Upper labial and buccal mucosa
Mandibular (V-3)	Lower lip and chin
	Mandibular teeth and gingiva
	Anterior 2/3 of the tongue
	Floor of mouth
	Portions of the ear and auditory canal

All peripheral branches of N5 are accessible to local infiltration or block anesthesia

proximate buccal mucosa, anterior two-thirds of the tongue, and the floor of the mouth. The various peripheral branches are easily accessible to local anesthetic blocks or infiltration which can provide excellent surgical anesthesia in a cooperative patient for most minor or localized surgical operations within the oral cavity and facial area [13]. Examples of such procedures include extraction of teeth, incision and drainage of localized abscesses, soft tissue biopsy, repair of soft tissue lacerations, and closed or open reductions of some fractures of the maxilla, nose, and mandible. Lidocaine or mepivacaine in suitable concentrations with small amounts of epinephrine to enhance and prolong the anesthetic effect is safe and effective for most pregnant patients [14].

Injection of the local anesthetic solution is always preceded by aspiration to ensure that an intravascular injection does not occur. Accidental intravascular injection of an epinephrine-containing solution can cause decreased placental blood flow with risk to the fetus. Small-bore needles are used for local anesthetic injection (gauge 27–30) so that with the application of topical lidocaine or benzocaine gel before injection, little or no pain is felt during insertion of the needle. If anxiety is an issue for the patient in an office procedure, inhalation of nitrous oxide/oxygen in 20/80 to 40/60 concentrations, respectively, provides acceptable relaxation or relief of anxiety for most patients before proceeding with the injections. At these levels, good oxygenation is provided, and the patient maintains consciousness so that airway integrity is not at risk.

Deep Sedation or General Anesthesia

In an office-based setting, urgent procedures on pregnant patients should preferably be done under local anesthesia, and a stress reduction protocol should be followed (see nitrous oxide/oxygen inhalation, above). If more complicated procedures require a deeper level of sedation or general anesthesia, the expertise of a nurse anesthetist or an anesthesiologist is highly desirable. The decision, jointly made between the OB-GYN and the OMFS, is then whether the patient is best treated in an office setting or in the hospital [11]. For more severe cases, such as maxillofacial trauma or dentoalveolar infections which have caused facial or neck cellulitis and compromise of the patient's airway, general endotracheal anesthesia in a hospital setting is the standard of care [15, 16]. The threshold for hospital admission of pregnant patients with a maxillofacial infection is lower than other patients as the need for supportive measures is higher in these patients. This is because fever, dehydration, inability to tolerate oral intake, and the side effects of various medications required for treatment (e.g., anesthetics, antibiotics, analgesics) are bigger risk factors for the pregnant patient and the fetus. Also, the risk of airway compromise is higher during pregnancy, especially when parapharyngeal tissues are involved. A preoperative MRI of the head and neck greatly assists the clinician in assessing the integrity of the upper airway, especially in patients with cellulitis from odontogenic infections or maxillofacial trauma.

These concerns are heightened in the presence of risk factors for premature contractions and preterm labor, such as twins or early sepsis [11].

Surgical Intervention

Dentoalveolar Surgeries

The most common surgical need of a pregnant patient referred to an OMFS is extraction of a nonrestorable, symptomatic tooth. The patient presents with localized jaw pain of varying duration and severity (as assessed on a "visual analog scale, 0 [no pain] to 10 [worst pain ever]"), tenderness to percussion of the involved tooth and to palpation of the adjacent soft tissue, and obvious tooth decay or a lost filling in the involved tooth. A brief history of the oral complaint, a review of the progress of the patient's pregnancy (and the name and contact information of her OB-GYN), a review of her medical history, an oral/head/neck examination (including vital signs, height, and weight), and appropriate imaging studies (patient protected with lead shield) provide the information to proceed expeditiously [16]. A telephone call from the OMFS to the OB-GYN ascertains whether or not the patient can tolerate removal of the offending tooth under local anesthesia, with or without mild nitrous oxide/oxygen sedation (see above under Local Anesthesia) as an office procedure.

The patient's tooth is then quickly removed in a brief procedure (usually 5–10 min or less), postoperative instructions are given, prescriptions are provided for antibiotics and/or analgesics as indicated, and the patient is reappointed for a postoperative visit within 1 week. This standard procedure has thus removed a nidus of localized infection (the tooth and any associated local pathology at the root ends, e.g., granuloma, dental cyst, etc.) and spared the patient progressive spread of infection to regional fascial spaces and lymph nodes, pain, difficulty chewing food and swallowing, airway obstruction, fever, and systemic illness from bloodstream invasion by the responsible bacteria. Such complications put the mother and fetus at considerable risk and require prompt hospitalization.

Oral Infections

Acute Odontogenic Infections

Decayed teeth or those with defective fillings may undergo infection and death of the pulpal tissue. The immediate symptom is a "toothache" with the pain intensified by chewing on the offending tooth. At this point, as noted above, the patient should seek immediate dental care and removal of the offending tooth. If this is done, the incipient infectious process in the dental pulp and immediate periapical (around the tooth root) tissues is usually halted, and no further definitive treatment is necessary. The extracted tooth can be replaced electively by the dentist (dental implant, fixed bridge, removable prosthesis) after successful delivery of the infant and postpartum recovery of the patient.

Unfortunately, either because of "dental neglect" due to fear of dental work by the patient or decreased immunity because of a comorbid condition (e.g., diabetes mellitus, connective tissue disease, steroid therapy) or changes in immunovigilance in some pregnant females, the infection spreads outside of local confines to fascial spaces adjacent to the maxilla (infratemporal space), the mandible (the masticator, submandibular, sublingual, submental spaces), or the pharynx (parapharyngeal and retropharyngeal spaces). Inflammation of these areas causes edema and erythema (cellulitis involving the face, tongue, and floor of mouth), spasticity of masticatory muscles (*trismus*, or restriction of jaw opening), and narrowing of the pharyngeal airway (dysphagia, dysphonia, dyspnea) (Figs. 20.1 and 20.2). For instance, Ludwig's angina is simultaneous infection of the submandibular, sublingual, and submental spaces bilaterally, with elevation and fixation of the tongue and floor of mouth and imminent airway obstruction [17]. The patient presents with pain, swelling of the upper neck, fever, malaise, dysphagia, and dyspnea. This is a surgical emergency, as are all other fascial space infections in which restricted jaw opening, airway compromise, and systemic effects of infection (elevated temperature, heart rate and respiratory rate, increased white blood cell count with predominance of polymorphonuclear leukocytes) predominate. In the pregnant female, these

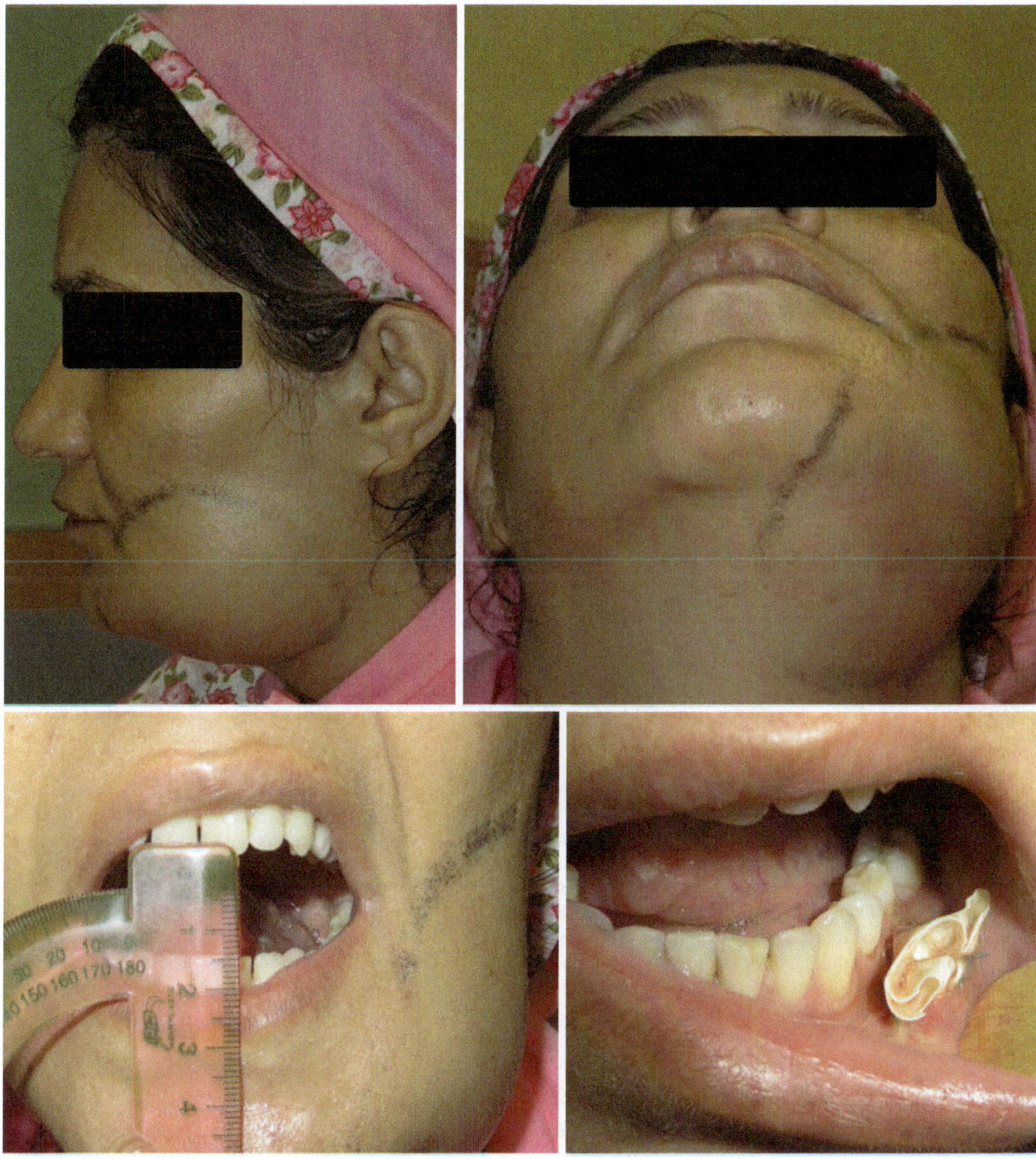

Fig. 20.1 A pregnant patient with a left perimandibular space odontogenic abscess. Clinical diagnosis is based on a recent history of a "bad tooth" with evidence of decay/ periodontal disease, possible recent ER or dentist visits, and relatively rapid-onset edema, erythema, tenderness to palpation, and a firm to doughy consistency. Difficulty opening (<35 mm) due to direct involvement of the masticatory muscles (trismus) or pain is seen. An incision and drainage of the left buccal space is performed in an outpatient setting

complications are all the more dangerous, due to the many anatomic and physiologic changes that are induced by the pregnancy and the developing fetus. Immediate hospitalization and securing of the airway are necessary, and the patient's obstetrician is consulted forthwith. Additional consultations with high-risk pregnancy specialists and others involved in infectious disease, anesthesiology, and critical care may be required acutely as well.

The goals of immediate care are to stabilize the patient, by securing the airway, placing

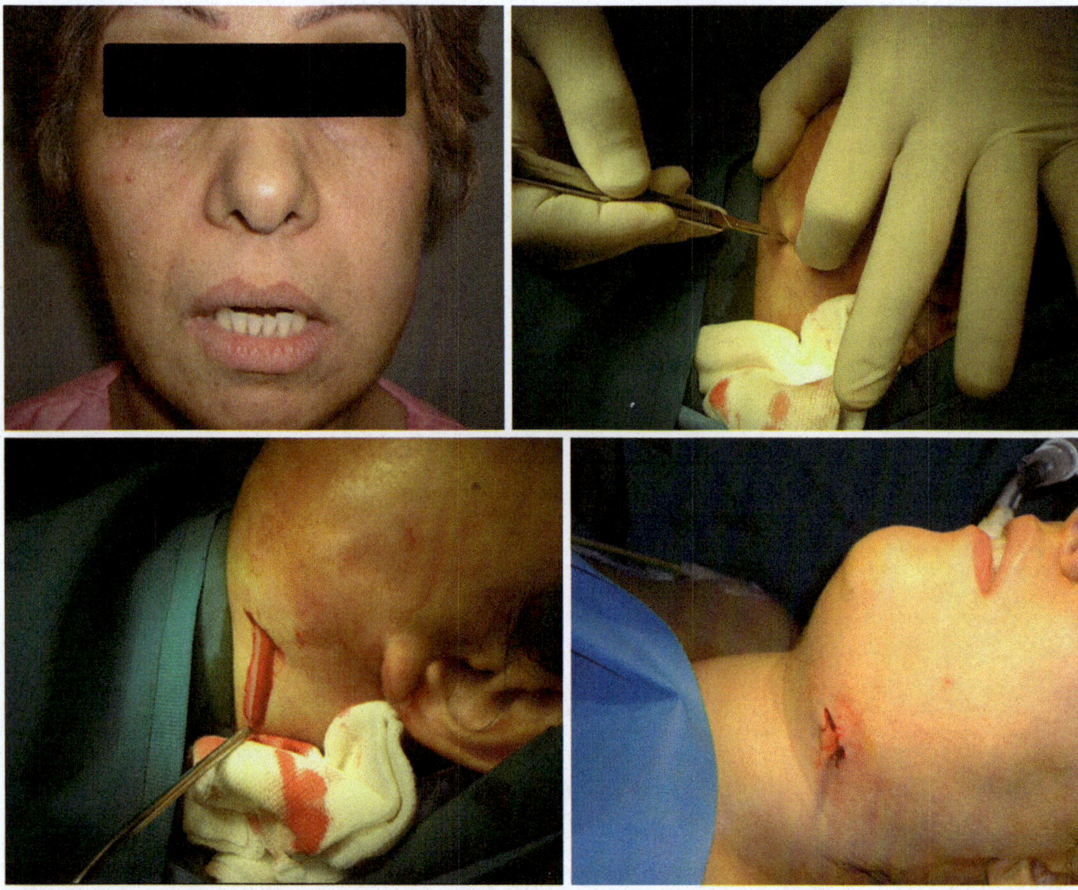

Fig. 20.2 The decision to take the patient to the operating room and perform a more aggressive treatment is based on presence of more ominous signs and symptoms such as difficulty breathing and/or swallowing due to possible involvement of the parapharyngeal spaces, severe trismus compromising the patient's ability to hydrate and nourish, and drooling due to tongue protrusion (emergency situation). The patient is followed up in 24 and 72 h and drain removed. Patient is seen again in a week to assure remission of the abscess. The edema and firm swelling might resist up to 6 weeks before completely resolving

intravenous lines, and administering adequate fluids. Imaging studies (panoramic, CT scan, and/or MRI) are obtained to delineate the causative pathology and evaluate the airway. If there is an obvious "pointing" abscess readily accessible to aspiration, a sample of pus is taken and sent to the laboratory for immediate Gram stain and culture/sensitivity. Initial decisions on choice of appropriate antibiotics are made based on appearance of the Gram stain. If such is not feasible at the onset of treatment, empirical antibiotics are administered (usually penicillin or clindamycin are the initial agents, as they are effective against the causative organisms in most odontogenic infections and pose little or no risk to the mother or fetus). Once these initial steps are completed, the decision is made to take the patient to the operating room for definitive treatment which usually includes removal of the involved tooth (or teeth), incision and drainage of any and all abscesses identified either by clinical examination or imaging studies, and definitive securing of the airway (endotracheal intubation or tracheostomy). Most such patients must be given general anesthesia because of the extent of their infection and the ineffectiveness of local anesthetics in the presence of widespread inflammation and infection. Intubation of the patient may involve an awake, fiber-optic technique requiring the services of a skilled endoscopist/anesthesiologist. If indicated, the patient is placed in a semi-supine position with a 15° tilt to the left to relieve compression of the vena cava and aorta and maintain adequate uterine and placental perfusion. If a nasal endotracheal intubation was accomplished, the tube can usually be left in place, and it is well-tolerated postoperatively in a sedated patient for several days, if needed. Patients who require a secured airway longer than 7–10 days usually have the endotracheal tube replaced with an elective tracheostomy. However, with removal of decayed teeth, drainage of abscesses, antibiotics, and supportive care, most acute oral/head/neck infections respond rapidly with resolution of cellulitis, restoration of jaw opening, return of adequate swallowing, and reversal of airway compromise, making long-term airway maintenance unnecessary in most patients. During recovery from an acute infection, the pregnant patient is at increased risk of deep vein thrombosis and pulmonary embolism, pulmonary edema and adult respiratory distress syndrome, and spontaneous abortion/fetal death. Appropriate preventive measures and monitoring by all involved specialists help to minimize the risks of these complications [15].

Osteomyelitis

Osteomyelitis (OMLTS) is an infection of the bone marrow [18]. Its occurrence is unusual in the highly vascularized maxilla, except in an immunocompromised patient. On the other hand, infection from abscessed teeth or an untreated fracture is more likely to progress to OMLTS in the mandible which is less well-perfused, albeit much more richly endowed with good circulation than the long bones, the most common site of OMLTS. OMLTS is classified as acute and chronic. Acute OMLTS may present similarly to an acute odontogenic infection (see above), and the evaluation and treatment are essentially the same, except that extensive debridement of the bone, in addition to tooth extraction and incision and drainage of abscesses, may be required. Long-term administration of antibiotics, based on culture and sensitivity results, is usually necessary. Chronic OMLTS is most often an urgent, but not life-threatening, condition. However, the additional risks of pregnancy require careful evaluation, surgical debridement, and monitoring of the mother and fetus during surgical treatment and prolonged antibiotic therapy.

OMS Trauma

As with all other patients sustaining traumatic injuries to the oral, head, and neck regions, pregnant patients sustaining maxillofacial trauma require initial evaluation and support of the airway, breathing, and circulation, which are the primary concern of first-responders in the hospital emergency department. Because of changes in blood flow due to hormonal effects and pressure on major blood vessels (vena cava, aorta), the pregnant female may experience syncope secondary to transient reduction of cerebral perfusion. "Falling out" (fainting spell) may cause the patient to strike her head, face, or jaw and sustain significant lacerations, dislocated teeth, or fracture of the maxilla, zygoma, nose, or mandible. Whenever possible, trauma victims are rapidly transported to the nearest Level I or II trauma center. Even seemingly minor injuries (abrasions, bruises, small lacerations, chipped or loosened teeth) require a thorough evaluation to determine the nature and extent of injuries, achieve stabilization of the patient, and make decisions about immediate surgical intervention. If there is suspicion of domestic violence, this should be reported immediately to social services and police authorities [19]; regardless of whether the cause of the injuries is a motor vehicle accident (MVA), interpersonal altercation, missile (gunshot wound), sharp penetration (knife), or other trauma, assessment (physical examination and imaging studies) of the entire patient (not just the head and neck area) is often necessary to rule out involvement of other locations or organs. In a patient with a penetrating wound of the neck, the status of the major blood vessels (carotid and jugular) must be ascertained. The cervical spine is evaluated for injury and instability. If there are avulsed or missing teeth, imaging studies are indicated to rule out swallowing or aspiration of these foreign objects. Or, a patient with obvious and extensive facial injuries may also have sustained blunt trauma to the abdomen during a MVA resulting in laceration of the liver or rupture of the spleen. OMFS will be consulted to evaluate and manage the oral and facial aspects of the patient's injuries. In some situations, airway embarrassment requires immediate endotracheal intubation or tracheostomy. Other consultants may be called, depending on the areas of the patient's injuries. The pregnant patient will, in addition, require timely evaluation by her OB-GYN or other readily available alternate and continuous monitoring of the mother and the fetus during hospitalization (Figs. 20.3 and 20.4).

Bone Injuries

Fractures of the facial bones (nose, zygoma, maxilla, mandible) can be open (compound, either through the skin or into the oral cavity) or closed, simple or comminuted, and displaced or non-displaced. Fractures that are open and comminuted are the most difficult to treat and the most likely to become infected, especially if not reduced and fixated promptly. The excellent

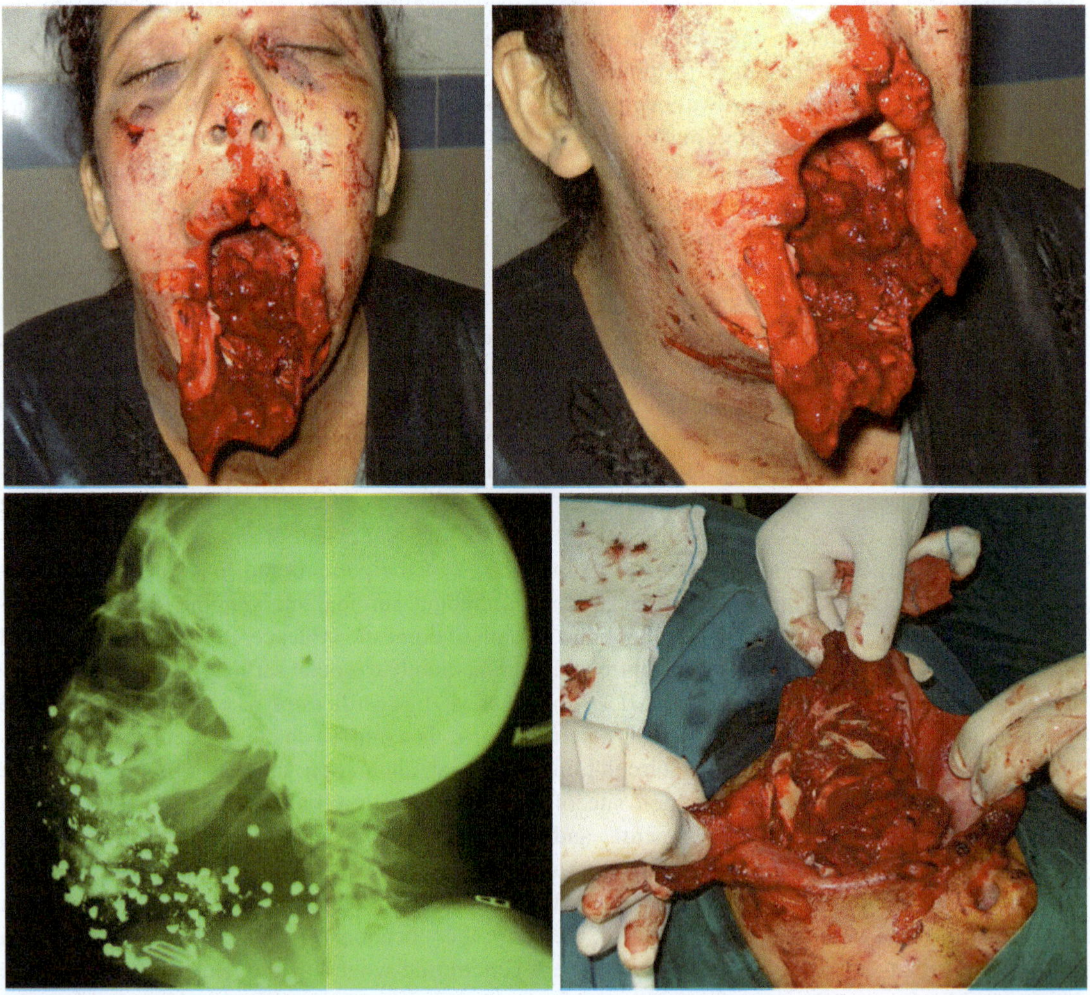

Fig. 20.3 A pregnant woman with a self-inflicted gunshot wound (GSW) is brought to the emergency room. The anterior part of the mandible and some of the anterior maxillary bony, dentition, and soft tissue are lost due to the trauma. The patient is taken to the operating room where copious irrigation and debridement are performed to further assess the extent of the trauma and plan the reconstruction

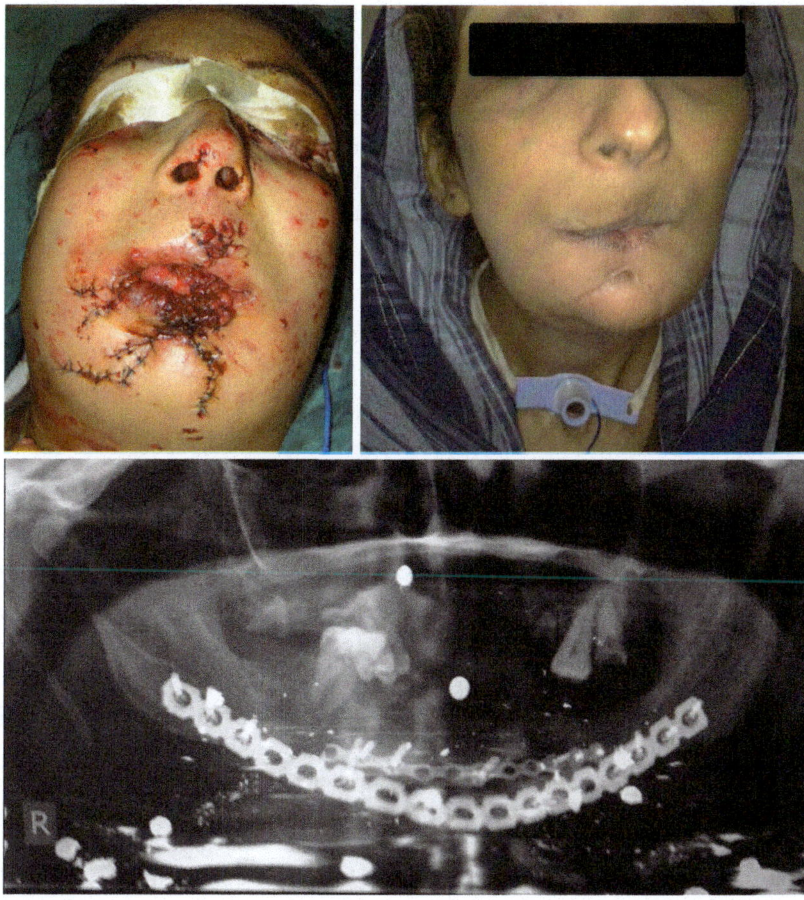

Fig. 20.4 The patient from Fig. 20.3 is shown after bony reconstruction with a bone graft and reconstruction plate and soft tissue primary closure

vascular supply of the head and neck regions likely limits the occurrence of infection in facial fractures versus that in fractures of the long bones.

Nasal packs and Epistats, among other similar hemostasis measures, are placed to control bleeding which mostly comes from the nasal septum injury. If hemostasis cannot be achieved using these primary measures, angiography with embolization of the injured arteries is indicated [20]. Nasal fractures can often be treated with closed reduction and splinting under local anesthesia. Localized, non-displaced, alveolar fractures of the maxilla or mandible with loosened teeth also can be reduced and fixated with dental arch bars under local anesthesia. Most other facial fractures require open reduction and internal fixation. Some maxillary and most mandibular fractures can be reduced and fixated via transoral incisions. Zygomatic and other periorbital fractures usually require cutaneous incisions for reduction/fixation. Nasal fractures that require open reduction often can be done with the same type of transfixion incision used for rhinoplasty. The rigid internal fixation plates used in maxillary and mandibular fracture stabilization frequently preclude the need for intermaxillary fixation (wiring of the upper and lower teeth together). The ability to open one's mouth makes it easier for the pregnant trauma patient to take adequate nourishment, breath without difficulty, and maintain oral hygiene (which also reduces the risk of infection of a healing, reduced, orally compounded fracture). Nutrition is usually provided in the form of liquid or pureed foods with attention to adequate caloric, protein, and vitamin intake.

Antibiotics are generally indicated preoperatively for compound fractures, and analgesics are usually necessary for the first few days following injury. The goals of facial fracture treatment are to reduce the fractured bone(s) into good anatomic alignment, to restore facial contour and appearance, and, in the case of fractures involving the tooth-bearing bones (maxilla, mandible), to restore the dental occlusion to its normal state to facilitate good chewing function [21]. Close follow-up during the postoperative period (4–8 weeks in most patients, depending on the location and severity of the injuries) is necessary to assure that adequate reduction and fixation are maintained, that the patient is taking adequate nutrition, and that good oral hygiene is practiced. The OB-GYN likewise maintains close monitoring of the status of the pregnant patient and fetus during this period.

Soft Tissue Injuries

Lacerations, abrasions, contusions, and other facial soft tissue injuries are assessed to determine possible involvement of important adjacent structures. Injuries to the cheek or face might have caused transection of a branch or branches of the facial nerve (VII), resulting in paresis or paralysis of the forehead, eyelids, and lips. The parotid gland Stenson's duct may have been torn or severed, which, if not repaired can lead to a sialocyst and/or infection. Penetrating neck wounds demand evaluation of the integrity of the carotid and jugular vessels, lest severe blood loss or interruption of cerebral circulation.

Most soft tissue injuries of the face, head, or neck are repaired under local or regional block anesthesia. Epinephrine in the local anesthetic solution aids in achieving hemostasis in the highly vascularized facial tissues. Wounds that are contaminated with foreign material are vigorously debrided and irrigated before repair. Conservative excision of ragged laceration margins is done, and the muscular layer is closed. Careful alignment of important anatomic landmarks (vermilion border of the lips, nasolabial fold, eyebrows, eyelid margins) before skin closure is critical essential in restoring normal facial appearance. Use of surgical loupes for accurate positioning of tissue margins and placement of sutures, eversion of skin margins, placement of fine sutures, and application of supportive adhesive strips gives the best cosmetic result with minimal risk of unsightly facial scarring. The African-American female (AAf) is at increased risk of developing a hypertrophic scar or keloid following cutaneous trauma. However, pregnant women of other races also occasionally develop a hypertrophic scar in a repaired laceration. Several factors contribute to hypertrophic scar or keloid formation, including race, tension on the repair margins, hormonal influences, infection, and patient age. Good surgical technique and postoperative local incision care maximize the chance of an acceptable scar. This situation can also be ameliorated by injection of a corticosteroid (e.g., triamcinolone) into the laceration margins in patients considered to be at high risk for keloid formation at the time of repair and periodically in the postoperative period as needed [22, 23].

Temporomandibular Disorders

The articulation of the condyle of the mandible with the temporal bone of the skull base forms the *temporomandibular joint* (the so-called TMJ). This is the only movable joint in the human body that has two movements (rotation and translation/sliding). Disorders of the TMJ are classified as *articular* and *nonarticular*. Nonarticular disorders are mainly those of the masticatory muscles (masseter, temporalis, internal and external pterygoid) origin. The myofascial pain dysfunction syndrome (MPDS) is caused by excessive, stress-related parafunctional jaw habits (jaw muscle clenching, tooth grinding, rigid jaw lower jaw posturing) that produce muscle fatigue, reduced muscle blood flow, and pain (around the TMJ) [24]. Patients are often not aware of their parafunctional jaw activity unless it is noticed by a bed partner or roommate. Temporal or frontal headaches are common in afflicted patients. The stress of pregnancy, other young children at home, and insufficient spousal support often precede the onset of MPDS. In some patients, an articular condition develops in which the position of the articular disc in the TMJ is altered, resulting in abnormal joint sounds (clicking or crepitus), decreased jaw opening or range of motion, and painful chewing. Treatment is usually nonsurgical and includes relaxation techniques to help the patient recognize and avoid tooth contact (except when chewing or swallowing), nonnarcotic analgesics, nighttime muscle relaxants, diet consistency modifications, physical therapy, wearing of an oral appliance to dampen the forces of parafunctional jaw activity, and, in selected instances, marital or psychological counseling.

The occasional patient develops a painful "closed lock" in which the displaced TMJ cartilage disc becomes nonreducing, jaw range of motion is severely limited, and effective chewing and swallowing and nutritional intake are compromised. This situation, fortunately rarely seen in pregnant females, requires surgical intervention, either arthrocentesis or arthroscopy or open-joint arthroplasty [25].

The TMJ can become involved with arthritis (degenerative, rheumatoid, gouty, infectious, etc.). Treatment may involve co-management with a rheumatologist. Fractures and dislocations of the TMJ are managed similarly to other traumatic injuries of the facial bones (see above).

Tumor Surgery

Oral pyogenic granuloma, commonly known as oral pregnancy tumor, mostly occurs in the second decade of life in response to various stimuli such as low-grade local irritation, traumatic injury, or hormonal factors (Fig. 20.5). Clinically, a small red-colored smooth or lobulated exophytic lesion usually non-tender and not painful is present. Excisional surgery is the treatment of choice [26].

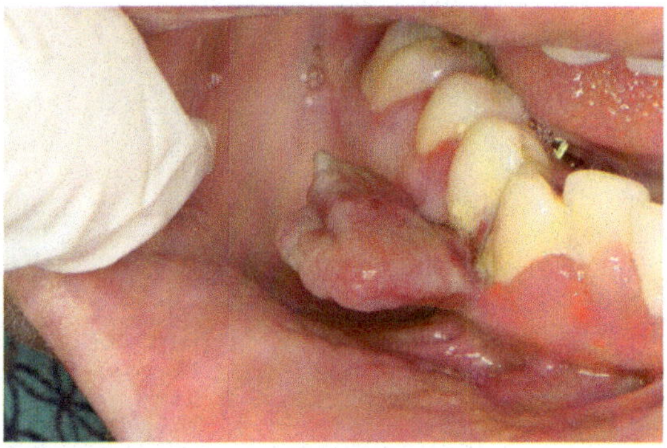

Fig. 20.5 This image shows a 27-year-old pregnant woman in the third trimester with a growth in the right lower mouth. The lesion is pedunculated to the marginal gingiva and has a smooth surface with small ulcerations caused by occlusal trauma. The lesion is excised under local anesthesia

Squamous cell carcinoma (SCC) of the oral cavity, once thought to be a disease predominantly affecting older patients of either gender, especially those who have abused alcohol or tobacco products for many years, is now being seen with increasing frequency in young women under the age of 30 who do not use tobacco or imbibe alcohol to excess [27–29] (Fig. 20.6). These cancers in younger patients are often highly anaplastic and, especially when they occur in the tongue, tend to metastasize early to regional lymph nodes in the neck. Malignancies other than SCC also occur in women of any age, including leukemias, lymphoma, and sarcomas, among others. Leukemia, for example, may present initially as enlargement and bleeding of the gingiva. Therefore, any suspicious ulceration or other lesion in the oral cavity that fails to heal in a reasonable period of time (e.g., 2 weeks) should be biopsied. This procedure, done under local anesthesia, should pose no significant risk to the pregnant patient or her fetus.

Women are increasingly delaying childbearing until their middle or late 30s and even early 40s. At that age, cancers of the breast, cervix, uterus, and ovaries are more likely to occur. Therefore, management of malignancies in pregnant females is becoming more frequent.

The pregnant patient with a diagnosed oral malignancy presents difficult challenges to the patient and the physicians caring for her and her fetus. The first decision to be made by the patient is whether to terminate her pregnancy or allow it to continue during treatment. Treatment should not be delayed until after delivery; the chance of long-term survival or cure would be adversely affected [27]. An exception to this might be a patient in which a malignancy is diagnosed in her third trimester. If a viable infant can be delivered prematurely, then postpartum cancer treatment can proceed forthwith. Ablative surgery (excision

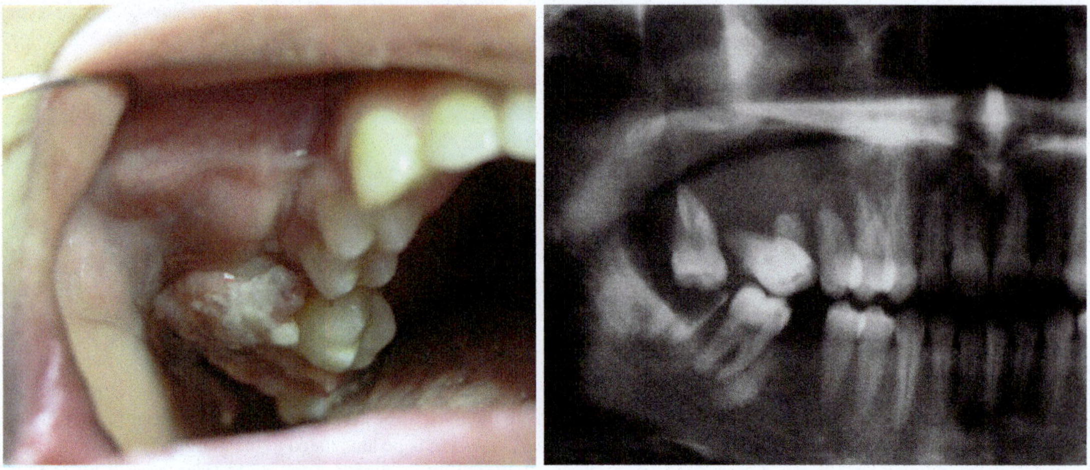

Fig. 20.6 A right posterior maxillary osteosarcoma in a 25-year-old primigravid woman in her 17th week of pregnancy is shown. A team including oncologist, OMFS, and OB-GYN was involved in treatment of this case. Management included resection, early termination of pregnancy, and the use of adjuvant systemic chemotherapy to prevent metastases

of the primary lesion and, in some patients with oral cancers, resection of an adjacent portion of the jaw and a neck dissection, all performed under general anesthesia), chemotherapy, and radiation pose significant risks to any patient, let alone one who is pregnant. Careful evaluation and tumor staging preoperatively and then continuous monitoring during surgery and the recovery period are essential to the best of care [30–32]. Provision of adequate nutrition is essential. Chewing and swallowing may be compromised by resection of a portion of the tongue and/or jaw; feeding tubes or parenteral administration may be required. Close communication and cooperation among all the clinicians (surgeon, OB-GYN, oncologist, radiation therapist, and others) caring for the pregnant patient are integral elements of cancer treatment. In fact, successful outcomes of oral cancer treatment (long-term survival or cure for the mother, delivery of a healthy infant) are being achieved with current treatment regimens [33, 34].

Reconstructive Surgery

Resection of oral malignancy involving portions of the tongue, jaw, palate, or neck creates significant defects in some patients. These defects leave the patient with alteration of facial appearance and, most importantly, difficulties with chewing food, drinking fluids, swallowing, speech, and airway maintenance.

Reconstructive procedures, including locally rotated flaps or osteomyocutaneous-free flaps from distant donor sites (e.g., forearm, hip, chest), are often necessary to replace ablated tongue, lip, jaw, or other tissues and restore important oral and respiratory functions [35, 36]. If essential to immediate recovery, they can be done at the time of ablative tumor surgery. In some patients, especially if done primarily for restoration of external appearance, reconstruction of ablative defects can be delayed until after the patient has delivered the infant and completed postpartum recovery.

Summary

Infections, tumors, injuries, or other conditions or diseases may develop in the oral cavity or jaws of a pregnant female. Some of these processes may pose urgent or life-threatening situations requiring prompt evaluation and treatment. Close cooperation and good communication between the patient's OB-GYN and the consultant OMFS will minimize risks and give the patient and fetus the best possible likelihood of continuing the pregnancy to term with the delivery of a healthy infant.

References

1. Moss KL, Ruvo AT, Offenbacher S, Beck JD, Mauriello SM, White RP Jr. Third molars and progression of periodontal pathology during pregnancy. J Oral Maxillofac Surg. 2007;65:106. https://doi.org/10.1016/j.joms.2006.10.074.
2. Turner M, Aziz SR. Management of the pregnant oral and maxillofacial surgery patient. J Oral Maxillofac Surg. 2002;60:1479. https://doi.org/10.1053/joms.2002.36132.
3. Bagheri SC, Bell RB, Khan HA. Current therapy in oral and maxillofacial surgery. Philadelphia: Elsevier/Saunders; 2012.
4. Council on Dental Education and Licensure ADA. Definitions of Recognized Dental Specialties. http://www.ada.org/en/education-careers/careers-in-dentistry/dental-specialties/specialty-definitions. Accessed 16 July 2017.
5. Guralnick WC. The combined oral surgery—MD program: the Harvard plan. J Oral Surg. 1973;31:271.
6. Dodson TB. A surge of surgeons. J Oral Maxillofac Surg. 2016;74:2333. https://doi.org/10.1016/j.joms.2016.09.042.
7. AAOMS. OMS Fellowship Opportunities. http://www.aaoms.org/education-research/oms-residents/oms-fellowship-opportunities. Accessed 16 July 2017.
8. Alling CC, Devlin DH, Connor FA, et al. The building of a specialty: oral and maxillofacial surgery in the United States, 1918–1998. J Oral Maxillofac Surg. 1998;56(suppl 3):1.
9. Lew D. A Historical Overview of AAOMS. AAOMS. 2013. http://www.aaoms.org/images/uploads/pdfs/historical_overview_aaoms.pdf. Accessed 16 July 2017.
10. AAOMS. OMS Procedures. AAOMS. http://www.aaoms.org/education-research/dental-students/oms-procedures. Accessed 16 July 2017.
11. Jo C, Jo J. Preoperative considerations for the pregnant patient. In: Bagheri SC, editor. Clinical review of oral and maxillofacial surgery: a case-based approach. 2nd ed. St. Louis: Elsevier/Mosby; 2014. p. 69–72.
12. Peterson LJ. Contemporary management of deep infections of the neck. J Oral Maxillofac Surg. 1993;51:226.
13. Malamed SF. Handbook of local anesthesia. 5th ed. Elsevier/Mosby: St. Louis, MO; 2004.
14. Becker DE, Reed KL. Essentials of local anesthetic pharmacology. Anesth Prog. 2006;53(3):98–109. https://doi.org/10.2344/0003-3006(2006)53[98:EOLAP]2.0.CO;2.
15. Lorenz DR, Whitley BD, Helfrick JF. Considerations in the management of maxillofacial infections in the pregnant patient. J Oral Maxillofac Surg. 1996;54:474.
16. American College of Obstetricians and Gynecologists' Committee on Obstetric Practice. Committee Opinion No. 656: Guidelines for diagnostic imaging during pregnancy and lactation. Obstet Gynecol. 2016;127(2):e75–80. https://doi.org/10.1097/AOG.0000000000001316.
17. Kao S, Girn J, Jo C, et al. Ludwig's Angina. In: Bagheri SC, editor. Clinical review of oral and maxillofacial surgery: a case-based approach. 2nd ed. St. Louis: Elsevier/Mosby; 2014. p. 96–1102.
18. Hudson JW. Osteomyelitis of the jaws: a 50-year perspective. J Oral Maxillofac Surg. 1993;51(12):1294–301.
19. Le BT, Dierks EJ, Ueeck BA, Homer LD, Potter BF. Maxillofacial injuries associated with domestic violence. J Oral Maxillofac Surg. 2001;59:1277–83. https://doi.org/10.1053/joms.2001.27490.
20. Cunningham LJH. RH. In: Miloro M, editor. Peterson's principles of oral and maxillofacial surgery. Toronto: BC Decker Inc; 2004.
21. O'Connor RC, Shakib K, Brennan PA. Recent advances in the management of oral and maxillofacial trauma. Br J Oral Maxillofac Surg. 2015;53:913. https://doi.org/10.1016/j.bjoms.2015.08.261.
22. Cohen KI, Diegelmann RF. The biology of keloid and hypertrophic scar and the influence of corticosteroids. Clin Plast Surg. 1977;4:297.
23. Ketchum LD. Hypertrophic scars and keloids. Clin Plast Surg. 1977;4:301.
24. Fricton J. Myofascial pain: Mechanisms to Management. Oral Maxillofac Surg Clin N Am. 2016;28:289–311. https://doi.org/10.1016/j.coms.2016.03.010.
25. Perez DE, Wolford LM. Contemporary management of temporomandibular joint disorders. Oral Maxillofac Surg Clin N Am. 2015;27(1):ix. https://doi.org/10.1016/j.coms.2014.10.001.
26. Aldulaimi S, Saenz A. A bleeding oral mass in a pregnant woman. JAMA. 2017;318(3):293–4. https://doi.org/10.1001/jama.2017.6901.
27. Terenzi V, Cassoni A, Della Monaca M, Priore P, De Felice F, Musio D, et al. Oral cancer during pregnancy. Oral Oncol. 2016;59:e1–3. https://doi.org/10.1016/j.oraloncology.2016.06.018.
28. Voulgaris E, Pentheroudakis G, Pavlidis N. Cancer and pregnancy: a comprehensive review. Surg Oncol. 2011;20(4):e175–85. https://doi.org/10.1016/j.suronc.2011.06.002.
29. Ward BB, Williams FC. Oral squamous cell carcinoma: epidemiology, clinical and radiographic evaluation, and staging. In: Bagheri SC, Bell RB, Khan HA, editors. Current therapy in oral and maxillofacial surgery. Philadelphia: Elsevier/Saunders; 2012. p. 414–22.
30. Hirsch DL, Spink MJ. Oral squamous cell carcinoma: Treatment. In: Bagheri SC, Bell RB, Khan HA, editors. Current therapy in oral and maxillofacial surgery. Philadelphia: Elsevier/Saunders; 2012. p. 422–34.
31. Bui TG, Bell RB. Oral squamous cell carcinoma: management of the neck. In: Bagheri SC, Bell RB, Khan HA, editors. Current therapy in oral and maxillofacial surgery. Philadelphia: Elsevier/Saunders; 2012. p. 435–44.
32. Ord RA. Oral squamous cell carcinoma: indications for adjuvant chemotherapy and radiation therapy. In: Bagheri SC, Bell RB, Khan HA, editors. Current therapy in oral and maxillofacial surgery. Philadelphia: Elsevier/Saunders; 2012. p. 445–9.

33. Murphy J, Berman DR, Edwards SP, Prisciandaro J, Eisbruch A, Ward BB. Squamous cell carcinoma of the tongue during pregnancy: a case report and review of the literature. J Oral Maxillofac Surg. 2016;74:2557. https://doi.org/10.1016/j.joms.2016.06.173.
34. Atabo A, Bradley PJ. Management principles of head and neck cancers during pregnancy: a review and case series. Oral Oncol. 2008;44(3):236–41. https://doi.org/10.1016/j.oraloncology.2007.02.003.
35. Potter JK. Mandibular reconstruction. In: Bagheri SC, Bell RB, Khan HA, editors. Current therapy in oral and maxillofacial surgery. Philadelphia: Elsevier/Saunders; 2012. p. 483–96.
36. Pirougsis P, Fernandes R. Contemporary methods in tongue reconstruction. In: Bagheri SC, Bell RB, Khan HA, editors. Current therapy in oral and maxillofacial surgery. Philadelphia: Elsevier/Saunders; 2012. p. 508–15.

21 Urologic Surgery During Pregnancy

Nancy N. Wang and Harcharan Gill

Stones

Etiology and Physiology

Pregnancy is associated with many physiologic changes that affect urinary composition, pH, and stasis; however, rates of kidney stone formation and renal colic are similar compared to nonpregnant females. Acute renal colic is reported in approximately 1 out of 1500 pregnancies [1, 2], and despite rising incidence of kidney stones in the overall population, the incidence among pregnant females have remained stable in the last two decades [3].

During pregnancy, several lithogenic factors are increased in the urine. Placental production of 1,25-dihydroxycholecalciferol increases intestinal calcium absorption, which leads to absorptive hypercalciuria [4]. Urinary levels of uric acid and oxalate also rise during this time, contributing to the risk of stone formation [5]. However, these are balanced out by concurrent increases of urinary citrate, magnesium, and glycosaminoglycan, which all help inhibit stone formation [4, 5].

Urine pH also tends to be more alkaline during pregnancy due to the increased urinary citrate [5]. While elevated urinary pH decreases risk of uric acid stone formation, it increases the risk of calcium phosphate stones. Indeed, calcium phosphate stones comprise up to 75% of stones reported in the pregnant population, whereas calcium oxalate stones are the most common culprit in the general population [5].

Another physiologic change that occurs during pregnancy is urinary stasis and hydronephrosis. This has been reported in up to 90% of pregnant women [6] and tends to be more pronounced as the uterus grows. Urinary stasis can encourage precipitation of stones and may contribute to the fact that 80–90% of acute kidney stone colic occurs during the second and third trimester [1, 5].

Diagnosis

Though the incidence of renal colic is no different in pregnant women, special consideration needs to be taken in the diagnoses and management in this population. Given the teratogenicity of radiation, ultrasound imaging is considered the gold standard for first-line diagnoses of kidney stones in pregnant females [5]. Sensitivity of ultrasound detection of kidney stones is operator-dependent and can be variable, with reported rates of 57% for the right kidney and 39% for the left kidney with an overall accuracy of up to 77% [7, 8] for experienced technicians and radiologist. Additionally, studies have shown that ultrasound sensitivity significantly drops when

N. N. Wang (✉) · H. Gill
Department of Urology, Stanford University School of Medicine, Stanford, CA, USA
e-mail: nwang4@stanford.edu; hgill@stanford.edu

C. H. Nezhat (ed.), *Non-Obstetric Surgery During Pregnancy*,
https://doi.org/10.1007/978-3-319-90752-9_21

evaluating stones <5 mm in size [9]. As such, MR urography is increasingly being used as a second-line evaluation, with good diagnostic success and tolerance reported [10].

Treatment

Medical Expulsive Therapy

As with management of kidney stones in the general population, imaging confirmation of a stone is not always required to start treatment. In pregnant patients without any signs of infection (clean urinary analysis and negative urine culture, no fevers, normal WBC) and who have appropriate renal function, medical expulsive therapy (MET) can be started empirically. MET includes hydration, IV if unable to tolerate oral intake, pain management, and either a calcium channel blocker such as nifedipine or an alpha-blocker such as tamsulosin. Both alpha-blockers and calcium channel blockers are category B drugs which are safe to give in pregnancy and can help with stone passage as well as renal colic symptoms. Tamsulosin is the more commonly prescribed expulsive therapy in the general population, and a recent retrospective study showed efficacy and safety when used in pregnant women with symptomatic renal colic [11].

One benefit of the associated hydroureteronephrosis seen in pregnancy is a higher rate of spontaneous stone passage with some studies reporting passage of 70–80% for stones <1 cm [5]. Furthermore, some studies show that up to half of the stones that do not pass during pregnancy will pass within the first month after delivery [12] without further intervention.

Interventions, however, are needed in cases where patients have refractory pain, urinary infection, solitary kidney, renal dysfunction from bilateral stones or a large obstructing stone, or preeclampsia. The decision to undergo a temporizing intervention, with the aim of decompression and drainage, versus a definitive intervention should be made by an interdisciplinary team with the aid of urologists.

Temporizing Interventions

Temporizing interventions include ureteroscopy with placement of an indwelling ureteral stent, which drains the urine around the stone, or percutaneous nephrostomy for direct drainage. Ureteroscopy is done in the operating room by urologists and usually requires general anesthesia, though they can sometimes be done with a spinal anesthetic. The stent is placed either using ultrasound guidance or, more commonly, limited pelvic fluoroscopy where a lead apron is used to minimize radiation to the fetus [5]. The stents can become a nidus for stone precipitation themselves, which is why they will need routine exchanges every 1–2 months. Additionally, the stents can cause their own set of ureteral colic and discomfort as well as bladder spasms and irritation. These symptoms can be treated with alpha-blockers such as tamsulosin, anticholinergic agents such as oxybutynin, or local analgesic medications such as phenazopyridine (Pyridium), all of which are category B drugs and safe to use during pregnancy [13].

Unlike stents, percutaneous nephrostomies can be placed under local and light sedation, oftentimes by interventional radiologists. They similarly need routine exchanges every 1–2 months as they can become encrusted in the renal pelvis. Though they do not cause ureteral colic, they can cause some pain and discomfort at the insertion site especially in patients who spend a lot of time lying on their backs.

The distinction between the need for an operating room procedure with anesthesia versus a procedure with light sedation may play an important role in decision-making as procedures requiring anesthesia are still discouraged during the first trimester due to anesthetic risks. Percutaneous nephrostomy drainage is also advantageous in cases where the stone may be too obstructed and not amenable to placement of a ureteral stent or in cases where the stone will need percutaneous nephrolithotomy for definitive treatment later on, which would require a percutaneous nephrostomy anyways [5].

Definitive Treatment

In recent decades, there has been much advancement in ureteroscopic equipment and treatments including the development of laser therapy for stone lithotripsy. Unlike previous lithotripsy treatments such as extracorporeal shock wave lithotripsy which is contraindicated as it can cause miscarriage, congenital malformation, and placental displacement [14], laser lithotripsy is safe for use during pregnancy as the light pulsations have only local penetrance that is precisely and directly applied to the stone with limited diffusion risk to the fetus. The use of both rigid and flexible ureteroscopy with laser lithotripsy has been shown to be safe in pregnancy and has been shown to be effective for stones found anywhere along the urinary tract including the upper ureter [15–18]. Reports of intraoperative complications are very rare. The procedure can be done under spinal anesthesia in some cases, which limits the general anesthetic risks. Additionally, the ureteroscopy portion of the procedure, which requires image guidance to establish the location of the wires and scope in the ureter, can be done using ultrasound guidance or very limited pelvic fluoroscopy [19].

Definitive treatment with laser lithotripsy has been increasingly used for patients who have failed symptomatic management, but given their safety profile, they are also being offered as an acceptable alternative to percutaneous nephrostomy or routine stent exchange in cases where the stones are amenable to a single lithotripsy procedure or in cases where patients have compromised renal status, such as a solitary kidney, and would benefit from early definitive treatment.

However, treatment with ureteroscopy and laser lithotripsy is not recommended in cases where the stone is >2–3 cm as success with ureteroscopy is limited and these patients will likely require percutaneous nephrolithotomy. Temporary percutaneous nephrostomy drainage is the recommended management as percutaneous nephrolithotomy is contraindicated during pregnancy due to the long operative time needed, prone position, complication rates, and high fluoroscopy radiation [5].

Patients who had good symptomatic control during pregnancy without any signs of infections or renal complications should be referred to a urologist for definitive care and stone workup after delivery. Though studies have shown rates of spontaneous passage as high as 47%, many women develop recurrent stones and would benefit from standard workup and prevention practices [20].

Obstructive Uropathy

Besides stone disease, there are several causes of obstructive uropathy that can occur during pregnancy. First, it is important to differentiate hydroureteronephrosis from obstructive uropathy. Hydroureteronephrosis is the radiographic finding of dilation of the ureters and/or kidney. This may or may not be associated with a pathologic issue. Obstructive uropathy, however, is the structural or functional blockage of urinary excretion from the kidney and ureters and implies a deviation from normal physiology.

Idiopathic Hydroureteronephrosis

Indeed, idiopathic hydronephrosis or hydroureteronephrosis has been incidentally seen and reported in up to 80–90% of pregnant patients in several studies [6]. The dilation develops during the second trimester and is believed to be due to anatomic compression of the ureters between the growing uterus and the linea terminalis [21, 22]. This is consistent with several large-scale analyses which have shown that the dilation is more pronounced above the pelvic brim, can be reduced by placing the woman in a lateral decubitus position or in the knee-elbow position, and self-resolves within a few weeks after delivery [6, 23].

Many studies have also shown that dilation of the right collecting system is more common and pronounced than the left, with one study reporting a 4–7 mm average increase in right renal pelvis dilation compared to the left [6]. Some studies also suggest that increased progesterone levels during pregnancy may contribute to increased smooth muscle relaxation of the ureters, allowing for notable dilation [22].

Though idiopathic hydroureteronephrosis is generally asymptomatic, there are reports of women with severe bilateral anatomic obstruction from the uterus with associated abdominal pain, increased incidence of UTI, and very rarely, an increased risk for preeclampsia [24]. In cases where women with radiographic hydroureteronephrosis report pain, infection, or other symptoms, it is important to complete a full workup to rule out other causes of obstructive uropathy that may require intervention.

Diagnosis

Women presenting with abdominal or flank pain should get a urinalysis with culture to evaluate for infection, chemistry to evaluate for renal dysfunction, and a renal bladder ultrasound to evaluate for anatomic obstruction, stone disease, or mass obstruction [25].

Some patients with abnormal urinary systems, such as a duplicated system, can have worsened dilation in the setting of increased circulatory volume associated with pregnancy [26]. Similar to idiopathic hydronephrosis, this should also resolve after delivery.

If there are signs of external mass compression on the ureters besides the gravid uterus, an MRI is recommended for further characterization given the risk of radiation associated with CT scans. External compression of the ureters can be caused by significant constipation, pelvic masses/tumors, primary ureteral tumors, or rarely ureteral endometriosis.

Management and Treatment

Urologic management in cases of pathologic obstructive uropathy during pregnancy is directed toward drainage and protection of renal function. Cystoscopy with placement of ureteral stents for drainage and interventional radiology with placement of nephrostomy drainage are both viable options during pregnancy if renal function is at risk. As discussed previously in the obstructive stone section, there are risks and benefits to each approach. However, the success of cystoscopy and stent drainage drops in the setting of external compression from pelvic cancers as these masses can preclude successful placement of the stents and can also compress the stents themselves even after they are placed. Nephrostomy drainage is recommended for management if external masses are expected to grow.

Ureteral Tumor

Though primary ureteral tumors are rare, accounting for up to 5% of urothelial cancer [27], patients can present with symptomatic obstructive uropathy. Workup once a ureteral mass is suspected involves evaluation of bilateral ureters for filling defects. During pregnancy, MR uropathy is recommended over CT IVP due to the radiation risks to the fetus.

Further treatment or management requires a multidisciplinary approach with careful assessment of risks depending on the size of the ureteral mass, grade of disease, degree of obstructive uropathy, and timing during pregnancy. As discussed previously in the stone section, ureteroscopy is safe during pregnancy and can be used for diagnostic biopsy as well as laser ablation for low-grade cancers. Management of high-grade ureteral tumors will require further discussion as standard treatment is radical nephroureterectomy.

Ureteral Endometriosis

Though endometriosis affects up to 15% of women, genitourinary involvement is rare with a reported incidence of 1.2% with the large majority involving the bladder [28, 29]. Ureteral endometriosis in particular requires a high index of suspicion as the majority of cases have been discovered incidentally during laparotomy for extensive disease [29] or during workup for a nonfunctioning kidney where the ureteral endometriosis was discovered as the cause of damaging silent obstruction [30]. Symptomatic patients who are not pregnant tend to present with dyspareunia, cyclical pain, menorrhagia, and cyclical hematuria due to intraluminal involvement [30].

Long-term treatment of ureteral endometriosis depends on the symptoms and reproductive desires of the patient as hysterectomy with bilateral salpingo-oophorectomy and ureteral resection has been offered in cases of severe pain and bleeding. During pregnancy, however, management would be focused on symptomatic control and renal protection.

Placenta Percreta

Placenta percreta, the most severe form of placental invasion, occurs in 1 out of 25,000 pregnancies and is defined as invasion through the myometrium of the uterus [31]. Once through the myometrium, the placental villi can invade the bladder or rectum, posing additional risks during delivery. In the last few years, the rate of placenta percreta has increased by 50 times, a rise that parallels the increased rate of cesarean sections [32]. Uterine scarring, either from cesarean sections, a history of placenta previa, uterine curettage, or Asherman syndrome, is the main risk factor for placenta percreta as the uterine myometrium is disrupted leaving it vulnerable to invasion by placental villi [31]. A history of endometriosis and grand multiparity are additional risk factors for all levels of placenta accreta [31].

Diagnosis can occur during antenatal ultrasound evaluation and should be followed by MRI for better evaluation. Patients with concern for bladder involvement should be sent to urology for clinic cystoscopy to directly evaluate the bladder without need for anesthesia [31]. Early and clear evaluation of the degree of placental invasion is important for appropriate delivery planning as placenta percreta is associated with significant obstetric hemorrhage that can be hard to temporize and can be life-threatening. Indeed, placenta percreta with involvement of the bladder has a reported mortality of up to 9.5% for the mother and 24% for the child [33].

When discovered prior to delivery, preparations include involvement of interventional radiology with placement of balloons for quick ligation/embolization of uterine vasculature, anticipated blood transfusion needs, and planned urologic interventions including cystoscopy and possible cystotomy with reconstruction. In addition to improved control and response to bladder bleeding, preoperative involvement of urology has been shown to decrease rates of ureteral or bladder injury compared to cases where urology was consulted intraoperatively or postoperatively [34].

However, many cases of placenta percreta are asymptomatic during pregnancy and aren't discovered until time of delivery despite antenatal imaging studies. One study reported that only 25% of patients with placenta percreta presented prior to delivery with painful gross hematuria [35]. The associated pain is important as it distinguishes from placenta previa, which is associated with painless gross hematuria. Given the high risks associated with this condition, we recommend a low threshold for urologic evaluation and involvement in patients with significant risk factors.

Iatrogenic Urologic Injury

Injury to the bladder and ureters can occur during both gynecologic and obstetric procedures. Gynecologic surgeries account for up to 52% of iatrogenic ureteral injuries [36] and have increased rates of bladder injury especially in gyn-onc cases where normal anatomy is distorted. For obstetrics, rates of bladder injuries vary with averages of 1 out of 10,000 vaginal deliveries and 14 out of 10,000 cesarean sections though some studies have shown incidence of up to 0.94% in cesarean sections [37]. Ureteral injuries are lower with rates of 0.3 per 10,000 vaginal deliveries and 2.7 per 10,000 cesarean sections [38].

Bladder Injuries

Bladder injuries include any full-thickness cystotomy or damage to the bladder. This can occur during entry into the peritoneal cavity, creation of a bladder flap, uterine incision and delivery, or closure [39]. Studies have shown that risk factors for bladder injury include an older age, adhesions, women with greater parity, and women with a history of prior cesarean section, which can cause scarring to the bladder [39]. When identified early and intraoperatively, urology can be consulted for primary repair with a two-layer vesicorrhaphy [39, 40]. Along with primary evaluation, the bladder can also be assessed by filling it with 300 cm^3 of methylene blue via urethral catheter to evaluate for extravasation; however, this is not always sensitive to small cystotomies. Urology consultation is recommended if there is concern for bladder injury. Following primary repair, the patient should then have an indwelling catheter for 10–14 days to allow for healing and evaluation with retrograde cystogram prior to removal of the Foley catheter.

While more bladder injuries are identified intraoperatively, some have a delayed presentation. Vesicouterine fistulas, also known as Youssef syndrome, can occur months after a cesarean section if the bladder wall is incorporated into the uterine suture line, as a complication of dilation and curettage procedures [41] or as a complication of pelvic irradiation, trauma, or bladder endometriosis [42]. Approximately 20% of women present with some combination of the classic Youssef triad of amenorrhea, urinary incontinence and hematuria associated with menses, also known as menouria. However, many others may only present with vague abdominal and pelvic discomfort, so a high level of suspicion is necessary. CT cystogram or hysterosalpingograms have the highest sensitivity for diagnosis, but given the intermittence of symptoms and varying fistula sizes, workup should include urologic cystoscopy for direct visual assessment if imaging is inconclusive [41]. Once the fistula is diagnosed, patients should also have a thorough upper tract evaluation with CT IVP to rule out any concurrent ureteral injuries.

Treatment of vesicouterine fistulas depends on timing of diagnosis as well as the patient's future fertility desires. If the fistula is found within 6 months of surgery and the patient desires more children in the future, conservative treatment with an indwelling catheter along with short-term endocrine suppression of menstruation can be attempted. This, however, is only successful approximately 50% of the time [41, 42]. If this fails or if the tract is found past 6 months and has been matured, the patient will require a transvaginal or transabdominal repair with omentum or a Martius flap. If the patient, however, does not desire further fertility, treatment with transabdominal hysterectomy and primary repair of the bladder is recommended [41].

Ureteral Injuries

Though less common, ureteral injuries can occur from direct ligation or from secondary thermal damage. Ligation often occurs in conjunction with ligation of the uterine artery, uterosacral/transverse uterine ligaments, or suspensory ligaments of the ovary [38]. The incidence of ureteral injury is higher in cases complicated by massive hemorrhage, which can impede visualization of structures and add an element of urgency, and in cases where adhesions can distort normal anatomy [43]. Early proactive identification of the ureters with careful dissection has been shown to decrease ureteral injury rates [44]. As such, urology consults for placement of ureteral stents prior to obstetric or gynecologic surgery have been increasing. Ureteral stents not only help with identification but can also straighten out otherwise tortuous ureters. Some newer stents are capable of lighting up which further aid with intraoperative identification [45]. Though many studies have shown that ureteral stents help reduce operative time spent identifying the ureters, there is still no clear data that shows a significant decrease in overall ureteral injury rates when stents are used [46].

Diagnosis and Evaluation

Unlike bladder injuries, iatrogenic ureteral injuries can have a delayed presentation. Though intraoperative ureteroscopy has been shown to have high sensitivity for identification of acute ligation injuries, they are not sensitive in recognizing thermal damage [47]. Secondary thermal damage can cause stricture and stenosis formation that can present with flank pain, fever, sepsis, ileus, and acute renal failure days to weeks following surgery [40]. A high suspicion for ureteral injury is necessary when patients present with delayed symptoms. Patients should be evaluated with labs including serum creatinine as well as a renal bladder ultrasound to evaluate for hydroureteronephrosis of the affected side. Further evaluations such as CT IVP or cystoscopy with retrograde pyelogram can help identify the area and extent of stenosis or injury.

Treatment

Treatment of ureteral injury depends on the type of injury, extent of damage, and if it is found intraoperatively or in a delayed fashion.

Suture ligations that are identified and removed intraoperatively without clear ureteral damage may be conservatively monitored and followed. If patients remain asymptomatic with stable renal function, a renal bladder ultrasound should be obtained a few weeks after surgery to evaluate for signs of silent stricture formation and, if negative, to document the post-op baseline so that any future changes can be better assessed.

If the ureter is transected sharply, with cautery or ligation, and identified intraoperatively, primary anastomosis may be attempted with placement of an indwelling ureteral stent. However, if the injury is found postoperatively, cystoscopy with placement of an indwelling ureteral stent will be attempted for realignment. If this is unsuccessful, the patient may need a nephrostomy tube for drainage and preservation of renal function on the affected side with plans for a delayed ureteral repair.

Pregnancy and Delivery in Patients with Urinary Diversions or Augmentations

Management of congenital urologic conditions has significantly improved in the last few decades, leading to a growing population of pregnant women with a history of bladder augmentation or urinary diversion. The majority of these patients are treated for non-cancerous pathologies such as bladder exstrophy, neurogenic bladder, or interstitial cystitis. However, the resulting changes in anatomy, especially in patients who have undergone cystectomy, raise concerns for increased risk of urinary tract infections, development of urinary incontinence, risk to the fetus, and increased risk of iatrogenic injuries during cesarean sections.

UTI

Patients with bladder augmentations or urinary diversions are at an increased risk for urinary tract infections at baseline. This is complicated by the fact that urine analysis and urine cultures can be misleading, with one study reporting up to 50–100% rates of asymptomatic bacteriuria, of which only 4–43% had a significant urinary tract infection [48]. Furthermore, diverted patients also have a higher risk for progression to pyelonephritis as most common diversions lead to ureteral reflux [49, 50].

Given the increased risk of premature labor in the setting of pyelonephritis, some practitioners recommend long-term prophylaxis during pregnancy especially in patients with known ureteral reflux [49]. Others, however, recommend close monitoring and early treatment of urinary tract infections with a low threshold for interventions such as nephrostomy tube drainage if there is no immediate improvement on antibiotics [50, 51].

Continence

Pregnancy alone increases the risk for development of urinary incontinence due to the effect of the gravid uterus weakening the pelvic floor. However, in patients with urinary diversions, the gravid uterus can also compress and strain the vascular supply of conduits and neobladders, increasing the risk of necrosis or stenosis, as well as directly impact the reservoirs themselves.

Some patients with catheterizable diversions experience increased retention and difficulty catheterizing as the gravid uterus stretches and distorts the conduit. This can generally be managed with an indwelling catheter, but on rare occasions the diversion may require repair after delivery or at the time of cesarean section [49]. On the other hand, some patients may experience increased urinary incontinence due to compression of the reservoir itself. Patients with stomas also have a slight increase risk for stomal prolapse. These cases, however, are rare as the progression of fetal growth is slow enough that the body generally can adapt and compensate without complications.

In addition to these gestational risks, there are concerns that patients with an artificial urinary sphincter or a history of vesical neck reconstruction could damage their continence mechanism during vaginal delivery [50, 51]. Though the traditional recommendation has been for these patients to undergo elective cesarean section to reduce these risks, recent studies have not shown a significant difference in outcomes [52, 53].

Anatomy Considerations for Cesarean Section

Indeed, recent studies have shown that there is no significant increased risk associated with vaginal delivery in women with a history of bladder augmentation or cystectomy with diversions [53]. However, for patients with a history of bladder exstrophy, there is a 25% chance of abnormal fetal presentation requiring cesarean section [54]. In these cases, there is an increase incidence of fetal demise seen when the cesarean sections are done emergently [54]. While this is due to a multitude of factors, the anatomic changes in these patients can pose significant vascular risks if they are unrecognized.

A high cesarean section approach or midline incision is recommended instead of the traditional low Pfannenstiel in order to avoid damaging the urinary reservoir and to allow for maximal visualization [49, 55]. In addition to distorted normal anatomy, these patients also have an increased risk for adhesions. It is especially important to identify both ureters as well as taking care to preserve the mesenteric vascular supply to augmentations and diversions. As locations of the ureters and reservoirs vary depending on the type of augmentation, diversion, or neobladder constructed, urology involvement in delivery planning is crucial and has been shown to decrease risk of urinary injury and complications [55].

Incidental Masses

With the rise of prenatal ultrasound and imaging, more women are being diagnosed with incidental adrenal and renal masses during pregnancy [56]. While the overall incidence still remains low, special considerations are needed for safe monitoring and management in the pregnant population.

Bladder Masses

Incidental masses in the bladder are uncommon and rarely malignancies due to the age group of pregnant patients. However, diagnostic workup with cystoscopy and possible biopsy is mandatory. Figure 21.1 shows a routine 8-week diagnostic ultrasound in a 35-year-old gravida 1 patient. An MRI was done at the end of the first trimester (Fig. 21.2), and due to concerns for a malignancy (transitional cell carcinoma or sarcoma), a diagnostic transurethral resection was done at 13 weeks of pregnancy. This returned as

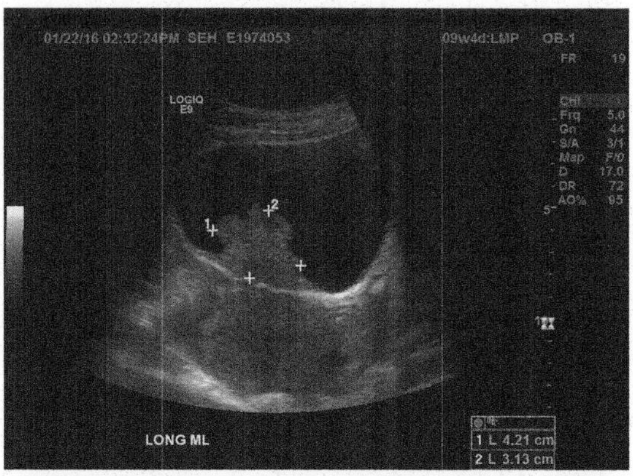

Fig. 21.1 Antenatal ultrasound at 8 weeks with a bladder mass

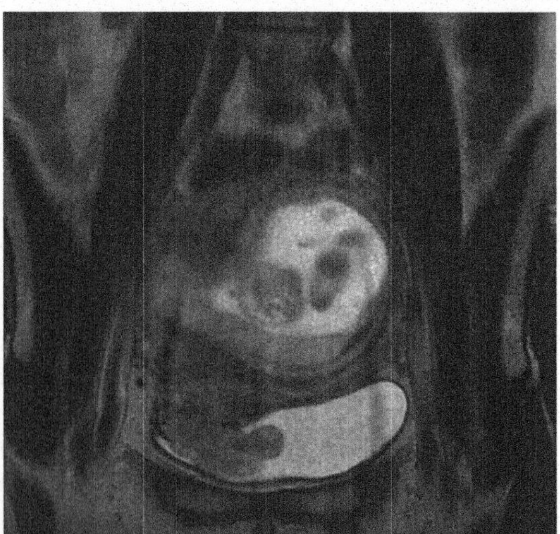

Fig. 21.2 MRI of pelvis at 12 weeks confirms the bladder mass and a gravid uterus

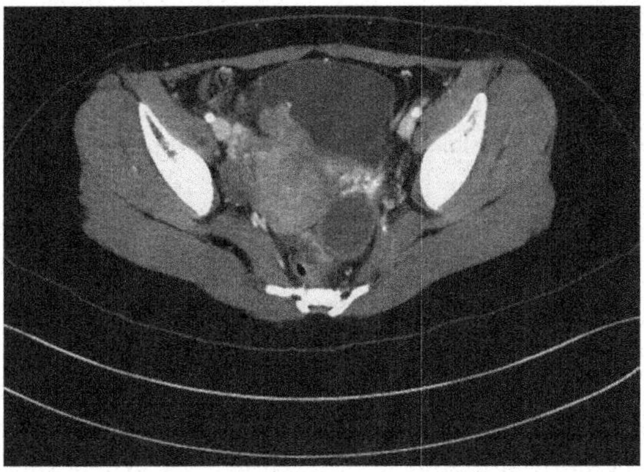

Fig. 21.3 Postpartum CT shows transmural endometriosis of the bladder wall

endometriosis and she had an uneventful pregnancy. Postpartum CT scan (Fig. 21.3) shows the extent of her endometriosis and this was managed medically.

Adrenal Masses

Though pheochromocytomas are rare, it is associated with fetal and maternal mortality rates as high as 50% when unrecognized [57, 58]. The incidence of pheochromocytoma in the general population is approximately 0.5–0.8% [59] and even lower in the pregnant population with reported rates of 0.002–0.007% [58, 60]. Diagnosis is often difficult given the variability of symptoms such as hypertension, headaches, dizziness, and palpitations. In the pregnancy population, this is made even more difficult as many symptoms can be confused with gestational hypertension or preeclampsia. A high level of suspicions is important especially in patients whose hypertension appears paroxysmal or patients who present with stories of associated paroxysmal symptoms.

Diagnosis is made based on elevated plasma metanephrines and urinary catecholamines. Renal ultrasounds and MRI can then be done to localize the mass without exposing the fetus to radiation with CT imaging. Functional MIBG scanning is contraindicated in pregnancy as the MBG molecules can cross the placenta and expose the fetus to radiation. MRI also has diagnostic sensitivities of 90–100% [58]. Once diagnosed, management and treatment of pheochromocytomas depend on the timing and patient preference.

Surgical resection after appropriate medical preparation with phenoxybenzamine, an alpha-blocker, and then beta-blockade is the gold standard treatment for pheochromocytomas. As with all surgeries during gestation, resection is ideally done during the second trimester while the gravid uterus is intermediate and the fetus has completed organogenesis. Thus, if the diagnosis is made during the first trimester, the option of termination should be discussed with the patient. If the patient chooses to proceed with the pregnancy, the recommendation is for medical management of the hypertension with an alpha-blocker until the second trimester when laparoscopic or open resection can be done safely [58, 61]. If discovered during the third trimester, the recommendation is for medical management and then elective cesarean section. Cesarean section not only allows for concurrent delivery and resection of the mass, but it is also associated with decreased maternal mortality rates. Vaginal deliveries have reported maternal mortality rates of up to 31% and are believed to be associated with a sudden androgen release that can occur in patients with pheochromocytomas [58].

Renal RCC

Renal solid masses are the most common urologic neoplasm discovered during pregnancy at a reported rate of 0.1% [62]. The large majority of masses are discovered incidentally as part of prenatal imaging, but some patients can present with flank pain, hematuria, hypertension, or a palpable mass [56].

If discovered on history and physical, a renal ultrasound should be done though sensitivity of detection is very poor for lesions <3 cm [63]. Additional imaging with MRI can be done as well as CT above the gravid uterus if needed [56]. Management of the mass depends on size, symptoms, and timing of diagnosis. Biopsies are not necessary for diagnosis of solid masses, but physicians should discuss the risks and benefits when masses are <4 cm and other treatment options such as cryoablation or surveillance are reasonable [56].

As overall incidence of renal cell carcinoma in pregnancy is low, management should always include a multidisciplinary team discussion of risks and benefits. Though previous recommendations have been for termination of pregnancy when diagnosed during the first trimester, recent studies have shown that patients without metastatic disease are able to have a smooth gestation and delivery when closely monitored and managed [56]. Given the slow growth rate of most renal cell carcinomas, close surveillance is a reasonable approach for smaller masses, usually <4 cm. Surgical resection, however, is still the gold standard of treatment for larger renal masses. A review of the literature shows reports of successful radical nephrectomies followed by vaginal deliveries and cesarean sections as well as simultaneous planned radical nephrectomies with cesarean sections, although a midline and large incision is required in these cases [64].

There is no clear guideline for the timing of surgery, though it is strongly recommended that surgery be delayed until after the 28th week of gestation if possible to allow for fetal lung maturity [56]. Of note, while the average renal cell carcinoma grows very slowly, there are reported cases of aggressive masses that have quickly doubled in size during gestation. Some studies suggest that this accelerated growth may be due to activation of estrogen and progesterone receptors in RCC during pregnancy [65] which is why some physicians recommend immediate resection even in the first trimester when discovered [56, 66].

Even more rarely, some women have been diagnosed with metastatic renal cell carcinoma during pregnancy. Again, a multidisciplinary approach is crucial, especially as many medical treatment have unknown pregnancy effects but include medications that are category D and should be avoided in pregnancy.

Renal Angiomyolipoma

Incidence of renal angiomyolipoma (AML) is approximately 0.3% in the general population and even more rare in pregnancy [67]. However, AMLs have been seen to have an accelerated rate of growth during pregnancy [68] and increased rate of spontaneous rupture especially when >4 cm [69].

Presentation can be similar to RCC; however, up to 10% of reported cases can present with rare hemorrhagic shock also known as Wunderlich syndrome [67]. Otherwise, renal AMLs are discovered during workup for a renal mass seen incidentally on ultrasound.

When asymptomatic, management is generally conservative with bed rest, repeat imaging, and close monitoring for symptoms. However, selective embolization can be done if there is growing concern for possible bleeding or in the case of bilateral AMLs. In rare cases of uncontrolled bleeding refractory to embolization, partial or radical nephrectomy can also be considered [67].

References

1. Maikranz P, Lindheimer MD, Coe FL. Nephrolithiasis in pregnancy. Baillieres Clin Obstet Gynaecol. 1994;8(2):375–86.
2. McAleer SJ, Loughlin KR. Nephrolithiasis and pregnancy. Curr Opin Urol. 2004;14(2):123–7.
3. Riley JM, Dudley AG, Semins MJ. Nephrolithiasis and pregnancy: has the incidence been rising? J Endourol. 2014;28(3):383–6.
4. Biyani CS, Joyce A. Urolithiasis in pregnancy. BJUI. 2002;89(8):811–23.
5. Semins MJ, Matlaga BR. Kidney stones during pregnancy. Nat Rev Urol. 2014;11(3):163–8.
6. Peake SL, Roxburgh HB, Langlois SH. Ultrasonic assessment of hydronephrosis of pregnancy. Radiology. 1983;146(1):167–70.
7. Ulusan S, Koc Z, Tokmak N. Accuracy of sonography for detecting renal stone: comparison with CT. J Clin Ultrasound. 2007;35(5):256–61.
8. Cosgrove DO, Meire HB, Lim A, Eckersley RJ. Ultrasound: general principles. In: Adam A, Dixon AK, Grainger RG, Allison DJ, editors. Grainger & Allison's diagnostic radiology. A textbook of medical imaging. Philadelphia, PA: Churchill Livingstone Elsevier; 2008.

9. Fowler KA, locken JA, Duchesne JH, Williamson MR. US for detecting renal calculi with nonenhanced CT as a reference standard. Radiology. 2002;222(1):109–13.
10. Spencer JA, Chahal R, Kelly A, Taylor K, Eardley I, Lloyd SN. Evaluation of painful hydronephrosis in pregnancy: magnetic resonance urographic patterns in physiological dilatation versus calculous obstruction. J Urol. 2004;171(1):256–60.
11. Baily G, Vaughan L, Rose C, Krambeck A. Perinatal outcomes with tamsulosin therapy in symptomatic urolithiasis. J Urol. 2016;195(1):99–103.
12. Stothers L, Lee LM. Renal colic in pregnancy. J Urol. 1992;148(5):1383–7.
13. Lee M, Bozzo P, Einarson A, Koren G. Urinary tract infections in pregnancy. Can Fam Physician. 2008;54(6):853–4.
14. Chaussy CG, Fuchs GJ. Current state and future developments of noninvasive treatment of human urinary stones with extracorporeal shock wave lithotripsy. J Urol. 1989;141(3 Pt 2):782–9.
15. Carringer M, Swartz R, Johansson JE. Management of ureteric calculi during pregnancy by ureteroscopy and laser lithotripsy. Br J Urol. 1996;77(1):17–20.
16. Akpinar H, Tufek I, Alici B, Kural AR. Ureteroscopy and holmium laser lithotripsy in pregnancy: stents must be used postoperatively. J Endourol. 2006;20(2):107–10.
17. Abedi AR, Allameh F, Razzaghi MR, Fadavi B, Qashqai H, Najafi S, Ranjbar A, Bashirian M. The efficacy and safety of laser lithotripsy in pregnancy. J Lasers Med Sci. 2017;Spring 8(2):84–7.
18. Adanur S, Ziypak T, Bedir F, Yapanoglu T, Aydin HR, Yilmaz M, Aksoy M, Ozbey I. Ureteroscopy and holmium laser lithotripsy: is this procedure safe in pregnant women with ureteral stones at different locations? Arch Ital Urol Androl. 2014;86(2):86–9.
19. Semins MJ, Trock BJ, Matlaga BR. The safety of ureteroscopy during pregnancy: a systematic review and meta-analysis. J Urol. 2009;181(1):139–43.
20. Burgess KL, Gettman MT, Rangel LJ, Krambeck AE. Diagnosis of urolithiasis and rate of spontaneous passage during pregnancy. J Urol. 2011;186(6):2280–4.
21. Rasmussen PE, Nielsen FR. Hydronephrosis during pregnancy: a literature survey. EurJ Obstet Gynecol Reprod Biol. 1988;27(3):249–59.
22. Fainaru O, Almog B, Gamzu R, Lessing JB, Kupferminc M. The management of symptomatic hydronephrosis in pregnancy. BJOG. 2002;109(12):1385–7.
23. Fried AM. Hydronephrosis of pregnancy: ultrasonographic study and classification of asymptomatic women. Am J Obstet Gynecol. 1979;135(8):1066–70.
24. Banon Perez VJ, Rigabert Montiel M, Nicolas Torralba JA, Valdelvira Nadal P, Lopez Cubillana P, Server Pastor G, Prieto Gonzalez A, Perez AM. Manejo de la uropatia obstructiva en el embarazo. [Management of obstructive uropathy in pregnancy]. Actas Urol Esp. 1999;23(3):227–31. Spanish.
25. McArthur T, Crystal CS, Miller MA. Hydronephrosis during pregnancy. Am J Emerg Med. 2007;25(4):482–3.
26. Lin YJ, Ou YC, Tsang LC, Lin H. Diagnostic value of magnetic resonance imaging for successful management of a giant hydronephrosis during pregnancy. J Obstet Gynaecol. 2013;33(1):91–3.
27. Siegel R, Ma J, Zou Z, Jemal A. Cancer statistics, 2014. CA Cancer J Clin. 2014;64(1):9–29.
28. Fisher JD. Urology in-service and board review. Corpus Christi: BMED Press; 2013.
29. Yohannes P. Ureteral endometriosis. J Urol. 2003;170(1):20–5.
30. Klein RS, Cattolica EV. Ureteral endometriosis. Urology. 1979;13(5):477–82.
31. Konijeti R, Rajfer J, Askari A. Placenta percreta and the urologist. Rev Urol. 2009;Summer 11(3):173–6.
32. Smith ZL, Sehgal SS, Van Arsdalen KN, Goldstein IS. Placenta percreta with invasion into the urinary bladder. Urol Case Rep. 2014;2(1):31–2.
33. Price FV, Resnik E, Heller KA, Christopherson WA. Placenta previa percreta involving the urinary bladder: a report of two cases and review of the literature. Obstet Gynecol. 1991;78(3):508–11.
34. Ng MK, Jack GS, Bolton DM, Lawrentschuk N. Placenta percreta with urinary tract involvement: the case for a multidisciplinary approach. Urology. 2009;74(4):778–82.
35. Takai N, Eto M, Sato F, Mimata H, Miyakawa I. Placenta percreta invading the urinary bladder. Arch Gynecol Obstet. 2005;271(3):274–5.
36. Schimpf MO, Gottenger EE, Wagner JR. Universal ureteral stent placement at hysterectomy to identify ureteral injury: a decision analysis. BJOG. 2008;115(9):1151–8.
37. Yossepowitch O, Baniel J, Livne PM. Urological injuries during caesarean section: intraoperative diagnosis and management. J Urol. 2004;172(1):196–9.
38. Rajasekar D, Hall M. Urinary tract injuries during obstetric intervention. Br J Obstet Gynaecol. 1997;104(6):731–4.
39. Gungorduk K, Asicioglu O, Celikkol O, Sudolmus S, Ark C. Iatrogenic bladder injuries during caesarean delivery: a case control study. J Obstet Gynaecol. 2010;30(7):667–70.
40. St Lezin MA, Stoller ML. Surgical ureteral injuries. Urology. 1991;38(6):497–506.
41. Rovner ES. Urinary tract fistulae. In: Win AJ, Kavoussi LR, Novick AC, Partin AW, Peters CA, editors. Campbell-Walsh urology, vol. 3. 10th ed. Philadelphia: Elsevier; 2012. p. 2246–68, Chapter 77.
42. Ikechebelu JI, Ugboaja JO, Okeke CF. Post-cesarean vesicouterine fistula (Youssef syndrome): report of two cases. J Obstet Gynaecol Res. 2011;37(7):912–5.
43. Rao D, Yu H, Zhu H, Duan P. The diagnosis and treatment of iatrogenic ureteral and bladder injury caused by traditional gynaecology and obstetrics operation. Arch Gynecol Obstet. 2012;285(3):763–5.
44. Neuman M, Eldelman A, Langer R, Golan A, Bukovsky I, Caspi E. Iatrogenic injuries to the ure-

ter during gynecologic and obstetric operations. Surg Gynecol Obstet. 1991;173(4):268–72.
45. Redan JA, McCarus SD. Protect the ureters. JSLS. 2009;13(2):139–41.
46. Lee Z, Kaplan J, Giusto L, Eun D. Prevention of iatrogenic ureteral injuries during robotic gynecologic surgery: a review. Am J Obstet Gynecol. 2016;214(5):566–71.
47. Gilmour DT, Da S, Flowerdew G. Rates of urinary tract injury from gynecologic surgery and the role of intraoperative cystoscopy. Obstet Gynecol. 2006;107(6):1366–72.
48. Khoury JM, Timmons SL, Corbel L, Webster GD. Complications of enterocystoplasty. J Urol. 1992;40(1):9–14.
49. Hautmann RE, Volkmer BG. Pregnancy and urinary diversion. Urol Clin N Am. 2007;34(1):71–88.
50. Taniguchi A, Kakizaki H, Murakumo M, Nonomura K, Koyanagi T. Management of pregnancy and delivery after augmentation cystoplasty. Nihon Hinyokika Gakkai Zasshi. 2002;93(1):39–43. Japanese.
51. Hill DE, Kramer SA. Management of pregnancy after augmentation cystoplasty. J Urol. 1990;144(2 Pt 2):457–9.
52. Quenneville V, Beurton D, Thomas L, Fontaine E. Pregnancy and vaginal delivery after augmentation cystoplasty. BJU Int. 2003;91(9):893–4.
53. Fenn N, Barrington JW, Stephenson TP. Clam enterocystoplasty and pregnancy. Br J Urol. 1995;75(1):85–6.
54. Clemetson CA. Ectopia vesicae and split pelvis. J Obstet Gynaecol Br Emp. 1958;65(6):973–81.
55. Hensle TW, Bingham JB, Reiley EA, Gleary-Goldman JE, Malone FD, Robinson JN. The urological care and outcome of pregnancy after urinary tract reconstruction. BJU Int. 2004;93(4):588–90.
56. Khaled H, Lahloubi NA, Rashad N. Review on renal cell carcinoma and pregnancy: a challenging situation. J Adv Res. 2016;7(4):575–80.
57. Schenker JG, Granat M. Pheochromocytoma and pregnancy: an updated appraisal. Aust N Z J Obstet Gynecol. 1982;22(1):1–10.
58. Lenders JW. Pheochromocytoma and pregnancy: a deceptive connection. Eur J Endocrinol. 2012;166(2):143–50.
59. Pace DE, Pm C, Schlachta CM, Mamazza J, Cadeddu MO, Poulin EC. Minimally invasive adrenalectomy for pheochromocytoma during pregnancy. Surg Lap Endos Perc Tech. 2002;12(2):122–5.
60. Mannelli M, Bemporad D. Diagnosis and management of pheochromocytoma during pregnancy. J Endocrinol Investig. 2002;25(6):567–71.
61. Dong D, Li H. Diagnosis and treatment of pheochromocytoma during pregnancy. J Matern Fetal Neonatal Med. 2014;27(18):1930–4.
62. Walker JL, Knight EL. Renal cell carcinoma in pregnancy. Cancer. 1986;58(10):2343–7.
63. Boussios S, Pavlidis N. Renal cell carcinoma in pregnancy: a rare coexistence. Clin Transl Oncol. 2014;16(2):122–7.
64. Pertia A, Managadze L, Chkhoutua A. Simultaneous nephron-sparing surgery and caesarian section for the treatment of renal cell carcinoma in pregnancy: case report and review of the literature. INTECH Open Access. 2012:436–42.
65. Chow W, McLaughlin JK, Mandel JS, Blot WJ, Niwa S, Fraumeni JF Jr. Reproductive factors and risk of renal cell carcinoma among women. Int J Cancer. 1995;60(3):321–4.
66. Loughlin KR. The management of urological malignancies during pregnancy. Br J Urol. 1995;76(5):639–44.
67. Dos Santos MM, Proenca SM, Res MI, Viana RM, Martins LM, Colaco JM, Nunes FM. Rotura espontanea de um angiomiolipoma durante a gravidez. [Spontaneous rupture of renal angiomyolipoma during pregnancy]. Rev Bras Ginecol Obstet. 2014;36(8):377–80. Portuguese.
68. Raft J, Lalot JM, Meistelman C, Longrois D. Role de la grossesse dans la rupture d'un angiomyolipome renal. [Influence of pregnancy on renal angiomyolipoma]. Gynecol Obstet Fertil. 2005;33(1):898–906. French.
69. Illescas Molina T, Montalvo Montes J, Contreras Cecilia E, Muñoz Muñiz M, González González A, Herraiz Martínez MA. Angiomiolipomas, esclerosis tuberosa y gestación: caso clínico. [Angiomyolipomas, tuberous sclerosis and pregnancy]. Ginecol Obstet Mex. 2009;77(8):380–6. Spanish.

22 Nonelective Orthopedic Procedures and Circumstances in Pregnant Patients

Annie Weber, Julie Yetso, and Farshad Adib

Pregnant Patients and Orthopedics

Pregnant patients present unique challenges to orthopedic physicians. While there are many orthopedic procedures that are not considered urgent, many injuries occur during pregnancy that need to be addressed in a timely manner. A recent American Congress of Obstetricians and Gynecologists (ACOG) committee on obstetric practice conceits that secondary to the difficulty of performing a large-scale randomized clinical trial, there are no data to allow for specific recommendations for non-obstetric surgery [1].

Recommendations made by the consensus of the committee include:

- A pregnant woman should never be denied indicated surgery, regardless of trimester.
- Elective surgery should be postponed until after delivery.
- If possible, nonurgent surgery should be performed in the second trimester when preterm contractions and spontaneous abortion are least likely.

Trauma affects 7% of pregnancies and requires admission in 4 of 1000 pregnancies. The incidence increases with advanced gestational age. Motor vehicle collisions are the most common cause of trauma, followed by falls and assault [2, 3]. Trauma is the leading non-obstetric cause of maternal death [4, 5]. Pregnant patients have both anatomic and physiologic changes that make treatment of musculoskeletal injuries more complex (Table 22.1). Pregnancy can also alter patient presentation. Physicians must also be aware of additional complications to the fetus including miscarriage, preterm labor, placental abruption, premature rupture of the membranes, fetal demise, and developmental delays [6–8].

The Eastern Association for the Surgery of Trauma (EAST) did a review of citations published between 1966 and 2003 and found 76 articles classified with both class II and class III research and came up with recommendations for diagnosis and management of injury in the pregnant patient, which are listed in Table 22.2 [4].

The initial primary management of a trauma patient should not be affected by pregnancy. Patients should be managed using advanced trauma life support algorithms, including assessing airway, breathing, and circulation [9]. Priority should be given to resuscitate the mother and stabilizing maternal vital signs because the mother's life has the greatest effect on the life of the fetus. If saving the fetus compromises the life of the mother, focus should be placed on the mother [4, 6, 10].

F. Adib (✉) · J. Yetso · A. Weber
Department of Orthopaedics, University of Maryland Medical Center, Baltimore, MD, USA
e-mail: Fadib1@umoa.umm.edu; jyetso@umoa.umm.edu; aweber@umoa.umm.edu

C. H. Nezhat (ed.), *Non-Obstetric Surgery During Pregnancy*,
https://doi.org/10.1007/978-3-319-90752-9_22

Table 22.1 Physiologic changes and related risk factors affecting diagnosis and treatment of pregnant patients with orthopedic injury [7, 8, 103]

Trimester	Physiologic change	Related risk factors
First	Major organogenesis Central nervous system development Increased WBC count Increased ESR	Radiosensitive development period Increased risk of teratogenesis Hypercoagulable state Increased risk of abortion with general anesthesia
Second	Relatively radioresistant fetal central nervous system Increased WBC count Increased ESR	Increased risk of supine aortocaval compression Hypercoagulable state Increased risk of abortion with general anesthesia Increased risk of seatbelt-related injury to the fetus
Third	Maternal blood volume increased by 40–50% Increased WBC count Increased ESR	Increased risk of supine aortocaval compression Increased risk of pregnancy-related osteoporosis Increased risk of seatbelt-related injury to the fetus

Table 22.2 The Eastern Association for the Surgery of Trauma (EAST) recommendations for diagnosis and management of injury in the pregnant patient [4]

Level	Recommendations
I	There are no level I standards
II	1. All pregnant women >20-week gestation who suffer trauma should have cardiotocographic monitoring for a minimum of 6 h. Monitoring should be continued, and further evaluation should be carried out if uterine contractions, non-reassuring fetal heart rate pattern, vaginal bleeding, significant uterine tenderness or irritability, serious maternal injury, or rupture of the amniotic membranes are present 2. Kleihauer-Betke analysis should be performed in all pregnant patients >12-week gestation
III	1. The best initial treatment for the fetus is the provision of optimum resuscitation of the mother and the early assessment of the fetus 2. All female patients of childbearing age with significant trauma should have a human chorionic gonadotropin (β-HCG) performed and be shielded for X-rays whenever possible 3. Concern about possible effects of high-dose ionizing radiation exposure should not prevent medically indicated maternal diagnostic X-ray procedures from being performed. During pregnancy, other imaging procedures not associated with ionizing radiation should be considered instead of X-rays when possible 4. Exposure to <5 rad has not been associated with an increase in fetal anomalies or pregnancy loss and is herein deemed to be safe at any point during the entirety of gestation 5. Ultrasonography and magnetic resonance imaging are not associated with known adverse fetal effects. However, until more information is available, magnetic resonance imaging is not recommended for use in the first trimester 6. Consultation with a radiologist should be considered for purposes of calculating estimated fetal dose when multiple diagnostic X-rays are performed 7. Perimortem cesarean section should be considered in any moribund pregnant woman of ≥24-week gestation 8. Delivery in perimortem cesarean sections must occur within 20 min of maternal death but should ideally start within 4 min of the maternal arrest. Fetal neurologic outcome is related to delivery time after maternal death 9. Consider keeping the pregnant patient tilted left side down 15° to keep the pregnant uterus off the vena cava and prevent supine hypotension syndrome 10. Obstetric consult should be considered in all cases of injury in pregnant patients

Imaging and Radiation

Multiple radiographic modalities are used for the diagnosis of musculoskeletal injuries. Many of the modalities including plain radiographs, CT scan, and fluoroscopy expose patients to ionizing radiation. Pregnant patients pose a dilemma to orthopedic surgeons as these modalities place both the mother and fetus at risk of ionizing radiation exposure, which can have both teratogenic and carcinogenic risks to a developing fetus [11]. It is well known that high levels of in utero radiation

Table 22.3 Summary of suspected in utero induced deterministic radiation effects[a] [104, 105]

Menstrual or gestational age	Conception age	mGy (<5 rad)	50–100 mGy (5–10 rad)	>100 mGy (>10 rad)
2 weeks (0–14 days)	Prior to conception	None	None	None
3rd and 4th weeks (15–28 days)	1st–2nd weeks (1–14 days)	None	Probably none	Possible spontaneous abortion
5th–10th weeks (29–70 days)	3rd–8th weeks (15–56 days)	None	Potential effects are scientifically uncertain and probably too subtle to be clinically detectable	Possible malformations increasing in likelihood as dose increases
11th–17th weeks (71–119 days)	9th–15th weeks (57–105 days)	None	Potential effects are scientifically uncertain and probably too subtle to be clinically detectable	Risk of diminished IQ or of mental retardation, increasing in frequency and severity with increasing dose
18th–27th weeks (120–189 days)	16th–25th weeks (106–175 days)	None	None	IQ deficits not detectable at diagnostic doses
>27 weeks (>189 days)	>25 weeks (>175 days)	None	None	None applicable to diagnostic medicine

[a]Stochastic risks are suspected, but data are not consistent [14]

exposure can result in deleterious developmental effects in the embryo and fetus [12, 13]. The likelihood of a harmful effect is proportional to the radiation dose and the gestational age of the embryo or fetus at the time of exposure [13, 14]. When diagnosing orthopedic conditions in pregnant patients, it is important to try and minimize radiation exposure to the fetus. Major organogenesis occurs during gestational weeks 3 through 8. The central nervous system is the most sensitive system to ionizing radiation. Because the risk to the fetus is based on both radiation dose and gestational age, the American College of Radiology (ACR) established guidelines for the management of pregnant patients. The American College of Radiology (ACR) and the Society for Pediatric Radiology (SPR) have practice parameters most recently updated in 2013, which describe the suspected radiation effects on the in utero fetus at predetermined ages depending on the radiation dose exposure (Table 22.3).

There are multiple factors that affect the exposure of a fetus to ionizing radiation during diagnostic imaging. Factors that affect the level of radiation include imaging protocol, imaging equipment, dose given, the mother's body habitus, and the distance between the fetus and the area that is being imaged [15]. As seen in Table 22.4, which lists the relative radiation exposure to the fetus during different radiographic modalities and for specified locations, the radiation exposure to the fetus during a plan radiograph of the upper extremity is ~300–600 times less than that of a plane radiograph of the lumbar spine [12, 16]. Careful shielding of the patient's abdomen and pelvis is recommended to reduce fetal radiation exposure for nonpelvic procedures [17].

According to the overall recommendations of the ACR and ACOG, when possible, ultrasound and MRI are the preferred imaging options for pregnant patients as they deliver nonionizing radiation to the patient and fetus and are not associated with known fetal effects [13].

Ultrasonography is commonly used for the diagnosis of multiple orthopedic conditions, including tendinosis and nerve compression, and evaluation of masses or foreign bodies [18–20]. Diagnostic ultrasound uses the production of sound waves to produce images of internal organs [21].

Magnetic resonance imaging (MRI) is frequently used as another noninvasive imaging method to diagnose a variety of musculoskeletal injuries. MRIs use a strong magnet to visualize soft tissue injuries such as meniscal, ligament, and tendon tears, as well as occult bone injuries [22]. MRI uses nonionizing radiation, and the

Table 22.4 Estimated radiation doses for common imaging modalities [12, 16]

Modality	Fetal dose (mGy)
Radiography	
Upper extremity	0.01
Lower extremity	0.01
Hips and femur	0.51–3.7
Pelvis	0.40–2.4
Abdomen	2.0–2.45
Chest	1
Lumbar spine	3.4–6.2
CT	
Pelvis	7.3–45
Chest	1–4.5
Lumbar spine	35
Head	0.5

The risk of major malformations is negligible in fetuses exposed to <50 mGy

American College of Radiology has no present data that has conclusively documented any deleterious effects of MR imaging exposure on the developing fetus. MR contrast agents should not be routinely used in pregnant patients as the risk to the fetus of gadolinium-based MR contrast agent administration remains unknown and may be harmful. Studies have demonstrated that gadolinium-based MR contrast agents readily pass through the placental barrier and enter the fetal circulation [23].

Non-traumatic Pelvic Injuries

Pubic symphysis separation can occur in pregnancy. The pubic symphysis is a synovial joint separated by a fibrocartilaginous disk and four pubic ligaments. Normal physiologic changes that occur during pregnancy to prepare for birth place a significant strain on the musculoskeletal system [24]. Widening of the pubic symphysis is considered normal during pregnancy, and 1- to 3-mm symphysis separation is usually asymptomatic. Pubic symphysis rupture is rare and can range in the literature from 1/300 to 1/30,000 pregnancies. Separation is considered pathologic at 10 mm. From an orthopedic standpoint, there are three categories of traumatic disruption of the pelvic ring: Type A pelvic lesion remains stable despite fracture. Type B lesion results from external and internal forces leading to "open-book" and "bucket-handle" fractures and is partially stable. Type C fractures from high-energy trauma lead to unstable fracture and complete disruption of pelvic ring. Pubic symphysis rupture is classified as a type B "open-book" lesion and treated according to staging, type, and associated musculoskeletal injuries of surrounding soft tissues.

Suggested risk factors associated with pubic symphysis separation include multiparity, macrosomia, cephalopelvic disproportion, joint laxity due to increased hormones in pregnancy, maternal connective tissue disorders, precipitous labor, malpresentation, prior pelvic trauma, McRoberts maneuver, and increased force on the pelvic ring, which can occur with a rapid second stage of labor or an intense uterine contraction [25–41]. However, there is some disagreement in the literature regarding the statistical significance of these factors [6, 9].

A clinical diagnosis of pubic symphysis rupture is often made with the following characteristics, which may include suprapubic pain, tenderness, and edema with pain radiating to the legs, hips, or back, a waddling gait, and sometimes having a palpable groove at the symphysis. Bone separation can be seen on a plain X-ray and can confirm diagnosis, but MRI can be a helpful adjunct.

Treatment for pubic symphysis rupture is usually conservative and has excellent outcomes in most cases. Treatment plans are typically based on the timing of diagnoses of the pubic symphysis rupture. If it is diagnosed during pregnancy, bed rest in lateral decubitus position with pelvic brace or girdle for support until delivery is recommended [6]. If diagnosed in the peripartum or postpartum period, it is recommended to try:

- Pelvic sling, belt, or binder.
- NSAIDs, narcotics, injection of steroid, chymotrypsin for pain control.
- Bed rest followed by PT.
- Open reduction and internal fixation with anterior plate for an intrapubic gap >25–40 mm. This has been shown to have less disadvantages than external fixator.

It is debated whether previous pubic symphysis separation changes the management of subsequent pregnancies [24]. Vaginal delivery is not contraindicated unless there has been fusion of the pubic symphysis, in which case cesarean delivery is the current recommendation.

Pelvic Fractures

A pelvic fracture during pregnancy is life-threatening to both the mother and the fetus [8]. There is limited literature addressing pelvic and acetabular fractures in pregnant women and equally limited publications regarding operative management of these injuries [8, 24, 42–45]. Pelvic fractures are usually caused by high-energy mechanisms, like motor vehicle accidents [8, 9, 42, 46]. Pelvic fracture can be an indicator of severe polytrauma, and there can be a high incidence of associated injuries, including head, thoracic, abdominal, and spinal injuries [8, 47]. Leggon et al. performed a literature review of pelvic fractures in pregnancy, including 101 cases analyzing factors influencing maternal and fetal mortality. The research concluded that pelvic and acetabular fractures in pregnant women are associated with a high maternal (9%) and fetal (35%) mortality rate. And fracture classification (simple vs. complex), fracture type (acetabular vs. pelvic), the trimester of pregnancy, and the era of literature reviewed did not influence mortality rates [42].

In the acute setting of a suspected pelvic fracture in a pregnant patient, standard ATLS protocols should be followed, and priority is given to resuscitation of the mother, which leads to better outcomes for the fetus [7–9]. Pelvic inlet and outlet radiographs can assess for and help differentiate fracture patterns in pelvic fractures. A Judet view of the pelvis is helpful if there is a questionable acetabular fracture [8]. Low-dose CT scan protocol may be helpful in diagnosis of fracture type and treatment plan, but the slot-scanning device (EOS system) is less irradiating than the CT exam [48, 49]. Emergent closed reduction of a type B (open book) pelvic fracture is performed by internally rotating the legs and compressing on the iliac wings to apply a pelvic sheet or binder. Taping the knees while the legs are internally rotated can also assist in holding the reduction [8]. Surgical indications for pelvic and acetabular fractures are the same for pregnant and nonpregnant patients [6–8]. If the fetus is determined to be viable and reduction and stability of the fracture are acceptable, the use of an external fixator may be a definitive treatment [8, 50]. Although no randomized control trial has been completed looking at preferred external fixation technique, the most common application appears to be in the supra-acetabular position [43]. As for all other procedures, operative positioning in a left lateral tilt position is preferred [51]. Application of the device should be done on a radiolucent table, and the use of image intensifier while taking intraoperative radiographs for pin positioning should be limited. In one case study examining a 29-year-old female 32 + 5wk pregnant with a closed anteroposterior type 2 pelvic fracture, the bars on the external fixation device were placed with the apex distal and deviated to the left side to allow the patient to sit up and avoid the gravid uterus [43, 51]. Temporary skeletal traction with elective delivery of the fetus at a more advanced gestational age is also an option if the fetus is close to 28 weeks, which would be followed by definitive operative treatment of the fracture [42]. It is more challenging to obtain adequate reduction during pelvic and acetabular fracture surgery when the injury is more than 3 weeks old [8, 52]. However, if the fetus is near term or full term, surgical fixation of a pubic symphysis injury can be performed at the same time as cesarean section by using the same Pfannenstiel incision [8, 53].

Musculoskeletal Tumors

Cancer is reported to occur in approximately 1 per 1000 pregnant women [54–56]. Because it is a rare occurrence, there is limited literature on how to treat musculoskeletal malignancy during pregnancy. One review of literature published by the Journal of Advanced Research in February 2016 reported only 137 well-documented bone or soft tissue sarcoma diagnoses in the English language between 1963 and 2014. Of those, 95 were variable soft tissue sarcomas, while 38 were osteosarcoma, chondrosarcoma, or Ewing's sarcoma [57]. Another retrospective study performed at one musculoskeletal tumor center treated 8 pregnant patients from a total of 240 soft tissue or bone sarcomas diagnosed between 2002 and 2010. Guidelines regarding the clinical diagnostics and acceptable as well as justifiable treatment of musculoskeletal tumors during pregnancy do not exist [58].

The clinical presentation of a musculoskeletal tumors most frequently presents with one or more of the five signs or symptoms, including soft tissue mass, painless bony mass, painful bone lesion, pathologic fracture, or as an incidental finding [59]. If a musculoskeletal tumor is suspected during pregnancy, imaging studies should be performed to aid in potential diagnosis. A potential delay in diagnosis may occur in pregnant patients secondary to concern about having diagnostic tests while pregnant [58]. The use of ultrasound for fetus screening in pregnancy is well established [60]. Therefore, its use in diagnostic imaging of soft tissue masses during pregnancy is preferred. In the *American College of Radiology Guidance Document for Safe MR Practices: 2007*, Kanal et al. state that if an MRI scan is necessary during pregnancy and the risk-benefit ratio is acceptable, it can be performed at any stage of pregnancy [61]. However, gadolinium is contraindicated during pregnancy since gadolinium-based MRI contrast agents diffuse across the placental barrier into the fetal circulation [16]. X-ray and CT scan radiation exposure should be avoided during pregnancy whenever possible, should be delayed until second trimester, and should be limited to <5 rad. A Consultation with a radiologist should be considered for purposes of calculating estimated fetal dose when multiple diagnostic X-rays are performed [4]. Nuclear medicine imaging should only be used in cases in which the results would change treatment management during pregnancy [62]. A biopsy can help confirm a diagnosis of cancer. Patients should always be referred to a specialist center prior to biopsy and that the biopsy should be carried out in the center where treatment is eventually going to be performed [63].

Once a diagnosis of musculoskeletal cancer is confirmed, a treatment plan should be discussed that is acceptable to both the mother and fetus [58]. Radiation is a treatment option, and many cancers can be treated with radiotherapy even during pregnancy [64]. Surgery can be considered but should be a multidisciplinary approach including obstetrics and anesthesia [65]. Chemotherapy, if recommended, is not advised to be withheld during pregnancy. Most chemotherapeutic drugs, however, are classified as category C and D. If diagnosed in the third trimester, chemotherapy may be held for several weeks until after delivery but is not recommended to be delayed for more than a few weeks [66]. Early delivery, if possible, is also a consideration to limit the exposure of the fetus to chemotherapeutic agents. The use of chemotherapeutic agents in the first trimester can have more severe fetal effect than the use in the second or third trimester. In these cases, termination of the pregnancy is a consideration. The use of chemotherapeutic agents in pregnancy may be modified from those used in a nonpregnant patient to reduce the adverse effects on the fetus [66].

Spinal Cord Compression and Thoracolumbar Spine Injury

As the female body changes in pregnancy and the body's center of gravity shifts anteriorly as the uterus enlarges, there is a change in the stresses applied to axial skeleton that predisposes women to increasing lordosis and sacroiliac joint laxity resulting in a high prevalence of back pain, especially in the lumbar spine [6]. One study showed that 61.8% of women reported at least moderately severe pregnancy-related back pain with 9% reporting complete disability secondary to their pain [6, 67]. Patient with prior back pain and multiparous women are at increased risk for pain during pregnancy. Although most women report a resolution of their back pain postpartum without any long-term effects, one study suggests that many women with chronic back pain report their initial symptoms during pregnancy [6, 68].

Although most back pain in pregnancy is benign and can be well controlled with noninvasive conservative measures, all back pains need to be fully evaluated with a thorough history and physical exam. Common symptomatic complaints associated with normal pregnancy can mask more ominous diagnoses, such as cauda equina syndrome, and lead to a delay in treatment. Cauda equina syndrome, the only absolute indication for spine surgery in pregnancy, is characterized by the compression of the lumbosacral nerve roots resulting in an acute or insidious onset of saddle anesthesia, urinary retention, urinary and bowel incontinence, radiating pain, numbness or paralysis in the lower extremities, and/or sexual dysfunction. Any suspicion of cauda equina syndrome warrants an immediate rectal exam and full motor sensory exam. With a concerning exam and history, an MRI should be performed as soon as possible to confirm diagnosis. MRI studies are level I supported in pregnancy, are not contraindicated in any stage of pregnancy, and should be the first-line imaging studies completed in pregnant women with concerning exams [69]. Although there are no general treatment guidelines specifically for spinal surgery in pregnant women, surgical intervention for the treatment of cauda equina syndrome should not be delayed, and indications for surgery on nonpregnant patients can typically be safely followed [69].

Less ominous than cauda equina syndrome but equally as important to evaluate for is lumbar back pain secondary to a herniated lumbar disk. Approximately 1:10,000 women during pregnancy experiences intractable pain in the sciatic nerve distribution secondary to herniated lumbar disk [69]. Patients report unilateral leg pain involving a dermatomal distribution with occasional associated paresthesia, reflex changes, muscle weakness, and/or positive straight leg raise depending on the nerve root being compressed [69]. This condition needs to be distinguished from pelvic girdle pain, which, unlike lumbar back pain, is not associated with a dermatomal distribution of pain and associated with the increased motion of the sacroiliac joints and pubic symphysis resulting in pain over these joints and occasional pain radiating down into the gluteal folds and thighs causing varying degrees of discomfort with standing, walking, or moving in bed, for example. Once, distinguished from pelvic girdle pain, an MRI can best help to define the degree of herniation. Conservative management is the first-line intervention and includes bed rest or decreased physical activity, footwear modification, analgesics such as acetaminophen (avoidance of NSAIDs—category C/D), muscles relaxants (cyclobenzaprine—only category B medication available), physical therapy, and/or lumbosacral brace. For continued uncontrolled pain after the implementation of noninvasive measures, the use of epidural steroid injections and nerve or regional blocks in the second and third trimesters can be considered. A short course of steroids may also have a role in the treatment of lumbar back pain, but long-term steroid use should be avoided in pregnancy due to its negative fetal effects [69]. Failure of conservative management resulting in severe debilitating pain and/or the association with progressive neurological deficits may be indicative of the need for surgical intervention and can be commonly safely performed.

Surgical intervention for cauda equina syndrome (CES) and for progressive motor weakness secondary to herniated lumbar disk is urgent and should not be delayed minimizing the risk of permanent neurological deficits [69, 70]. Complete CES is defined by painless urinary retention and overflow incontinence with loss of executive bladder control, usually associated with extensive saddle or genital sensory deficit as well [71]. This is compared to incomplete CES in which the patient has altered urinary sensation, loss of desire to void, poor urinary stream, and need to strain during voids. Incomplete CES has a better prognosis than complete CES, but urgent treatment in both cases is warranted [71]. Studies have shown even with complete CES cases can have around 70% socially acceptable long-term outcome [71].

Surgical intervention on the spine in women after their 34th–36th week of gestation can safely follow an induction of labor or cesarean section [69]. However, women of a younger gestational age should not wait until 34 weeks of gestation to undergo surgical intervention for urgent spine conditions. Surgical planning should encompass decreasing radiation exposure, optimizing surgical positioning, and administering the safest form of analgesic [69, 72]. The most common surgical intervention undergone in pregnancy for the above conditions is a laminectomy and microdiscectomy, with some case reports for endoscopic discectomy [69, 72–74]. Positioning of the pregnant patient needs to also be considered. During the first trimester and beginning of the second, a prone position continues to be safe. However, after the beginning of the second trimester, the lateral decubitus position or prone position on a specialized frame, such as the Relton-Hall laminectomy frame, is preferred to avoid pressure on the IVC and uterus [69, 72, 75]. Epidural anesthesia is the safest at any stage of gestation [69, 72, 73]. Monitoring of the fetal heart rate is recommended after 23 weeks but is controversial in younger than the 23rd week and contraindicated in younger than the 20th week.

As with many orthopedic conditions in pregnancy, there are no current guidelines to direct definitive care for spine trauma resulting in thoracolumbar spine fractures, and most surgical guidance are case report based, which have commented on various treatment plans that weigh the risk and benefits of surgical vs. nonsurgical intervention on a case-by-case basis. Surgical intervention exposes the mother and fetus to risks associated with positioning, blood loss, anesthesia, and radiation [76]. However, nonoperative management for unstable spine fractures until the patient is postpartum can preclude early immobilization and increase the risk for deep vein thrombosis, which is already elevated in pregnancy, pulmonary complications, and risk of neurologic decline [76]. Most agree that an unstable spinal column injury and incomplete neurological deficits are injuries warranting deeper consideration of acute surgical intervention. A study by Goller et al. showed that patients with spinal trauma and resulting paraplegia had a higher rate of fetal malformations and disabilities after birth secondary to (1) the trauma itself (i.e., direct trauma to the abdomen or indirect trauma from a flexion injury), (2) the immediate posttraumatic stress state of the patient, and (3) the resulting chronic infections and anemia in paraplegic pregnant patient (urinary tract infections, sacral decubitus infections) [77].

When planning surgery on the thoracolumbar spine, positioning for an anterior vs. posterior approach to the spine needs to be carefully evaluated. An anterior approach will allow the surgeon to avoid positioning that increases intraoperative pressure on the gravid uterus and IVC, but in women of later gestational age, the uterus can reach the xiphisternum making exposure of the thoracolumbar spine difficult [76]. A posterior approach can also be safely completed with the use of specialized frames, such as the Toronto frame and Relton-Hall laminectomy frame, to relieve extrinsic pressure off the IVC [78].

Extremity Injuries

Trauma resulting in extremity fractures is not unique to pregnant women, but there are several biologic and social considerations to keep in mind. In the general population, 1 in 6 women who present to fracture clinics has experienced intimate partner violence in the past year, and 1 in 50 women presents to fracture clinics with intimate partner violence-related injuries [79]. Pregnant women are at high risk for being or becoming a victim of domestic violence. Studies have shown that an upward of 40–60% of women are abused during pregnancy and many note that the abuse started when the patient discovered she was pregnant [79]. Physicians should be aware of the significance of inmate partner violence and screen at risk patients. Red flags include but are not limited to [79]:

- Concerning injury characteristics
  - Injury patterns inconsistent with history
  - Multiple injuries
  - Injuries at various stages of healing
  - Substantial delay between injury and presentation

- Concerning patient characteristics
  - Flat affect
  - Need for partner approval before answering questions
  - Partner answering for the patient
  - Uneasiness about leaving care facility
- Concerning partner characteristics
  - Partners that are overly attentive
  - Reluctance to allow for private discussion or exam of patient
  - Aggressive behavior
  - Speaking for the patient

Active intervention and care should be taken with all patients where intimate partner violence is a concern. It is important to be aware of the local resources available and refer patients as needed [79, 80].

The biological changes in the female body during pregnancy affect the level of circulating steroid hormones, which alter bone healing potential. In the first trimester, there is an increase in progesterone, followed by an increase in estrogens and prolactin in the second and third trimesters. It has been shown that progesterone alone and in combination with estradiol increases bone mineralization and formation [81], which has been shown to lead to early or accelerated union rates during pregnancy [82].

The changes in hormones and the potential for increased healing rates must be kept in mind for fracture management. When evaluating and treating tibial fractures in pregnant patients, the risks and benefits for nonoperative vs. operative management need to be weighed in each patient. Operative management with intramedullary nails (IMN), external fixation, or plating associated with surgical, anesthetic, positioning, and radiation risks needs to be discussed with the patient. Pregnant patients should be placed in the left lateral decubitus position for surgery or with a 15-degree bump under the right hip to allow the uterus to be displaced and offset the pressure from the IVC [9]. IMN have increased the risk of embolic events during surgery and radiation exposure that can reach ~50% of the total exposure for the case during the placement of the distal interlocks [83, 84] but have the highest union rates and allow the patient to immediately weight bear. External fixation, primarily used for damage control orthopedics, increases the difficulty of having a natural delivery and limits weight-bearing status [85]. Plating requires a period of partial weight bearing until union, increasing risks associated with immobilization. Similarly, nonoperative management with casting can have increased risks associated with the patient's non-weight-bearing status resulting in a higher risk of DVT, the innate nature of the cast making it difficult for the mother in positioning for a natural delivery, and can result in a cumbersome pre- and postdelivery immobilization scenario. Additionally, as discussed above, closed fractures managed initially nonoperatively with the intent of delayed surgical management until postpartum can become more difficult to treat due to the accelerated time to union and quicker callous formation [86].

Like most other non-axial fractures and sprains, the research is limited, and no definitive guidelines have been published. There have been several case reports on locked knees during pregnancy and on the treatment of ankle fractures and/or dislocations. An acutely locked knee, most commonly secondary to a bucket handle meniscus tear or loose body, is frequently considered to be of surgical urgency requiring a timely diagnostic and therapeutic arthroscopy [87–89]. Flik et al. reported two cases of women in their 7th month of a high-risk pregnancy with previous cerclage of the cervix and 16th week of an uncomplicated pregnancy, respectively, with an acutely locked knee. Both patients underwent evaluation by their obstetrician and anesthesiologist before proceeding with a knee arthroscopy under spinal anesthesia to treat the underlying lesions (loose body and bucket handle meniscal tear). Both women underwent an uncomplicated procedure, regained mobility of their knee, and proceeded with an uncomplicated pregnancy. As in all procedures, additional considerations need to be broached before proceeding with surgery on a pregnant female. In these cases, spinal anesthetic was used, which requires a smaller dose of anesthetic, provides a more generalized area of coverage, and allows for muscle relaxation, which can prove to be superior to a local injection or nerve block alone [89, 90]. Additionally, it should be noted that radiographic evaluation was not undergone prior to surgery and is not deemed necessary in these case as the physiologic mechanism of locking is associated with an intra-articular pathology in greater than 90% of all cases [87, 89].

Surgical management as seen in the case examples above can be safe for both the fetus and mother, but discussions and plans need to be in place with the team and patient for alternative interventions. For example, when looking at a case report of treatment of ankle fractures in a pregnant female reported by Schwarzkopf et al., they depict a case that required emergent obstetric intervention. As in ankle fractures in nonpregnant females, ankle fractures in pregnant females are addressed first with closed reduction and splinting at the initial encounter. The mortis and reduction are then analyzed for alignment and stability. A well-aligned, stable fracture can then be treated conservatively in a splint or cast [91, 92]. However, if the fracture is highly unstable on exam and there is incomplete mortis restoration or talar subluxation, surgery is recommended, and discussion with the patient and obstetrician should be had. In the Schwarzkopf et al. case report, they discussed a 36-week pregnant 39-year-old female that sustained a trimalleolar left ankle fracture dislocation (supination external rotation type IV) after ground-level fall. Her neurovascular exam was intact, initially closed reduced and splinted at the initial encounter. The reduction was highly unstable with incomplete mortis reduction and talar subluxation. She was taken to the operative room for open reduction internal fixation of her left ankle. She was placed in the left lateral decubitus position for spinal anesthesia and then repositioned supine with a bump under her right side to off-load the uterus from the IVC. The fetus was monitored with fetal heart rate monitoring, which began to show decelerations to 50–60 bpm even with positional changes. The decision was made to do an emergent cesarean section, which was safely performed, with the delivery of a healthy baby and then followed by ORIF of the left ankle and final splint placement. The splint was changed to a cast on postoperative day 4, and the patient was doing well through her 12 weeks follow-up [91]. This example shows that although surgery can be done in the pregnant patient, plans are required to be in place and obstetricians need to be readily available for emergent interventions.

Neuropathies

Carpal tunnel syndrome is the most common mononeuropathy in pregnancy thought to be secondary to increased fluid retention in the carpal tunnel, hypersensitivity of the median nerve, or progesterone hyperemia. The incidence has been reported anywhere from 2 to 60% in pregnant women, with approximately 85–95% of cases resolved 2–4 weeks after delivery or cessation of breastfeeding [6] and 4–6 months after presentation [9]. Therefore, carpal tunnel syndrome can be managed primarily in nonoperative, conservative manner. Conservative options mimic those in the nonpregnant population with night splints, simple analgesia, and cortisone injections. Only for severe, refractory cases is operative release of the carpal tunnel considered and is then performed under local anesthesia with or without a tourniquet [6, 9].

Cubital tunnel syndrome, much like carpal tunnel syndrome, is thought to be associated with fluid retention within the cubital tunnel causing extrinsic compression on the nerve. The McLennan et al. study of 1216 pregnancies reported a cubital tunnel syndrome incidence of 12% during pregnancy, with most symptoms appearing in the third trimester and resolving shortly after delivery [9, 93].

Meralgia paresthetica is also a well-recognized compressive neuropathy in pregnancy, where the lateral femoral cutaneous nerve is compressed by the increased abdominal girth of the pregnant female resulting in burning and/or tinging of the lateral thigh. Conservative treatment is the mainstay of treatment (analgesics, compression relief with position changes, or loose-fitting clothes), with ~85% of cases resolving within 4–6 months of presentation and most cases resolving after delivery with decreased abdominal girth and uterine size. Occasionally, severe symptoms may require local anesthetic injections or transdermal lidocaine patches [9].

Acute Septic Arthritis

Acute septic arthritis (SA) or infectious arthritis is uncommon in pregnancy but is an orthopedic emergency and is one of the most devastating and costly complications during pregnancy [94]. The most common cause is *Staphylococcus aureus* [94, 95], and large joints (hip, knee, and shoulder) are the most involved [94–96]. Significant risk factors for SA include diabetes mellitus, rheumatoid arthritis, drug abuse, a prior intra-articular steroid injection, and trauma [97]. Several case reports have also shown urinary tract infections to be another potential source of infection, resulting in SA after potential micro-trauma to the joint and subsequent seeding of the joint [98].

There is no "gold standard" for diagnosis of SA. Red flags include a history of acute onset of pain in the involved joint and a physical examination of the joint concerning for decreased range of motion, pain with range of motion, swelling, and redness [99, 100]. Diagnostic tests that increase the suspicion for septic arthritis in a native joint include increased erythrocyte sedimentation rate (ESR) and C-reactive protein (CRP) in the serum plus an elevated white blood cell (WBC) count >50,000/mm^3 and polymorphonuclear (PMN) leukocyte percentage of >70% in the aspirated synovial fluid [101]. Gram stain and cultures of the aspirated synovial fluid are often requested, but the treatment should not be delayed if the clinical suspicion for infection is high. Additionally, if the gram stain is negative, but the suspicion for bacterial arthritis is high, antibiotics should still be given [101]. Radiographs of the joint are neither sensitive nor specific in the acute phase but can reveal an acute effusion. As the disease progresses, radiographs of late or inadequately treated septic arthritis can show generalized joint destruction. Treatment includes arthroscopic or open irrigation and debridement plus intravenous antibiotic. Early diagnosis with safe and urgent irrigation and debridement of the involved joint [101] plus the multidisciplinary approach can help to decrease the mortality and morbidity of this devastating complication.

Diagnosis and management of septic arthritis in a native joint are challenging, and misdiagnosis can quickly lead to irreversible cartilage damage and arthropathy as well significant complications during pregnancies [95, 98]. Diagnosis can be difficult as joint pain during pregnancy can be secondary to a wide variety of pathologies, such as trauma, bacterial or viral arthropathy, collagen vascular diseases, or enteropathic arthritis, but due to the destructive nature of septic arthritis and the associated risks to the mother and fetus, SA must be ruled out [98]. Raiser et al. reported a case of left shoulder septic arthritis in a 30-year-old female at 28 weeks pregnant. This patient had asymptomatic bacteriuria at her initial prenatal visit and presented to the hospital at 28 weeks with persistent back pain, fever, positive urine analysis, and left shoulder pain. The patient was diagnosed with pyelonephritis, and the left shoulder joint aspiration cultures were significant for *Staphylococcus aureus*. The patient was treated with IV antibiotics, but ultimately her pregnancy was complicated by a preterm premature rupture of membranes and preterm labor. On postpartum day 5, the patient required an incision and drainage of the glenohumeral joint and distal clavicle resection for septic arthritis and osteomyelitis [98].

O'Leary et al. reported a case on a 23-year-old female who was 30 weeks pregnant with a 1-week history of pain and swelling over her left clavicle. On evaluation, her serum WBC was within normal limits and her ESR was elevated to 52 mm 1 h, and repeat labs revealed an increase in ESR to 87 mm 1 h and a CRP of 132.7 mg/L. MRI was obtained of her sternoclavicular joint, which revealed fluid within the joint. Concern for septic arthritis was high, an aspiration was obtained, and cultures were positive for *Neisseria gonorrhoeae*, which was sensitive to cefotaxime. Patient was treated with 1 week of intravenous antibiotics and then transitioned to oral antibiotics without difficulty and with full resolution of her symptoms without further complications

[102]. As seen in these two case studies, the outcomes of septic arthritis in pregnant patients can be very different depending on the source of the infection, the joint involved, and the timing of treatment.

Summary

Pregnancy presents a unique physiologic status for the female patient that guides but does not dictate patient care. Most orthopedic conditions in the pregnant female can be postponed until postpartum for definitive treatment and care, such as most peripheral neuropathies. For urgent or emergent conditions, however, treatment of the pregnant patient is guided by unique patient positioning on the operating table, radiation considerations, drug alternatives, anesthesia considerations, and biologic changes in the pregnant female.

References

1. ACOG Committee on Obstetric Practice. Committee Opinion No. 696: Nonobstetric surgery during pregnancy. Obstet Gynecol. 2017;129:777–8.
2. Mendez-Figueroa H, Dahlke JD, Vrees RA, Rouse DJ. Trauma in pregnancy: an updated systematic review. Am J Obstet Gynecol. 2013;209(1):1–10.
3. Murphy NJ, Quinlan JD. Trauma in pregnancy: assessment, management, and prevention. Am Fam Physician. 2014;90(10):717–22.
4. Barraco RD, Chiu WC, Clancy TV, Como JJ, Ebert JB, Hess LW, et al. Practice management guidelines for the diagnosis and management of injury in the pregnant patient: the EAST practice management guidelines work group. J Trauma. 2010;69(1):211–4.
5. Fildes J, Reed L, Jones N, Martin M, Barrett J. Trauma: the leading cause of maternal death. J Trauma. 1992;32(5):643–5.
6. Matthews LJ, McConda DB, Lalli TA, Daffner SD. Orthostetrics: management of orthopedic conditions in the pregnant patient. Orthopedics. 2015;38(10):e874–80.
7. Tejwani N, Klifto K, Looze C, Klifto CS. Treatment of pregnant patients with orthopaedic trauma. J Am Acad Orthop Surg. 2017;25(5):e90–e101.
8. Amorosa LF, Amorosa JH, Wellman DS, Lorich DG, Helfet DL. Management of pelvic injuries in pregnancy. Orthop Clin North Am. 2013;44(3):301–15, viii.
9. McGoldrick NP, Green C, Burke N, Quinlan C, Mccormack D. Pregnancy and the orthopaedic patient. Orthop Traumatol. 2012;26(3):212–9.
10. Petrone P, Marini CP. Trauma in pregnant patients. Curr Probl Surg. 2015;52(8):330–51.
11. Oxford CM, Ludmir J. Trauma in pregnancy. Clin Obstet Gynecol. 2009;52(4):611–29.
12. Groen RS, Bae JY, Lim KJ. Fear of the unknown: ionizing radiation exposure during pregnancy. Am J Obstet Gynecol. 2012;206(6):456–62.
13. Matzon JL, Lutsky KF, Ricci EK, Beredjiklian PK. Considerations in the radiologic evaluation of the pregnant orthopaedic patient. J Am Acad Orthop Surg. 2015;23(8):485–91.
14. Wang PI, Chong ST, Kielar AZ, Kelly AM, Knoepp UD, Mazza MB, et al. Imaging of pregnant and lactating patients: part 1, evidence-based review and recommendations. AJR Am J Roentgenol. 2012;198(4):778–84.
15. Lowe SA. Diagnostic radiography in pregnancy: risks and reality. Aust N Z J Obstet Gynaecol. 2004;44(3):191–6.
16. Chen MM, Coakley FV, Kaimal A, Laros RK Jr. Guidelines for computed tomography and magnetic resonance imaging use during pregnancy and lactation. Obstet Gynecol. 2008;112(2 Pt 1):333–40.
17. ACOG Committee on Obstetric Practice. ACOG Committee Opinion. Number 299, September 2004 (replaces No. 158, September 1995). Guidelines for diagnostic imaging during pregnancy. Obstet Gynecol. 2004;104(3):647–51.
18. Adelman S, Fishman P. Use of portable ultrasound machine for outpatient orthopedic diagnosis: an implementation study. Perm J. 2013;17(3):18–22.
19. Freire V, Guerini H, Campagna R, Moutounet L, Dumontier C, Feydy A, et al. Imaging of hand and wrist cysts: a clinical approach. AJR Am J Roentgenol. 2012;199(5):W618–28.
20. Sato J, Ishii Y, Noguchi H, Takeda M. Sonographic appearance of the flexor tendon, volar plate, and A1 pulley with respect to the severity of trigger finger. J Hand Surg [Am]. 2012;37(10):2012–20.
21. National Institute of Health. Ultrasound National Institute of Biomedical Imaging and Bioengineering 2016:1–2.
22. Crues J, Bydder G. Frontiers in musculoskeletal imaging. J Magn Reson Imaging. 2007;25(2):232–3.
23. Expert Panel on MR Safety, Kanal E, Barkovich AJ, Bell C, Borgstede JP, Bradley WG Jr, et al. ACR guidance document on MR safe practices: 2013. J Magn Reson Imaging. 2013;37(3):501–30.
24. Shnaekel KL, Magann EF, Ahmadi S. Pubic symphysis rupture and separation during pregnancy. Obstet Gynecol Surv. 2015;70(11):713–8.
25. Culligan P, Hill S, Heit M. Rupture of the symphysis pubis during vaginal delivery followed by two subsequent uneventful pregnancies. Obstet Gynecol. 2002;100(5, Part 2):1114–7.
26. Osterhoff G, Ossendorf C, Ossendorf-Kimmich N, Zimmermann R, Wanner GA, Simmen HP, et al.

Surgical stabilization of postpartum symphyseal instability: two cases and a review of the literature. Gynecol Obstet Investig. 2012;73:1–7.
27. Niederhauser A, Magann EF, Mullin PM, Morrison JC. Resolution of infant shoulder dystocia with maternal spontaneous symphyseal separation: a case report. J Reprod Med. 2008;53(1):62–4.
28. Kurzel RB, Au AH, Rooholamini SA, Smith W. Magnetic resonance imaging of peripartum rupture of the symphysis pubis. Obstet Gynecol. 1996;87(5 Pt 2):826–9.
29. Smith MW, Marcus PS, Wurtz LD. Orthopedic issues in pregnancy. Obstet Gynecol Surv. 2008;63(2):103–11.
30. Yoo JJ, Ha YC, Lee YK, Hong JS, Kang BJ, Koo KH. Incidence and risk factors of symptomatic peripartum diastasis of pubic Symphysis. J Korean Med Sci. 2014;29(2):281–6.
31. Wurdinger S, Humbsch K, Reichenbach JR, Peiker G, Seewald HJ, Kaiser WA. MRI of the pelvic ring joints postpartum: normal and pathological findings. J Magn Reson Imaging. 2002;15(3):324–9.
32. Valsky DV, Anteby EY, Hiller N, Amsalem H, Yagel S, Hochner-Celnikier D. Postpartum pubic separation associated with prolonged urinary retention following spontaneous delivery. Acta Obstet Gynecol Scand. 2006;85(10):1267–9.
33. Bhardwaj A, Nagandla K. Musculoskeletal symptoms and orthopaedic complications in pregnancy: pathophysiology, diagnostic approaches and modern management. Postgrad Med J. 2014;90(1066):450–60.
34. Kharrazi FD, Rodgers WB, Kennedy JG, Lhowe DW. Parturition-induced pelvic dislocation: a report of four cases. J Orthop Trauma. 1997;11(4):277–81; discussion 281–2.
35. Gräf C, Sellei RM, Schrading S, Bauerschlag DO. Treatment of parturition-induced rupture of pubic Symphysis after spontaneous vaginal delivery. Case Rep Obstet Gynecol. 2014;2014:3.
36. McElin TW, Scott R. Rupture of the symphysis pubis during spontaneous labor. Obstet Gynecol. 1965;25:401–4.
37. Luger EJ, Arbel R, Dekel S. Traumatic separation of the symphysis pubis during pregnancy: a case report. J Trauma. 1995;38(2):255–6.
38. Snow RE, Neubert AG. Peripartum pubic symphysis separation: a case series and review of the literature. Obstet Gynecol Surv. 1997;52(7):438–43.
39. Jain N, Sternberg LB. Symphyseal separation. Obstet Gynecol. 2005;105(5 Pt 2):1229–32.
40. Phupong V, Sudjai D. Vaginal delivery with intrapartum pubic symphysis separation. A case report. J Reprod Med. 2003;48(4):296–8.
41. Dunivan GC, Hickman AM, Connolly A. Severe separation of the pubic symphysis and prompt orthopedic surgical intervention. Obstet Gynecol. 2009;114(2 Pt 2):473–5.
42. Leggon RE, Wood GC, Indeck MC. Pelvic fractures in pregnancy: factors influencing maternal and fetal outcomes. J Trauma. 2002;53(4):796–804.
43. Pape HC, Pohlemann T, Gansslen A, Simon R, Koch C, Tscherne H. Pelvic fractures in pregnant multiple trauma patients. J Orthop Trauma. 2000;14(4):238–44.
44. Dunlop DJ, McCahill JP, Blakemore ME. Internal fixation of an acetabular fracture during pregnancy. Injury. 1997;28(7):481–2.
45. Yosipovitch Z, Goldberg I, Ventura E, Neri A. Open reduction of acetabular fracture in pregnancy. A case report. Clin Orthop Relat Res. 1992;282:229–32.
46. Atkinson A, Sherlock D, Hux C. Pelvic fracture in the pregnant patient. J Med Cases. 2013;4(4):201–3.
47. Papadopoulos IN, Kanakaris N, Bonovas S, Triantafillidis A, Garnavos C, Voros D, et al. Auditing 655 fatalities with pelvic fractures by autopsy as a basis to evaluate trauma care. J Am Coll Surg. 2006;203(1):30–43.
48. Abdennebi BA, Aubry S, Ounalli L, Fayache MS, Delabrousse E, Petegnief Y. Comparative dose levels between CT-scanner and slot-scanning device (EOS system) in pregnant women pelvimetry. Phys Med. 2017;33:77–86.
49. Ramac JP, Vidjak V, Skegro D, Duic Z, Blaskovic D, Erdelez L, et al. Low-dose computed tomography in a pregnant woman with a ruptured pseudoaneurysm of the abdominal aorta. Coll Antropol. 2015;39(3):785–90.
50. Mattox KL, Goetzl L. Trauma in pregnancy. Crit Care Med. 2005;33(10 Suppl):S385–9.
51. Stohlner V, Gill JR, Murphy CG, Carrothers AD. Definitive use of external fixation for pelvic ring injuries (open book/APC2) in pregnancy. BMJ Case Rep. 2015. https://doi.org/10.1136/bcr-2015-212690.
52. Letournel E, Judet E, editors. Fractures of the acetabulum. 2nd ed. New York: Springer; 1993.
53. Almog G, Liebergall M, Tsafrir A, Barzilay Y, Mosheiff R. Management of pelvic fractures during pregnancy. Am J Orthop (Belle Mead NJ). 2007;36(11):E153–9.
54. Cardonick E, Usmani A, Ghaffar S. Perinatal outcomes of a pregnancy complicated by cancer, including neonatal follow-up after in utero exposure to chemotherapy: results of an international registry. Am J Clin Oncol. 2010;33(3):221–8.
55. Brewer M, Kueck A, Runowicz CD. Chemotherapy in pregnancy. Clin Obstet Gynecol. 2011;54(4):602–18.
56. Donegan WL. Cancer and pregnancy. CA Cancer J Clin. 1983;33(4):194–214.
57. Zarkavelis G, Petrakis D, Fotopoulos G, Mitrou S, Pavlidis N. Bone and soft tissue sarcomas during pregnancy: a narrative review of the literature. J Adv Res. 2016;7(4):581–7.
58. Postl LK, Gradl G, von Eisenhart-Rothe R, Toepfer A, Pohlig F, Burgkart R, et al. Management of musculoskeletal tumors during pregnancy: a retrospective study. BMC Womens Health. 2015;15:48-015-0204-3.
59. OrthopaedicsOne—The Orthopaedic Knowledge Network. Musculoskeletal Tumors—The Five

Presenting Complaints. 2011. http://www.orthopaedicsone.com/x/toAaB. Accessed 19 Nov 2017.
60. Siddique J, Lauderdale DS, TJ VW, Lantos JD. Trends in prenatal ultrasound use in the United States: 1995 to 2006. Med Care. 2009;47(11):1129–35.
61. Molho RB, Kollender Y, Issakov J, Bickels J, Flusser G, Azem F, et al. The complexity of management of pregnancy-associated malignant soft tissue and bone tumors. Gynecol Obstet Investig. 2008;65(2):89–95.
62. Maxwell C, Barzilay B, Shah V, Wunder JS, Bell R, Farine D. Maternal and neonatal outcomes in pregnancies complicated by bone and soft-tissue tumors. Obstet Gynecol. 2004;104(2):344–8.
63. Grimer R, Carter S, Spooner D, Sneath R. Diagnosing musculoskeletal tumours. Sarcoma. 2001;5(2):89–94.
64. Kal HB, Struikmans H. Radiotherapy during pregnancy: fact and fiction. Lancet Oncol. 2005;6(5):328–33.
65. Ni Mhuireachtaigh R, O'Gorman DA. Anesthesia in pregnant patients for nonobstetric surgery. J Clin Anesth. 2006;18(1):60–6.
66. Leslie KK, Koil C, Rayburn WF. Chemotherapeutic drugs in pregnancy. Osdtet Gynecol Clin N Am. 2005;32:627–40.
67. Stapleton DB, MacLennan AH, Kristiansson P. The prevalence of recalled low back pain during and after pregnancy: a South Australian population survey. Aust N Z J Obstet Gynaecol. 2002;42(5):482–5.
68. Ostgaard HC, Andersson GB, Karlsson K. Prevalence of back pain in pregnancy. Spine (Phila Pa 1976). 1991;16(5):549–52.
69. Di Martino A, Russo F, Denaro L, Denaro V. How to treat lumbar disc herniation in pregnancy? A systematic review on current standards. Eur Spine J. 2017;26(Suppl 4):496–504.
70. LaBan MM, Perrin JC, Latimer FR. Pregnancy and the herniated lumbar disc. Arch Phys Med Rehabil. 1983;64(7):319–21.
71. Gardner A, Gardner E, Morley T. Cauda equina syndrome: a review of the current clinical and medico-legal position. Eur Spine J. 2011;20(5):690–7.
72. Han IH, Kuh SU, Kim JH, Chin DK, Kim KS, Yoon YS, et al. Clinical approach and surgical strategy for spinal diseases in pregnant women: a report of ten cases. Spine (Phila Pa 1976). 2008;33(17):E614–9.
73. Brown MD, Brookfield KF. Lumbar disc excision and cesarean delivery during the same anesthesia. A case report. J Bone Joint Surg Am. 2004;86-A(9):2030–2.
74. Brown MD, Levi AD. Surgery for lumbar disc herniation during pregnancy. Spine (Phila Pa 1976). 2001;26(4):440–3.
75. Kathirgamanathan A, Jardine AD, Levy DM, Grevitt MP. Lumbar disc surgery in the third trimester–with the fetus in utero. Int J Obstet Anesth. 2006;15:181–2.
76. Sonawane DV, Nemade PS, Chandanwale A, Pawar E, Jagtap SA. Management of fracture dorso-lumbar spine in a pregnant female by surgery in prone position. Eur Spine J. 2017. https://doi.org/10.1007/s00586-017-5127-2.
77. Goller H, Paeslack V. Pregnancy damage and birth-complications in the children of paraplegic women. Paraplegia. 1972;10(3):213–7.
78. Relton JE, Hall JE. An operation frame for spinal fusion. A new apparatus designed to reduce haemorrhage during operation. J Bone Joint Surg (Br). 1967;49(2):327–32.
79. Zillmer DA. Domestic violence: the role of the orthopaedic surgeon in identification and treatment. J Am Acad Orthop Surg. 2000;8(2):91–6.
80. Madden K, Bhandari M. Cochrane in CORR(Â®): screening women for intimate partner violence in healthcare settings (review). Clin Orthop Relat Res. 2016;474(9):1897–903.
81. Burnett CC, Reddi AH. Influence of estrogen and progesterone on matrix-induced endochondral bone formation. Calcif Tissue Int. 1983;35(4–5):609–14.
82. Ahmad MA, Kuhanendran D, Kamande IW, Charalambides C. Accelerated tibial fracture union in the third trimester of pregnancy: a case report. J Med Case Rep. 2008;2:44.
83. Sugarman ID, Adam I, Bunker TD. Radiation dosage during AO locking femoral nailing. Injury. 1988;19(5):336–8.
84. Levin PE, Schoen RW Jr, Browner BD. Radiation exposure to the surgeon during closed interlocking intramedullary nailing. J Bone Joint Surg Am. 1987;69(5):761–6.
85. Rudge W, Newman K, Trompeter A. Fractures of the tibial shaft in adults. Orthop Traumatol. 2014;28(4):243–55.
86. Bozkurt C, Report SBC. A surgical opinion in a 36-week pregnant with tibia fracture: intramedullary nailing. Case Rep Orthop. 2016;2016:1–4.
87. Allum RL, Jones JR. The locked knee. Injury. 1986;17(4):256–8.
88. Critchley IJ, Bracey DJ. The acutely locked knee—is a manipulation worth while? Injury. 1985;16(4):281–3.
89. Flik K, Anderson K, Urmey W, Wickiewicz T. Locked knee during pregnancy. Arthroscopy. 2004;20(2):191–5.
90. Steinberg ES, Santos AC. Surgical anesthesia during pregnancy. Int Anesthesiol Clin. 1990;28(1):58–66.
91. Schwarzkopf R, Gross SC, Coopersmith A, Gidumal R. Ankle fracture surgery on a pregnant patient complicated by intraoperative emergency caesarian section. Case Rep Orthop. 2013;2013:1–4.
92. Isik C, Tahta M, Isik D, Ustu Y, Ugurlu M, Bozkurt N, et al. Management of ankle sprains during pregnancy: evaluation of 96 cases. Ulus Travma Acil Cerrahi Derg. 2014;20(4):275–80.
93. McLennan HG, Oats JN, Walstab JE. Survey of hand symptoms in pregnancy. Med J Aust. 1987;147(11–12):542–4.

94. Karaaslan F, Mermerkaya MU, Yurdaku E, Tanin O. Bilateral septic knee arthritis after treatment of an ectopic pregnancy with methotrexate. Int Med Case Rep J. 2015;13(8):33–5.
95. Sharff KA, Richards EP, Townes JM. Clinical management of septic arthritis. Curr Rheumatol Rep. 2013;15:6(332).
96. DeNoble PH, Gonzalez D. Septic arthritis of the shoulder following elective termination of pregnancy. J Shoulder Elb Surg. 2009;18(5):e5–e6.
97. Almoujahed MO, Khatib R, Baran J. Pregnancy-associated pyogenic sacroiliitis: case report and review. Infect Dis Obstet Gynecol. 2003;11:53–7.
98. Raiser S, Davidson K, Walsh A, Egerman R. Septic arthritis of the shoulder complicating pregnancy. Case Rep Obstet Gynecol. 2014;2014:1–3.
99. Parvizi J, Gehrke T. Definition of Periprosthetic joint infection. J Arthroplast. 2014;29(7):1331.
100. Parsaei S, Lane MA, Marschall J. Prosthetic joint infection: diagnosis and treatment. Inf Dis Board Rev Manual. 2014;15(3):1–18.
101. Shirtliff ME, Mader JT. Acute septic arthritis. Clin Microbiol Rev. 2002;15(4):527–44.
102. O'Leary AJ, Tejura H, Latibeaudiere M, Edwards G. Gonorrhoea infection presenting in pregnancy with septic arthritis of the sternoclavicular joint. J Obstet Gynaecol. 2006;26(4):373–4.
103. Flik K, Kloen P, Toro JB, Urmey W, Nijhuis JG, Helfet DL. Orthopaedic trauma in the pregnant patient. J Am Acad Orthop Surg. 2006;14(3):175–82.
104. Valentin J. Biological effects after prenatal irradiation (embryo and fetus). ICRP. 2003;90:1–200.
105. International Commission on Radiological Protection. Pregnancy and medical radiation. ICRP. 2000;84:1–43.

Part IV

Gynecological Surgery During Pregnancy

Myomas and Pregnancy

23

Tracy Nicole Hadnott and William Parker

Epidemiology

Uterine fibroids are the most common benign tumor in women of reproductive age and have been identified in up to 50% of women in this population [1–3]. Myomas are observed in 5–10% of women with infertility [1, 4, 5], and 2–13% of pregnancies are affected by fibroids [6]. As such, in-depth understanding of the pathophysiology and clinical manifestations of fibroids is integral to the care of women before, during, and after pregnancy.

Myomas and Fertility

The International Federation of Gynecology and Obstetrics (FIGO) has standardized fibroid classification based upon anatomic location (Table 23.1). Submucosal fibroids can be Type 0, 1, or 2, with Type 0 fibroids localized completely within the endometrial cavity. Type 1 fibroids have less than 50% extension into the myometrium, while Type 2 fibroids extend more than 50% into the myometrium. FIGO Type 5, 6, and 7 fibroids have similar classification relative to the subserosal, while Types 3 and 4 are intramural. Extrauterine fibroids are classified as Type 8.

T. N. Hadnott
Division of Reproductive Endocrinology and Infertility, Department of Reproductive Medicine, University of California, San Diego, La Jolla, CA, USA

W. Parker (✉)
Department of Ob Gyn and Reproductive Sciences, UC San Diego, La Jolla, CA, USA
e-mail: wparker@ucla.edu

Fibroid Location

The presence of submucosal fibroids decreases fertility rates, and removal of submucosal fibroids improves fertility. Subserosal fibroids do not affect fertility rates, and removal does not increase fertility. Intramural fibroids may slightly decrease fertility rates, but removal has not been shown to increase fertility. A systemic review of 23 studies of the relationship between fibroids

Table 23.1 FIGO fibroid location classification system

FIGO type	Location
0	Intracavitary
1	Submucosal with less than 50% myometrial extension
2	Submucosal with more than 50% myometrial extension
3	Intramural with endometrial contact, no extension into cavity
4	Intramural without endometrial/serosal contact
5	Subserosal with more than 50% myometrial extension
6	Subserosal with less than 50% myometrial extension
7	Subserosal, pedunculated

C. H. Nezhat (ed.), *Non-Obstetric Surgery During Pregnancy*,
https://doi.org/10.1007/978-3-319-90752-9_23

and infertility assessed the effect of submucosal and non-submucosal fibroids on implantation rate, clinical pregnancy rate, ongoing pregnancy/live birth rate, and spontaneous abortion rates [7]. This study found that clinical pregnancy rates were decreased 65–70% among women with submucosal myomas as compared to those with non-submucosal myomas. There was no evidence for significant effect of intramural and subserosal fibroids on fertility, as there was no difference in clinical pregnancy rate of women with non-submucosal fibroids as compared to controls without fibroids. It is important to note, however, that this review is limited by the imaging modalities used to document the location of fibroids. Only four of the included studies used careful inspection with saline infusion sonography or hysteroscopy to diagnose presence of fibroids with a submucosal component. All other studies utilized less accurate methods of assessment, such as transvaginal sonography or hysterosalpingogram alone.

A retrospective study of 369 women, including 94 with non-submucosal fibroids, found no difference in implantation rate, clinical pregnancy rate, spontaneous abortion, or ectopic pregnancy following in vitro fertilization in women with non-submucosal fibroids versus those without fibroids [8]. Therefore, until intramural fibroids are shown to decrease fertility rate, or myomectomy to improve fertility, surgical management of asymptomatic intramural myomas should be approached with caution.

Myomas and Endometrial Receptivity

Endometrial expression of transcription factors required for normal embryo implantation is altered in the presence of submucosal fibroids. Several studies have described the role of homeobox domain-containing transcription factors HOXA10 and HOXA11 on uterine factor infertility associated with endometrial receptivity [9–14]. HOXA10 and HOXA11 in humans, and analogously Hoxa10 and Hoxa11 in mice, are expressed in mid-secretory-phase endometrium in response to estrogen and progesterone expression. This expression has been shown to be altered in several conditions associated with diminished fertility, including polycystic ovary syndrome, endometriosis, hydrosalpinges, and submucosal fibroids.

In normal endometrium, BMP-2 upregulates HOXA10 expression. This process is absent in endometrial cells of women with submucosal fibroids. In vitro studies have demonstrated that TGF-β 3 (transforming growth factor beta 3) is overexpressed in myoma cells as compared to myometrium and TGF-β 3 downregulates expression of receptors for BMP-2 with a resultant decrease in HOXA10 expression. Endometrial expression of HOXA10 and HOXA11 in particular has been shown to be reduced throughout the endometrial cavities of humans with submucosal myomas, while intramural myomas were not associated with altered expression [15]. The result is altered decidualization and inhibition of embryo implantation and decreased uterine factor fertility [16–18].

Myomas and Pregnancy

Prevalence

Myomas are observed in 2–13% of pregnancies [6]. In one prospective cohort of 4271 women with first-trimester or post-miscarriage sonograms, the prevalence of fibroids among pregnant women was 18% in African-American women, 8% in white women, and 10% in Hispanic women [19]. The mean size of the fibroids was 2.5 cm. Clinical exam detects 42% of fibroids greater than 5 cm during pregnancy but only 12.5% when they are less than 5 cm [20].

Natural History of Myomas During Pregnancy

Pathophysiology

Uterine fibroids are benign, monoclonal tumors arising from the smooth muscle of the uterine myometrium. Growth of myomas is stimulated by sex steroid hormones estrogen and progesterone, in addition to local growth factors and angiogenesis that may all be upregulated during pregnancy.

Fibroid Growth During Pregnancy

Most fibroids do not increase in size during pregnancy. Pregnancy has a variable and unpredictable effect on fibroid growth, likely dependent upon individual differences in gene expression, circulating growth factors, and fibroid-localized receptors. A prospective study of 36 pregnant women with a single fibroid discovered during routine first trimester sonographic screening found that 69% of the women had no increase in fibroid volume when followed sonographically throughout pregnancy at 2–4-week intervals [21]. In the 31% of women noted to have an increase in volume, the greatest increase occurred before the tenth week of gestation. There was no relationship between initial fibroid volume and fibroid growth during gestational periods. A reduction in fibroid size was observed 4 weeks after delivery.

Degeneration During Pregnancy

Degeneration is the most common myoma-related complication in pregnancy but only occurs in about 5% of pregnant women based on clinical symptoms and sonographic evidence of fibroid degeneration [22]. Among 113 women followed during pregnancy with serial sonography, 10 (9%) developed anechoic spaces or coarse heterogeneous patterns consistent with fibroid degeneration. Seven of ten women also had severe abdominal pain requiring hospitalization, consistent with clinical symptoms of degeneration. No sonographic changes were noted in the other 103 women. A small study of women with fibroid-associated pain during pregnancy identified a shortened hospital stay and decreased rate of readmission in those who utilized ibuprofen [23].

Pregnancy Outcomes in Women with Fibroids

Obstetric Outcomes

The majority of women with myomas have no adverse pregnancy outcomes related to having fibroids [24]. Two studies report large populations of pregnant women examined with routine second trimester sonography with follow-up care and delivery within the same institution. In one study of 12,600 pregnant women, including 167 with fibroids, only cesarean delivery was more common among women with fibroids compared to those with no fibroids (23% vs. 12%). Incidence of preterm delivery, premature rupture of membranes, fetal growth restriction, placenta previa, placental abruption, postpartum hemorrhage, or retained placenta was not significantly different in the two groups [25].

The second study of 15,104 pregnancies, including 401 women with fibroids, found no increased risk of premature rupture of membranes, operative vaginal delivery, chorioamnionitis, or endomyometritis [26]. However, there were slight increases in the absolute risks of preterm delivery (19.2% vs. 12.7%), placenta previa (3.5% vs. 1.8%), and postpartum hemorrhage (8.3% vs. 2.9%). Cesarean section was again found to be more common (49.1% vs. 21.4%).

Numerous studies have reported that antepartum bleeding is more common in pregnancies with fibroids [20, 27–29]; however, several studies have subsequently been unable to confirm this association [6, 22, 30]. Pooled cumulative data suggest the risk of abruption is increased threefold (3.0% vs. 0.9%) in women with fibroids. Fibroid proximity to the placenta may be a significant factor in risk of bleeding and/or abruption during pregnancy.

While the relative risk of adverse outcomes including preterm delivery, placenta previa, and postpartum hemorrhage may be slightly increased in the setting of fibroids, the absolute risk of these outcomes remains low. In addition, the risks should be weighed with regard to the risks of myomectomy, including risks of surgery and anesthesia, infection, discomfort, time away from work or family during recovery, and expense.

Fetal Outcomes

Fetal injury attributed to mechanical compression by fibroids has been reported to occur very infrequently. A search of the PubMed database from 1980 to 2010 revealed one case of fetal head anomalies with fetal growth restriction [31], one case of a postural deformity [32], one case of a limb reduction [33], and one case of fetal head deformation with torticollis [34].

Surgical Management of Women with Myomas

Any decision to perform a myomectomy in order to prevent adverse pregnancy outcomes should take into account the risks of surgery, anesthesia, postoperative adhesions, increased likelihood of subsequent cesarean delivery, and concerns about discomfort, expense, and time away from work or family.

Preconception Myomectomy

Evaluation

While history and physical examination remain the gold standard for evaluation of any medical condition, imaging modalities including magnetic resonance imaging (MRI) and saline infusion sonography (SIS) are of particular utility in the diagnosis of uterine fibroids.

Transvaginal pelvic ultrasound is the first-line imaging modality for clinical diagnosis of uterine fibroids with sensitivity of 95–100% in uteri less than 10 weeks gestational size [35]. However, MRI and SIS offer theoretical improvements in the evaluation of Type 0 and Type 1 myomas. In preparation for minimally invasive myomectomy including robotic, laparoscopic, or hysteroscopic myomectomy with limited intraoperative tactile sensation, MRI helps determine the appropriateness of minimally invasive approach and may help the surgeon avoid missing any myomas during surgery.

When compared with hysterectomy specimens, a study of transvaginal ultrasonography, saline infusion ultrasonography, hysteroscopy, and MRI found that MRI had superior sensitivity in detecting myomas [36]. MRI more accurately identified submucosal myomas with 100% sensitivity and 91% specificity, compared with transvaginal ultrasonography (sensitivity 83%, specificity 90%), SIS (sensitivity 90%, specificity 89%), and hysteroscopy (sensitivity 82%, specificity 87%). The improved sensitivity and specificity of MRI and SIS as compared to transvaginal ultrasonography are integral to the accurate evaluation of myoma size and location relative to the endometrium, thus guiding preoperative planning and choice of surgical approach.

Surgical Approach

Abdominal Myomectomy: Surgical Technique

Abdominal myomectomy can usually be performed via a vertical midline or low transverse incision. For a large uterus, a transverse fascial incision may be extended cephalad at the lateral borders of the rectus increasing pelvic access while also avoiding transection of the ilioinguinal nerve. Midline separation of the fascia away from rectus muscles to the level of the umbilicus also allows for more space to exteriorize the uterus.

Several perioperative techniques have been described to minimize intraoperative blood loss at the time of abdominal myomectomy. First, a tourniquet may be placed around the lower uterine segment and infundibulopelvic ligaments after exteriorizing the uterus. Such a tourniquet may be released and replaced intermittently to allow reperfusion of the uterus and ovaries and to allow for assessment of hemostasis intraoperatively. Secondly, injection of dilute vasopressin (20 U diluted in 100 mL of saline) into the pseudo-capsule of each fibroid just prior to each serosal incision may be utilized, with monitoring of cardiovascular status. Additional pharmacologic techniques to minimize intraoperative blood loss involve administration of a preoperative vaginal misoprostol dose of 400 μg and tranexamic acid 10 mg/kg intravenously at the time of incision. A Cochrane review of randomized, controlled trials found significant reductions in blood loss with each of these techniques [37].

On rare occasions, for women with low preoperative hemoglobin levels and the possibility of greater than 500 mL operative blood loss due to numerous fibroids, an autologous blood recovery system may be considered. Such devices suction blood from the operative field, combine the recovered whole blood with heparinized saline, and store the solution for potential reinfusion. If necessary, the system filters and centrifuges the solution of heparinized saline and whole blood to a hematocrit of approximately 50% for delivery back to the patient intravenously. Use of blood collected as opposed to non-autologous blood transfusion may thus avoid risks of infection and transfusion reaction. Importantly, the oxygen transport capacity of salvaged red blood cells is equal to, or better than, stored allogeneic red cells, and the survival of red blood cells appears to be at least as good as transfused allogeneic red cells [38].

Uterine incisions can be made in coronal, transverse, or sagittal plane. Because fibroids distort the normal vascular architecture of the uterus, attempts to avoid arcuate vessels of the uterus are futile [39]. However, careful planning and placement of uterine incisions can avoid inadvertent extension of the incision to the uterine cornua, ascending uterine vessels, or visible large arteries and veins. Extension of uterine incisions through the myometrium and the entire pseudo-capsule until the fibroid is clearly seen assists in identification of a less vascular surgical plane. Further, placement of uterine incisions to facilitate removal of multiple fibroids through each incision while avoiding tunneling through the myometrium to distant fibroids may both maximize hemostasis and minimize postoperative adhesion formation.

Another method for adhesion prevention during abdominal myomectomy involves use of solid barriers, such as the sodium hyaluronate-based Seprafilm (carboxymethylcellulose). One prospective study randomized 127 women undergoing abdominal myomectomy to treatment or no treatment with Seprafilm [40]. During second-look laparoscopy, women treated with Seprafilm had significantly fewer adhesions and lower adhesion severity scores than untreated women.

Laparoscopic Myomectomy: Outcomes in Comparison to Abdominal Myomectomy

Currently available instruments make laparoscopic myomectomy feasible, although the wide application of this approach is limited by the size and number of fibroids and by the technical difficulty of the procedure and of laparoscopic suturing. While robotic myomectomy may obviate some of these technical problems, the added cost and longer operating times associated with this approach must be considered.

A systematic review of randomized controlled trials of laparoscopic versus open myomectomy included six studies with a total of 576 patients [41]. Laparoscopic myomectomy was associated with longer operating times but reduced operative blood loss, less postoperative decline in hemoglobin levels, reduced postoperative pain, more patients fully recuperated at day 15, and fewer overall complications. Major complications, pregnancy rates, and new appearance of fibroids were comparable in the two groups.

Case series without controls show the feasibility of laparoscopic surgery in women with large fibroids. In a series of 144 women with mean fibroid diameter of 7.8 cm (range, 5–18 cm), only 2 women required conversion to laparotomy [42]. In another series of 332 consecutive women undergoing laparoscopic myomectomy for symptomatic fibroids as large as 15 cm, only 3 women required conversion to laparotomy [43].

Laparoscopic Myomectomy: Surgical Technique

Port placement should be based on the position and size of the fibroids to be removed. Laparoscopic suturing may be more ergonomic if there are two ports on either the patient's right side for right-handed surgeons or on the left side of the patient for left-handed surgeons. A 12-mm port is placed approximately 2 cm medial to the iliac crest for suture access, and another 5-mm lateral port near the level of the umbilicus [44]. A left upper quadrant approach may be used for initial access when uterine size is near or above the umbilicus [45].

As with abdominal myomectomy, vasopressin may be injected into the fibroid. Transverse uterine incisions may permit more ergonomic suturing. After incision over the fibroid is carried through the pseudo-capsule down to the myoma, the fibroid can be grasped with a tenaculum for traction and the plane between the myometrium and fibroid dissected until the fibroid is free. Bleeding vessels in the myometrial defect may be desiccated sparingly with bipolar electrosurgical devices taking care to avoid devascularization of the myometrium and thereby compromising wound healing. Delayed absorbable sutures should be placed in one, two, or three layers, as needed, adhering to accepted surgical technique for abdominal myomectomy. Morcellation of the fibroid with an electromechanical device may be accomplished under direct visualization. Interceed, an oxidized regenerated cellulose barrier for adhesion prevention that can be used laparoscopically, has been associated with significantly reduced risk of adhesions in a Lancet meta-analysis [46].

Hysteroscopic Myomectomy: Surgical Technique

Resection of Type 0 and Type 1 fibroids can be accomplished under direct visualization using a hysteroscope and continuous flow of distension fluid through the uterine cavity. The electrosurgical working element of a hysteroscopy may utilize an oscillating blade or electrodes for monopolar or bipolar electrosurgery. Monopolar electrodes require nonconducting distending solution (sorbitol 5%, sorbitol 3% with mannitol 0.5%, or glycine 1.5%), while bipolar electrodes can be used with saline.

Cervical dilation is usually required prior to insertion of the hysteroscope. Preoperative misoprostol may facilitate easier dilation [44]. With electrosurgery, a cutting loop is passed beyond the fibroid and cutting activated only when the loop is moving toward the surgeon and in direct view. When using an oscillating hysteroscopic morcellator, the device may be applied directly to the endometrium overlying the pathology for resection. Fibroids should be resected down to the level of the surrounding myometrium, and, if fertility is desired, care should be taken to avoid excessive electrosurgical damage to normal myometrium. Often, the remaining portion of the fibroid will be expressed into the uterine cavity by uterine contractions, allowing further resection. Flow of distension fluid may also be reduced to decrease intrauterine pressure and facilitate delivery of any remaining intramural component of a myoma into the endometrial cavity. Fragments of fibroid may be removed from the cavity automatically with use of a hysteroscopic morcellator, and in the case of fibroids removed using electrosurgery, fragments may be removed with grasping forceps or by capturing the fragments with the loop and extracting them through the cervix.

Cervical dilatation or insertion of the hysteroscope can cause uterine perforation, as can deep myometrial resection. The risk of perforation increases with deeper myometrial involvement of the fibroid [47]. Often the first sign of perforation is a rapid increase in the fluid deficit. Careful inspection of the uterine cavity should be undertaken to look for brisk bleeding or bowel injury. If no injury is apparent, the procedure should be terminated, and the patient should be observed and may be discharged if stable [48]. In some cases, repeat resection may be required after a few weeks, as the remaining portion of the fibroid is expressed into the uterine cavity by uterine contractions. If a perforation occurs during activation of the electrode, then laparoscopy should be performed to carefully inspect for bowel or bladder injury.

Intravascular absorption of distending media is a potentially dangerous complication which can result in pulmonary edema, hyponatremia, heart failure, cerebral edema, and even death [49]. Careful monitoring of the fluid deficit is important, and a fluid deficit of 750 mL during surgery should serve as a warning sign, with planned termination of the procedure. The American Association of Gynecologic Laparoscopists guidelines recommend a maximum fluid deficit of 2500 mL for isotonic media in healthy adults, 1000 mL for hypotonic solution in healthy adults, and a universal maximum of 750 mL in elderly patients or those with cardiovascular disease [49]. Electrolytes should be assessed and corrected if necessary and diuretics considered. Risk factors for fluid overload include resection of fibroids with deep intramural extension or prolonged operating time. The use of normal saline combined with bipolar energy reduces the risk of hyponatremia, but a fluid deficit over 1500 mL can lead to cardiac overload [50].

Uterine Rupture After Preconception Myomectomy

Two studies comprising 236,454 deliveries reported 209 instances of uterine rupture, with only 4 cases attributable to prior myomectomy [51, 52]. Since the number of women who had a previous myomectomy was not known, the incidence of rupture in these studies could not be determined. One retrospective study of 412 women who had abdominal myomectomies reported only 1 woman with uterine rupture (0.2%) [53]; however, this study is limited by absence of information on the size and position of fibroids removed at the time of myomectomy.

Operative technique, instrument selection, and energy source used during laparoscopic myomectomy may differ from those employed during laparotomy and thus may have differing effects on pregnancy outcome. A study of 19 cases of uterine rupture during pregnancy following laparoscopic myomectomy found that almost all cases involved deviations from standard surgical technique as described for abdominal myomectomy [54]. In seven cases, the uterine defect was not repaired, in three cases it was repaired with a single suture, in four cases it was repaired with only one layer of suture, and in one case, only the serosa was closed. In only three cases was a multilayered closure employed. In 16 of the cases, monopolar or bipolar energy was used for hemostasis.

While definite conclusions and recommendations regarding appropriate technique for laparoscopic myomectomy must await proper study of myometrial wound healing, it appears prudent for surgeons to adhere to time-tested techniques developed for abdominal myomectomy, including multilayered closure of myometrium (for other than superficial uterine defects) and limited use of electrosurgery for hemostasis. However, even with ideal surgical technique, individual wound healing characteristics may predispose to uterine rupture.

Fertility Outcomes Following Preconception Myomectomy

A systematic review found no difference in clinical pregnancy rate, spontaneous abortion, or the combined outcome of ongoing pregnancy/live birth rate among women with intramural fibroids that did and did not undergo myomectomy [7]. The same study did find a twofold increase in relative risk of clinical pregnancy in those who underwent myomectomy for submucosal myomas vs. those who did not undergo myomectomy. Although the numbers are small, the ongoing pregnancy/live birth rate and spontaneous abortion rate did not differ between those who underwent surgical management for submucosal fibroids and those with submucosal myomas left in situ.

Myomectomy During Pregnancy

Myomectomy Prior to Delivery

Given risk of rare but clinically significant complications, uterine surgery during pregnancy should be avoided if possible. However, the available literature suggests that myomectomy during pregnancy may be considered in limited situations of refractory pain and/or undesired pregnancy.

A limited number of case studies and case series exist in the literature to describe technique, risks, and benefits of myomectomy during pregnancy, but prior to delivery. The largest case series available includes 18 patients who underwent abdominal myomectomy between 6 and 24 weeks gestation. One woman was lost to follow-up, and one suffered a miscarriage. The remaining 16 patients delivered healthy babies between the 36th and 41st week, 14 delivered by cesarean section and 2 vaginally [55]. Another case series of women undergoing abdominal myomectomy during pregnancy reported six antepartum abdominal myomectomies for evaluation and management of abdominal masses with refractory pain [56]. The report also described three gravid hysterectomies for women with undesired pregnancy and known symptomatic fibroids during their preconception state. Surgical morbidity in this series was reported as being minimal, with five of six patients delivering at term following antepartum myomectomy.

One series of laparoscopic myomectomy during pregnancy describes three cases occurring at 19–20 weeks' gestation for symptomatic, torsed, pedunculated myomas which were refractory to conservative management. All procedures were uncomplicated and followed by subsequent full-term deliveries (two vaginal and the remaining via cesarean) [57]. The limited remaining data consists of single case reports of laparoscopic myomectomies performed between 10 and 25 weeks' gestation [58–66]. While most published cases were uncomplicated, one case at 17 weeks' gestation was complicated by septic necrosis of the myometrium, with a 7 × 2 cm area of exposed amniotic membranes noted during a second look exploratory laparotomy on postoperative day 6. The patient eventually underwent elective cesarean delivery at 37 weeks, with incidental placenta accreta noted adjacent to the myomectomy site [63].

Myomectomy During Cesarean Delivery

Myomectomy at the time of cesarean delivery is traditionally avoided due to associated risk of intraoperative hemorrhage; however, some limited data suggest that the procedure may be safely considered under specific circumstances. One retrospective cohort study compared 111 who underwent cesarean myomectomy to 257 women with documented fibroids during an index pregnancy who underwent cesarean delivery alone and found similar rates of obstetric hemorrhage in the two groups (12.8% vs. 12.6%). There were no identified differences in risk of operative time, postoperative length of stay, or postpartum fever [67].

A longitudinal panel study followed 63 women who underwent trans-endometrial myomectomy during an index cesarean delivery with an elective cesarean delivery with the subsequent pregnancy [68]. This study found similar composite outcomes of surgical blood loss, blood transfusion, postoperative fever, length of hospital stays, and mean adhesion scores across the two cesarean deliveries. Rates of uterine rupture, placental abruption, placenta previa, and placenta accrete were similar across deliveries. The mean gestational age at birth and newborn weight were increased in the second pregnancy following cesarean myomectomy at the first.

These studies suggest that, contrary to current dogma, myomectomy at the time of cesarean delivery may be considered in the appropriately selected patient without clinically significant impact on surgical outcome.

References

1. Buttram VC Jr, Reiter RC. Uterine leiomyomata: etiology, symptomatology, and management. Fertil Steril. 1981;36(4):433–45.
2. Wallach EE, Vlahos NF. Uterine myomas: an overview of development, clinical features, and management. Obstet Gynecol. 2004;104(2):393–406.
3. Practice Committee of American Society for Reproductive Medicine in Collaboration with Society of Reproductive, S. Myomas and reproductive function. Fertil Steril. 2008;90(5 Suppl):S125–30.
4. Donnez J, Jadoul P. What are the implications of myomas on fertility? A need for a debate? Hum Reprod. 2002;17(6):1424–30.
5. Verkauf BS. Myomectomy for fertility enhancement and preservation. Fertil Steril. 1992;58(1):1–15.
6. Klatsky PC, Tran ND, Caughey AB, Fujimoto VY. Fibroids and reproductive outcomes: a systematic literature review from conception to delivery. Am J Obstet Gynecol. 2008;198(4):357–66.
7. Pritts EA, Parker WH, Olive DL. Fibroids and infertility: an updated systematic review of the evidence. Fertil Steril. 2009;91(4):1215–23.
8. Klatsky PC, Lane DE, Ryan IP, Fujimoto VY. The effect of fibroids without cavity involvement on ART outcomes independent of ovarian age. Hum Reprod. 2007;22(2):521–6.
9. Taylor HS. The role of HOX genes in human implantation. Hum Reprod Update. 2000;6(1):75–9.
10. Taylor HS, Vanden Heuvel GB, Igarashi P. A conserved Hox axis in the mouse and human female reproductive system: late establishment and persistent adult expression of the Hoxa cluster genes. Biol Reprod. 1997;57(6):1338–45.
11. Bagot CN, Kliman HJ, Taylor HS. Maternal Hoxa10 is required for pinopod formation in the development of mouse uterine receptivity to embryo implantation. Dev Dyn. 2001;222(3):538–44.
12. Bagot CN, Troy PJ, Taylor HS. Alteration of maternal Hoxa10 expression by in vivo gene transfection affects implantation. Gene Ther. 2000;7(16):1378–84.
13. Taylor HS, Daftary GS, Selam B. Endometrial HOXA10 expression after controlled ovarian hyperstimulation with recombinant follicle-stimulating hormone. Fertil Steril. 2003;80(Suppl 2):839–43.
14. Satokata I, Benson G, Maas R. Sexually dimorphic sterility phenotypes in Hoxa10-deficient mice. Nature. 1995;374(6521):460–3.
15. Rackow BW, Taylor HS. Submucosal uterine leiomyomas have a global effect on molecular determinants of endometrial receptivity. Fertil Steril. 2010;93(6):2027–34.

16. Lee KY, Jeong JW, Wang J, Ma L, Martin JF, Tsai SY, et al. Bmp2 is critical for the murine uterine decidual response. Mol Cell Biol. 2007;27(15):5468–78.
17. Paria BC, Ma W, Tan J, Raja S, Das SK, Dey SK, et al. Cellular and molecular responses of the uterus to embryo implantation can be elicited by locally applied growth factors. Proc Natl Acad Sci U S A. 2001;98(3):1047–52.
18. Sinclair DC, Mastroyannis A, Taylor HS. Leiomyoma simultaneously impair endometrial BMP-2-mediated decidualization and anticoagulant expression through secretion of TGF-beta3. J Clin Endocrinol Metab. 2011;96(2):412–21.
19. Laughlin SK, Baird DD, Savitz DA, Herring AH, Hartmann KE. Prevalence of uterine leiomyomas in the first trimester of pregnancy: an ultrasound-screening study. Obstet Gynecol. 2009;113(3):630–5.
20. Muram D, Gillieson M, Walters JH. Myomas of the uterus in pregnancy: ultrasonographic follow-up. Am J Obstet Gynecol. 1980;138(1):16–9.
21. Rosati P, Exacoustos C, Mancuso S. Longitudinal evaluation of uterine myoma growth during pregnancy. A sonographic study. J Ultrasound Med. 1992;11(10):511–5.
22. Lev-Toaff AS, Coleman BG, Arger PH, Mintz MC, Arenson RL, Toaff ME. Leiomyomas in pregnancy: sonographic study. Radiology. 1987;164(2):375–80.
23. Katz VL, Dotters DJ, Droegemeuller W. Complications of uterine leiomyomas in pregnancy. Obstet Gynecol. 1989;73(4):593–6.
24. Segars JH, Parrott EC, Nagel JD, Guo XC, Gao X, Birnbaum LS, et al. Proceedings from the Third National Institutes of Health International Congress on Advances in Uterine Leiomyoma Research: comprehensive review, conference summary and future recommendations. Hum Reprod Update. 2014;20(3):309–33.
25. Vergani P, Ghidini A, Strobelt N, Roncaglia N, Locatelli A, Lapinski RH, et al. Do uterine leiomyomas influence pregnancy outcome? Am J Perinatol. 1994;11(5):356–8.
26. Qidwai GI, Caughey AB, Jacoby AF. Obstetric outcomes in women with sonographically identified uterine leiomyomata. Obstet Gynecol. 2006;107(2 Pt 1):376–82.
27. Exacoustos C, Rosati P. Ultrasound diagnosis of uterine myomas and complications in pregnancy. Obstet Gynecol. 1993;82(1):97–101.
28. Coronado GD, Marshall LM, Schwartz SM. Complications in pregnancy, labor, and delivery with uterine leiomyomas: a population-based study. Obstet Gynecol. 2000;95(5):764–9.
29. Winer-Muram HT, Muram D, Gillieson MS, Ivey BJ, Muggah HF. Uterine myomas in pregnancy. Can Med Assoc J. 1983;128(8):949–50.
30. Roberts WE, Fulp KS, Morrison JC, Martin JN Jr. The impact of leiomyomas on pregnancy. Aust N Z J Obstet Gynaecol. 1999;39(1):43–7.
31. Chuang J, Tsai HW, Hwang JL. Fetal compression syndrome caused by myoma in pregnancy: a case report. Acta Obstet Gynecol Scand. 2001;80(5):472–3.
32. Joo JG, Inovay J, Silhavy M, Papp Z. Successful enucleation of a necrotizing fibroid causing oligohydramnios and fetal postural deformity in the 25th week of gestation. A case report. J Reprod Med. 2001;46(10):923–5.
33. Graham JM Jr. The association between limb anomalies and spatially-restricting uterine environments. Prog Clin Biol Res. 1985;163C:99–103.
34. Romero R, Chervenak FA, DeVore G, Tortora M, Hobbins JC. Fetal head deformation and congenital torticollis associated with a uterine tumor. Am J Obstet Gynecol. 1981;141(7):839–40.
35. Dueholm M, Lundorf E, Hansen ES, Ledertoug S, Olesen F. Accuracy of magnetic resonance imaging and transvaginal ultrasonography in the diagnosis, mapping, and measurement of uterine myomas. Am J Obstet Gynecol. 2002;186(3):409–15.
36. Dueholm M, Lundorf E, Hansen ES, Ledertoug S, Olesen F. Evaluation of the uterine cavity with magnetic resonance imaging, transvaginal sonography, hysterosonographic examination, and diagnostic hysteroscopy. Fertil Steril. 2001;76(2):350–7.
37. Kongnyuy EJ, Wiysonge CS. Interventions to reduce haemorrhage during myomectomy for fibroids. Cochrane Database Syst Rev. 2011;(11):CD005355.
38. Ansell J, Parrilla N, King M, Fournier L, Szymanski I, Doherty P, et al. Survival of autotransfused red blood cells recovered from the surgical field during cardiovascular operations. J Thorac Cardiovasc Surg. 1982;84(3):387–91.
39. Discepola F, Valenti DA, Reinhold C, Tulandi T. Analysis of arterial blood vessels surrounding the myoma: relevance to myomectomy. Obstet Gynecol. 2007;110(6):1301–3.
40. Diamond MP. Reduction of adhesions after uterine myomectomy by Seprafilm membrane (HAL-F): a blinded, prospective, randomized, multicenter clinical study. Seprafilm Adhesion Study Group. Fertil Steril. 1996;66(6):904–10.
41. Jin C, Hu Y, Chen XC, Zheng FY, Lin F, Zhou K, et al. Laparoscopic versus open myomectomy—a meta-analysis of randomized controlled trials. Eur J Obstet Gynecol Reprod Biol. 2009;145(1):14–21.
42. Malzoni M, Rotond M, Perone C, Labriola D, Ammaturo F, Izzo A, et al. Fertility after laparoscopic myomectomy of large uterine myomas: operative technique and preliminary results. Eur J Gynaecol Oncol. 2003;24(1):79–82.
43. Andrei B, Crovini G, Rosi A. Uterine myomas: pelviscopic treatment. Clin Exp Obstet Gynecol. 1999;26(1):44–6.
44. Koh C, Janik G. Laparoscopic myomectomy: the current status. Curr Opin Obstet Gynecol. 2003;15(4):295–301.
45. Agarwala N, Liu CY. Safe entry techniques during laparoscopy: left upper quadrant entry using the ninth intercostal space—a review of 918 procedures. J Minim Invasive Gynecol. 2005;12(1):55–61.
46. Ten Broek RPG, Stommel MWJ, Strik C, van Laarhoven CJHM, Keus F, van Goor H. Benefits

and harms of adhesion barriers for abdominal surgery: a systematic review and meta-analysis. Lancet. 2014;383(9911):48–59.
47. Murakami T, Hayasaka S, Terada Y, Yuki H, Tamura M, Yokomizo R, et al. Predicting outcome of one-step total hysteroscopic resection of sessile submucous myoma. J Minim Invasive Gynecol. 2008;15(1):74–7.
48. Indman PD. Hysteroscopic treatment of submucous myomas. Clin Obstet Gynecol. 2006;49(4):811–20.
49. AAGL Advancing Minimally Invasive Gynecology Worldwide, Munro MG, Storz K, Abbott JA, Falcone T, Jacobs VR, et al. AAGL practice report: practice guidelines for the Management of Hysteroscopic Distending Media: (replaces Hysteroscopic Fluid Monitoring Guidelines. J Am Assoc Gynecol Laparosc. 2000;7:167–168.). J Minim Invasive Gynecol. 2013;20(2):137–48.
50. Murakami T, Tamura M, Ozawa Y, Suzuki H, Terada Y, Okamura K. Safe techniques in surgery for hysteroscopic myomectomy. J Obstet Gynaecol Res. 2005;31(3):216–23.
51. Palerme GR, Friedman EA. Rupture of the gravid uterus in the third trimester. Am J Obstet Gynecol. 1966;94(4):571–6.
52. Garnet JD. Uterine rupture during pregnancy. An analysis of 133 patients. Obstet Gynecol. 1964;23:898–905.
53. Obed JY, Omigbodun A. Rupture of the uterus in patients with previous myomectomy and primary caesarean section scars: a comparison. J Obstet Gynaecol. 1996;16(1):16–21.
54. Parker WH, Einarsson J, Istre O, Dubuisson JB. Risk factors for uterine rupture after laparoscopic myomectomy. J Minim Invasive Gynecol. 2010;17(5):551–4.
55. De Carolis S, Fatigante G, Ferrazzani S, Trivellini C, De Santis L, Mancuso S, et al. Uterine myomectomy in pregnant women. Fetal Diagn Ther. 2001;16(2):116–9.
56. Burton CA, Grimes DA, March CM. Surgical management of leiomyomata during pregnancy. Obstet Gynecol. 1989;74(5):707–9.
57. Maccio A, Madeddu C, Kotsonis P, Caffiero A, Desogus A, Pietrangeli M, et al. Three cases of laparoscopic myomectomy performed during pregnancy for pedunculated uterine myomas. Arch Gynecol Obstet. 2012;286(5):1209–14.
58. Pelosi MA, Pelosi MA 3rd, Giblin S. Laparoscopic removal of a 1500-g symptomatic myoma during the second trimester of pregnancy. J Am Assoc Gynecol Laparosc. 1995;2(4):457–62.
59. Ardovino M, Ardovino I, Castaldi MA, Monteverde A, Colacurci N, Cobellis L. Laparoscopic myomectomy of a subserous pedunculated fibroid at 14 weeks of pregnancy: a case report. J Med Case Rep. 2011;5:545.
60. Son CE, Choi JS, Lee JH, Jeon SW, Bae JW, Seo SS. A case of laparoscopic myomectomy performed during pregnancy for subserosal uterine myoma. J Obstet Gynaecol. 2011;31(2):180–1.
61. Fanfani F, Rossitto C, Fagotti A, Rosati P, Gallotta V, Scambia G. Laparoscopic myomectomy at 25 weeks of pregnancy: case report. J Minim Invasive Gynecol. 2010;17(1):91–3.
62. Melgrati L, Damiani A, Franzoni G, Marziali M, Sesti F. Isobaric (gasless) laparoscopic myomectomy during pregnancy. J Minim Invasive Gynecol. 2005;12(4):379–81.
63. Sentilhes L, Sergent F, Verspyck E, Gravier A, Roman H, Marpeau L. Laparoscopic myomectomy during pregnancy resulting in septic necrosis of the myometrium. BJOG. 2003;110(9):876–8.
64. Saccardi C, Visentin S, Noventa M, Cosmi E, Litta P, Gizzo S. Uncertainties about laparoscopic myomectomy during pregnancy: a lack of evidence or an inherited misconception? A critical literature review starting from a peculiar case. Minim Invasive Ther Allied Technol. 2015;24(4):189–94.
65. Currie A, Bradley E, McEwen M, Al-Shabibi N, Willson PD. Laparoscopic approach to fibroid torsion presenting as an acute abdomen in pregnancy. JSLS. 2013;17(4):665–7.
66. Kosmidis C, Pantos G, Efthimiadis C, Gkoutziomitrou I, Georgakoudi E, Anthimidis G. Laparoscopic excision of a pedunculated uterine leiomyoma in torsion as a cause of acute abdomen at 10 weeks of pregnancy. Am J Case Rep. 2015;16:505–8.
67. Roman AS, Tabsh KM. Myomectomy at time of cesarean delivery: a retrospective cohort study. BMC Pregnancy Childbirth. 2004;4(1):14.
68. Huang SY, Shaw SW, Su SY, Li WF, Peng HH, Cheng PJ. The impact of a novel transendometrial approach for caesarean myomectomy on obstetric outcomes of subsequent pregnancy: a longitudinal panel study. BJOG. 2018;125(4):495–500. https://doi.org/10.1111/1471-0528.14798. [Epub ahead of print].

Adnexal Mass in Pregnancy

24

Farr Nezhat, Pengfei Wang, and Andrea Tinelli

Introduction

The increasing use of antenatal ultrasound and screening during the first trimester of pregnancy has led to an increased incidence of adnexal pathology diagnosis. Even though adnexal pathology is most commonly associated with masses of ovarian origin (Fig. 24.1), it can also include causes of tubal and paratubal pathology (Fig. 24.2) as well as pedunculated fibroids (Fig. 24.3) that in imaging may appear to be extrauterine. Occasionally non-gynecological pathology such as dilated loops of bowel or bowel tumors sitting in the pelvic can be mistaken as an adnexal mass. The incidence of an adnexal mass in pregnancy ranges in the literature from 1 to 10% depending on the patient population, the frequency of ultrasound use, and the gestational age at the time of the ultrasound exam [1–3]. The incidence of adnexal masses is higher in the first trimester (Fig. 24.4) because most of them are of benign functional ovarian cysts and approximately two-thirds will resolve spontaneously later in pregnancy [3]. The risk of malignancy of an adnexal mass is very low. A population-based study of more than 4 million obstetrical patients reported that the incidence of ovarian cancer is as low as 0.93% [4]. Another report of 130 cases of adnexal masses, which were managed surgically, estimated a higher risk of invasive or borderline malignancy at 6.1% [5]. Other risks associated with adnexal masses during pregnancy that contribute to maternal morbidity include torsion, rupture, bleeding,

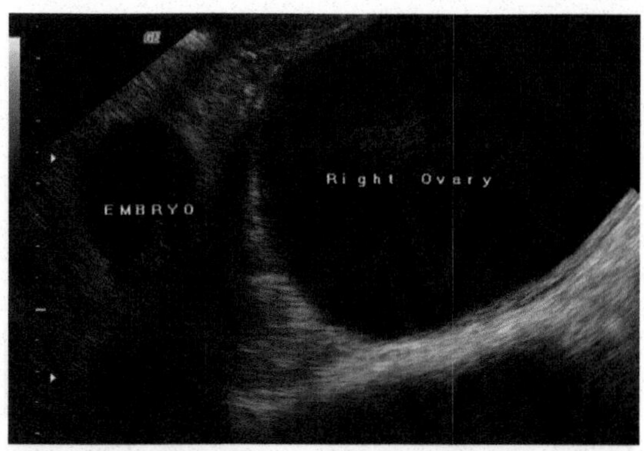

Fig. 24.1 Ultrasonographic image showing a right ovarian cyst in pregnancy at 6 week and 5 days of pregnancy

F. Nezhat (✉)
Department of Obstetrics and Gynecology, Weill Cornell Medical College of Cornell University, New York, NY, USA
e-mail: farr@farrnezhatmd.com

P. Wang
Department of Obstetrics and Gynecology, NYU-Winthrop Hospital, Mineola, NY, USA

A. Tinelli
Department of Obstetrics and Gynecology, Division of Experimental Endoscopic Surgery, Imaging, Technology and Minimally Invasive Therapy, Vito Fazzi Hospital, Lecce, Italy

C. H. Nezhat (ed.), *Non-Obstetric Surgery During Pregnancy*,
https://doi.org/10.1007/978-3-319-90752-9_24

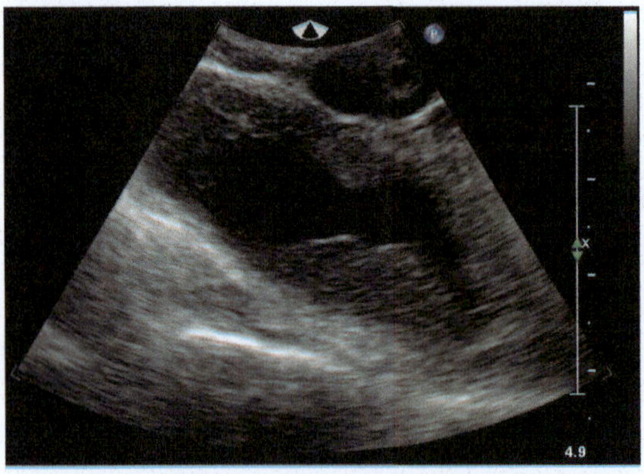

Fig. 24.2 Ultrasonographic image showing a left sactosalpinx in early pregnancy

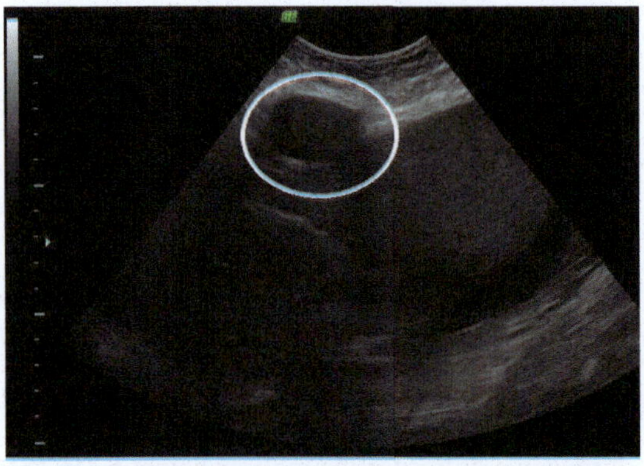

Fig. 24.3 Ultrasonographic image showing a pedunculated anterior fibroid of 4 cm of diameter (in the with ring), in a pregnant at 30 weeks of pregnancy

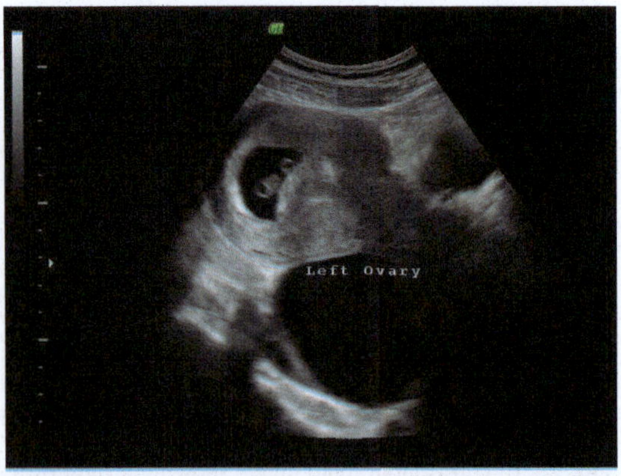

Fig. 24.4 Ultrasonographic image showing a left ovarian cyst in a pregnant woman at 9 weeks

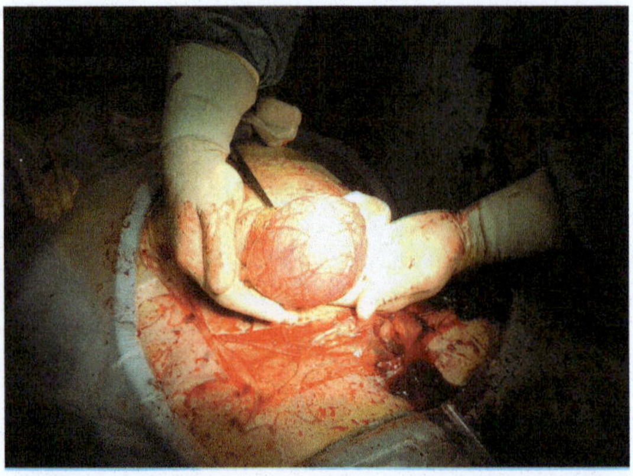

Fig. 24.5 A left ovarian mucinous cystadenoma removed during cesarean section, causing labor obstruction

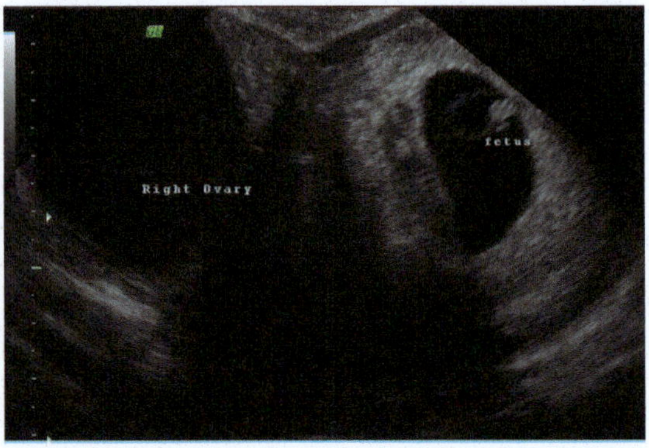

Fig. 24.6 A right serous adnexal cyst discovered occasionally during a first trimester scanning

infection, and labor obstruction (Fig. 24.5) [3]. It should be noted that the overwhelming majority of patients are asymptomatic at the time that an adnexal mass is discovered by ultrasound (Fig. 24.6). However, in some cases, it presents with abdominal pain secondary to rupture, torsion infection, or bleeding [6–9].

Most first trimester cystic adnexal masses will resolve spontaneously during the second trimester. However, controversy exists regarding the diagnosis and management of a persistent adnexal mass since the risks and benefits of certain diagnostic and surgical options should be carefully balanced.

Causes of Adnexal Pathology in Pregnancy

The most common causes of adnexal pathology in pregnancy are functional or hemorrhagic cysts (Fig. 24.7), which usually resolve later in pregnancy (Fig. 24.8). However, the differential diagnosis should also include nonfunctional benign ovarian masses such as dermoids (Fig. 24.9), serous and mucinous cystadenoma, endometrioma, fibroids, and adenofibroma (Fig. 24.10) [5, 10]. Adnexal masses specific to pregnancy include luteomas, hyperreactio luteinalis, and theca lutein cysts, especially in the presence of a molar pregnancy or hyperstimula-

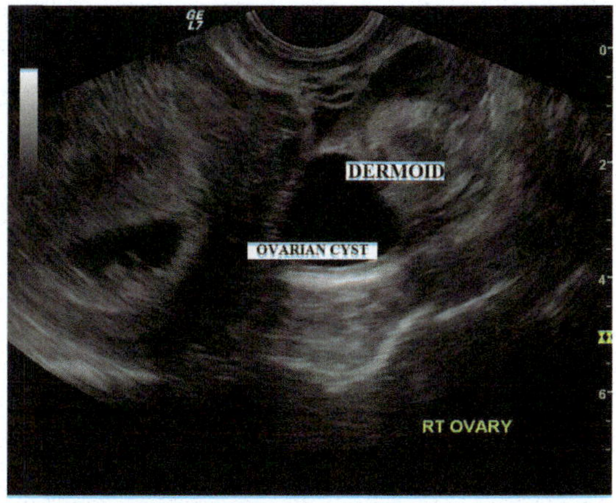

Fig. 24.9 A right ovarian cyst in pregnancy, with a dermoid mass inside

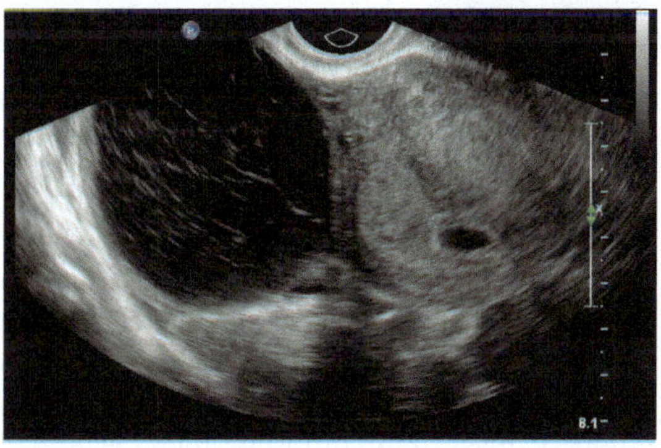

Fig. 24.7 A left hemorrhagic cyst detected in the first trimester of pregnancy

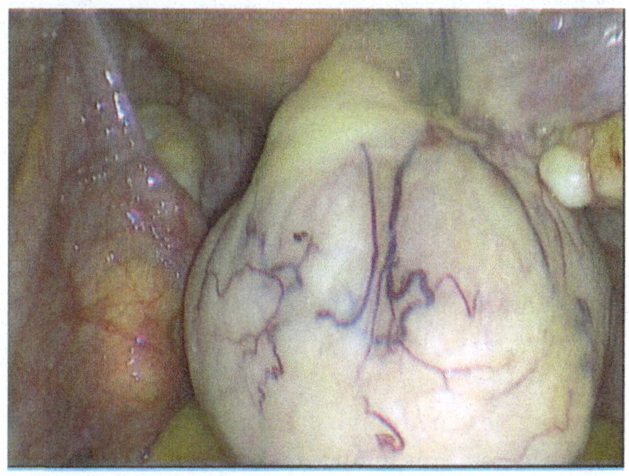

Fig. 24.10 A laparoscopic image of a right twisted ovarian adenofibroma in a pregnant woman at 9 weeks of pregnancy

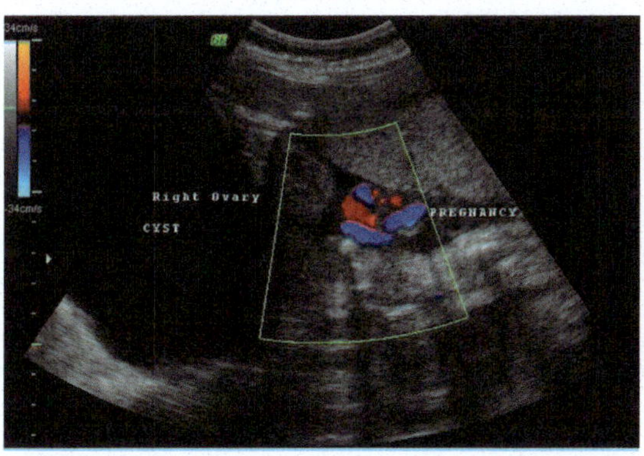

Fig. 24.8 Right functional cyst reducing in diameter at 30 weeks of pregnancy (disappeared at term of pregnancy)

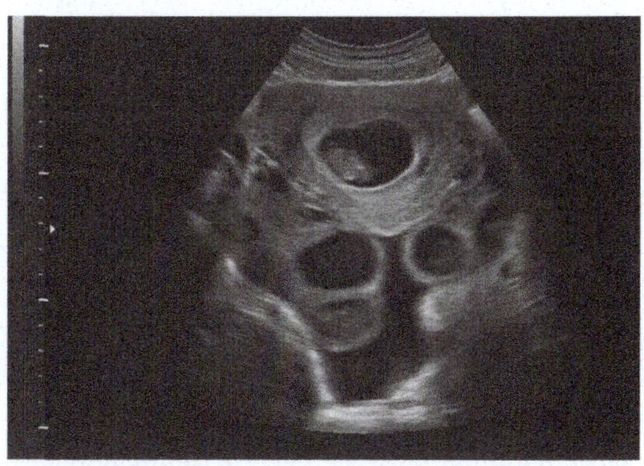

Fig. 24.11 An ovarian hyperstimulation at 9 weeks of pregnancy

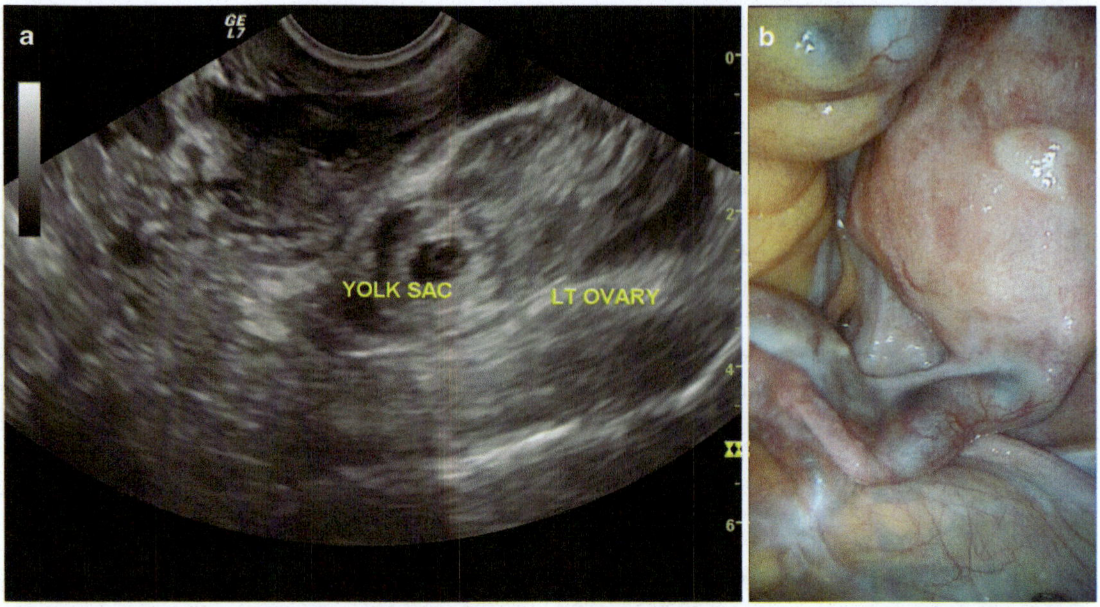

Fig. 24.12 (**a**) An ultrasonographic image showing a left heterotopic tubaric pregnancy. (**b**) A laparoscopic image of a right tubal pregnancy

tion (Fig. 24.11) secondary to infertility treatment [11]. Tubal pathology includes heterotopic pregnancy (Fig. 24.12a, b), tubo-ovarian abscess, hydrosalpinx, and paratubal cysts. Uterine fibroids can also appear as adnexal masses in imaging. Even though the incidence of malignancy is low, epithelial tumors, germ cell tumors, and sex stromal tumors should be included in the differential diagnosis. A study of Leiserowitz et al., which examined pathologically cases of ovarian cancer in pregnancy in a large cohort of obstetrical population, showed that the majority of cases were epithelial, both malignant and borderline (51%) [4]. Germ cell tumors were the second most common malignancy, with predominance of dysgerminomas and malignant teratomas.

Ovarian Pathology

Simple and Hemorrhagic Cysts

Most common ovarian cyst in premenopausal women is functional cysts: follicular cysts and corpus luteum cyst. Simple and corpus luteum hemorrhagic cysts account for the majority of adnexal masses in pregnancy, and usually they regress spontaneously in the second trimester [12]. A simple ovarian cyst usually presents as a simple anechoic adnexal mass, whereas a hemorhagic corpus luteum cyst presents as a complex mass with diffusely thick wall and peripheral vascularity. Up to 70% of cysts identified in the first trimester resolved spontaneously by 18–20 weeks gestation. The best predictors for persistence of these masses are complex appearance on sonography and the size of the mass [13]. Masses with diameter larger than 5 cm have higher likelihood to persist during pregnancy. Matured cystic teratoma and serocystadenoma followed by borderline ovarian tumor are the most common histological diagnosis among persistent mass [14].

Endometrioma

An endometrioma is a rare entity in pregnancy (Fig. 24.13) [15, 16]. It usually presents as a unilocular cyst with diffuse homogeneous groundglass echoes. Complications during pregnancy, such as rupture, have been reported in the literature [17]. However, it is not clear whether endometrioma in general is associated with

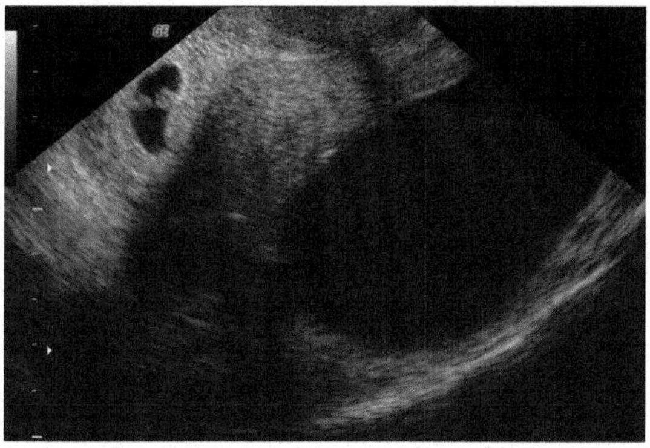

Fig. 24.13 A small right ovarian endometrioma in a pregnant woman at 7 weeks

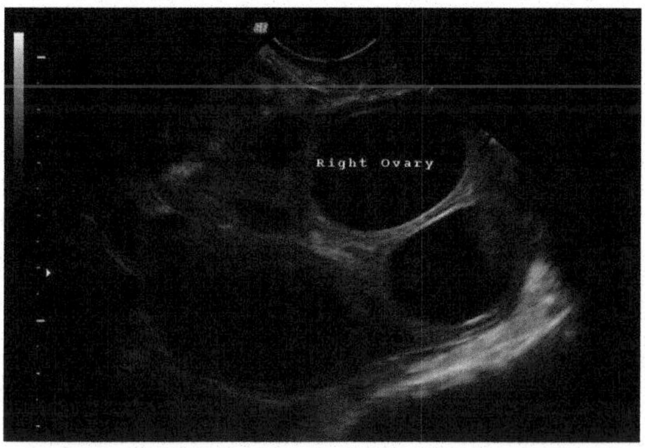

Fig. 24.14 A right enlarged ovary hyperstimulated, with multiple peripherally located cysts

adverse obstetrical outcomes. Some studies have suggested that the presence of endometriomas during pregnancy is associated with complications such as preterm birth, antepartum hemorrhage, and preeclampsia [18, 19], whereas other investigations have failed to show increased risk for obstetrical complications [20].

Ovarian Hyperstimulation

Ovarian hyperstimulation during in vitro fertilization-embryo transfer is a risk factor for developing adnexal torsion in pregnancy. The syndrome presents with enlarged ovaries with multiple peripherally located cysts (Fig. 24.14) and in the majority of the cases is self-limited. However, there have been reports in the literature of adnexal complications during pregnancy such as hemorrhage and torsion [11, 21, 22].

Leiomyomas

Uterine fibroids are very common findings in women of reproductive age. In pregnancy, solid adnexal masses very commonly present as subserous (Fig. 24.15), intramural (Fig. 24.16), pedunculated fibroids, or fibroids located in broad ligament. Approximately one-third will increase in size, whereas a small percentage will undergo red/carneous degeneration secondary to hemorrhagic infarction with subsequent acute abdominal pain [23].

Luteoma

Luteomas constitute a rare adnexal mass specific to pregnancy which usually regress in the postpartum period and can be hormonally active. The condition is not a true neoplasm but rather a specific, benign, hyperplastic reaction of ovarian theca lutein cells. These nodules do not arise from the corpus luteum of pregnancy.

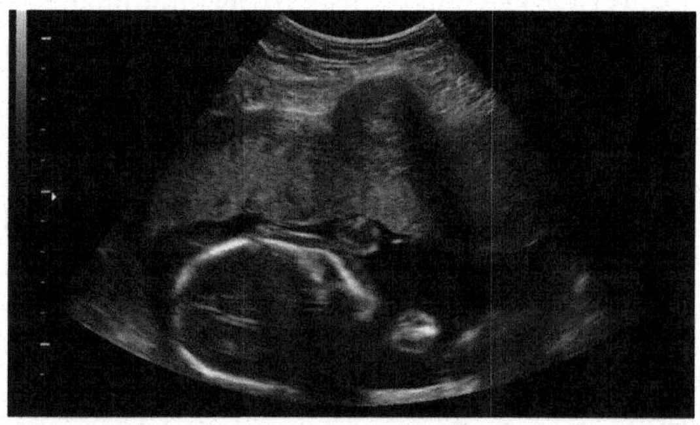

Fig. 24.15 An anterior subserous uterine body fibroid in a pregnant at 20 weeks of pregnancy

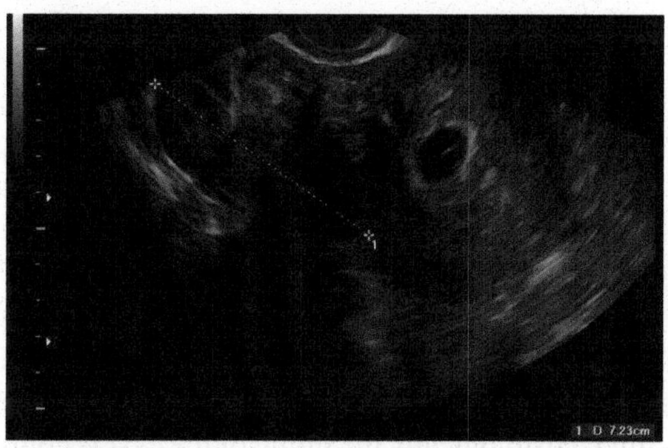

Fig. 24.16 A left transmural uterine fibroid of 7 cm of diameter in a pregnant woman at 6 weeks of pregnancy

Most cases have been reported in multiparous African-American women. Luteomas most commonly present in the second half of pregnancy as bilateral solid or mixed ovarian masses associated with elevated testosterone levels [24, 25], which can also be found in normal pregnancy. They are usually asymptomatic, but they may present with signs and symptoms of virilization of the mother or infant or with complications such as torsion. Due to the commonly seen solid nature of this entity, the differentiation from an ovarian neoplasm can be challenging.

Hyperreactio Luteinalis

The condition of ovarian enlargement secondary to the development of multiple luteinized follicular cysts is termed hyperreactio luteienalis. It is a rare entity usually associated with trophoblastic disease, high-order multiple pregnancy, and fertility treatment. It is caused by increased levels of β-hCG and is usually asymptomatic or presents with abdominal pain or signs and symptoms of torsion. In one-fourth of the cases, it can be associated with hyperandrogenism. Large adnexal masses consisting of many thin-walled small cysts can be seen in ultrasound similar to ovarian hyperstimulation syndrome. The majority of these lesion resolve spontaneously after delivery [26].

Theca Lutein Cysts

Theca lutein cysts are almost always bilateral and produce moderate to massive enlargement of the ovaries. The individual cyst varies in size from 1 cm to 10 cm or more in diameter. These cysts arise from either prolonged or excessive stimulation of the ovaries by endogenous or exogenous gonadotropins or increased ovarian sensitivity to gonadotropin. The bilateral enlargement is secondary to hundreds of thin-walled locules or cysts, producing a honeycombed appearance. Grossly the external surface of the ovary appears lobulated. The small cysts contain a clear to straw-colored or hemorrhagic fluid. Histologically the lining of the cyst is composed of theca lutein cells [27].

The presence of theca lutein cysts is established by palpation and often confirmed by ultrasound examination. Treatment is conservative because these cysts gradually regress. If these cysts are discovered incidentally at cesarean section, they should be handled delicately. No attempt should be made to drain or puncture the multiple cysts because of the possibility of hemorrhage. Bleeding is difficult to control in these cases because of the thin walls that constitute the cyst.

Dermoid Cysts

Dermoid cysts constitute the most common diagnosis of surgically removed adnexal masses in pregnancy (see Fig. 24.9) [28]. Sonographic findings of dermoid cysts may include a cystic or a combined cystic and solid component. Some mature teratomas (10–20%) are cystic in nature, and they may be indistinguishable from other cystic masses. However, the most common ultrasound appearance is combined both solid and cystic (Fig. 24.17) with the following characteristics: (1) a solid spherical component, representing hair and sebum, may occupy part of the cyst; (2) echogenic lines and dots, representing floating hair, dispersed throughout the cyst; and (3) shadowing from the echogenic portion of the tumor due to calcifications from bone or adipose tissue. Many studies in the literature have reported complications secondary to rupture,

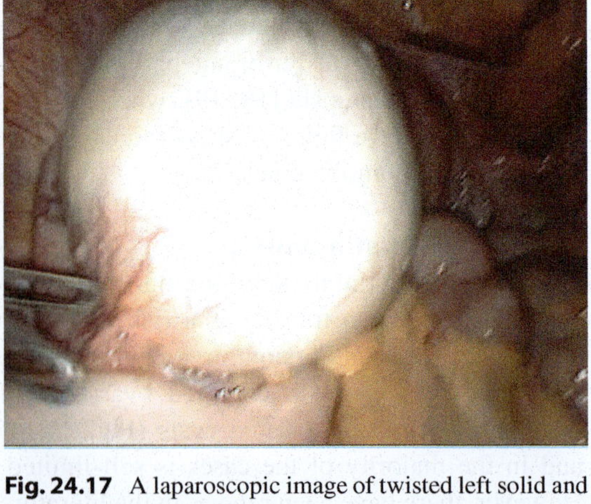

Fig. 24.17 A laparoscopic image of twisted left solid and cystic ovarian dermoid pregnancy in a pregnant woman at 9 weeks

torsion, or labor dystocia of dermoid cysts in pregnancy [29, 30]. However a study by Caspi et al. has demonstrated that ovarian dermoid cysts <6 cm are not expected to grow or to cause complications during pregnancy or labor [31].

Cystadenomas

Cystadenomas are benign tumors and constitute the most common ovarian neoplasm. There have been many reports in the literature of both serous (Fig. 24.18) and mucinous (Fig. 24.19) cystadenomas in pregnancy [32, 33]. In the cohort of Goh et al. which included patients with persistent ovarian masses during pregnancy that underwent surgical treatment, almost one-third of the cases were serous and mucinous cystadenomas [28]. In the retrospective study by Gordon et al., benign cystedenomas comprised one-fifth of all surgically resected ovarian neoplasms [34]. During ultrasonography they present as simple cysts, or they may contain septations. Mucinous cystadenomas tend to be larger at presentation compared to serous. The presence of irregular septations and nodules increases the risk of malignancy.

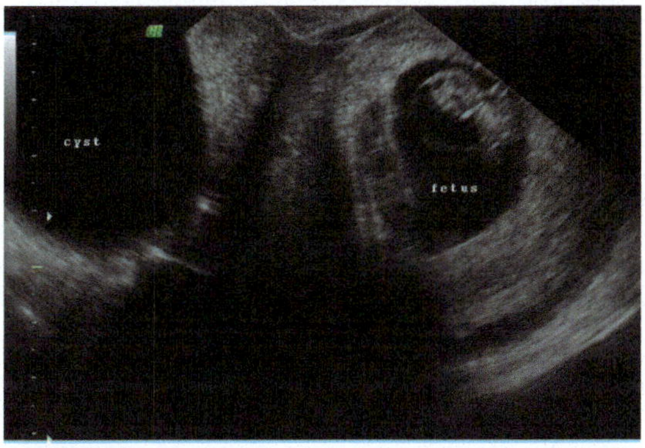

Fig. 24.18 An ovarian left serous cystadenomas at 8 weeks of pregnancy

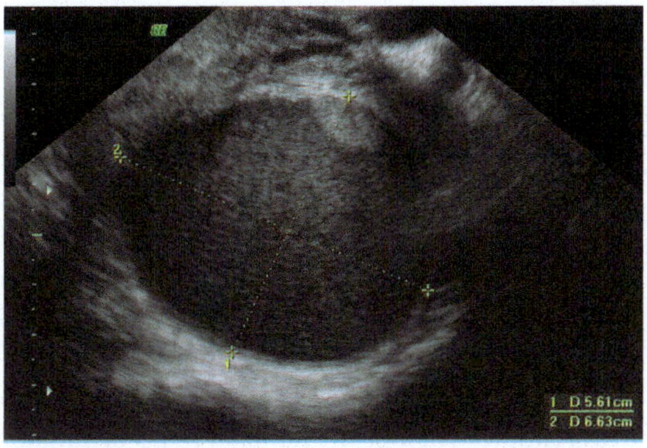

Fig. 24.19 A right ovarian mucinous cystadenomas at 7 weeks of pregnancy

Ovarian Malignancy

The incidence of ovarian malignancy during pregnancy is very low. Sonographic features suggestive of malignancy include a complex cyst with thickened walls, septations, papillary solid components, and increased blood flow detected by color Doppler. Rarely pelvic ascites present that can be confused with amniotic fluid. Most of the ovarian cancers diagnosed during pregnancy are epithelial and low-malignant-potential tumors. Most malignancies are diagnosed at earlier stages [35]. This can be explained by the younger age of pregnant women. For the same reason, it appears that there is an increased incidence of germ cell tumors during pregnancy.

Tubal Pathology

Tubal pathology can present during pregnancy as hydrosalpinx, tubo-ovarian abscess (TOA), or heterotopic pregnancy. Hydrosalpinx commonly associated with pelvic inflammatory disease (PID) appears at sonographic imaging as an anechoic tubular or elongated fluid-filled structure, and its morphology remains unchanged during pregnancy. Tubo-ovarian abscess (Fig. 24.20) is a very uncommon entity in pregnancy and most often arises as a consequence of PID. However,

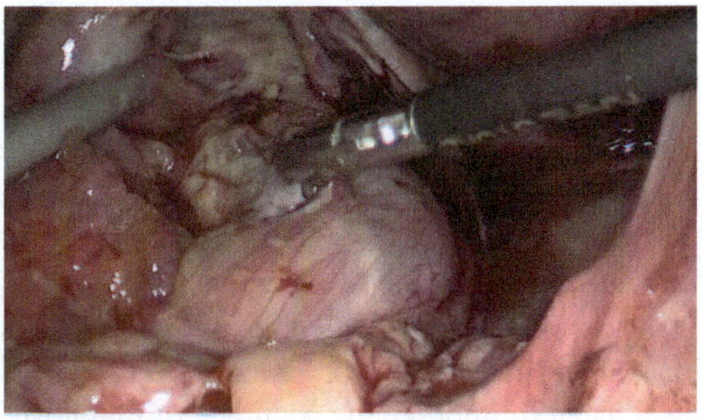

Fig. 24.20 A laparoscopic image of a tubo-ovarian abscess in pregnancy

TOA can be also associated with recent pelvic surgery of intra-abdominal infectious process such as appendicitis. Also, there have been case reports of TOA in pregnancy after oocyte retrievals in women with preexisting endometriomas [36, 37]. TOAs usually present with signs and symptoms of pelvic infection and in ultrasound imaging as one or more multilocular complex cysts. Heterotopic pregnancy, even though extremely rare, should be included in the differential diagnosis especially in patients with history of IVF or ovulation induction [38]. The ultrasound may reveal features of concomitant ectopic and intrauterine pregnancy.

Diagnosis

Ultrasound

Most of the adnexal masses in pregnancy are incidental findings during antenatal ultrasound evaluation. If a mass is clinically palpated during pregnancy, ultrasonography is the initial imaging modality of choice because of its low cost, safety, high resolution, and noninvasive nature.

Features suggestive of malignancy include a solid component within a cystic mass papillary projections, excrescences, vegetation, and nodules, peritoneal metastasis, and pelvic lymphadenopathy that can be seen sometimes by ultrasound. Septations in a cystic ovarian mass may indicate the presence of a malignant neoplasm especially if greater than 2–3 mm in thickness; other ultrasound signs suggestive of malignancy include ascites, increased thickness of the cyst wall, and a very large size of the mass [13, 39]. Conventional ultrasonography has been shown in many studies to be helpful in characterizing the nature of adnexal lesions and identifying the cases with possible malignancy [5, 10, 40, 41]. Although the accuracy of conventional ultrasound in differentiating malignant from benign neoplasms has been questioned and color Doppler has been suggested as a mean to improve the accuracy of diagnosis, the high incidence of false-positive results up to 49% provided by color Doppler makes unclear at this time if it adds any further information to the conventional sonogram [39, 42]. The IOTA (International Ovarian Tumor Analysis) studies are established to develop rules and models to characterize ovarian pathology and to demonstrate their utility in the hands of examiners with different levels of ultrasound expertise. The "simple rules" can be used to classify 75% of all ovarian masses [43] (Table 24.1).

Table 24.1 IOTA simple rules

Ultrasonic features
For predicting a malignant tumor (M features)
M1—irregular solid tumor
M2—presence of ascites
M3—at least four papillary structures
M4—irregular multilocular solid tumor with largest diameter ≥ 100 mm
M5—very strong blood flow (color score 4)
For predicting a benign tumor (B features)
B1—unilocular
B2—presence of solid components, of which largest solid component has largest diameter < 7 mm
B3—presence of acoustic shadows
B4—smooth multilocular tumor with largest diameter < 100 mm
B5—no blood flow (color score 1)
Rule 1: If one or more M features are present in absence of B feature, mass is classified as malignant Rule 2: If one or more B features are present in absence of M feature, mass is classified as benign Rule 3: If both M features and B features are present or if no M features or B features are present, result is inconclusive, and second stage test is recommended

MRI

Many studies have evaluated the role of MRI in the diagnosis of adnexal masses in pregnant populations as it is generally considered a safe modality during pregnancy. MRI is a useful adjunct when sonography is inconclusive and can be used to guide management of adnexal masses especially due to its ability to evaluate tissue contrast [44]. MRI imaging may help the physician differentiate whether the adnexal mass originates from the uterus, the ovary, or the tube and also identify specific characteristics of the morphology of the mass such as degenerating leiomyoma

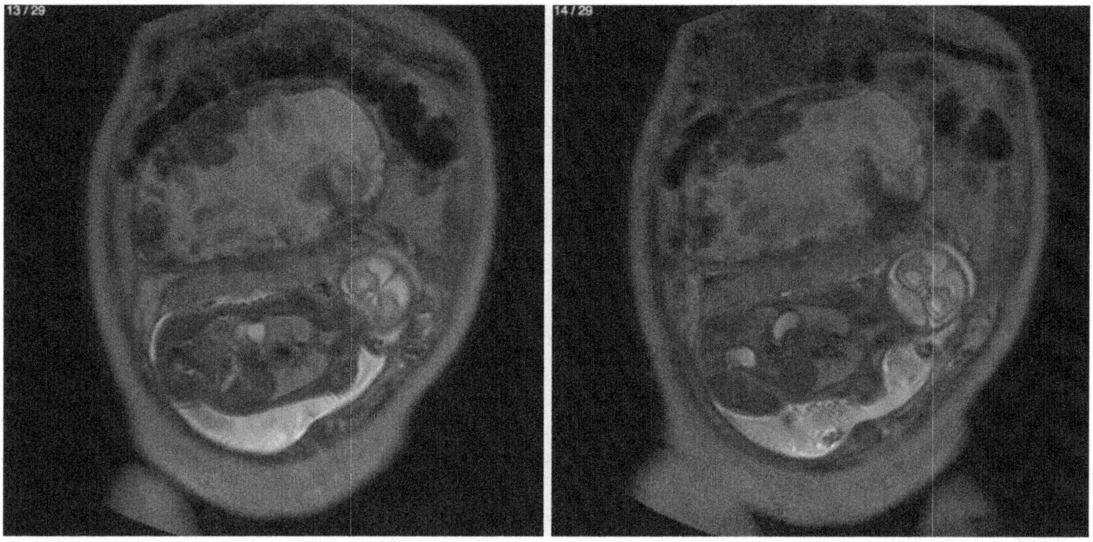

Fig. 24.21 A MRI coronal scan showing a huge subserous leiomyoma in degeneration in a pregnant woman at 25 weeks

d (Fig. 24.21), decidualization of endometrioma, and presence of massive ovarian edema [45]. Additionally, in cases of malignancy, the MRI can define the extent of the disease and possible metastases [46].

CT Scan

CT scan of the abdomen and pelvis is another imaging modality that can be used in the evaluation of maternal adnexal masses. Even though CT scan is considered relatively safe during pregnancy since the typical fetal radiation dose for a routine CT of the abdomen and pelvis is only 25 mGy [47], it should be kept in mind that the contrast material, if needed, can cross the placenta. CT scan is also very useful in identifying other intra-abdominal pathology in a pregnant woman such as appendicitis or diverticulitis.

Tumor Markers

The interpretation of tumor markers during pregnancy can be very challenging.

CA 125 is a glycoprotein that holds an important role in monitoring patients with certain ovarian cancer. However, its levels can be elevated in early pregnancy and during the early postpartum period, thus making its interpretation very difficult in the presence of suspicious adnexal masses [48]. AFP (a fetoprotein) which is typically used as part of antenatal screening can be elevated in endodermal sinus tumors, and elevated lactate dehydrogenase levels may be associated with dysgerminomas. However, the levels of these tumor markers can vary in pregnancy, thus limiting their use; additionally, normal levels of tumor markers cannot exclude malignancy. As a result, the decision to pursue surgical versus conservative management should be in general based on the symptomatology, physical examination, and imaging findings rather than the level of the tumor markers.

Management of Adnexal Mass in Pregnancy: Observation Versus Surgery

Controversy exists regarding the management of adnexal mass in pregnancy. Some studies recommend conservative management and observation, whereas other investigations favor surgical intervention [10, 49]. The majority of simple cysts that are less than 5 cm in diameter will resolve spontaneously during the course of pregnancy [13]. Thus, many observational studies support close monitoring during pregnancy in selected cases as an alternative to antepartum surgery [10, 50]. Surgical management is warranted when the patient is symptomatic and when complications such as adnexal torsion, rupture, or enlargement enough to cause possible labor obstruction occur. If an adnexal mass is suspicious of malignancy with sonographic evidence of solid component(s), nodules, thick septations, and size greater than 5 cm, surgical management should be strongly considered, ideally during the second trimester of pregnancy [35, 51]. Figure 24.22 presents the flowchart to aid the decision-making for optimal management of an adnexal mass during the pregnancy.

Studies in the literature have shown the advantages of surgical management during the second trimester of pregnancy. The intervention at this time of pregnancy is associated with reduction of obstetrical complications such as miscarriage and preterm labor or birth with the absolute risk being very small. The theory behind this recommendation is that the developing pregnancy is dependent on the corpus luteum during the first trimester and much less in the second trimester [52]. Generally, surgeons operating on pregnant patients must be familiar with the following specific pathophysiologic aspects of pregnancy: (1) elevated hemostatic capacity, (2) reduced anticoagulation activity and major alterations in the fibrinolytic systems, (3) cardiovascular changes specific to each trimester during pregnancy, and (4) change in surgical incision site to conform to the size of gravid uterus to maximize exposure and displacement of other pelvic and extra-pelvic organs. If surgery is indispensable during the first trimester, progestin support should be provided postoperatively. Corticosteroids for fetal lung maturation should be given at least 48 h before surgery between 24 and 34 weeks whenever possible. Prophylactic perioperative tocolytic therapy is controversial. Intrauterine asphyxia is one of the most serious fetal risks during maternal

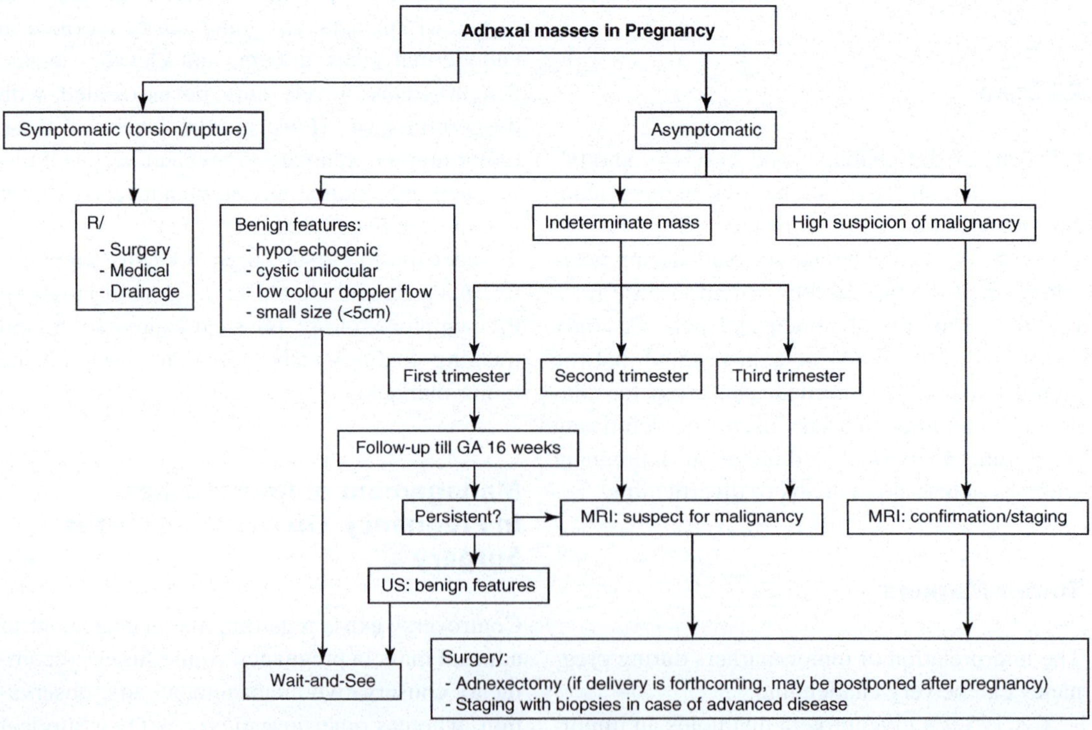

Fig. 24.22 Optimal management of an adnexal mass during the pregnancy

surgery, which may be minimized by maintaining hemodynamic stability. Surgery should be performed at an institution with neonatal and pediatric services. Before the age of fetal viability, it may be sufficient to ascertain the fetal heart rate before and after the procedure. If the fetus is considered to be viable, simultaneous electronic fetal heart rate and contraction monitoring should be performed before and after the procedure. Before induction of anesthesia, the patient should be placed in a left lateral oblique position to prevent inferior vena cava compression and supine hypotension syndrome as well as to improve the uterine blood flow. Proper precautions against maternal aspiration must be ensured. Kleihauer–Betke (KB) test, measuring fetal hemoglobin in the maternal blood, should be performed in the postoperative period, and all Rhesus-negative patients should receive Rh immune globulin (RhIG) at the recommended doses within 72 h after surgery. For women with positive KB test, more RhIG can be administered according to the measurable extent of fetomaternal hemorrhage. The need of thromboprophylaxis should be individualized; the hypercoagulable state during pregnancy may increase the risk of thromboembolic events in the postsurgical period. Subcutaneous enoxaparin 40 mg can be used perioperatively and is listed by the FDA in pregnancy as category B [14].

The surgical approach for the management of adnexal mass during pregnancy can be via a laparotomy or laparoscopy. Even though until the 1990s, pregnancy had been considered a contraindication to use of laparoscopy, many observational studies have shown that laparoscopy in the second trimester for the management of adnexal mass can be safe and technically feasible in the hands of a skilled laparoscopic surgeon [53–56]. The frequency of obstetric complications, such as low birth weight, preterm delivery, use of tocolytics for preterm labor, low Apgar score, and fetal anomaly, is quite acceptable [56].

Laparoscopy in pregnancy can provide accurate diagnosis, faster recovery, minimal risk for thromboembolic disease, less fetal depression secondary to decreased narcotic use, fewer incisional hernias, and fewer postoperative adhesions. However, the risks related to pregnancy should always be taken into account [57, 58]. The trocar placement can lead to uterine injuries due to the enlarged uterine size; therefore, trocar placement under direct visualization rather than insufflation with Veress needle, left upper quadrant entry instead of transumbelical site, or open laparoscopic approach using the Hasson cannula is suggested. An additional concern is that increased intra-abdominal pressure can decrease cardiac output in pregnancy; thus, left lateral position of the mother is of utmost importance. Finally, the potential risk of hypercarbia and acidosis can be decreased by maintaining the intra-abdominal pressure, preferably between 12 and 15 mmHg.

Even though observational studies have provided overwhelming evidence for the safety of laparoscopy and the advantages in postoperative course during the second trimester of pregnancy, the decision regarding laparotomy versus laparoscopic approach should be tailored on each case individually based on the preference and experience of the surgeon.

Adnexal mass can be detected for the first time during cesarean section in 0.3–0.0.5% of cases, and up to 5% can be bilateral [59, 60]. The options include conservative management for simple small cysts and excision for larger heterogenous complex cysts so that further surgical intervention after cesarean section is avoided and malignancy is excluded [1, 46, 52, 59].

Same principles of management of adnexal mass during nonpregnant condition (through evaluation of abdominal and pelvic cavity for any sign of peritoneal metastasis, peritoneal washing, biopsy of any suspicious lesion) have to be performed and documented. Cystectomy or salpingo-oophorectomy has to be performed based on the possible pathology, size of the mass, patient's age, etc. If spillage of the cyst content occurred, thorough irrigation, preferably with warm irrigation should be performed. If in case malignancy was found intraoperatively, we recommend only limited staging (peritoneal washing, multiple peritoneal biopsies, and infracolic omentectomy) be performed to limit the operating time and possible complications.

Step-by-Step Techniques in Laparoscopy Surgery in Pregnancy [61–63]

1. Patients are placed in the supine lithotomy position with the table tilted to the left side.
2. Sequential pneumatic compression is used for deep vein thrombosis prophylaxis.
3. A Foley catheter is placed.
4. The pneumoperitoneum is established by either Veress needle at palmer's site or the Hasson technique at umbilical site.
5. A carbon dioxide (CO_2) pneumoperitoneum of 12 mmHg is obtained. The pressure can be increased to 15 mmHg if deemed necessary during the operation.
6. A 5-mm port is inserted for a 0° 5-mm laparoscope. Subsequent ports are placed under laparoscopic vision.
7. The position of these ports is determined by the gestational age, the position of the uterine fundus, and the surgical procedure. In most cases, the periumbilical port needs to be placed in a more cephalad position.
8. Ovarian cystectomy, salpingo-oophorectomy, or other procedures are performed accordingly.

Conclusion

The extensive use of ultrasound for antenatal screening has led to an increased frequency of incidental adnexal masses diagnosis during pregnancy. Thus, is it of utmost importance that the physician is familiar with the modes of accurate diagnosis and management of this entity? Other than ultrasound, MRI and CT scan can be employed for better characterization of the morphology of the mass and for evaluation of other intra-abdominal pathology. In terms of management of adnexal mass in pregnancy, observation can be a viable option in cases of small masses with no signs of possible malignancy. Surgical intervention is recommended for larger persistent complex masses as the risks of complications such as torsion or rupture as well as the risk of malignancy is increased. Given the benefits of laparoscopy versus laparotomy, laparoscopy should be preferred as a surgical option in the hands of a skilled laparoscopic surgeon.

References

1. Schwartz N, Timor-Tritsch IE, Wang E. Adnexal masses in pregnancy. Clin Obstet Gynecol. 2009;52(4):570–85.
2. Nelson MJ, Cavalieri R, Graham D, Sanders RC. Cysts in pregnancy discovered by sonography. J Clin Ultrasound. 1986;14(7):509–12.
3. Condous G, Khalid A, Okaro E, Bourne T. Should we be examining the ovaries in pregnancy? Prevalence and natural history of adnexal pathology detected at first-trimester sonography. Ultrasound Obstet Gynecol. 2004;24(1):62–6.
4. Leiserowitz GS, Xing G, Cress R, Brahmbhatt B, Dalrymple JL, Smith LH. Adnexal masses in pregnancy: how often are they malignant? Gynecol Oncol. 2006;101(2):315–21.
5. Whitecar MP, Turner S, Higby MK. Adnexal masses in pregnancy: a review of 130 cases undergoing surgical management. Am J Obstet Gynecol. 1999;181(1):19–24.
6. Yen CF, Lin SL, Murk W, Wang CJ, Lee CL, Soong YK, et al. Risk analysis of torsion and malignancy for adnexal masses during pregnancy. Fertil Steril. 2009;91(5):1895–902.
7. Krissi H, Shalev J, Bar-Hava I, Langer R, Herman A, Kaplan B. Fallopian tube torsion: laparoscopic evaluation and treatment of a rare gynecological entity. J Am Board Fam Pract. 2001;14(4):274–7.
8. Morice P, Louis-Sylvestre C, Chapron C, Dubuisson JB. Laparoscopy for adnexal torsion in pregnant women. J Reprod Med. 1997;42(7):435–9.
9. Matsunaga Y, Fukushima K, Nozaki M, Nakanami N, Kawano Y, Shigematsu T, et al. A case of pregnancy complicated by the development of a tubo-ovarian abscess following in vitro fertilization and embryo transfer. Am J Perinatol. 2003;20(6):277–82.
10. Schmeler KM, Mayo-Smith WW, Peipert JF, Weitzen S, Manuel MD, Gordinier ME. Adnexal masses in pregnancy: surgery compared with observation. Obstet Gynecol. 2005;105(5 Pt 1):1098–103.
11. Mashiach S, Bider D, Moran O, Goldenberg M, Ben-Rafael Z. Adnexal torsion of hyperstimulated ovaries in pregnancies after gonadotropin therapy. Fertil Steril. 1990;53(1):76–80.
12. Hogston P, Lilford RJ. Ultrasound study of ovarian cysts in pregnancy: prevalence and significance. Br J Obstet Gynaecol. 1986;93(6):625–8.
13. Bernhard LM, Klebba PK, Gray DL, Mutch DG. Predictors of persistence of adnexal masses in pregnancy. Obstet Gynecol. 1999;93(4):585–9.
14. Mukhopadhyay A, Shinde A, Naik R. Ovarian cysts and cancer in pregnancy. Best Pract Res Clin Obstet Gynaecol. 2016;33:58–72.
15. Pateman K, Moro F, Mavrelos D, Foo X, Hoo WL, Jurkovic D. Natural history of ovarian endometrioma in pregnancy. BMC Womens Health. 2014;14:128.
16. Barbieri M, Somigliana E, Oneda S, Ossola MW, Acaia B, Fedele L. Decidualized ovarian endometriosis

in pregnancy: a challenging diagnostic entity. Hum Reprod. 2009;24(8):1818–24.

17. Garcia-Velasco JA, Alvarez M, Palumbo A, Gonzalez-Gonzalez A, Ordas J. Rupture of an ovarian endometrioma during the first trimester of pregnancy. Eur J Obstet Gynecol Reprod Biol. 1998;76(1):41–3.
18. Stephansson O, Kieler H, Granath F, Falconer H. Endometriosis, assisted reproduction technology, and risk of adverse pregnancy outcome. Hum Reprod. 2009;24(9):2341–7.
19. Fernando S, Breheny S, Jaques AM, Halliday JL, Baker G, Healy D. Preterm birth, ovarian endometriomata, and assisted reproduction technologies. Fertil Steril. 2009;91(2):325–30.
20. Benaglia L, Bermejo A, Somigliana E, Scarduelli C, Ragni G, Fedele L, et al. Pregnancy outcome in women with endometriomas achieving pregnancy through IVF. Hum Reprod. 2012;27(6):1663–7.
21. Tsai HC, Kuo TN, Chung MT, Lin MY, Kang CY, Tsai YC. Acute abdomen in early pregnancy due to ovarian torsion following successful in vitro fertilization treatment. Taiwan J Obstet Gynecol. 2015;54(4):438–41.
22. Munshi S, Patel A, Banker M, Patel P. Laparoscopic detorsion for bilateral ovarian torsion in a singleton pregnancy with spontaneous ovarian hyperstimulation syndrome. J Hum Reprod Sci. 2014;7(1):66–8.
23. Lee HJ, Norwitz ER, Shaw J. Contemporary management of fibroids in pregnancy. Rev Obstet Gynecol. 2010;3(1):20–7.
24. Masarie K, Katz V, Balderston K. Pregnancy luteomas: clinical presentations and management strategies. Obstet Gynecol Surv. 2010;65(9):575–82.
25. Choi JR, Levine D, Finberg H. Luteoma of pregnancy: sonographic findings in two cases. J Ultrasound Med. 2000;19(12):877–81.
26. Van Holsbeke C, Amant F, Veldman J, De Boodt A, Moerman P, Timmerman D. Hyperreactio luteinalis in a spontaneously conceived singleton pregnancy. Ultrasound Obstet Gynecol. 2009;33(3):371–3.
27. Montz FJ, Schlaerth JB, Morrow CP. The natural history of theca lutein cysts. Obstet Gynecol. 1988;72(2):247–51.
28. Goh WA, Rincon M, Bohrer J, Tolosa JE, Sohaey R, Riano R, et al. Persistent ovarian masses and pregnancy outcomes. J Matern Fetal Neonatal Med. 2013;26(11):1090–3.
29. Maiti S, Fatima Z, Anjum ZK, Hopkins RE. Ruptured ovarian cystic teratoma in pregnancy with diffuse peritoneal reaction mimicking advanced ovarian malignancy: a case report. J Med Case Rep. 2008;2:203.
30. Stuart GC, Smith JP. Ruptured benign cystic teratomas mimicking gynecologic malignancy. Gynecol Oncol. 1983;16(1):139–43.
31. Caspi B, Levi R, Appelman Z, Rabinerson D, Goldman G, Hagay Z. Conservative management of ovarian cystic teratoma during pregnancy and labor. Am J Obstet Gynecol. 2000;182(3):503–5.
32. Yenicesu GI, Cetin M, Ozdemir O, Cetin A, Ozen F, Yenicesu C, et al. A prospective case-control study analyzes 12 thrombophilic gene mutations in Turkish couples with recurrent pregnancy loss. Am J Reprod Immunol. 2010;63(2):126–36.
33. Antoniou N, Varras M, Akrivis C, Demou A, Bellou A, Stefanaki S. Mucinous cystadenoma of the ovary with functioning stroma and virilization in pregnancy: a case report and review of the literature. Clin Exp Obstet Gynecol. 2003;30(4):248–52.
34. Sherard GB 3rd, Hodson CA, Williams HJ, Semer DA, Hadi HA, Tait DL. Adnexal masses and pregnancy: a 12-year experience. Am J Obstet Gynecol. 2003;189(2):358–62. discussion 62-3
35. Garite TJ, Kurtzman J, Maurel K, Clark R, Obstetrix Collaborative Research N. Impact of a 'rescue course' of antenatal corticosteroids: a multicenter randomized placebo-controlled trial. Am J Obstet Gynecol. 2009;200(3):248e1–9.
36. Kim JW, Lee WS, Yoon TK, Han JE. Term delivery following tuboovarian abscess after in vitro fertilization and embryo transfer. Am J Obstet Gynecol. 2013;208(5):e3–6.
37. Andrikopoulou MADR, Becker A, Nezha FR. Tubo-ovarian abscess in second trimester of pregnancy after transvaginal oocyte retrieval: challenges in management. Int Arch Urol Complications. 2016;2(1):016.
38. Habana A, Dokras A, Giraldo JL, Jones EE. Cornual heterotopic pregnancy: contemporary management options. Am J Obstet Gynecol. 2000;182(5):1264–70.
39. Brown DL, Dudiak KM, Laing FC. Adnexal masses: US characterization and reporting. Radiology. 2010;254(2):342–54.
40. Bromley B, Benacerraf B. Adnexal masses during pregnancy: accuracy of sonographic diagnosis and outcome. J Ultrasound Med. 1997;16(7):447–52. quiz 53-4
41. Kumari I, Kaur S, Mohan H, Huria A. Adnexal masses in pregnancy: a 5-year review. Aust N Z J Obstet Gynaecol. 2006;46(1):52–4.
42. Wheeler TC, Fleischer AC. Complex adnexal mass in pregnancy: predictive value of color Doppler sonography. J Ultrasound Med. 1997;16(6):425–8.
43. de Haan J, Verheecke M, Amant F. Management of ovarian cysts and cancer in pregnancy. Facts Views Vis Obgyn. 2015;7(1):25–31.
44. Saini A, Dina R, McIndoe GA, Soutter WP, Gishen P, deSouza NM. Characterization of adnexal masses with MRI. AJR Am J Roentgenol. 2005;184(3):1004–9.
45. Telischak NA, Yeh BM, Joe BN, Westphalen AC, Poder L, Coakley FV. MRI of adnexal masses in pregnancy. AJR Am J Roentgenol. 2008;191(2):364–70.
46. Goh W, Bohrer J, Zalud I. Management of the adnexal mass in pregnancy. Curr Opin Obstet Gynecol. 2014;26(2):49–53.
47. McCollough CH, Schueler BA, Atwell TD, Braun NN, Regner DM, Brown DL, et al. Radiation exposure and pregnancy: when should we be concerned? Radiographics. 2007;27(4):909–17. discussion 17-8
48. Spitzer M, Kaushal N, Benjamin F. Maternal CA-125 levels in pregnancy and the puerperium. J Reprod Med. 1998;43(4):387–92.

49. Giuntoli RL 2nd, Vang RS, Bristow RE. Evaluation and management of adnexal masses during pregnancy. Clin Obstet Gynecol. 2006;49(3):492–505.
50. Hoover K, Jenkins TR. Evaluation and management of adnexal mass in pregnancy. Am J Obstet Gynecol. 2011;205(2):97–102.
51. Marret H, Lhomme C, Lecuru F, Canis M, Leveque J, Golfier F, et al. Guidelines for the management of ovarian cancer during pregnancy. Eur J Obstet Gynecol Reprod Biol. 2010;149(1):18–21.
52. Spencer CPRP. Management of adnexal masses in pregnancy. The Obstetrician & Gynaecologist. 2006;8(1):14–9.
53. Yuen PM, Ng PS, Leung PL, Rogers MS. Outcome in laparoscopic management of persistent adnexal mass during the second trimester of pregnancy. Surg Endosc. 2004;18(9):1354–7.
54. Moore RD, Smith WG. Laparoscopic management of adnexal masses in pregnant women. J Reprod Med. 1999;44(2):97–100.
55. Nezhat CSS, Evans D. Ovarian cancer diagnosed during operative laparoscopy. South Med J. 1991;84(1):101.
56. Ko ML, Lai TH, Chen SC. Laparoscopic management of complicated adnexal masses in the first trimester of pregnancy. Fertil Steril. 2009;92(1):283–7.
57. Nezhat FR, Tazuke S, Nezhat CH, Seidman DS, Phillips DR, Nezhat CR. Laparoscopy during pregnancy: a literature review. JSLS. 1997;1(1):17–27.
58. Guidelines Committee of the Society of American G. Endoscopic S, Yumi H. Guidelines for diagnosis, treatment, and use of laparoscopy for surgical problems during pregnancy: this statement was reviewed and approved by the Board of Governors of the Society of American Gastrointestinal and Endoscopic Surgeons (SAGES), September 2007. It was prepared by the SAGES guidelines committee. Surg Endosc. 2008;22(4):849–61.
59. Ulker V, Gedikbasi A, Numanoglu C, Saygi S, Aslan H, Gulkilik A. Incidental adnexal masses at cesarean section and review of the literature. J Obstet Gynaecol Res. 2010;36(3):502–5.
60. Koonings PP, Platt LD, Wallace R. Incidental adnexal neoplasms at cesarean section. Obstet Gynecol. 1988;72(5):767–9.
61. Buser KB. Laparoscopic surgery in the pregnant patient: results and recommendations. JSLS. 2009;13(1):32–5.
62. Upadhyay A, Stanten S, Kazantsev G, Horoupian R, Stanten A. Laparoscopic management of a nonobstetric emergency in the third trimester of pregnancy. Surg Endosc. 2007;21(8):1344–8.
63. Nezhat FNC, Silfen SL, Fehnel SH. Laparoscopic ovarian cystectomy during pregnancy. J Laparoendosc Surg. 1991;1(3):161–4.

25 Ovarian Cancer in Pregnancy

Benedict B. Benigno

Introduction

Ovarian cancer is an avaricious tumor, and its domain is nothing less than the entire abdominal cavity. It can extend from the deepest part of the pelvis up to the diaphragm, to the right and left of the colon, and on everything in between. It can appear after only a few weeks of the mildest symptoms, and by then it has already declared *open season* on the body of a woman. It is fiendishly difficult to treat and unrelenting in its destructive ambition. It is a modern-day scourge, casting a narrow and selective net, forever changing the lives of its victims. Because most patients turn to the Internet at the first hint of ovarian cancer, and because what they learn is so dreadful and depressing, these people arrive at the oncologist's office in a state of terror and disbelief.

Ovarian cancer robs a woman of both health and dignity, and presents her with a playing field that is far from level. Women in their 80s are devastated by this diagnosis, and women in their 30s frequently refuse to believe what they are being told. However, when a 30-year-old woman is pregnant and is told that she has ovarian cancer, she becomes a tightrope walker above the abyss of terror. A gynecologic cancer is very rare in pregnancy, occurring in approximately 4–6 times in every 100,000 pregnancies. It can be difficult to diagnose, as the principle symptom, abdominal distention, is frequently attributed to the expanding uterus. Ovarian cysts are common in pregnancy, and to know when to intervene surgically and when to merely observe, is as much art as it is science, since less than 5% of ovarian tumors in pregnancy represent a cancer. In fact, it is an ovarian cyst itself, the corpus luteum, which sustains an early pregnancy until the placenta takes over. It is not unusual for these cysts to persist into the second trimester, thus making the use of ultrasound so critical in the management of these patients.

Ovarian cancer occurs in 14 of every 1000 American women and is the most lethal of the common gynecologic cancers. It is most prevalent in the Scandinavian countries and is rarest in the Orient. There is no pap smear for this tumor, and despite what you may have heard, there is no way to screen for this disease. I have seen ovarian cancer in its most advanced stages where the pelvic examination and ultrasound, as well as the CA 125 blood test, are negative. This *screening test* is negative in up to 20% of patients with ovarian cancer! There are usually no symptoms in early-stage disease, and the most common symptoms, abdominal cramping and distention, represent a partial, intermittent small bowel obstruction secondary to the numerous metastatic

B. B. Benigno
Ovarian Cancer Institute, Northside Hospital, Atlanta, GA, USA

Gynecologic-Oncology, Northside Hospital, Atlanta, GA, USA
e-mail: benedict.benigno@ugynonc.com

C. H. Nezhat (ed.), *Non-Obstetric Surgery During Pregnancy*,
https://doi.org/10.1007/978-3-319-90752-9_25

nodules present on the wall of the bowel. It is very common to hear this complaint, "My jeans don't fit any more and I am not gaining weight!" A modern symptom for a modern age—ovarian cancer is not known for its subtlety.

There are more than 30 different kinds of ovarian cancer, and they are classified according to the type of cell from which they arise:

Surface epithelium—cells covering the outer layer of the ovary
Germ cells—cells that are destined to form eggs
Stromal cells—cells that hold the structure of the ovary together and produce hormones

Ultrasonography remains the major diagnostic tool, as the CT scan should be avoided in pregnancy unless absolutely necessary, especially in the first trimester. The presence of ascites and extra-ovarian nodularity frequently indicate a cancer, and invite an earlier surgical intervention. Simple cysts can be followed with repetitive ultrasounds, even when they are quite large. Many of these cysts are functional and will get smaller as the pregnancy progresses. Excessive size and pain are the major reasons for surgery. The CA 125 diagnostic test can be slightly elevated in pregnancy, and this can be a source of confusion.

As is true in all cancers, the cure rate diminishes exponentially as the stage increases. The ovary is the only organ in the body that has its functioning cells facing the interior of the abdomen. Long before a tumor forms, the malignant cells detach themselves from the surface of the ovary, and implant along peritoneal surfaces, especially the serosal surface of the bowel. This explains why this cancer is almost always diagnosed in late stages. Indeed, a stage I cancer is frequently a serendipitous event, discovered when the surgeon is operating for another reason. The staging system for ovarian cancer is described in Table 25.1.

Table 25.1 Ovarian cancer staging system

Stage I: Tumor confined to ovaries	
IA	Limited to one ovary, capsule intact, no tumor on surface, negative washings
IB	Tumor involves both ovaries, capsule intact, no tumor on surface, negative washings
IC	Tumor limited to one or both ovaries
IC1	Surgical spill
IC2	Capsule rupture before surgery or tumor on ovarian surface
IC3	Malignant cells in the ascites or pelvic washings
Stage II: Tumor involves one or both ovaries with pelvic extension (below the pelvic brim)	
IIA	Extension to the uterus or fallopian tube(s)
IIB	Extension to other pelvic intraperitoneal tissues
Stage III: Spread to the peritoneum outside the pelvis and/or metastasis to the retroperitoneal lymph nodes	
IIIA	Positive retroperitoneal lymph nodes and/or microscopic metastasis beyond the pelvis
IIIA1	Positive retroperitoneal nodes only
	IIIA1(i) Metastasis < 10 mm
	IIIA1(ii) Metastasis > 10 mm
IIIA2	Microscopic extra-pelvic peritoneal involvement with or without positive retroperitoneal nodes
IIIB	Macroscopic extra-pelvic peritoneal metastasis, 2 cm or less, with or without + nodes. Includes extension to the capsule of the liver/spleen
IIIC	Macroscopic extra-pelvic peritoneal metastasis >2 cm with or without positive nodes and also includes extension to the capsule of the liver/spleen
Stage IV: Distant metastasis	
IVA	Pleural effusion with positive cytology
IVB	Hepatic and/or splenic parenchymal metastasis, metastasis to extra-abdominal organs
(including inguinal and extra-abdominal lymph nodes)	

Surgery

The operating room is the proper domain of the gynecologic oncologist, and unfortunately, it is the *stopping-off place*, at least once, for all patients with ovarian cancer. Whenever possible, surgical intervention should be delayed until the second trimester, allowing the best chance for the preservation of the pregnancy. Whenever there is the suspicion of an ovarian cancer, a gynecologic oncologist should be available. The extent of the surgical procedure when a cancer is encountered is not set in stone. Debulking is the unfortunate noun that has become attached to the surgical procedure for cancer of the ovary. Ideally, all visible tumors should be removed, but this frequently involves a degree of surgical intervention that is quite dangerous in pregnancy. There are very few instances in gynecologic oncology where wisdom and experience are more important. The involved tube and ovary as well as the omentum can usually be removed quite easily, allowing for a complete staging procedure at the conclusion of chemotherapy and after the baby is born. We need to remember that most cancers of the ovary are diagnosed in advanced stages, and that, unfortunately, can be true in pregnancy.

The extent of surgery for cancer of the breast has diminished over the years, from the ultraradical mastectomy with removal of the pectoral muscles, to the modern lumpectomy and sentinel node removal. Surgery for cancer of the ovary, on the other hand, seems to jump in intensity logarithmically with each passing decade. The extent of the surgical procedure will, of course, depend on the findings at the time of surgery, as well as the tumor type. The following is a list of what could happen to such a patient:

- Removal of the uterus tubes, ovaries, and omentum
- Pelvic and para-aortic lymphadenectomy
- Resection of the rectosigmoid colon with trans-anal anastomosis
- Multiple small bowel resections
- Distal pancreatectomy
- Splenectomy
- Resection of portions of the liver and diaphragm

Such extensive surgery in someone who is pregnant is extremely dangerous, requiring great skill, wisdom, and frequently restraint, on the part of an extremely experienced gynecologic oncologist! It must be remembered that a full staging procedure can always be done at the time of a cesarean section or at an appropriate time following a vaginal delivery.

Ideally, the surgery can be performed laparoscopically. If an open procedure is necessary, the placement of the incision varies with the presentation. Some tumors are enormous and require a midline incision. In some cases, a transverse incision is all that is required. Blood should be available, and fetal monitoring should be performed during and after surgery. Excessive blood loss sometimes accompanies surgery performed during pregnancy. All patients undergoing such surgery should be advised of the possibility of preterm labor.

Postoperative complications can be especially serious when the patient is pregnant, and she should be placed on a ward where the nurses are well trained in the care of such patients. All such patients, of course, should have a fetal monitor. If any risks of preterm labor develop, prompt administration of betamethasone is recommended for fetal lung maturation, certainly between viable gestational ages and 34 weeks, as well as between 34 and 36 weeks in certain clinical scenarios. Similarly, magnesium sulfate should be administered if the fetus is viable and <32 weeks, unless the patient is at risk of developing pulmonary edema. Oral indomethacin may also be used to help prevent preterm labor, but should not be used after 32 weeks because of the theoretical risk of the premature closure of the patent ductus arteriosus. Such patients are at risk for all the complications encountered after such surgery, but they are at greater risk for thromboembolic events. Sequential compression devices are especially important, and prophylactic intravenous heparin should be used. A CBC should be ordered daily for the first few days to monitor blood loss and to check for heparin-induced thrombocytopenia. Special attention should be paid to early and frequent ambulation, and I would also recommend occasional Doppler ultrasound examination of the lower extremities.

Chemotherapy

Chemotherapy is the glove on the hand of surgery, as it is very unusual for a patient with ovarian cancer to be told that she does not need chemotherapy, and this is equally true for patients who are pregnant. In order to avoid chemotherapy, the tumor would need to be confined to one ovary, removed without rupture, and a full staging procedure would need to be negative for metastatic disease. In addition to this, all high-grade tumors would need to be excluded. For the last 32 years, all patients have received a combination of carboplatin and paclitaxel following surgery.

There has been nothing new in almost a third of a century, and this, of course, is quite disgraceful! It is all about division! Cells divide and produce new daughter cells along strict guidelines and according to an internal timetable. Chemotherapy drugs work by inhibiting DNA synthesis and slowing down mitotic division. If cancer cells were to acquire a slogan, I am sure it would be *divide and conquer*!

The management of a patient with ovarian cancer in pregnancy is an extremely complex issue on many levels, and the decisions should be shared among an experienced team, including a gynecologic oncologist, a maternal fetal medicine specialist, and a pediatrician. Concerns about the administration of cytotoxic chemotherapy during pregnancy arise because chemotherapy preferentially destroys rapidly proliferating cells, and the fetus represents a rapidly proliferating mass of cells. Fetal exposure to chemotherapy has theoretical risks, such as growth restriction, preterm delivery, fetal anomalies, and bone marrow suppression. Most case reports describing the use of chemotherapy during pregnancy show a good outcome for the baby. In fact, evidence thus far demonstrates that preterm deliveries, congenital anomalies, and growth limitations do not appear to be increased in babies exposed to chemotherapy in utero, provided that the chemotherapy is started in the second trimester. Since the workup, counseling, and surgery take up so much time, it would be most unusual for a patient to be ready for chemotherapy until well into the second trimester.

Chemotherapy with a platinum agent has been the standard of care for patients with ovarian cancer for decades. In addition to bone marrow suppression, patients can experience renal toxicity and damage to the eighth cranial nerve. Paclitaxel has been combined with platinum since the 1980s and is associated with the additional complications of peripheral neuropathy and alopecia. All patients who receive chemotherapy should receive extensive counseling, and this, of course, is especially true in pregnancy. They should attend a class where all possible complications and their treatment are explained in detail. A class has the additional value of the presence of other patients in similar situations, allowing a feeling of not being alone to devolve on them. It is extremely important that the healthcare team involved in the care of patients with ovarian cancer has all aspects of management reduced to a routine schedule, so that errors are reduced to the barest minimum. On the other hand, these patients must also be made to feel that they are very special and unique to the practice. This is especially important when the patient is pregnant, as an extra level of terror devolves on all aspects of treatment.

Let's try for a moment to place ourselves into the mindset of one of these patients. She is in the first trimester of a much-desired pregnancy, and she is told that the ultrasound has revealed a tumor on one of the ovaries. In addition to this, there is a disturbing amount of fluid present in the pelvis along with some nodularity. She is told by her obstetrician that a consultation has been arranged with a gynecologic oncologist for the next morning. Confusion! Fear! Distance from all shades of reality! After all attempts are made to properly communicate this information to the patient, this is what is processed:

- There is a good chance that this tumor is malignant.
- I recommend that you have surgery between week 14 and 16 of your pregnancy.
- If it is an ovarian cancer, you will lose the involved tube and ovary.
- Ovarian cancer is famous for metastasizing.
- Other operations may be necessary, including a bowel resection.
- There may be more blood loss than usual because you are pregnant.
- Complications may occur, sometimes requiring additional surgery.
- The surgery may cause you to go into labor and lose your baby.
- You may need chemotherapy **WHILE YOU ARE PREGNANT.**
- It is unlikely, but possible, that chemotherapy will damage your baby.
- I would like to suggest that you attend a chemotherapy teaching class in the morning.

The term *surreal experience* does not do justice to the mindset of a patient stumbling home from such an encounter. Chemotherapy teaching class! I would rather study the bassoon! But she arrives on time for the class the next morning, and these are some of the things that she is told:

- You will need to have a chest port so that the chemotherapy can be safely administered.
- You will need to see a genetic counselor and be tested for a mutation on the BRCA gene.
- You will lose your hair, so here is a prescription for a wig.
- Here is a prescription for nausea, which almost always accompanies chemotherapy.
- We have to watch you carefully for a drop in the hemoglobin, white blood cells and platelets.
- You will have fatigue and need to pay attention to nutrition and exercise.

Obviously, these terrifying messages are delivered with considerable compassion and over a long period of time and not in the terse sentences that were just relayed. However, those sentences are what the patient takes home with her. One of the best ways to help a patient begin this most dreadful of journeys is an encounter with a patient who had an identical problem many years ago and who is doing very well. That is worth ten visits to a physician and many hours of counseling. Once the first course of chemotherapy has been given, the patient has crossed the Rubicon, a metaphor for not being able to turn back. It does not mean that she cannot choose to stop the treatment at this point; rather, it simply means that almost all patients choose to continue. There is an enormous difference in the patient's psyche between the first and the second round of chemotherapy. Even though the hair is falling out and nausea is rearing its ugly head, the whole process finally appears to be *doable*.

Patients with epithelial cancers of the ovary are treated with a combination of carboplatin and paclitaxel for six cycles in the following manner. These are the same drugs and dosages that would be used were she not pregnant. The following represents one cycle, and there are no time breaks between cycles:

Dexamethasone sodium phosphate 10 mg IV days 1, 8, and 15
Famotidine 20 mg IV days 1, 8, and 15
Diphenhydramine HCL 25 mg IV days 1, 8, and 15
Emend 150 mg IV day 1
Ondansetron HCL 16 mg IV day 1
Palonosetron HCL 0.25 mg IV day 1
Paclitaxel 80 mg/m^2 IV over 1 h days 1, 8, and 15
Carboplatin AUC 6 IV over 1 h day 1
Sodium chloride 1000 mL IV over 2 h day 1
Sodium chloride 500 mL over 1 h days 8 and 15

Some oncologists prefer to give paclitaxel every 3 weeks instead of weekly. In that case, it is given in a dose of 175 mg/m^2 IV over 3 h so that both carboplatin and paclitaxel are given on the same day, and the regimen is repeated every 3 weeks. Appropriate dose reductions are made based on tolerance and side effects. Drugs administered for problems associated with chemotherapy should be administered with the safety of the fetus in mind. It is possible that all six regimens of chemotherapy will be administered prior to the birth of the baby. In that case, the treatment will be discontinued as it would without the presence of the pregnancy. If a cesarean section is required, a gynecologic oncologist should be in attendance to assess the tumor status and to perform additional surgery as required by the operative findings. If an incomplete staging procedure was performed at the original operation, the additional procedures can be performed at this time. If a cesarean section is not done in a patient who had an incomplete staging procedure, then a decision must be made to perform this at an appropriate time in the postpartum period. Yet another cause for alarm and depression!

In addition to epithelial cancers, patients who are pregnant can also develop germ cell tumors. These tumors are rarely bilateral, allowing for the preservation of the uterus and contralateral tube and ovary, thus making additional pregnancies possible. Most germ call tumors are benign teratomas which are rarely associated with malignant degeneration.

Germ cell tumors of the ovary are derived from primordial ovarian germ cells and may be benign or malignant. The benign teratoma can be managed laparoscopically with a simple cystectomy, allowing the ovary to be preserved. Ultrasonography can predict such tumors with high accuracy and can allow the clinician to manage these patients conservatively during pregnancy, unless the size of the tumor is causing problems. There is, however, always the possibility of torsion, which would require emergency surgery, but this is quite rare. Malignant germ cell tumors of the ovary include dysgerminomas, immature teratomas, embryonal cell carcinomas, endodermal sinus (yolk sac) cancers, and primary ovarian (non-gestational) choriocarcinomas. Many of these tumors produce serum markers, such as alpha fetoprotein (AFP), human chorionic gonadotropin (hCG), and lactate dehydrogenase (LDH). The presence of these markers is amazingly specific for certain tumor types (Table 25.2).

The surgical management of these cancers during pregnancy is identical to the management of epithelial ovarian cancer, except that the uterus and contralateral tube and ovary are conserved. Ovarian germ cell tumors are exquisitely sensitive to chemotherapy, and so every effort should be made to remove all visible tumors at the initial surgery when feasible. If the surgeon feels that a complete staging procedure is unwise, it can be performed robotically after delivery or at the time of cesarean section.

Table 25.2 Tumor markers in unusual ovarian cancers

	AFP	hCG	LDH
Dysgerminoma	–	±	+
Embryonal cell carcinoma	±	+	±
Immature teratoma	±	–	±
Endodermal sinus tumor	+	–	+
Choriocarcinoma	–	+	±

The most popular chemotherapy regimen for germ cell cancers of the ovary involves the use of Bleomycin, etoposide, and cisplatin (BEP). Numerous case reports describe the use of these drugs in pregnancy, usually with no harm to the fetus. Four cycles of this regimen are usually given, and there is an excellent survival rate, even in advanced disease. Follow-up visits should include the tumor markers described, as they are an excellent harbinger of recurrent disease.

Stromal tumors of the ovary are even rarer than germ cell tumors, they may be malignant, and they can complicate a pregnancy. The two types of stromal tumors include the granulosa cell tumors and the very rare Sertoli-Leydig cell tumors. These tumors are usually treated only with surgery when metastases are absent. Metastatic granulosa cell tumors are treated with bleomycin, etoposide, and cisplatin (BEP). Sertoli-Leydig tumors do not need chemotherapy unless the tumor is high grade, and then there is no unanimity of opinion as to the proper regimen. The following is a detailed description of the BEP regimen. The duration of each cycle is 21 days and four cycles are given:

Emend 150 mg IV days 1, 3, and 5.
Palonosetron HCL 0.25 mg IV day 5.
Ondansetron HCL 16 mg IV days 1, 3, and 4.
Dexamethasone sodium phosphate 10 mg IV days 1, 2, 3, 4, and 5.
Acetaminophen 650 mg oral tablet days 1, 8, and 15.
Bleomycin sulfate 30 IU days 1, 8, and 15—give test dose 1 mg IVP; if no reaction, infuse the remaining dose.
Etoposide 100 mg/m^2 over 1 h days 1, 2, 3, 4, and 5.
Furosemide 20 mg IV days 1, 2, 3, 4, and 5.
Cisplatin 20 mg/m^2 IV over 1 h days 1, 2, 3, 4, and 5.
Potassium chloride 10 meq and magnesium sulfate 2 G in 1000 mL sodium chloride IV over 2 h.
Sodium chloride 1000 mL IV over 2 h on days 1, 2, 3, 4, and 5.
Neulasta 6 mg subcutaneously day 6.

Discussion

There is no reason why a pregnant patient with ovarian cancer should not have the same outcome as a patient who is not pregnant. Poorer outcomes arise when surgery and chemotherapy are delayed until after delivery. Indeed, since the use of pelvic ultrasound is so standard in the management of patients in the first trimester of pregnancy, it is possible that cancers of the ovary will be diagnosed earlier, auguring for a better prognosis. Certain aphorisms have been created to guide the healthcare team during the management of such high profile and difficult patients:

- Treat the patient as though she is not pregnant.
- Delay surgery until the mid-trimester.
- The management team should include a surgeon, maternal fetal medicine specialist, and a pediatrician.
- The extent of surgery should be dictated by the operative findings and the wisdom to know when to stop.

Following surgery and chemotherapy, patients go into a follow-up mode with a CA 125 and an office visit every 3 months and get an occasional CT scan. Since the recurrence rate is so high, a predictable level of anxiety devolves on these women, and it is not uncommon to hear them say that they are waiting for the other shoe to drop. However, when the chemotherapy is stopped in the immediate postpartum period and they are involved in the care of the baby, anxiety may reach another level altogether. I would suggest that it might be a form of post-traumatic stress disorder and may require a special form of counseling and treatment.

The presence of an ovarian cancer in pregnancy represents a jousting between the joy of an anticipated life and the dread of an unimaginable death. I would like to summarize the approach to the management of such a patient with several axioms:

- Cystic masses in the ovary during pregnancy are common.
- Watchful waiting and surgical intervention are a blend of art and science.
- Ultrasound findings of extra-ovarian nodularity and ascites are strong indicators of cancer.
- The surgeon must always anticipate ovarian cancer.
- A gynecologic oncologist must always be in attendance.
- A full staging procedure should be performed when feasible.
- Chemotherapy should be given during pregnancy.
- If a cesarean section is performed, the abdomen should be explored for residual tumor.
- The principles of management are identical to those that devolve on patients who are not pregnant.

Chemotherapy for ovarian cancer is given with the same drugs and dosages well into the twenty-first century. Slash, burn, and poison remain oncology's ignoble triad: slash referring to the scalpel, burn being the province of the radiation oncologist, and poison, of course, the dreadful and correct noun associated with chemotherapy. With rare exception, radiation therapy has no place in the management of patients with ovarian cancer. However, surgery has a rich history, extending back to Ephraim McDowell's historic operation in 1809, and the modern age of chemotherapy emerged from Sidney Farber's groundbreaking work in childhood leukemia in the 1940s. For the past 32 years, carboplatin and paclitaxel are the drugs of choice following surgery for cancer of the ovary. Things are changing, slowly, of course. Trials using immunotherapy drugs have appeared, and there will soon be trials using PARP inhibitor drugs as maintenance therapy following first-line chemotherapy. These represent a variation on an existing theme and are incremental at best. Where is the *sea change* we have been waiting for all these years?

Full fathom five thy father lies.
Of his bones are coral made.
Those are pearls that were his eyes.
Nothing of him that doth fade,
But doth suffer a sea change.
Into something rich and strange.

–William Shakespeare, *The tempest*
Ariel's Song

Ectopic and Heterotopic Pregnancies

26

Mehmet Cihat Unlu and Gazi Yildirim

Introduction

Ectopic pregnancy is an abnormal gestation in which the fertilized ovum is implanted outside the uterine cavity; the ampulla region of the fallopian tube is the most common site of implantation [1]. Pregnancies in the fallopian tube account for 97% of ectopic pregnancies: 55% in the ampulla, 25% in the isthmus, 17% in the fimbria, and 3% in the abdominal cavity, ovary, and cervix [2]. The incidence of ectopic pregnancy is approximately 1–2% of all pregnancies, with implantation in the fallopian tubes being the most common site. Nontubal ectopic pregnancies are those that implant in sites other than the fallopian tubes, accounting for <10% of ectopic pregnancies [3]. There has been an increased incidence of these rare pregnancies, especially cesarean scar ectopic pregnancies [4].

Previously, ectopic pregnancy was a significant cause of maternal morbidity and mortality, as well as fetal loss. Ruptured ectopic pregnancy accounts for 10–15% of all maternal deaths [5]. The widespread use of transvaginal USG with high-resolution probes, accurate and rapid serum beta-human chorionic gonadotrophin (b-hCG) assays, and the establishment of dedicated early pregnancy units have allowed for early diagnosis [3]. This has resulted in a decrease in both maternal morbidity and mortality. Fifteen to twenty percent of ectopic gestations will present as surgical emergencies. Clinical outcomes have improved, and costs associated with emergency surgery have been reduced because therapeutic intervention is often possible before the patient's condition deteriorates and tubal integrity is lost. Moreover, conservative surgery has become an option in patients who desire future fertility.

Etiology

The etiology of ectopic pregnancy is not well understood. Several risk factors have been found to be associated with ectopic pregnancy (Table 26.1). However, more than half of identified ectopic pregnancies are in women without known risk factors [6]. In women with ectopic pregnancies, up to 50% will have had salpingitis previously, and in most of these patients, the uninvolved tube is also abnormal. Previous tubal surgery including tubal ligation has a 16–50% ectopic pregnancy rate if pregnancy occurs after tubal ligation. Adhesions from infection or previous

Electronic Supplementary Material The online version of this chapter (https://doi.org/10.1007/978-3-319-90752-9_26) contains supplementary material, which is available to authorized users.

M. C. Unlu (✉)
Department of Obstetrics and Gynecology, Bakirkoy Hospital, Acibadem University, Istanbul, Turkey

G. Yildirim
Department of Obstetrics and Gynecology, Yeditepe University Hospital, Istanbul, Turkey

C. H. Nezhat (ed.), *Non-Obstetric Surgery During Pregnancy*,
https://doi.org/10.1007/978-3-319-90752-9_26

Table 26.1 Risk factors for ectopic pregnancy[a]

Risk factor	Odds ratio (%)
High risk	
Previous tubal surgery	21
Sterilization	9.3
Previous ectopic pregnancy	8.3
In utero diethylstilbestrol exposure	5.6
Previous intrauterine device (IUD) use	4.2–45
Documented tubal pathology	3.8–21
Moderate risk	
Infertility	2.5–21
Previous genital infections	2.4–3.7
Multiple sexual partners	2.1
Slight risk	
Previous abdominal/pelvic surgery	0.9–3.8
Current smoking	2.3–2.5
Vaginal douching	1.1–3.1
Early age at first intercourse (<18 years)	1.6

[a]Adapted from [59]

abdominal surgery, endometriosis, and even leiomyomas have been associated with ectopic pregnancy. Abnormal hormonal stimulation and/or exogenous hormones may play a role in ectopic gestation. For example, of the pregnancies in women taking progestin-only oral contraceptives, 4–6% are ectopic pregnancies. Intrauterine device (IUD) users are also at risk for ectopic pregnancy if pregnancy occurs, although the risk of ectopic pregnancy is still lower than if no contraceptive method is used. Smoking and increasing age are also associated with ectopic pregnancy. Multiple previous elective abortions are also felt to be a risk factor for ectopic pregnancy.

Clinical Findings

No specific symptoms or signs are pathognomonic for ectopic pregnancy. Normal pregnancy, threatened or incomplete abortion, rupture of an ovarian cyst, ovarian torsion, gastroenteritis, and appendicitis can all be confused for ectopic pregnancy (Table 26.2). Pain, bleeding, amenorrhea, and syncope are the usual symptoms of an ectopic pregnancy. Generalized tenderness, especially in the pelvis, is present in approximately

Table 26.2 Differential diagnosis of ectopic pregnancy

Differential diagnosis
Acute appendicitis
Miscarriage
Ovarian torsion
Pelvic inflammatory disease
Ruptured corpus luteum cyst or follicle
Tubo-ovarian abscess
Urinary calculi

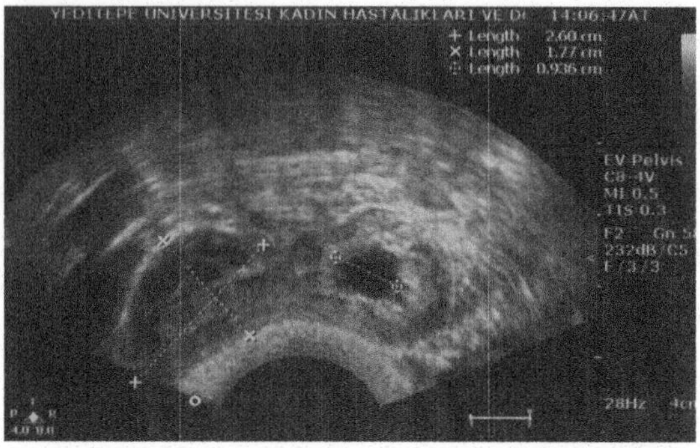

Fig. 26.1 Tubal ectopic pregnancy sac on the right tuba uterine in the view of transvaginal ultrasonography

80% of patients. Adnexal or cervical motions are very disturbing. There is usually an adnexal mass, but its palpation is generally limited because of severe tenderness and pain.

Diagnosis

In up to half of all women with ectopic pregnancies who present to an emergency department, the condition is not identified at the initial medical assessment [7]. Although the incidence of ectopic pregnancy in the general population is about 2%, the prevalence among pregnant patients presenting to an emergency department with first-trimester bleeding or pain, or both, is 6–16% [8]. Accordingly, greater suspicion and a lower threshold for investigation are justified [9].

An ectopic pregnancy can be diagnosed through noninvasive methods due to sensitive pregnancy tests (in urine and serum) and high-resolution transvaginal sonography (Fig. 26.1). Due to noninvasive early diagnosis, the clinical presentation of ectopic pregnancy has changed

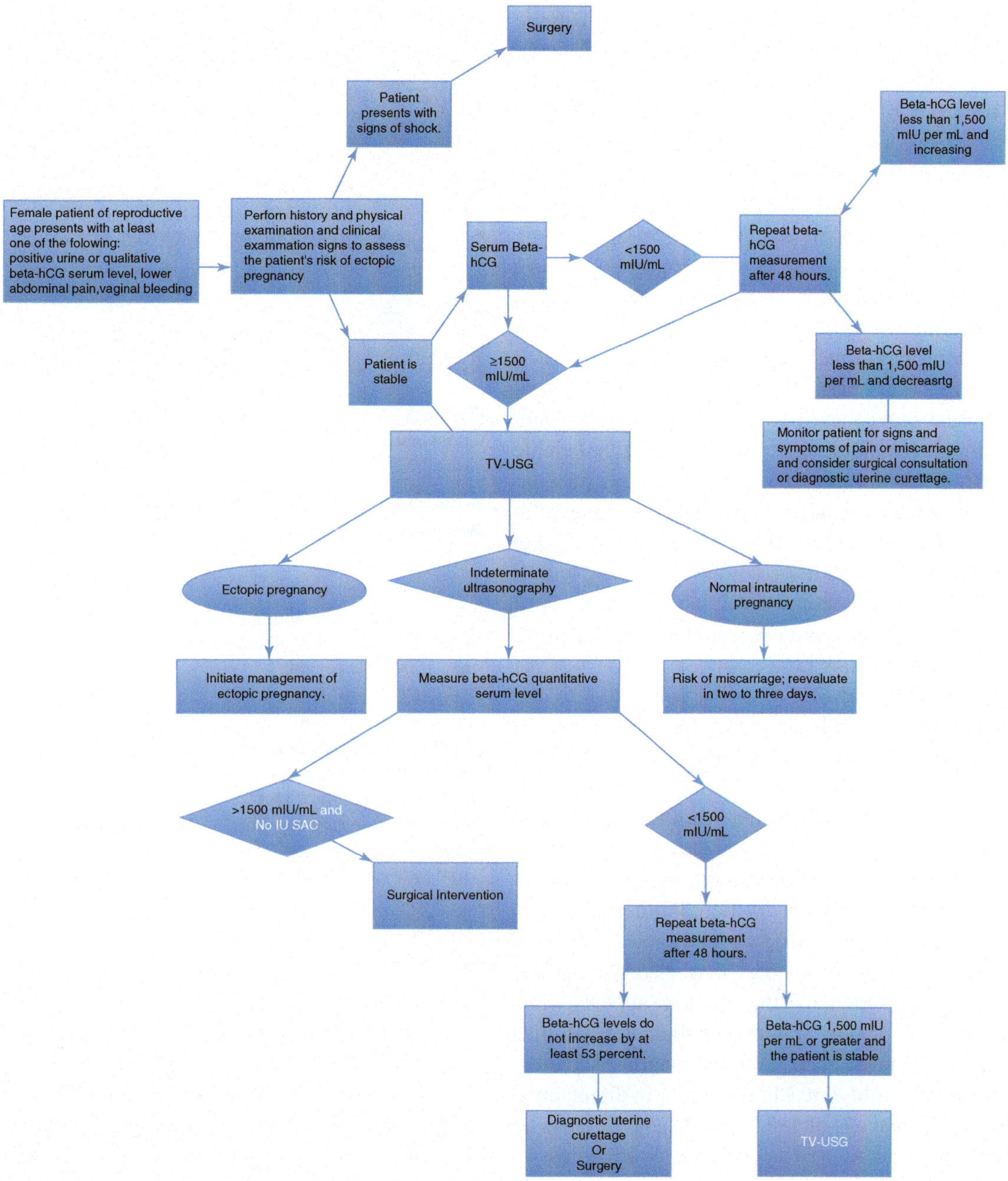
Surgery
Patient presents with signs of shock.
Beta-hCG level less than 1,500 mIU per mL and increasing
Female patient of reproductive age presents with at least one of the folowing: positive urine or qualitative beta-hCG serum level, lower abdominal pain,vaginal bleeding
Perform history and physical examination and clinical exammation signs to assess the patient's risk of ectopic pregnancy
Serum Beta-hCG
<1500 mIU/mL
Repeat beta-hCG measurement after 48 hours.
Patient is stable
≥1500 mIU/mL
Beta-hCG level less than 1,500 mIU per mL and decreasrtg
Monitor patient for signs and symptoms of pain or miscarriage and consider surgical consultation or diagnostic uterine curettage.
TV-USG
Ectopic pregnancy
Indeterminate ultrasonography
Normal intrauterine pregnancy
Initiate management of ectopic pregnancy.
Measure beta-hCG quantitative serum level
Risk of miscarriage; reevaluate in two to three days.
>1500 mIU/mL and No IU SAC
<1500 mIU/mL
Surgical Intervention
Repeat beta-hCG measurement after 48 hours.
Beta-hCG levels do not increase by at least 53 percent.
Beta-hCG 1,500 mIU per mL or greater and the patient is stable
Diagnostic uterine curettage Or Surgery
TV-USG

Fig. 26.2 Algorithm for the initial diagnosis of suspected ectopic pregnancy

from a life-threatening disease to a more benign condition [7]. Nonsurgical conservative strategies, i.e., medical treatment and expectant management, have become a focus of research because laparoscopy is no longer needed for the diagnosis of ectopic pregnancy [7]. There are several diagnostic processes with which ectopic pregnancy can be diagnosed. Using a combination of β-hCG titers with USG findings, an ectopic pregnancy can often be differentiated from an intrauterine pregnancy (Fig. 26.2). Serum testing detects levels as low as 5 IU/L, whereas urine testing detects levels as low as 20–50 IU/L [7]. A single serum β-hCG measurement cannot exclude ectopic pregnancy or predict the risk of rupture unless it is less than 5 IU/L. Serial β-hCG measurements are often used for women with first-trimester bleeding. In a normal pregnancy, the first-trimester β-hCG concentration rapidly increases, doubling about every 2 days. An increase over 48 h of at least 66% has been used as a cutoff point for viability [9].

Measurements of serum progesterone have been investigated as a potentially useful adjunct to serum β-hCG measurement. A stable patient with progesterone levels above 22 ng/mL has a high (but not certain) likelihood of viable intrauterine pregnancy; patients with levels of 5 ng/mL or less almost certainly have a nonviable pregnancy. Invasive diagnostic testing (e.g., dilation and curettage [D&C]) could be postponed in patients with progesterone levels above 22 ng/mL but offered to those with levels of 5 ng/mL or less, as could treatment with methotrexate, without fear of interrupting a potentially viable intrauterine pregnancy [9].

Transvaginal USG is a very useful tool to distinguish a normal intrauterine pregnancy from a blighted ovum, incomplete abortion, or complete abortion. Transvaginal USG has reported sensitivities of 87.0–99.0% and specificities of 94.0–99.9% for the diagnosis of ectopic pregnancy [10]. A normal gestational sac, an ovoid collection of fluid adjacent to the endometrial stripe, can be visualized using a transvaginal probe at a gestational age of about 4–5 weeks. The earliest embryonic landmark, the yolk sac, appears when the sac is 8 mm or more in diameter. Cardiac activity can be seen with endovaginal scanning when the embryo reaches 2–3 mm in diameter, at a gestational age of 5–5.5 weeks [11]. There is no specific endometrial appearance or thickness to support a diagnosis of tubal ectopic pregnancy. In up to 20% of cases, a collection of fluid may be seen within the uterine cavity, classically referred to as a "pseudosac" (Fig. 26.3). An intrauterine sac should be visible using transvaginal USG when the β-hCG is approximately 1000 mIU/mL (the discriminatory threshold) and through transabdominal USG approximately 1 week later, when the β-hCG is 3600 mIU/mL. The universally accepted discriminatory threshold is 6500 IU/L with the transabdominal approach and between 1000 and 2000 IU/L with transvaginal imaging [9]. Thus, when an empty uterine cavity is seen with a β-hCG titer above this threshold, the patient is likely to have an ectopic pregnancy, but it may also be seen with an early IUP (Table 26.3).

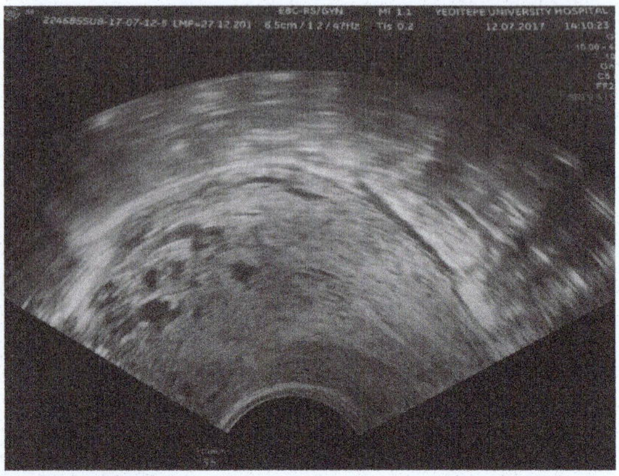

Fig. 26.3 A "pseudo sac" could be seen by transvaginal ultrasound

Table 26.3 Diagnostic tests for detecting ectopic pregnancy[a]

Diagnostic test	Sensitivity (%)	Specificity (%)
Transvaginal ultrasonography with beta-hCG level greater than 1500 mIU per mL	67–100	100
Beta-hCG levels do not increase appropriately	36	63–71
Single progesterone level to distinguish ectopic pregnancy from nonectopic pregnancy	15	>90
Single progesterone level to distinguish pregnancy failure from viable intrauterine pregnancy	95	40

[a]Adapted from [19]

A diagnosis can often be established even in the subgroup of patients with β-hCG levels below the discriminatory threshold. In some studies, transvaginal scanning identified up to one-third of patients with below-threshold β-hCG levels who had ectopic pregnancy [7]. Given the likelihood of a definitive diagnosis, even with below-threshold β-hCG levels, USG is the best initial investigation in problematic early pregnancy. Transvaginal

USG should therefore be the initial investigation for pregnant patients who present to the emergency department with first-trimester bleeding or pain. It is highly accurate in identifying ectopic pregnancy, and it offers patients what they are most expecting from their visit: information about the health and viability of their pregnancy.

As previously described, USG is the first-line imaging modality for obstetric imaging and diagnosing ectopic pregnancy. In addition to the limitation of operator dependence, USG is also limited by bowel gas interference, obesity or large body habitus, and small field of view. Another important limitation relative to diagnosis of ectopic pregnancy is USG's inability to differentiate hemorrhage from other fluids. As such, magnetic resonance imaging (MRI) plays an important role in the early diagnosis and management of ectopic pregnancy. MRI has gained popularity as an imaging tool for evaluating pregnant patients, and it is used as a problem-solving tool in special circumstances, including ectopic pregnancy. MRI can confirm abnormal implantation site and distinguish rupture from nonrupture cases before management. Other benefits include absence of ionizing radiation, superb soft tissue contrast, and sensitivity sufficient for identifying hemorrhage and its stages [12]. A non-contrast technique should be used because gadolinium crosses the placenta and is relatively contraindicated in pregnancy. If a viable intrauterine pregnancy has not been conclusively ruled out, administration of gadolinium should not be performed.

Treatment

Expectant Management

It may be reasonable to manage an asymptomatic, compliant patient expectantly if β-hCG titers are low (<200 mIU/mL) or decreasing, and the risk of rupture is low because many ectopic pregnancies resolve spontaneously. However, about 90% of women with ectopic pregnancy and serum β-hCG levels greater than 2000 IU/L require surgical intervention owing to increasing symptoms or tubal rupture [13]. Tubal rupture can also occur when serum β-hCG levels are low or declining or both. Expectant management should be offered only when transvaginal USG fails to show the location of the gestational sac and the serum levels of β-hCG and progesterone are low and declining. These patients must be carefully monitored until the serum β-hCG concentration falls below 15 IU/L because of the possibility of tubal rupture. At this point, almost all ectopic pregnancies resolve spontaneously, without rupture [9].

Medical Treatment

Methotrexate (MTX) inhibits DNA synthesis in actively dividing cells, including trophoblasts. MTX is the drug of choice in the treatment of ectopic pregnancy. This drug is the most commonly known and has been widely used in clinical practice. MTX treatment in selected patients with ectopic pregnancy was as effective as laparoscopic treatment. Treatment with MTX is less expensive than laparoscopic surgery.

A good candidate for MTX has the following characteristics:

- Hemodynamic stability
- Low serum β-hCG, ideally less than 1500 IU/L, but can be up to 5000 IU/L
- No fetal cardiac activity seen on USG
- Certainty that there is no intrauterine pregnancy
- Willingness to attend follow-up
- No known sensitivity to MTX

The National Institute for Health and Care Excellence (NICE) [14] recommends that methotrexate should be the first-line treatment in the management of women who are able to return for follow-up and have:

- No significant pain
- An unruptured ectopic pregnancy with a mass smaller than 35 mm with no visible heartbeat
- A serum β-hCG between 1500 and 5000 IU/L
- No intrauterine pregnancy (as confirmed on USG)

Exclusion criteria include:

- A noncompliant patient
- Peptic ulcer disease
- Immunodeficiency
- Pulmonary disease
- Liver disease
- Renal disease
- Blood dyscrasias
- Hemodynamic instability
- Free fluid in the cul-de-sac plus
- Pelvic pain
- Known sensitivity to MTX

Relative contraindications include:

- An adnexal mass ≥ 3.5 cm
- An extrauterine gestation with fetal heart motion because of the higher failure rate

Success rates are higher with lower β-hCG levels. Success rates of 81–98% have been reported if serum β-hCG levels are less than 1000 IU/L, compared with only 38% if β-hCG levels are more than 5000 IU/L [15].

Protocols vary from single to multiple injections, typically given systemically (Table 26.4). The dose of MTX depends on the patient's body surface area, and nomograms are available for determining the correct dose. In select cases, approximately 90% of ectopic pregnancies resolve, taking on average just under 1 month. The overall success rate is greater with multiple-dose MTX therapy than with single-dose therapy (93% vs. 88%); however, single-dose therapy is less expensive, has a lower rate of adverse effects (29% vs. 48%), requires less intensive monitoring, does not require rescue with folinic acid, and is effective for most women [16]. The success in ectopic pregnancy depends mainly on β-hCG concentration: a meta-analysis of data for 1327 women with ectopic pregnancies treated with MTX showed that resolution was inversely associated with β-hCG levels and that increasing levels were significantly correlated with treatment failure (Table 26.5). Fetal cardiac activity was also associated with MTX treatment failure [16].

Table 26.4 Methotrexate therapy protocols[a]

Protocol	Single dose	Multiple dose
Medication	50 mg per square meter of body surface methotrexate IM	Alternate every other day: 1 mg per kg methotrexate IM and 0.1 mg per kg leucovorin
Laboratory values	LFTs, CBC, and renal function at baseline and beta-hCG at baseline, day 4 and day 7	LFTs, CBC, and renal function at baseline and beta-hCG at baseline, day 1, day 3, day 5, and day 7 until levels decrease
Repeat medication	Repeat regimen if beta-hCG level does not decrease by 15% between day 4 and day 7	Repeat regimen (for up to four doses of each medication) if beta-hCG level does not decrease by 15% with each measurement
Follow-up	Beta-hCG level weekly, and continue regimen until no longer detected	Beta-hCG level weekly, and continue regimen until no longer detected

IM intramuscular, *LFT* liver function test, *CBC* complete blood count, *beta-hCG* beta subunit of human chorionic gonadotropin

[a]Adapted from [19]

Table 26.5 Methotrexate therapy success rate at different baseline beta-hCG levels[a]

Initial beta-hCG level (mIU per mL)	Success rate (%)
Less than 1000 (1000 IU per L)	98
1000 to 1999 (1000 to 1999 IU per L)	93
2000 to 4999 (2000 to 4999 IU per L)	92
5000 to 9999 (5000 to 9999 IU per L)	87
10,000 to 14,999 (10,000 to 14,999 IU per L)	82
15,000 or greater (15,000 or greater IU per L)	68

[a]Adapted from [59]

Follow-up β-hCG levels, along with a complete blood count, serum creatinine, and serum aspartate transaminase, are obtained, for a comparison with baseline values. β-hCG levels should decrease by at least 15% 4–7 days after MTX administration. Patients treated with MTX should be closely monitored. Severe abdominal pain can be a sign of tubal rupture. The serum β-hCG concentration should be measured weekly; if serum β-hCG concentration has not declined by at least 25% 1 week after MTX administration, a second dose should be given. In general, a second dose is needed in 15–20% of patients [7]. Only 1% of patients need more than two doses. The time for the serum β-hCG concentration to decline to less than 15 IU/L is 33.6 days on average but may be up to 109 days [9].

Failure of MTX therapy is suggested by a persistent rise or plateau in the β-hCG titer, worsening pain in conjunction with a hemoperitoneum on USG, and/or hemodynamic instability, and demands either another dose of MTX or surgery.

Rho (D) immune globulin should be given to any Rh-negative mother who has been diagnosed as having an ectopic pregnancy because sensitization can occur just as with intrauterine pregnancy.

Local Injections

Local administration of drugs into the gestational sac transvaginally under USG guidance or under laparoscopic guidance has recently been introduced in selected patients with an unruptured ectopic pregnancy without active bleeding. The selection criteria used were as follows: ectopic pregnancy size, maximum serum hCG concentrations, and fetal cardiac activity [7].

Various protocols exist for local treatment with MTX administered into the gestational sac transvaginally under sonographic or laparoscopic guidance [17]. The results of an updated study showed that transvaginal administration of MTX under sonographic guidance was significantly less successful than laparoscopic salpingotomy in the elimination of tubal pregnancies (RR 0.83, 95% CI: [0.68–1.0]). This was mainly the result of the higher persistent trophoblastic disease (PTD) rate (RR 4.2, 95% CI: [0.88–20]) for which additional systemic MTX injections were necessary. Various protocols for local treatment were administered into the gestational sac transvaginally under sonographic or under laparoscopic guidance with methotrexate [18], prostaglandins [19], or hyperosmolar glucose [20] to attain maximal efficacy while minimizing or eliminating adverse effects.

The results of a small study that involved 36 hemodynamically stable women with a small unruptured ectopic pregnancy [21] showed that the treatment success of MTX administered transvaginally under USG guidance was significantly better than "blind" intra-tubal injections under laparoscopic guidance (RR 1.6, 95% CI [1.0–2.5]). In addition, the mean serum hCG clearance time was significantly shorter in women treated through this administration route (17 vs. 29 days). However, compared with laparoscopic salpingotomy, local MTX given transvaginally under USG guidance is less effective in the elimination of tubal pregnancy. Compared with the local routes of administration, systemic MTX is more practical, easier to administer, and less dependent on clinical skills. Most importantly, in combination with noninvasive diagnostic tools, systemic MTX offers complete noninvasive outpatient management.

Surgical Treatment

Surgical management of ectopic pregnancy should be reserved for patients who refuse or have contraindications to medical treatment, those in whom medical treatment has failed, and those who are hemodynamically unstable. Immediate surgery is indicated when the diagnosis of ectopic pregnancy with hemorrhage is made. There is no place for conservative therapy in a hemodynamically unstable patient. Laparoscopic treatment is the standard for diagnosis and therapy in patients with conditions from acute abdomen to asymptomatic hemoperitoneum. Salpingotomy (Video 26.1) or salpingectomy (Videos 26.2 and 26.3) are the surgical treatments. Laparoscopic surgery is the cornerstone of treatment in the majority of women with tubal pregnancy. If the physician is competent in operative laparoscopy, both of these procedures (salpingotomy or salpingectomy) can be performed through the laparoscope. In stable patients, laparoscopy is preferred over laparotomy because of the associated reduction in morbidity and cost. Operation time, perioperative blood loss, analgesic requirements, duration of hospital stay, and convalescence time were significantly shorter or less with the laparoscopic surgical approach [7]. Based on the available evidence, laparoscopic surgery appears to be the treatment of choice.

Conservative surgery (i.e., preservation of the fallopian tube) may be indicated in hemodynamically stable patients with an ampullary pregnancy who wish to preserve fertility. A linear salpingotomy may be performed with small (< 3 cm), intact ampullary pregnancies. Subsequent reproductive performance is comparable, with intrauterine pregnancy rates of 40–90%, but recurrent ectopic rates may be higher, up to 16%. A small study involving 40 hemodynamically stable women with small unruptured ectopic pregnancies [22] reported that prophylactic vasopressin injections significantly reduced the need for electrocoagulation for hemostasis (RR 0.36, 95% CI: [0.14–0.95]) without adverse effects, resulting in a significantly shorter operation time (68 vs. 88 min). These positive effects of prophylactic vasopressin, however, were not reflected in primary treatment success (RR 1.3, 95% CI: [0.90–1.9]) and tubal preservation (RR 1.1, 95% CI: [0.84–1.3]), because the number of conversions to open surgery and salpingectomy between the two treatment groups for uncontrollable bleeding did not differ. With laparoscopic salpingotomy, the risk of PTD will always remain present.

Salpingectomy may be necessary for women with uncontrolled bleeding, recurrent ectopic pregnancy in the same tube, a severely damaged tube, or a tubal gestational sac greater than 5 cm in diameter [23]. In the presence of a healthy contralateral tube, salpingectomy should be performed in preference to salpingotomy [24].

"Milking" the pregnancy out of the distal end of the tube is often tempting, but this has been associated with PTD and need for re-exploration, as well as increased risks of recurrent ectopic pregnancy. With an isthmic ectopic pregnancy, segmental resection with subsequent anastomosis (usually at a later date) is typically recommended. As opposed to ampullary ectopic pregnancies, the muscularis is well-developed, forcing the pregnancy to grow in the lumen. More conservative treatment such as salpingotomy would likely cause scarring and compromise of the lumen. Furthermore, a tubal fistula may result if the tube is allowed to heal by secondary intention.

Based on the available evidence, laparoscopic surgery appears to be the treatment of choice. Although laparoscopic conservative surgery was less successful than the open surgical approach in the elimination of tubal pregnancy, this technique, which seemed feasible in virtually all patients, has proven to be safe and less costly due to the higher PTD rate of laparoscopic surgery. Long-term follow-up showed a comparable intrauterine pregnancy rate and a lower repeat ectopic pregnancy rate.

With both salpingotomy and salpingectomy, a β-hCG titer should be obtained weekly after surgery to ensure adequate removal of trophoblast and rule out a persistent ectopic pregnancy.

Surgical Techniques for Tubal Ectopic Pregnancies

Laparoscopic treatment is the standard for therapy for patients with conditions ranging from acute abdomen to asymptomatic hemoperitoneum. Salpingotomy and salpingectomy are the surgical treatments. At present, laparotomy is an exceptional procedure for salpingectomy or salpingotomy. Laparotomy should be performed only when laparoscopy is not possible for technical, logistical, or medical reasons. Laparoscopy is today the method of choice for diagnosis and usually also for treatment of nearly all clinical presentations of EUP, even (and especially) in clinically critical situations because it offers the fastest access to the abdomen [25].

When the surgical decision was made, patients must be informed about the situation and the general risks of the procedure such as hemorrhage or injury to neighboring organs. The problem of tube-preserving surgery vs. salpingectomy must also be discussed.

Surgical Steps for Salpingotomy

- The routine steps of any diagnostic laparoscopy are followed: inspection of the entire abdomen, photo documentation, search for the tubal pregnancy (Fig. 26.4), and assessment of the antimesenteric border.

- Linear, antimesenteric salpingotomy, ideally made with a monopolar needle, is the classic operation technique for EUP in the ampullary part of the tube (Fig. 26.5).
- Injection of a vasoconstrictor substance in the region of the mesosalpinx can reduce the number of bleeding points requiring coagulation after removal of the EUP and forms part of the atraumatic surgical approach.

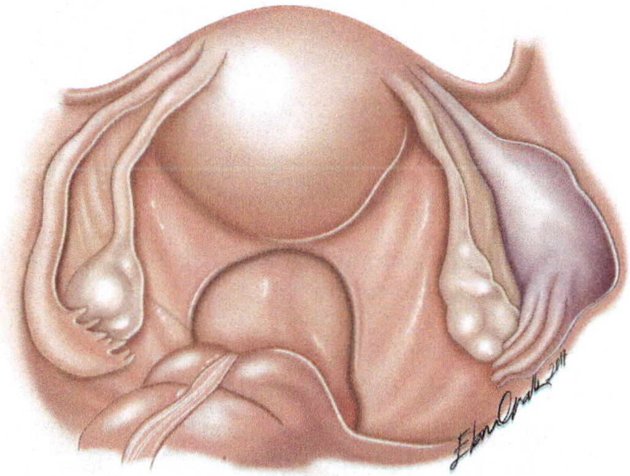

Fig. 26.4 Classic appearance of a nonruptured tubal pregnancy in the ampullary part of the right tube. Figure created by Gazi Yildirim and Ebru Oralli

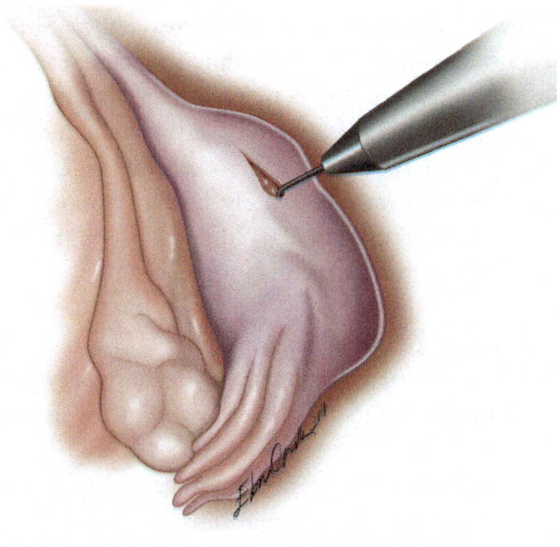

Fig. 26.5 A linear, antimesenteric salpingotomy, ideally made with a monopolar needle. Figure created by Gazi Yildirim and Ebru Oralli

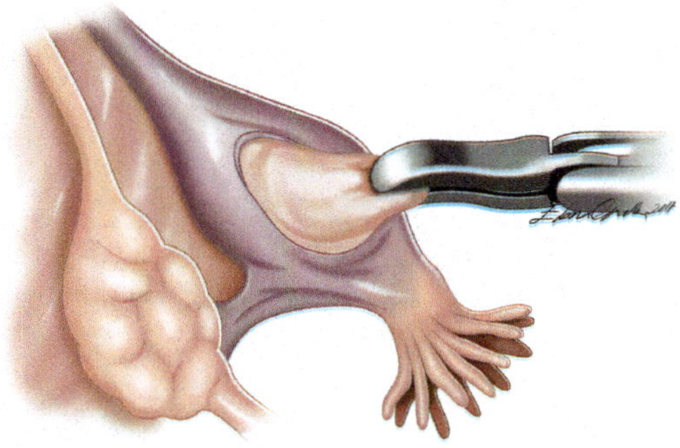

Fig. 26.6 Removal of the entire tubal pregnancy with an atraumatic grasping forceps. Figure created by Gazi Yildirim and Ebru Oralli

- The tubal pregnancy is removed from the tube with light pressure from the outside (Fig. 26.6) or alternatively by using hydrodissection with irrigation. The gestational tissue can usually be removed in this way because the tube and trophoblast have already separated somewhat.
- As much trophoblastic tissue as possible must be removed, but, critically, none of the tube should be removed. Copious irrigation helps to differentiate between gestational tissue and regressive tube wall.
- After the conceptus has been removed, hemostasis must be achieved with as little electrocoagulation as possible. Careful irrigation helps in identifying bleeding points and coagulating them accurately.
- After optimal hemostasis, the tube can remain open for secondary healing (see Video 26.1). Reapproximation of the opened tube does not appear to improve the chances of successful pregnancy or reduce the risk of recurrent tubal pregnancy (Fig. 26.7).
- Insertion of a drain is optional after unruptured EUP.

Surgical Steps for Salpingectomy

- When the patient's family is complete and at her express wish, salpingectomy can be performed as definitive treatment of tubal pregnancy. Technically, salpingectomy can be performed faster and more easily than linear salpingotomy.

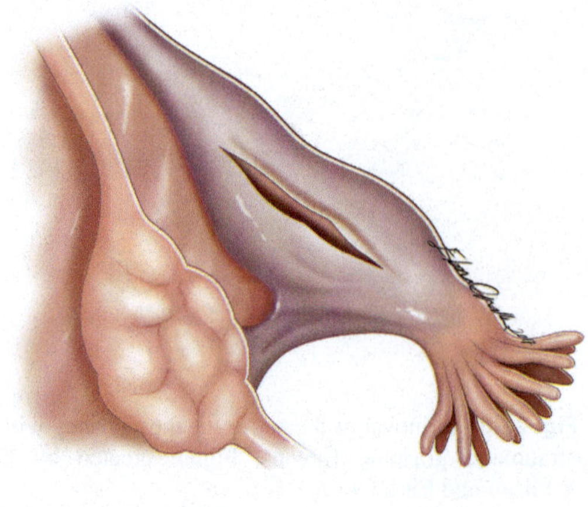

Fig. 26.7 Suture closure is not necessary. Figure created by Gazi Yildirim and Ebru Oralli

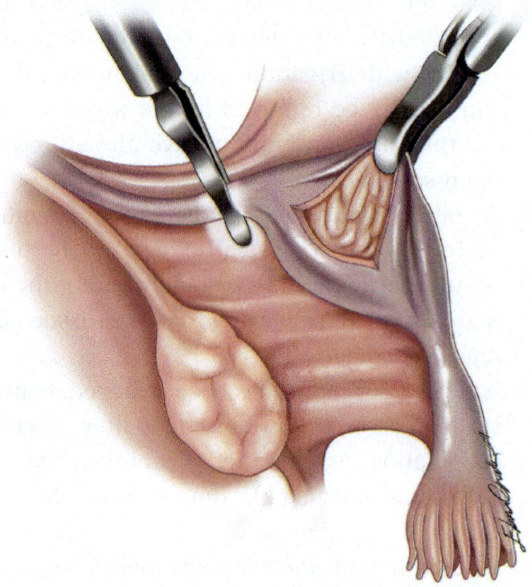

Fig. 26.8 Salpingectomy after coagulation. Figure created by Gazi Yildirim and Ebru Oralli

- A clear field of vision should be obtained, especially if a hemoperitoneum is present; widespread aspiration may be necessary to achieve clear exposure.
- The tube is elevated with an instrument at the fimbrial end, and the mesosalpinx is clamped from the fimbrial side with traditional or advanced bipolar forceps (Fig. 26.8). Ensure that the clamps are placed close to the base of the tube so as not to interfere with the ovarian vessels along the mesovarium (Fig. 26.9).

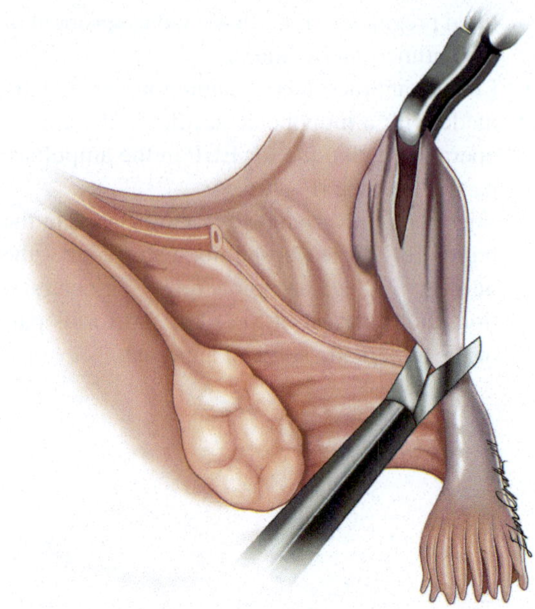

Fig. 26.9 Salpingectomy is completed. Figure created by Gazi Yildirim and Ebru Oralli

- Alternatively, the tube is simply excised somewhat distal to the uterus, depending on the location of the tubal pregnancy (see Videos 26.2 and 12.3).

Nontubal Ectopic Pregnancies

Cornual/interstitial pregnancies have been reported as 2–4% of all ectopic pregnancies. The associated morbidity is much higher with mortality rates of 2–2.5%, two to five times the mortality rate associated with other tubal ectopic pregnancy locations, largely due to hemorrhage [2]. Timor–Tritsch et al. [26] put forward the following criteria for the diagnosis of IP:

- An empty uterine cavity
- A gestational sac located eccentrically and 1 cm from the most lateral wall of the uterine cavity and
- A thin (less than 5 mm) myometrial layer surrounding the gestational sac

Medical treatment is not recommended for large cornual ectopic pregnancies or those with a heartbeat [27]. Injections of potassium chloride and MTX have both been reported as successful treatments of cornual pregnancy, with no difference in efficacy of either method [28]. Medical treatment carries the possible risk of uterine rupture and hemorrhage. It requires at least a corneal wedge resection, with uterine reconstruction and sometimes salpingectomy on the affected side [29].

If there has been extensive tissue damage or if the patient is unstable, a hysterectomy may be needed. Classically, these have been managed by hysterectomy or cornual resection during laparotomy. The desire for fertility has meant that more conservative approaches are now being considered. Laparoscopic surgery is fast becoming the gold standard for the surgical management of cornual and interstitial ectopic pregnancies [30]. Advanced laparoscopic skills are essential because of the potential for hemorrhage. It is possible to perform these procedures without hemostatic agents. Hysteroscopic resection may be appropriate in selected cases; Nezhat and Dun described a combined laparoscopically assisted, hysteroscopic removal of an unruptured interstitial pregnancy [31]. With this technique, the authors completely removed the pregnancy in one attempt with no injury to the uterus or ipsilateral fallopian tube. The patient required no pre- or postoperative MTX and had a normal hysterosalpingogram 2 months after the procedure.

Cervical ectopic pregnancy (CEP) is defined as an implantation of a fertilized ovum within the cervical canal. Risk factors include previous cesarean section (CS), induced abortion, Asherman's syndrome, leiomyomas, presence of an IUD, in vitro fertilization (IVF), and prior in utero exposure to diethylstilbestrol; however, a history of previous D&C is described in more than 70% of cases [2]. It is important to differentiate cervical ectopic pregnancies from an incomplete or inevitable miscarriage. The advent of more advanced USG, as well as other imaging modalities including MRI, has led to earlier diagnosis. This makes more conservative options possible with the aim of uterine or fertility preservation.

Options of treatment described in the literature include the use of systemic MTX, intra-amniotic administration of potassium chloride, prostaglandins or MTX under USG guidance, as well as the combination of both systemic and local (intra-amniotic) use of MTX. There are suggestions that patient factors such as crown-rump length > 10 mm in transvaginal ultrasound, gestational age > 9 weeks, and the presence of fetal cardiac activity may be associated with treatment failure with systemic MTX.

Early diagnosis of CEP has led to a shift away from hysterectomy to more conservative techniques aimed at uterine or fertility preservation. Techniques described include D&C and hysteroscopic resection of CEP. Researchers have also described surgical techniques with the aim of minimizing operative vaginal bleeding, including UAE, ligation of the cervical branches of the uterine arteries, a Shirodkar-type cerclage, balloon tamponade, and local injection of vasopressin to the cervix. Many of the surgical approaches to treatment involve a combination of evacuation of CEP and one or two techniques at minimization of bleeding.

Ovarian pregnancy accounts for 0.5–3% of all ectopic pregnancies. The main risk factors are the use of an IUD, assisted reproductive techniques, endometriosis, and pelvic inflammatory disease. Intraoperatively, ovarian ectopic pregnancies (OEP) can be misdiagnosed as hemorrhagic corpus luteum or ovarian cysts. The diagnosis of ovarian pregnancy is made surgically using Spiegelberg's criteria [32]:

- Fallopian tube entirely normal
- Gestational sac anatomically located in the ovary
- Ovary and gestational sac connected to the uterine ovarian ligament
- Placental tissue mixed with ovarian cortex

There have been successful reports of medical management with MTX, but mostly it requires oophorectomy and sometimes salpingectomy on the affected side. Ovarian preservation is the cornerstone of management; thus, the common procedures are ovarian wedge resection, partial oophorectomy, or blunt dissection of the trophoblastic tissue using diathermy forceps, which has been shown to successfully provide ovarian hemostasis. Oophorectomy should only be used in advanced gestation or if bleeding from the ovary becomes uncontrollable. Surgery is the mainstay of treatment, and operative laparoscopy should be the gold standard approach because in most cases, laparoscopy is required for a definitive diagnosis. Postoperative MTX is indicated in the presence of residual PTD.

Abdominal pregnancy is defined as a pregnancy that occurs in the peritoneum of the abdomen outside the reproductive tract. The incidence of abdominal pregnancy is extremely rare at 1.3%. It is associated with high maternal and perinatal mortality. Maternal mortality is 7.7 times higher in an abdominal ectopic than tubal pregnancy, most likely due to the diagnostic challenge they present [2]. Sites of implantation recorded in the literature in order of descending frequency include (but are not limited to) pouches around the uterus, multiple abdominal organs, omentum, bowel, liver, spleen, and abdominal wall [33]. There are reports of maternal and fetal survival from advanced abdominal pregnancies [34].

USG scans remain the choice investigation for the diagnosis of abdominal ectopic pregnancies. Gerli et al. [35] stated that major sonographic features included:

- The absence of an intrauterine gestation sac
- The absence of both an evident dilated tube and a complex adnexal mass
- A gestational cavity surrounded by loops of bowel and separated by peritoneum
- A wide mobility-like fluctuation of the sac particularly evident with pressure of the transvaginal probe toward the posterior cul-de-sac

MRI has also been shown to be valuable for the diagnosis. MRI can accurately locate both the fetus and placenta and also assess the degree of vascular adherence to surrounding tissues [36].

Medical management is most often used when there is risk of massive hemorrhage, for example, if the abdominal ectopic pregnancy has implanted on a highly vascular site such as the liver or spleen. Use of both systemic and local MTX has been reported. The risk of massive hemorrhage means that maternal mortality can be as high as 11% [2]. Most abdominal ectopic pregnancies are managed with surgery. It is likely this is so high partially because of the number of patients who present with intra-abdominal bleeding. Managing these patients expectantly, particularly in the second trimester, carries a risk of catastrophic intra-abdominal hemorrhage. Due to the seriousness of this complication, it is recommended that when diagnosed, these women undergo surgery [37]. Classically, these pregnancies are managed with laparotomy, but in a 12-year study that began in 2000, Shaw et al. [38] managed all their cases by means of operative laparoscopy. Several methods have been used to control hemorrhage laparoscopically including electrocauterization, harmonic ultrasonic device, hemostatic sealant agents, vasopressin analogues, oxidized cellulose, or a combination of the above.

Usually, abdominal pregnancy diagnosed at a late gestation may frequently present with shock. If an abdominal pregnancy is diagnosed during third trimester, and the patient is stable, the management involves delivery of the fetus with ligation of the umbilical cord close to the placenta. The placenta is usually left in place to avoid hemorrhage following removal.

Cesarean scar pregnancy (CSP) is a relatively new type of ectopic pregnancy. Early diagnosis and treatment is important for the best outcome. This is related to the increasing number of cesarean deliveries and to advances in imaging. Although the exact mechanism of scar implantation is not well understood, the most probable mechanism is that there is invasion of the myometrium between the endometrial canal and cesarean scar through a small tract [39].

There are two types of CSP: CSP with progression to the cervico-isthmic space or uterine cavity (type I, endogenic type) or with deep invasion of the scar defect with progression toward the bladder and abdominal cavity (type II, 25 exogenic type). The endogenic type of CSP could result in a viable pregnancy, yet with a high risk of bleeding at the placental site. The exogenic type could be complicated with uterine rupture and bleeding early in pregnancy [40]. Diagnosis can be achieved with USG. On Doppler imaging, the gestational sac embedded in a scar defect is surrounded by vascular flows characterized by high-velocity and low-impedance blood flow. The USG criteria [41, 42] of CSP are as follows:

- Absence of intrauterine gestation and empty cervical canal with clearly visible endometrium
- A gestational sac located in the anterior isthmus, surrounded by cesarean scar tissue, separated from the uterine cavity, and with or without the presence of a thin myometrial layer between the bladder and the gestation sac
- Gestational sac with or without fetal pole in presence or absence of cardiac activity
- Negative "sliding organs sign," which is defined as the inability to displace the gestational sac from its position at the level of the internal os using gentle pressure applied by the transvaginal probe

All CSPs carry a high risk of uterine rupture and uncontrollable hemorrhage. Expectant management could be dangerous in cesarean scar pregnancies. Women need to be made aware of the morbidity and mortality associated with such pregnancies [24].

Treatment options are expectant, medical (local potassium chloride injection, systemic or local administration of MTX), and surgical intervention with or without extra hemostatic procedures (D&C, hysteroscopy, uterine artery embolization (UAE), laparoscopy, laparotomy, or hysterectomy). In any event, early treatment provides the best results. Medical treatment of previous cesarean scar pregnancy (PCSP) has become an attractive alternative, especially for patients with a maximum PCSP mass diameter of <3.5 cm [39]. Ultimately, management should be with the aim to preserve fertility. Besides systemic single- or multiple-dose MTX injections, local MTX has been described. The success rates of local MTX (with or without potassium chloride) are as high as 80% [43]. Uterine artery embolization (UAE) is an adjuvant treatment of CSP. It minimizes bleeding particularly in cases when trophoblasts are deeply embedded in the myometrium. When β-hCG levels do not decline and where the patient reports continuous vaginal bleeding, a secondary intervention may be necessary after medical management, which can be achieved through operative laparoscopy [44]. In a recent study, the authors used the Cook Cervical Ripening Balloon as an adjuvant treatment method to prevent bleeding in patients who were diagnosed as having CSP and subject to USG-guided suction curettage and found that it effectively reduced bleeding during treatment for CSP [45].

The surgical approach for the management of CSP depends on local expertise. Careful attention needs to be made to prevent potential catastrophic hemorrhage [2]. Hysteroscopy can be performed as a primary treatment especially for type I CSP, as well as for follow-up [46]. Laparoscopic removal of CSP is applicable when an ectopic gestation is growing toward the bladder and abdominal cavity (type II CSP) [47].

Rudimentary horn pregnancy is a rare condition. The diagnosis is challenging, and such anomalies can be frequently overlooked during routine gynecologic evaluation, especially when a communicating horn without any symptoms is present. It might be misdiagnosed as an ectopic, cornual, or isthmic pregnancy [48]. Rudimentary horns tend to rupture between the 10th and 20th gestational weeks because of the weak musculature. Thus, if pregnancy in a rudimentary horn is diagnosed, excision of the pregnant horn is of crucial importance, which can be performed either through laparotomy of laparoscopy. Systemic MTX administration and feticide with intracardiac potassium chloride were also used as alternatives or adjuncts to surgery in early gestation; however, a small number of reported cases preclude making a direct comparison of the feasibility and effectiveness of medical treatment with that of surgical resection. Nevertheless, when a rudimentary horn is diagnosed, the suggested treatment is excision of the rudimentary horn to prevent associated complications.

Heterotopic Pregnancy

Heterotopic pregnancy is defined as the coexistence of intrauterine pregnancy and ectopic pregnancy. The incidence of heterotopic pregnancy is estimated to be 1/30,000 but much higher at

1/100 when associated with in vitro fertilization [49, 50]. Diagnosis is intrinsically difficult as the presence of an intrauterine pregnancy leads many physicians to disregard the symptoms and signs of a parallel pregnancy. Instead, the symptoms are readily attributed to a spectrum of normal and pathologic intrauterine pregnancy manifestations. Heterotopic pregnancy should be kept in mind even if an intrauterine twin pregnancy is diagnosed [51].

Most heterotopic pregnancies are diagnosed after tubal heterotopic rupture, acute abdomen, and hemoperitoneum. In patients who present with pelvic pain, hemoperitoneum, and intrauterine pregnancy, USG adnexal site examination should be recommended for the possibility of heterotopic pregnancy, especially in patients with risk factors (tubal factor infertility, pelvic infections, in vitro fertilization, more embryos transfer, and use of pharmacologic ovulation induction). Biology, and especially monitoring serum β-hCG level, is not helpful for this diagnosis.

Heterotopic pregnancy is a dangerous condition. The management approach adopted for heterotopic pregnancy should incorporate the prognosis of the intrauterine pregnancy and the wishes of the woman regarding its final outcome. After diagnosis of hemoperitoneum with a high suspicion index of heterotopic pregnancy has been made, the management is primarily surgical [52]. Medical modalities have been reported in the literature (transvaginal ultrasound guided injection of potassium chloride, MTX, and/or hyperosmolar glucose into the gestational sac) with a high risk of subsequent emergency salpingectomy. Parenteral injection of MTX is effective for ectopic pregnancy but is not compatible with the continuation of the intrauterine pregnancy. Nonsurgical interventions also have some limitations such as systemic adverse effects and the possible adverse effect on a live fetus [53].

Laparoscopy approaches are recommended. However, heterotopic pregnancies frequently present with hemodynamic instability. Given the effective role of laparotomy in the emergency setting, it is therefore unlikely, at least in the near future, to be eliminated from the management repertoire. Thus, trans-umbilical Veress needle insufflation is contraindicated, and two-trocar insertion techniques are thus recommended: open laparoscopy (using the trans-umbilical or supra-umbilical routes, depending on the volume of the uterus) or micro-laparoscopy via the left upper quadrant. After 24 weeks of gestation, it is recommended to apply open laparoscopy, above the level of the umbilicus [54]. The insufflation pressure must be adapted and maintained at a maximum of 12 mmHg in the case of laparoscopy during pregnancy. If the patient wants to preserve the intrauterine pregnancy, salpingectomy should be performed to ensure the efficacy of the treatment.

Impact of Ectopic Pregnancy for Reproductive Prognosis in Next Generation

The impact of an ectopic pregnancy in the next generation is unknown. We know that daughters of mothers with ectopic pregnancy have a 50% higher risk of ectopic pregnancy and a 30% increased risk of induced abortions than daughters of women with no such history [55]. The increased risk is not necessarily due to a genetically transmitted disposition but could also be influenced by similar lifestyles in mother and daughter, for example, in sexual and contraceptive practices. Behavioral patterns, such as smoking and alcohol, are socially transmitted, and children of smokers or alcohol users are more likely to smoke or drink than children of non-smokers or those who do not drink alcohol [55]. Therefore, other behavioral patterns might also be affected by social heritage.

Conclusion and Future Research

In summary, many treatment options are now available to the physician in the treatment of tubal pregnancy:

- Expectant management
- Medical treatment with a variety of drugs that can be administered systemically and/or

locally by different routes (transvaginally under sonographic guidance or under laparoscopic guidance)

- Surgical treatment, which can be performed radically or conservatively, either laparoscopically or by an open surgical procedure

Laparoscopic surgery is the cornerstone of treatment in the majority of women with tubal pregnancy. This technique is feasible in virtually all patients, is safe, and is less costly compared with the open surgical approach. Also, minimally invasive approaches are safe and effective treatment options for nontubal ectopic pregnancies in women who wish to conserve fertility. Ideally, the operating physician should have the skills to perform the appropriate surgical treatment, i.e., salpingectomy and salpingotomy. If not, there should be on-call support available in the event that other procedures be necessary and to provide on-the-job training. Studies have shown that virtual reality simulators offer realistic training for surgical procedures such as salpingectomy [56].

Around 10% of women with a single previous EP, regardless of choice of management, have a second EP as their subsequent pregnancy. Consequently, all women who have been previously affected by EP are offered pre-booked USG around 6–9 weeks after the onset of their last menstrual period for pregnancy localization. Following an EP, women who have a viable intrauterine pregnancy have similar reproductive outcomes compared with women without prior EP as their first pregnancy. However, women with previous EP have a higher rate of repeat EP and miscarriage in their second pregnancy.

Active research into improvements in diagnosis and management of EP is in progress. A single serum biomarker for EP remains elusive [57]. A randomized controlled trial of placebo or gefitinib (an oral anti-epidermal growth factor receptor agent [EGFR]) used in combination with MTX to hasten resolution of ectopic pregnancy is underway). The rationale is based on evidence that EGFR is highly expressed on placental tissue from EPs, and encouraging results from early clinical trials have shown it to be safe and tolerated well by women with EP [58].

Psychological sequelae from pregnancy loss with an ectopic pregnancy can be prolonged and as severe as post-traumatic stress disorder. Subfertility and EP share common risk factors, which may only have partly been overcome with assisted reproductive technology. The absence of additional risk factors for women with subfertility means that they can be advised that future rates of intrauterine pregnancy and EP are similar between surgical, medical, and expectant management for tubal EP [59].

References

1. King L, Nezhat C, Nezhat F, et al. Laparoscopic access. In: Nezhat C, Nezhat F, Nezhat C, editors. Nezhat's video-assisted and robotic-assisted laparoscopy and hysteroscopy, 4th ed. New York, NY: Cambridge University Press; 2013.
2. Alalade AO, Smith FJE, Kendall CE, Odejinmi F. Evidence-based management of non-tubal ectopic pregnancies. J Obstet Gynaecol. 2017;37(8):982–91.
3. Ramkrishna J, Kan GR, Reidy KL, Ang WC, Palma-Dias R. Comparison of management regimens following ultrasound diagnosis of nontubal ectopic pregnancies: a retrospective cohort study. BJOG. 2017. https://doi.org/10.1111/1471-0528.14752. [Epub ahead of print]
4. Riaz RM, Williams TR, Craig BM, Myers DT. Cesarean scar ectopic pregnancy: imaging features, current treatment options, and clinical outcomes. Abdom Imaging. 2015;40:2589–99.
5. Tenore JL. Ectopic pregnancy. Am Fam Physician. 2000;61:1080–8.
6. Dart RG, Kaplan B, Varaklis K. Predictive value of history and physical examination in patients with suspected ectopic pregnancy. Ann Emerg Med. 1999;33:283–90.
7. Hajenius PJ, Mol F, Mol BW, Bossuyt PM, Ankum WM, van der Veen F. Interventions for tubal ectopic pregnancy. Cochrane Database Syst Rev 2007;(1):CD000324.
8. Spandorfer SD, Barnhart KT. Role of previous ectopic pregnancy in altering the presentation of suspected ectopic pregnancy. J Reprod Med. 2003;48:133–6.
9. Murray H, Baakdah H, Bardell T, Tulandi T. Diagnosis and treatment of ectopic pregnancy. CMAJ. 2005;173(8):905–12.
10. Condous G, Okaro E, Khalid A, Lu C, Van Huffel S, Timmerman D, et al. The accuracy of transvaginal ultrasonography for the diagnosis of ectopic pregnancy prior to surgery. Hum Reprod. 2005;20:1404–9.
11. Preisler J, Kopeika J, Ismail L, Vathanan V, Farren J, Abdallah Y, et al. Defining safe criteria to diagnose miscarriage: prospective observational multicentre study. BMJ. 2015;h4579:351.

12. Srisajjakul S, Prapaisilp P, Bangchokdee S. Magnetic resonance imaging in tubal and non-tubal ectopic pregnancy. Eur J Radiol. 2017;93:76–89.
13. Elson J, Tailor A, Banerjee S, Salim R, Hillaby K, Jurkovic D. Expectant management of tubal ectopic pregnancy: prediction of successful outcome using decision tree analysis. Ultrasound Obstet Gynecol. 2004;23:552–6.
14. National Institute for Health and Care Excellence. Ectopic pregnancy and miscarriage: diagnosis and initial management in early pregnancy of ectopic pregnancy and miscarriage. NICE clinical guideline 154. Manchester: NICE; 2012.
15. Kirk E, van Calster B, Condous G, Papageorghiou AT, Gevaert O, van Huffel S, et al. Ectopic pregnancy: using the b-hCG ratio to select women for expectant or medical management. Acta Obstet Gynecol Scand. 2011;90:264–72.
16. Barnhart KT, Gosman G, Ashby R, Sammel M. The medical management of ectopic pregnancy: a meta-analysis comparing "single dose" and "multidose" regimens. Obstet Gynecol. 2003;101:778–84.
17. Pansky M, Bukovsky I, Golan A, et al. Local methotrexate injection: a nonsurgical treatment of ectopic pregnancy. Obstet Gynecol. 1989;161:393–6.
18. Fernandez H, Baton C, Beniflan JL, Frydman R, Lelaidier C. Methotrexate treatment of ectopic pregnancy: 100 cases treated by primary transvaginal injection under sonographic control. Fertility & Sterility. 1993;59:773–7.
19. Egarter C, Husslein P. Treatment of tubal pregnancy by prostaglandins. Lancet. 1988;14:1104–5.
20. Lang P, Weiss PAM, Mayer HO. Local application of hyperosmolar glucose solution in tubal pregnancy. Lancet. 1989;2(8668):922–3.
21. Tzafettas J, Anapliotis S, Zournatzi V, Boucklis A, Oxouzoglou N, Bondis J. Transvaginal intra amniotic injection of methotrexate in early ectopic pregnancy. Advantages over the laparoscopic approach. Early Hum Dev. 1994;39:101–7.
22. Ugur M, Yesilyurt H, Soysal S, Gokmen O. Prophylactic vasopressin during laparoscopic salpingotomy for ectopic pregnancy. J Am Assoc Gynecol Laparosc. 1996;3:365–8.
23. Yao M, Tulandi T. Current status of surgical and nonsurgical management of ectopic pregnancy. Fertil Steril. 1997;67:421–33.
24. Elson CJ, Salim R, Potdar N, Chetty M, Ross JA, Kirk EJ. Diagnosis and Management of Ectopic Pregnancy: green-top guideline no. 21. BJOG. 2016;123(13):e15-e55.
25. Laparoscopic removal of an ectopic pregnancy. In: Wallwiener D, Becker S. Atlas of gynecologic surgery. 4th ed. Stuttgart: Thieme; 2009.
26. Timor-Tritsch IE, Monteagudo A, Matera C, Veit CR. Sonographic evolution of cornual pregnancies treated without surgery. Obstet Gynecol. 1992;79:1044–9.
27. Faraj R, Steel M. Management of cornual (interstitial) pregnancy. Obstet Gynaecol. 2007;9:249–55.
28. Monteagudo A, Minior VK, Stephenson C, Monda S, Timor-Tritsch IE. Non-surgical management of live ectopic pregnancy with ultrasound- guided local injection: a case series. Ultrasound Obstet Gynecol. 2005;25:282–8.
29. Damario M, Rock J. Chapter 34: ectopic pregnancy. In: Rock JJ, Jones HI, editors. TeLInde's operative gynecology. 10th ed. Philadelphia: Lippincott Williams & Wilkins; 2011. p. 798–824.
30. Cucinella G, Calagna G, Rotolo S, Granese R, Saitta S, Tonni G, et al. Interstitial pregnancy: a road map of surgical treatment based on a systematic review of the literature. Gynecol Obstet Investig. 2014;78:141–9.
31. Nezhat CH, Dun EC. Laparoscopically-assisted, hysteroscopic removal of an interstitial pregnancy with a fertility-preserving technique. J Minim Invasive Gynecol. 2014;21(6):1091–4.
32. Spiegelberg O. The casuistry of ovarian pregnancy. Archiv Fur Gynaekologie. 1878;13:73–6.
33. Poole A, Haas D, Magann EF. 2012. Early abdominal ectopic pregnancies: a systematic review of the literature. Gynecol Obstet Investig. 2012;74:249–60.
34. Hailu FG, Yihunie GT, Essa AA, Tsega WK. Advanced abdominal pregnancy, with live fetus and severe preeclampsia, case report. BMC Pregnancy Childbirth. 2017;17(1):243.
35. Gerli S, Rossetti D, Baiocchi G, Clerici G, Unfer V, Di Renzo GC. Early ultrasonographic diagnosis and laparoscopic treatment of abdominal pregnancy. Eur J Obstet Gynecol Reprod Biol. 2004;113:103–5.
36. Lockhat F, Corr P, Ramphal S, Moodley J. The value of magnetic resonance imaging in the diagnosis and management of extra-uterine abdominal pregnancy. Clin Radiol. 2006;61:264–9.
37. Agarwal N, Odejinmi F. Early abdominal ectopic pregnancy: challenges, update and review of current management. Obstet Gynaecol. 2014;16:193–8.
38. Shaw SW, Hsu JJ, Chueh HY, Han CM, Chen FC, Chang YL, et al. Management of primary abdominal pregnancy: twelve years of experience in a medical Centre. Acta Obstet Gynecol Scand. 2007;86:1058–62.
39. Ying X, Zheng W, Zhao L, Zhou M, Chen Z. Clinical characteristics and salvage management of persistent cesarean scar pregnancy. J Obstet Gynaecol Res. 2017;43(8):1293–8.
40. Gonzalez N, Tulandi T. Cesarean scar pregnancy: a systematic review. J Minim Invasive Gynecol. 2017;24(5):731–8.
41. Rheinboldt M, Osborn D, Delproposto Z. Cesarean section scar ectopic pregnancy: a clinical case series. J Ultrasound. 2015;18:191–5.
42. Huanxiao Z, Shuqin C, Hongye J, Hongzhe X, Gang N, Chenkag X, et al. Transvaginal hysterotomy for cesarean scar pregnancy in 40 consecutive cases. Gynecol Surg. 2015;12:45–51.
43. Ko JK, Li RH, Cheung VY. Caesarean scar pregnancy: a 10-year experience. Aust N Z J Obstet Gynaecol. 2015;55:64–9.

44. Agarwal N, Shahid A, Odejinmi F. Caesarean scar pregnancy (CSP): a rare case of complete scar dehiscence due to scar ectopic pregnancy and its management. Arch Gynecol Obstet. 2013;288:231–2.
45. Wu C, Li Y, Ye W, Ma W, Zhao D. Cook cervical ripening balloon successfully prevents excessive hemorrhage combined with ultrasound-guided suction curettage in the treatment of cesarean scar pregnancy. J Obstet Gynaecol Res. 2017;43(6):1043–7.
46. Mollo A, Alviggi C, Conforti A, Insabato L, De Placido G. Intact removal of spontaneous twin ectopic cesarean scar pregnancy by office hysteroscopy: case report and literature review. Reprod Biomed Online. 2014;29:530–3.
47. Litwicka K, Greco E. Cesarean scar pregnancy: a review of management options. Curr Opin Obstet Gynecol. 2013;25:456–61.
48. Sönmezer M, Taskin S, Atabekoğlu C, Güngör M, Unlü C. Laparoscopic management of rudimentary uterine horn pregnancy: case report and literature review. JSLS. 2006;10(3):396–9.
49. Fernandez H, Gervaise A. Ectopic pregnancies after infertility treatment: modern diagnosis and therapeutic strategy. Hum Reprod Update. 2004;10(6):503–13.
50. Tal J, Haddad S, Gordon N, Timor-Tritsch I. Heterotopic pregnancy after ovulation induction and assisted reproductive technologies: a literature review from 1971 to 1993. Fertil Steril. 1996;66:1–12.
51. Bataille P, Reynard A, Ducarme G. Spontaneous heterotopic triplets—a review of literature. J Gynecol Obstet Hum Reprod. 2017. pii: S2468-7847(17)30140-X.
52. Talbot K, Simpson R, Price N, Jackson SR. Heterotopic pregnancy. J Obstet Gynaecol. 2011;31(1):7–12.
53. Habana A, Dokras A, Giraldo JL, Jones EE. Cornual heterotopic pregnancy: contemporary management options. Am J Obstet Gynecol. 2000;182(5):1264–70.
54. Deffieux X, Ballester M, Collinet P, Fauconnier A. Pierre F; French National College of gynaecologists and obstetricians. Risks associated with laparoscopic entry: guidelines for clinical practice from the French college of gynaecologists and obstetricians. Eur J Obstet Gynecol Reprod Biol. 2011;158(2):159–66.
55. Kårhus LL, Egerup P, Skovlund CW, Lidegaard Ø. Impact of ectopic pregnancy for reproductive prognosis in next generation. Acta Obstet Gynecol Scand. 2014;93(4):416–9.
56. Hessel M, Buzink SN, Schoot D, Jakimowicz JJ. Face and construct validity of the SimSurgery SEP VR simulator for salpingectomy in case of ectopic pregnancy. J Gynecol Surg. 2012;28:411–7.
57. Tong S, Skubisz MM, Horne AW. Molecular diagnostics and therapeutics for ectopic pregnancy. Mol Hum Reprod. 2015;21(2):126–35.
58. Capmas P, Fernandez H. Effectiveness of gefitinib in combination with methotrexate in the treatment of ectopic pregnancy. Int J Womens Health. 2015;7:673–6.
59. Lozeau AM, Potter B. Diagnosis and management of ectopic pregnancy. Am Fam Physician. 2005;72(9):1707–14.

Part V

Surgical Management of Obstetric Complications

Molar Pregnancy

27

Meaghan E. Tenney

Introduction

Molar pregnancy (hydatidiform mole, mole) is a subset of gestational trophoblastic disease (GTD), a spectrum of benign and malignant disorders [invasive molar pregnancy, choriocarcinoma, placental site trophoblastic tumor (PSTT), and epithelioid trophoblastic tumor (ETT)] arising from abnormal placental trophoblastic tissue [1, 2] (Fig. 27.1). Gestational trophoblastic neoplasia (GTN) refers to the entire group of malignant GTD. Reportedly first described by Hippocrates as "dropsy of the uterus" in relation to "unwholesome" water in 400 BC in *On Airs, Waters, and Places* [3–6], hydatidiform mole exists in two distinct forms, complete hydatidiform mole and partial hydatidiform mole. Complete and partial moles differ in their epidemiology, pathology, cytogenetics, clinical presentation, and outcome [7–13].

Epidemiology and Risk Factors

Wide variety exists in the reported regional incidence of hydatidiform mole, and numerous factors likely play a role [8, 14–16]. At baseline, GTD and hydatidiform mole are very rare conditions and the population at risk is hard to define [17]. Both hospital-based and population-based data are often used and the denominator varies between total number of pregnancies, live births, or deliveries [14, 15, 17–20]. The availability of centralized review, radiography, and cytogenetics varies greatly worldwide, often within the same population, contributing to the varied incidence rates [17]. Recent trends have shown stable to slightly increased incidence rates in many countries, potentially due to increasing maternal age [19, 21, 22].

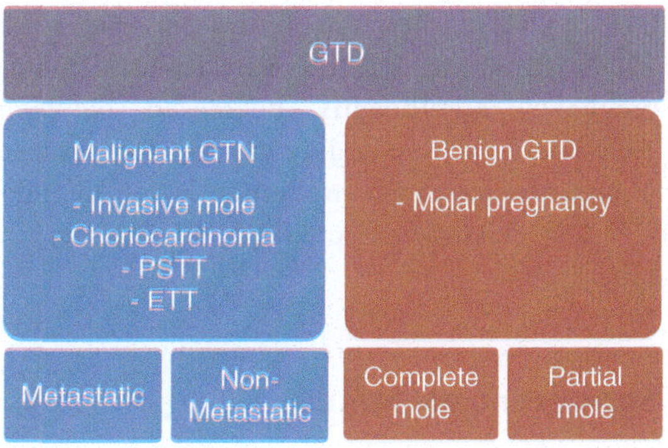

Fig. 27.1 Spectrum of gestational trophoblastic disease

M. E. Tenney
University Gynecologic Oncology, Northside Hospital, Atlanta, GA, USA
e-mail: meaghan.tenney@northside.com

C. H. Nezhat (ed.), *Non-Obstetric Surgery During Pregnancy*,
https://doi.org/10.1007/978-3-319-90752-9_27

Geography, Race, and Ethnicity

Asian countries have long reported much higher rates of molar pregnancy than European or North American countries, and significant variation exists within geographic regions and even within the same country [5, 8, 17]. One study in Japan reported an incidence of molar pregnancy of 2.0 per 1000 pregnancies [16]; however, another Japanese study reported a range of 2.83–3.05 per 1000 live births [23]. These rates are two to three times higher than the reported incidence in Europe or North America (0.6–1.1 per 1000 pregnancies) [16]. Rates in Nigeria and Pakistan are reported to be 4/1000 deliveries and 5.1/1000 pregnancies, respectively [24, 25]. Some of the highest incidence rates have been reported in China and Indonesia, at 6.7 and 11.5 per live birth, respectively [17]. In New Mexico, American Indian women are at significantly higher risk than non-Hispanic and Hispanic white women with age-adjusted incidence rates of 11.16%, 3.57%, and 5.32%, respectively [26].

Recently, rates in Asian countries and Asian women have decreased to be more similar to those in Europe and North America. In the 1990s in South Korea, the incidence of molar pregnancy decreased to 1.6 per 1000 births from a much higher 4.4 per 1000 births in the 1960s, while in Italy, the overall rate of molar pregnancy significantly decreased between 1996 and 2008, due largely in part to a decrease in pregnancies in Asian women living in Italy [27, 28]. A similar decrease has been seen in Japan [29].

Socioeconomic Status

Socioeconomic factors may play a role in the wide range of incidence rates. In Nepal, the 5-year annual rate of molar pregnancy was 4.17 per 1000 live births with the majority of patients being of Hindu religion [30]. In Iran, 7/1000 pregnancies are molar which was associated with a significantly higher rate of prior molar pregnancy, oral contraceptive use, abortion, and ovulation induction [31]. A 5-year prospective study in Hawaii showed a significantly increased rate of complete mole in Filipino women and, however, showed no difference in maternal age, race, place of birth, or socioeconomic status for women with partial mole [32].

Diet and Nutrition

Dietary and nutritional factors have been associated with molar pregnancy. Vitamin A deficiency is associated with spontaneous abortion in female rhesus monkeys and abnormal spermatogenesis in male rhesus monkeys [33]. In areas with a high frequency of vitamin A deficiency, high incidence of molar pregnancy is seen [34]. Low dietary intake of carotene (vitamin A precursor) and animal fat is potentially associated with increased risk of complete mole in case-control studies [35, 36]. A recent randomized, double-blind placebo-controlled clinical trial in Indonesia, an area with one of the highest reported rates of molar pregnancy [17], demonstrated a significantly lower rate of postmolar GTN in women with complete mole randomized to high doses of vitamin A (200,000 IU/day) compared to placebo (6.3% vs. 28.6%, respectively) further supporting an association between vitamin A and GTD [37]. In Senegal and Morocco, nutritional deficiency in the mother leads to a higher incidence of complete mole in their daughters' pregnancies, potentially due to effects on normal oocyte development in the daughters during fetal development [38]. Unlike complete mole, the risk of partial mole does not seem to be associated with dietary factors [8].

Maternal Age

Extremes of maternal age have consistently been shown to increase the risk for molar pregnancy, particularly complete mole, and areas seeing increasing numbers of molar pregnancies suspect this is due to more advanced maternal age [21, 32, 39–42]. In a series of 7916 molar pregnancies, median age at presentation was 27 years old. The highest risk was seen in women ≤15 years old or ≥45 years old [43]. In women over age 35, the risk of complete mole is two times higher, and is increased 7.5-fold for women over age 40 [44]. An updated series out of Charing Cross in the UK reported a risk for complete mole of <1/1000 conceptions in women age 18–40, compared to 1/156 for those age 45 and an impressive 1/8 for women age 50 and older [45]. A more contemporary series out of Brigham and Women's Hospital confirms these earlier observations and demonstrated a sevenfold increase in complete mole in adolescents under age 20 and a twofold increase in women age 40 and over compared to average age women (aged 20–39). The age-related risk of molar pregnancy does not seem to be associated with partial mole [46].

Reproductive History

Recurrent Molar Pregnancy

History of molar pregnancy is the second consistent risk factor for molar pregnancy. The risk of developing a subsequent molar pregnancy after a first episode is approximately 1–2% and rises to 15–20% after two molar pregnancies [47–53]. These rates remain consistent in updated series from Charing Cross in London and the New England Trophoblastic Disease Center, two of the largest referral centers worldwide [54, 55].

Spontaneous Abortion and Infertility

Women with prior spontaneous abortions appear to be at risk for both complete and partial molar pregnancy. When comparing women with two or more spontaneous abortions to women with no previous miscarriage, the risk for complete and partial mole was three and two times higher, respectively, in those with prior miscarriage [56]. Previously, the same group reported a 32-fold increase in complete mole in women with two consecutive spontaneous abortions [57].

Women with infertility may have an increased risk of both molar pregnancy and "twin pregnancies" made up of one or more normal fetuses and a molar pregnancy. Women with difficulty conceiving or with history of infertility have a 2.4 and 3.2 times increased risk of complete and partial mole, respectively [56]. In Iran, ovulation induction is associated with risk of molar pregnancy [31]. Women undergoing ovulation induction, intrauterine insemination, in vitro fertilization, and/or intracytoplasmic sperm injection have been reported to have twin, triplet, and even quadruplet pregnancies consisting of one to three normal fetuses and a molar pregnancy [58–61]. Ectopic ovarian molar pregnancy has been reported after in vitro fertilization [62].

Familial Recurrent Hydatidiform Mole

A rare autosomal recessive familial disorder, familial recurrent hydatidiform mole syndrome (FRHM), leads to repetitive diploid molar pregnancies of biparental origin. Outcome is independent of male partner, and live birth of a normal fetus is rare. Egg donation from a normal donor may be the best option for these women to achieve a successful pregnancy [1, 63–65]. The majority (80%) of women with FRHM have a mutation in the leucine-rich region of the NLRP7 gene on chromosome 13, and another 5% have a mutation in the KHDC3L gene [66–69].

Other Possible Risk Factors

Data is inconsistent on other potential risk factors such as oral contraceptive use, irregular menstruation, consanguinity, and ABO blood group [16, 31, 70–72].

Pathology and Cytogenetics

Molar pregnancy is separated into two distinct entities, complete and partial mole, which are easily distinguishable from each other based on their pathologic features and cytogenetics (Table 27.1) [10–13, 73–75].

Pathology

Molar pregnancies originate from placental trophoblastic tissue, specifically, the cytotrophoblast and syncytiotrophoblast [15]. Complete molar pregnancies are characterized by marked villous edema (hydropic villi) and trophoblastic proliferation (hyperplasia or hypertrophy), central cistern formation, and an absence of fetal red blood cells, amnion, or fetal parts (Fig. 27.2). Hydropic villi are easily identified grossly (Fig. 27.3) [10, 11, 13]. Partial molar pregnancies have focal villous edema and minimal trophoblastic proliferation and lack central cisterns (Fig. 27.4). Fetal vessels, red blood cells, and amnion are usually present. Grossly, fetal parts, umbilical cord, and an amniotic membrane are often identified [10, 11, 13].

Table 27.1 Pathologic and cytogenetic features of complete and partial hydatidiform moles (Adapted from [2, 6, 166])

	Partial mole	Complete mole
Pathology		
Fetus	Often present	Absent
Amnion, fetal RBC	Usually present	Absent
Villous edema	Focal	Diffuse
Trophoblastic proliferation	Focal	Diffuse
Karyotype	Triploid: 69,XXY (majority) 69,XXX and 69,XYY	Diploid: 46,XX (majority) 46,XY
	Paternal and maternal origin	All paternal origin

Cytogenetics

The cytogenetic makeup of complete and partial moles is similarly distinct. Complete moles are diploid, with the majority being 46,XX and the result

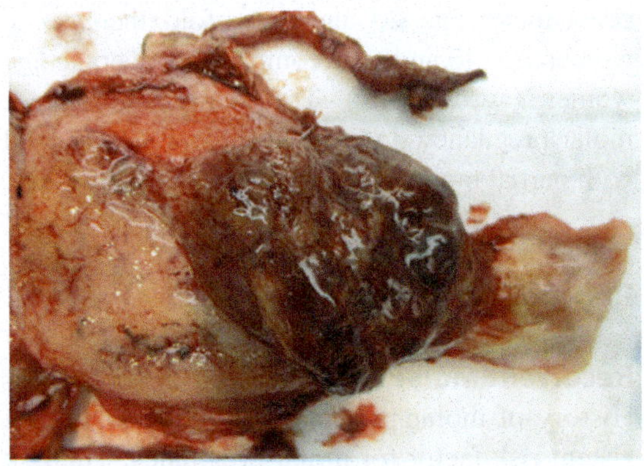

Fig. 27.3 Complete molar pregnancy in hysterectomy specimen with grossly enlarged hydropic villi. Photo courtesy of Ralph Sams, MD

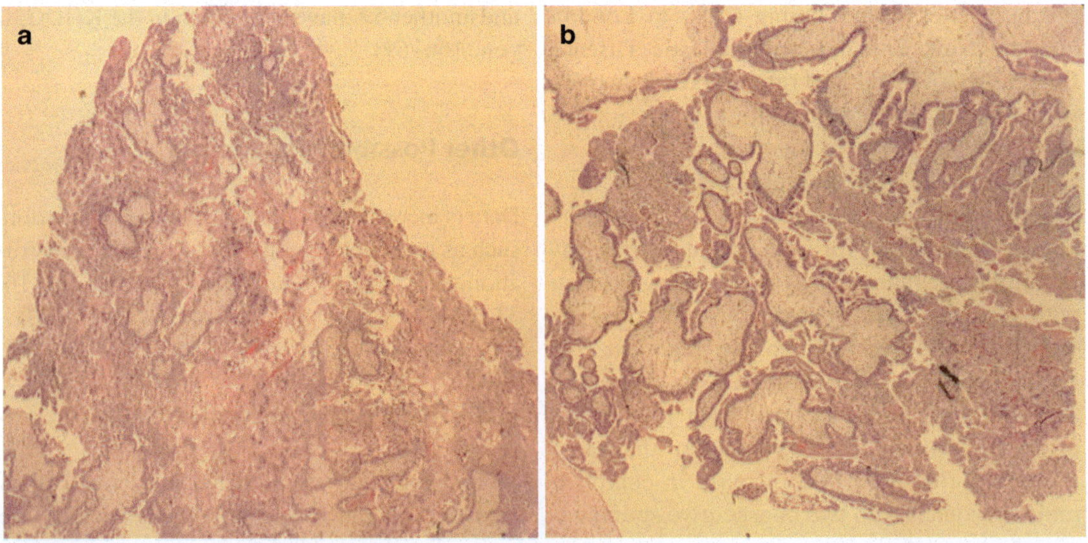

Fig. 27.2 (**a**, **b**) Complete molar pregnancy with large hydropic villi, trophoblastic proliferation, and central cistern formation. Photos courtesy of Ralph Sams, MD

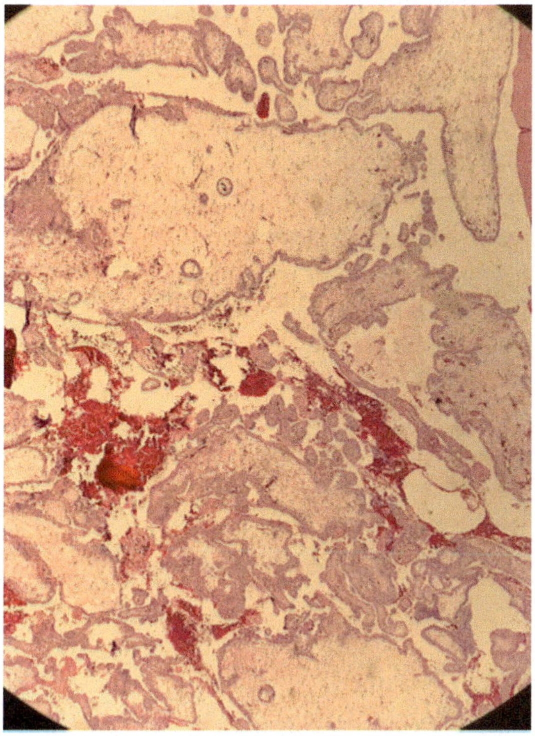

Fig. 27.4 Partial molar pregnancy. Photo courtesy of Ralph Sams, MD

of fertilization of an empty egg with a haploid sperm and subsequent duplication of the paternal chromosomes after fertilization [10, 11, 13, 73, 76]. Approximately 10% of complete moles are 46,XY or 46,XX and dispermic in origin, resulting from the fertilization of an empty egg with two haploid sperm (Fig. 27.5) [15, 74, 75, 77]. Despite complete paternal origin of the chromosomes in a complete mole, the mitochondrial DNA is maternal in origin [78]. Dispermic 46,XY complete moles may have a higher risk of postmolar GTN compared to 46,XX [75, 79]. Partial moles are triploid, usually 69,XXY but also 69,XXX and 69,XYY. They result from either the fertilization of a haploid egg with a haploid sperm and subsequent duplication of the paternal chromosomes after fertilization or the fertilization of a haploid egg with two haploid sperm (Fig. 27.6) [10, 11, 77, 80].

Diagnostic Challenges

Molar pregnancy is now frequently diagnosed in the first trimester due to greater availability of early ultrasonography and quantitative human

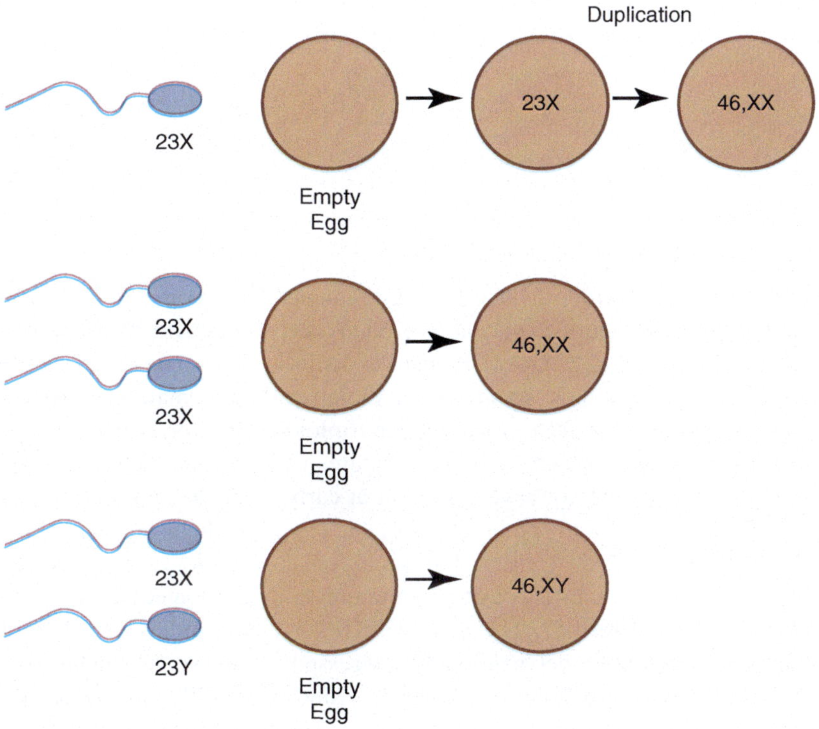

Fig. 27.5 Karyotypes of complete hydatidiform mole. Reproduced from Schink JC, Lurain JR. Gestational trophoblastic disease: molar pregnancy and gestational trophoblastic neoplasia. In: Barakat RR, Berchuck A, Markman M, Randall ME, editor. Principles and practice of gynecologic oncology, 6th ed. Philadelphia: Lippincott Williams & Wilkins; 2013. p. 889. With permission from Wolters Kluwer

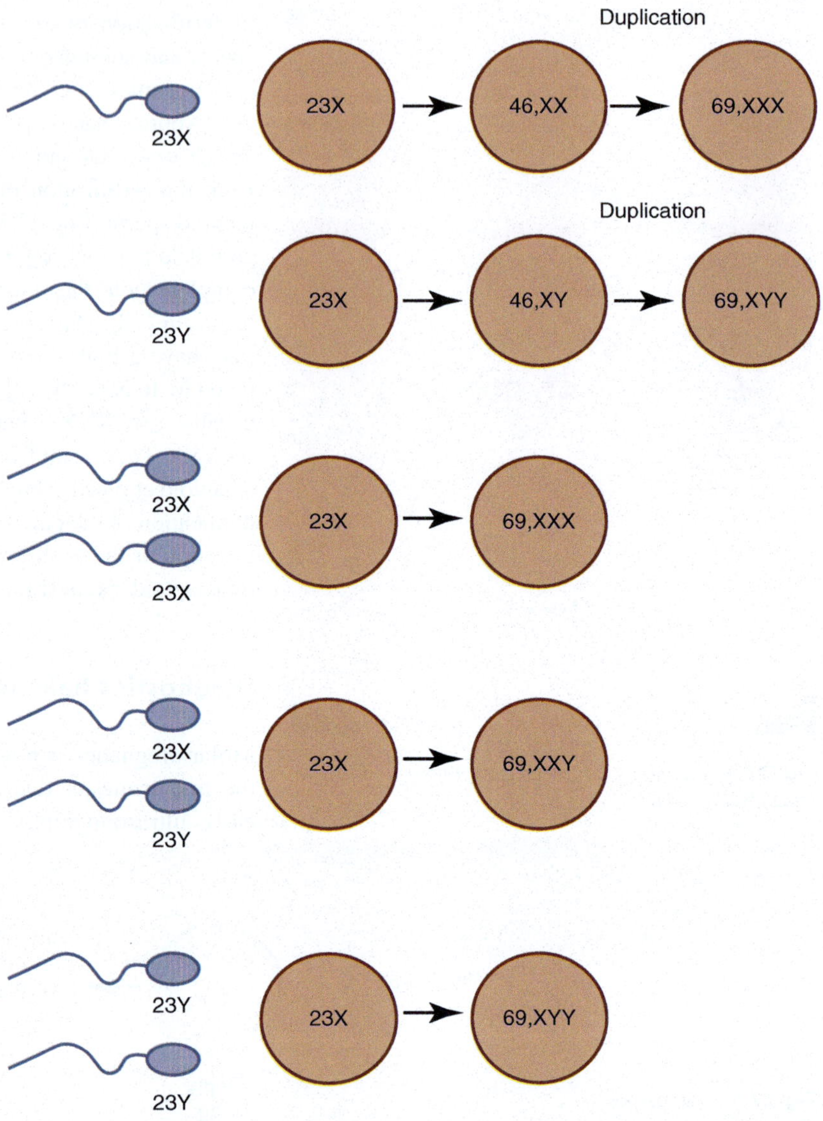

Fig. 27.6 Karyotypes of partial hydatidiform mole. Reproduced from Schink JC, Lurain JR. Gestational trophoblastic disease: molar pregnancy and gestational trophoblastic neoplasia. In: Barakat RR, Berchuck A, Markman M, Randall ME, editor. Principles and practice of gynecologic oncology, 6th ed. Philadelphia: Lippincott Williams & Wilkins; 2013. p. 889. With permission from Wolters Kluwer

chorionic gonadotropin (hCG) measurement, leading to earlier uterine evacuation [81]. When this occurs, pathologists face challenges in distinguishing complete mole from partial mole, as well as partial mole from a non-molar triploid pregnancy because the characteristic features of molar pregnancy are not always present at early gestations [82, 83]. Early complete mole can easily be distinguished from partial mole or a hydropic non-molar abortus using immunohistochemistry (IHC) for p57. The gene p57KIP2 is paternally imprinted, yet maternally expressed, so IHC of a complete mole will be negative since it is completely paternal in origin, while partial mole and hydropic non-molar abortus will have positive staining since they contain both paternal and maternal tissue (Fig. 27.7) [84–86]. Differentiating between partial mole and a hydropic abortus is a bit more challenging and can be impossible based on histology or morphology alone [87]. A combination of histopathology and molecular genotyping of placental and maternal tissue to determine parental origin and ploidy can definitively distinguish between the two yet can be cost prohibitive and is not universally available [88–90]. When available,

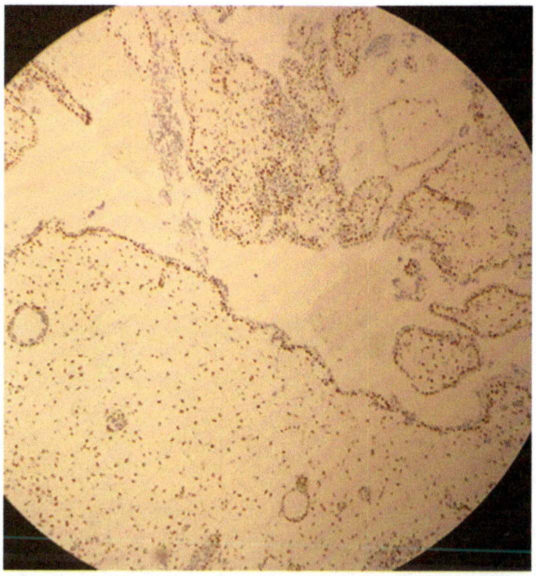

Fig. 27.7 Partial mole and positive p57 stain. Photo courtesy of Ralph Sams, MD

genotyping should be done to evaluate the presence of partial mole when any of the following histologic features are seen: villous size ≥ 2.5 mm, cistern formation, two populations of villi, or round or oval pseudoinclusions [87]. When genotyping was not available, a combination of large trophoblastic inclusions, multifocal trophoblast proliferation, and cistern formation correctly identified over 90% of partial moles in one study [91].

Clinical Presentation

The clinical presentation of hydatidiform mole has changed in recent decades with the widespread use of early ultrasonography and serum hCG testing (Table 27.2) [9, 82, 92–94].

Complete Mole

Historically, complete molar pregnancy was typically diagnosed in the second trimester due to consequences of abnormally elevated hCG and advanced disease, such as uterine size greater than dates, hyperemesis gravidarum, hemoptysis from trophoblastic embolization, hyperthyroidism, theca lutein cysts, and early-onset preeclampsia. Reports from multiple centers demonstrate that these clinical features are now seen much less with earlier diagnosis [82, 92–94]. In two series of patients seen for complete molar pregnancy at the New England Trophoblastic Disease Center, the changing trends for some clinical features can be seen across three cohorts of patients from 1965 to 1975, 1988 to 1993, and 1994 to 2013 (Table 27.3) [82, 94, 95]. When comparing patients who presented between 5 and 9 weeks gestation to those who presented at 10 and 22 weeks gestation, those who presented later were more likely to have higher hCG, pre-evacuation diagnosis of complete mole, hyperemesis, biochemical hyperthyroidism, anemia, and theca lutein cysts [82]. Because of the earlier presentation, the typical "snowstorm pattern" (Fig. 27.8) and theca lutein cysts (Fig. 27.9) seen on imaging studies of complete moles are often not present, and the diagnosis is only made on pathologic evaluation of uterine contents after a dilation and curettage for a presumed spontaneous abortion [96]. Despite earlier diagnosis, the risk of developing postmolar gestational trophoblastic neoplasia has remained relatively constant over the past 50 years at the New England Trophoblastic Disease Center (Table 27.3) and other centers worldwide [22, 82, 93, 95].

Partial Mole

The presentation of partial hydatidiform mole differs quite significantly from complete molar pregnancy. Women with partial molar pregnancy are less likely to have uterine size greater than dates, abnormally elevated serum hCG, vaginal bleeding, biochemical hyperthyroidism, hyperemesis, theca lutein cysts, or preeclampsia compared to those with complete mole [94, 97]. Because of this, over 90% of women with partial molar pregnancy have an initial diagnosis of missed or incomplete abortion and are only found to have a mole after the pathologic evaluation of uterine contents after a dilation and curettage [97].

Table 27.2 Clinical features of complete and partial hydatidiform moles (Adapted from [2, 6, 166])

	Partial mole	Complete mole
Diagnosis	Missed abortion	Molar gestation
hCG	Usually < 100,000 mIU/mL	Often > 100,000 mIU/mL
Uterine size	Small for dates	Large for dates
Theca lutein cysts	Rare	15–30%
Medical complications	Rare	10–25%
Postmolar malignant risk	<5%	6–32%

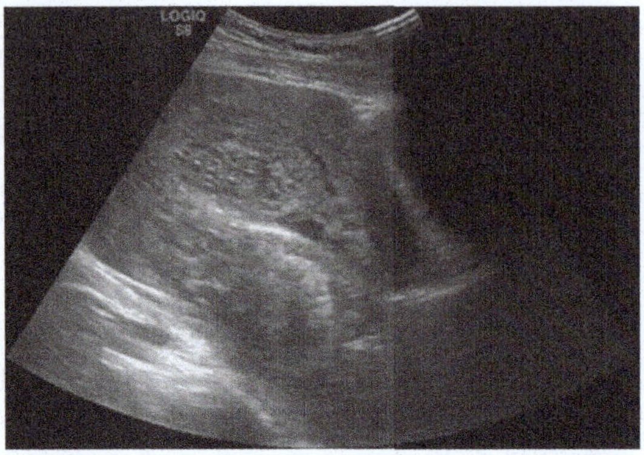

Fig. 27.8 “Snowstorm” ultrasound appearance of classic complete hydatidiform mole. Photo courtesy of Meaghan Tenney, MD

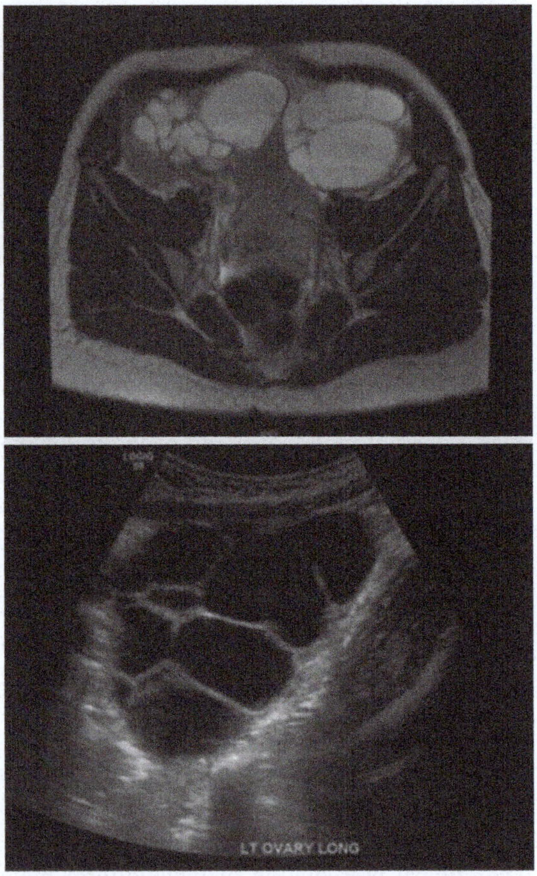

Fig. 27.9 Theca lutein cysts in complete molar pregnancy on MRI (upper) and ultrasound (lower). Photos courtesy of Meaghan Tenney, MD

Diagnosis

As previously mentioned, the diagnosis of molar pregnancy is frequently not made until after uterine evacuation is performed for an abnormal pregnancy; however, this diagnosis should be suspected in any woman of reproductive age with abnormal vaginal bleeding. The index of suspicion should be raised if any of the classic clinical features for molar pregnancy are present such as uterine size greater than dates, hyperemesis gravidarum, early preeclampsia, theca lutein cysts, or abnormally high serum hCG for presumed gestational age [2].

Ultrasonography

Transvaginal pelvic ultrasound is the preferred imaging study for the preoperative evaluation and diagnosis of both complete and partial molar pregnancy but is often incorrect or indeterminate at early gestational age [15, 95, 98–101]. Fowler et al. reported a series of over 1000 cases referred to Charing Cross, a major trophoblastic center in the UK, and found that molar pregnancies were correctly identified on routine pre-evacuation ultrasound less than 50% of the time and more frequently appeared to have the sonographic appearance of missed or incomplete abortion. Ultrasound was significantly better at detecting

Table 27.3 Changing clinical presentation of complete molar pregnancy at the New England Trophoblastic Disease Center from 1965 to 2013 (Adapted from [82, 94, 95])

	1965–1975 (*n* = 306)	1988–1993 (*n* = 74)	1994–2013 (*n* = 180)
Vaginal bleeding	297 (97%)	62 (84%)	80 (46%)
Anemia	165 (54%)	4 (5%)	7 (4%)
Size greater than dates	156 (51%)	21 (28%)	34 (24%)
Preeclampsia	83 (27%)	1 (1%)	2 (1%)
Hyperemesis	80 (26%)	6 (8%)	25 (14%)
Postmolar GTN	57 (18.6%)	15 (23%)	33 (23%)

complete versus partial mole (79% vs. 29%, $p < 0.0001$). Increasing gestational age correlated with improved ultrasound detection rates after 14 weeks' gestation (35–40% vs. 60% before and after 14 weeks, respectively) [101].

Complete Mole

Complete molar pregnancy can be identified on ultrasound by a lack of fetal parts, an abnormal gestational sac, and a central heterogeneous placental mass containing multiple anechoic spaces or holes (see Fig. 27.8). The anechoic spaces seen within the placenta are due to the hydropic swelling of the villi [15, 96]. With earlier diagnosis, this "snowstorm" pattern of the placenta is often not seen in the first trimester, leading to the high rates of incorrect or missed pre-evacuation diagnosis [96]. Theca lutein cysts (see Fig. 27.9, lower) can be seen with more advanced gestational age but are often not seen in early complete molar pregnancy given lower hCG levels at diagnosis.

Partial Mole

While the pre-evacuation ultrasound of partial mole is less likely to diagnose the pregnancy correctly as a molar pregnancy, there are certain ultrasound findings that can be predictive of the diagnosis [101]. In addition to an often growth-restricted fetus, the combination of focal cystic placental changes and a ratio of transverse to anteroposterior dimension of the gestation sac > 1.5 is predictive of partial molar pregnancy 87% of the time. When neither of the latter criteria is seen, there is a 90% chance of missed abortion [99, 102].

Human Chorionic Gonadotropin (hCG)

hCG is a glycoprotein produced by the placenta consisting of two unique subunits: the α subunit that is similar to pituitary glycoprotein hormones, such as thyroid-stimulating hormone (TSH) and luteinizing hormone (LH), and the β subunit that is unique to the placenta. The β subunit exists in at least six different subtypes and tends to be degraded more often in GTD compared to normal pregnancy. It is therefore imperative that the hCG assay used to diagnose and follow molar pregnancy and GTD patients is able to detect all forms of hCG and its degradation products equally well [5, 15, 96]. One case report described a woman with a partial hydatidiform mole who had a negative urine qualitative hCG and a serum quantitative hCG of 1,094,950 mIU/mL because the urine qualitative test was unable to detect degradation products [103]. If physicians do not understand the limitations of commercially available assays, the diagnosis of molar pregnancy can be delayed, affecting patient outcomes.

Serum hCG levels above 100,000 mIU/mL are seen in nearly 50% of complete molar pregnancies, and an hCG level > 100,000 mIU/mL can help distinguish a missed abortion from a complete molar pregnancy [104–106]. In contrast, less than 10% of partial molar pregnancies present with an hCG greater than 100,000 mIU/mL, and one must be sure that the pregnancy is not just an early normal intrauterine pregnancy prior to proceeding with uterine evacuation [97]. The combined use of ultrasound and hCG has been shown to significantly increase the correct pre-evacuation diagnosis of molar pregnancy. In one series, only 58% of molar pregnancies were successfully identified using ultrasound alone; however, when an hCG level in excess of two standard deviations above the mean for gestational age was used in addition to ultrasound, 89% of molar pregnancies were correctly identified ($p \leq 0.005$) [107].

False-Negative hCG: The "Hook Effect"

When serum levels of hCG are extremely high, typically above 500,000 mIU/mL, a phenomenon known as the "hook effect" can be seen. The "hook effect" occurs when the excess hCG saturates the detection antibodies in the assay resulting in a false-negative or falsely low serum hCG. This can lead to a delay in the diagnosis of molar pregnancy, which can delay appropriate care and lead to complications or mismanagement [108–110].

Pathology

The definitive diagnosis of hydatidiform mole is made pathologically on the specimen obtained at uterine evacuation or hysterectomy and was previously discussed in the pathology section.

Treatment

Initial Evaluation

When the diagnosis of molar pregnancy is suspected prior to uterine evacuation, the following tests are recommended by the American College of Obstetricians and Gynecologists (ACOG) [2]:

- Complete blood count
- Clotting studies
- Renal and liver function studies
- Blood type and antibody screen
- Serum hCG level
- Chest X-ray
- Thyroid-stimulating hormone (if hyperthyroidism clinically suspected)
- Coagulopathy studies (if coagulopathy suspected)

Any medical complications should be stabilized as quickly as possible, and once the patient is medically and hemodynamically stable, uterine evacuation should occur [2, 15, 111]. In women who are not suspected to have a molar gestation prior to uterine evacuation, a baseline chest X-ray and hCG can be obtained once the diagnosis has been made. All women should be serially monitored as outlined in the section on postmolar surveillance [2].

Uterine Evacuation

Suction curettage is the recommended method of uterine evacuation, independent of uterine size, in women who wish to maintain fertility [111, 112]. Induction of labor with oxytocin or prostaglandin and hysterotomy have a significantly higher risk of bleeding, infection, and retained molar tissue compared to suction curettage [2, 111, 112] and also increase the risk of dissemination of trophoblastic tissue and the development of postmolar GTN [2, 15, 113]. To appropriately address any medical or surgical complications of uterine evacuation and molar pregnancy, immediate access to anesthesiology services, a blood bank, and an intensive care unit should be available [2]. Once adequate intravenous access and anesthesia have been obtained, the cervix should be serially dilated to allow a 12–14 mm cannula. Ultrasound guidance can facilitate complete uterine evacuation and decrease the risk of uterine perforation. Intravenous oxytocin should be started after cervical dilation and continued postoperatively for several hours to prevent uterine atony and decrease bleeding [2, 15]. Some authors suggest gentle sharp curettage after suction evacuation [15]. Women who are Rh-negative should be given Rh immunoglobulin at the time of uterine evacuation because Rh D factor is expressed on the trophoblast [2, 5, 111].

Significant pulmonary complications requiring invasive monitoring or ventilator support can occur during the time of molar evacuation including trophoblastic embolization and high output congestive heart failure from anemia, hyperthyroidism, iatrogenic fluid overload, or preeclampsia [2, 114, 115]. Medical complications such as hyperthyroidism and preeclampsia typically resolve soon after molar evacuation and rarely require extended therapy [2]. Theca lutein cysts that form from hCG stimulation of the ovaries often do not resolve for months, and surgical intervention is not required except in the rare case of torsion or rupture [2, 116].

Hysterectomy

Hysterectomy with adnexal preservation can be considered for women who have completed childbearing or in the case of life-threatening hemorrhage [5, 111, 117, 118]. It is important for these women to know that they are still at risk for the development of postmolar GTN because hysterectomy does not eliminate the risk for metastasis, and they should undergo standard post-evacuation hCG monitoring [47, 111, 119]. In a small group of women over age 50 treated at the New England Trophoblastic Disease Center ($N = 22$), hysterectomy was shown to reduce the risk of postmolar GTN compared to D&C, 0% vs. 60%, respectively; however, given the small numbers, this is not generalizable to the general population [117].

Minimally Invasive Hysterectomy

Historically, hysterectomy was performed via an open abdominal approach, as the uterus was often large and vascular, sometimes requiring ligation of the hypogastric vessels [118, 120]. With the increasing availability of laparoscopic and robotic surgery and earlier diagnosis of molar pregnancy, a minimally invasive approach can be safely undertaken in many women with molar pregnancy or GTN who undergo hysterectomy [120–123]. A robotic or laparoscopic approach allows for complete evaluation of the abdomen and pelvis, and patients recover much quicker compared to laparotomy [121–123]. For those with GTN, this allows them to safely begin or resume chemotherapy, if necessary, immediately after the procedure.

Prophylactic Chemotherapy

The use of prophylactic chemotherapy with either methotrexate or actinomycin D after uterine evacuation remains controversial. Toxicities such as stomatitis, nausea, vomiting, hair loss, and oral ulcers have been reported to occur in nearly 30% of women undergoing prophylactic chemotherapy and are typically mild [124, 125]. Multiple studies have consistently shown that the administration of a single dose of prophylactic chemotherapy decreases the rate of postmolar GTN in high-risk women (older age, markedly elevated hCG, uterine size > dates, enlarged theca lutein cysts) with complete molar pregnancy. This may be especially useful in resource-poor settings where hCG follow-up is unreliable or unavailable or when patient compliance is a concern [124–129]. A recent meta-analysis of 613 patients from three randomized trials reported a 63% reduction in the risk of postmolar GTN with the use of prophylactic chemotherapy; however, the time to diagnosis of subsequent GTN was longer in those who received prophylactic chemotherapy, and they also required more cycles of chemotherapy to obtain a cure. Because of these findings, the poor methodological quality of the studies, small sample sizes, and the exposure to potentially unnecessary toxic chemotherapy, the authors ultimately concluded that the use of prophylactic chemotherapy is not recommended [130]. Trophoblastic referral centers in the United States, however, continue to recommend and administer prophylactic chemotherapy in select high-risk patients [15, 126]. For compliant, low-risk patients who have access to reliable hCG monitoring, prophylactic chemotherapy does not decrease the risk of developing postmolar GTN, and chemotherapy should only be administered to these patients at the time of GTN diagnosis [128].

Postmolar Surveillance

Serum hCG Monitoring

Frequency and Duration of Monitoring

The American College of Obstetricians and Gynecologists recommends serial quantitative hCG monitoring in all patients with molar pregnancy at the following intervals [2]:

- Within 48 h of uterine evacuation
- Every 1–2 weeks while elevated
- Every month for an additional 6 months once normalized (typically <5 mIU/mL)

Patients who have not undergone hysterectomy should use a reliable form of hormonal contraception, and all patients should have frequent pelvic exams during the period of hCG elevation to evaluate for vaginal metastases [2].

Recently, data from over 20,000 women treated for molar pregnancy at Charing Cross has questioned the need for prolonged monitoring after normalization of hCG, particularly for those with partial mole [9, 131]. Women with partial mole had only a 0.03% risk (1 in 3195) of developing postmolar GTN after hCG normalization, and the authors recommend only a single confirmatory urine hCG 1 month after normalization. Those with complete mole continue to have higher risk of developing postmolar GTN; therefore, standard monitoring should still be followed [131]. Some authors suggest that since the risk of progression to postmolar GTN after hCG normalization is less than 1% in complete mole, these patients can also likely be monitored for a shorter period of time without compromising outcome; however, this has not been accepted as an official recommendation [9].

False-Positive hCG

False-positive or "phantom" hCG results can occur, leading to the unnecessary treatment of healthy women with either chemotherapy or surgery [1, 15, 132, 133].

Heterophile antibodies. False-positive hCG results are most often due to nonspecific human anti-mouse heterophile antibodies that cross-react with the hCG assay resulting in a positive test when no hCG is present. These antibodies are present in a large percentage of the general population, and can occur from incidental or occupational exposure to mice, or in patients who have been treated with monoclonal mouse antibodies for various medical conditions [15, 134, 135]. Levels of false-positive hCG are usually low; however, values of 300 mIU/mL and even as high as 800 mIU/mL have been reported [15, 133, 134, 136]. When phantom hCG is suspected (such as with plateau of hCG at low levels), confirmatory tests should be done to ensure the hCG elevation is real prior to initiating chemotherapy or proceeding with further surgery. Three fairly easy confirmatory tests can be done at most laboratories or an hCG reference lab [15]:

1. Urine pregnancy test—Heterophile antibodies are large, filtered out at the glomerulus, and not excreted in urine. A negative urine pregnancy test in the setting of a positive serum test suggests a false-positive hCG due to heterophile antibodies [1, 5, 15].
2. Serial serum dilutions—Heterophile antibodies do not dilute whereas true hCG does. Serial dilution of the patient's serum will not affect false-positive hCG assays and true hCG will be diluted along with the serum [2, 15].
3. Multiple assays—While some variation is expected in hCG values run with different assays, false-positive hCG assays will have markedly different results when using different techniques [2, 134].

Cross-reactivity with LH. As previously mentioned in the section on human chorionic gonadotropin (hCG), hCG shares the α subunit with LH. If LH cross-reacts with the hCG assay, it can lead to low levels of false-positive hCG. An elevated serum level of LH can suggest this, and a trial of oral contraceptive pills to suppress LH can resolve the false-positive results [15, 137].

Contraception

It is extremely important for women and their partners to use reliable contraception during the postmolar surveillance period since a new pregnancy would interfere with hCG monitoring [111]. It was previously thought that the use of oral contraceptive pills (OCPs) both increased the risk of postmolar GTN and delayed the fall in hCG after uterine evacuation [138]. A randomized trial by the Gynecologic Oncology Group comparing OCP to barrier methods after molar evacuation demonstrated 50% fewer intercurrent pregnancies in those using OCP compared to barrier methods as well as a lower incidence of postmolar GTN and a faster return to normal hCG [139]. These findings continue to be confirmed in retrospective studies and a recent meta-analysis. OCPs are the preferred method of contraception during the postmolar surveillance period [140–142].

Postmolar Gestational Trophoblastic Neoplasia

Postmolar GTN occurs in less than 6% of partial molar pregnancies and up to 30% of complete molar pregnancies [2, 8, 15, 45, 111, 143–146]. Despite earlier diagnosis of molar pregnancy, the current rates of postmolar GTN have not changed compared to historical studies [82, 92]. The obstetrician-gynecologist should be aware of the diagnostic criteria for postmolar GTN as defined by the International Federation of Gynecology and Obstetrics (FIGO) and recommended by ACOG in order to promptly refer to a gynecologic oncologist or trophoblastic referral center [2, 147]:

1. Plateau of hCG of four values ± 10% over a 3-week time frame (days 1, 7, 14, and 21)
2. Increase of hCG of more than 10% of three values over a 2-week time frame (days 1, 7, and 14)
3. Persistent elevation of hCG for more than 6 months after molar evacuation

This last FIGO criterion has been challenged in a recent report from the trophoblastic center in Brazil where 81 women with raised but falling hCG levels at 6 months were not given chemotherapy and were expectantly managed. Eighty percent of these women achieved spontaneous remission and avoided chemotherapy. There were no differences in the need for multiagent chemotherapy, relapse, or death in those who developed GTN after expectant management compared to those who were treated immediately at the 6-month mark [148].

Risk Factors for the Development of Postmolar GTN

In women with complete mole and signs of extensive trophoblastic proliferation (hCG > 100,000 mIU/mL, uterine size greater than dates, theca lutein cysts > 6 cm), the risk of postmolar GTN can be as high as 41–57% [8, 111, 143, 149, 150]. Age also significantly affects the risk of postmolar GTN in complete molar pregnancy. In women with complete mole age 40–49 or 50 and older, postmolar GTN developed in 53% and 60% of women after uterine evacuation. Hysterectomy appears to decrease the risk of developing postmolar GTN and should be considered in these women [117, 151]. Adolescents with complete mole, on the other hand, have a much lower risk of developing postmolar GTN compared to adults (hazard ratio 0.67, 95% CI 0.48–0.93) [39]. Repetitive molar pregnancy increases the risk of postmolar GTN three to four times compared to women who have only had one molar pregnancy [53, 152]. Unlike complete mole, there do not appear to be any clinical or pathologic features unique to women with partial mole who develop GTN compared to those who do not [146, 153].

Special Considerations

Future Fertility and Subsequent Pregnancies

Because of the increased risk of recurrent molar pregnancy, women with a history of molar pregnancy should undergo early obstetric ultrasound to confirm a normal pregnancy and pathologic evaluation of all subsequent placentas and products of conception [15, 111]. Women with prior molar pregnancy should be reassured that they will have obstetric outcomes roughly similar to the general population, even if they have gone on to receive chemotherapy for GTN [55, 154, 155]. There appear to be no adverse maternal outcomes. Some, but not all, studies have shown a very low increased risk of stillbirth [55, 155, 156].

Coexistence of Molar Pregnancy and Normal Fetus

A “twin” pregnancy with a normal fetus and a molar pregnancy is very rare, estimated to occur in only 1 in every 22,000–100,000 pregnancies

[15, 157]. These patients have a higher risk of medical complications of molar pregnancy such as preeclampsia, hyperthyroidism, and hemorrhage, which often requires early termination of pregnancy [2, 157, 158]. Patients should be counseled that they may have an increased risk of persistent GTN compared to singleton molar pregnancy, especially if they require termination due to medical complications. This risk was reported to be as high as 46% in the most recent series from two trophoblastic centers [158, 159]. In patients who do not terminate the pregnancy, either electively or due to medical comorbidities, 38%–60% of women will go on to deliver a viable infant [159–161].

Psychosocial Issues

Women with a diagnosis of molar pregnancy or gestational trophoblastic neoplasia have to deal with delays in future pregnancy, the loss of a pregnancy, and a potentially life-threatening illness [162]. Despite favorable reproductive outcomes, survivors of gestational trophoblastic disease continue to have significant effects on long-term quality of life (QOL) [162–164]. Significant predictors of long-term QOL include sexual functioning, reproductive concerns, gynecologic pain, cancer-specific distress, spiritual well-being, and social support; young women and those without children appear to be most affected [162, 164]. Male partners of women with molar pregnancy have high persisting levels of anxiety [165]. Patients and their partners should receive care from a multidisciplinary team that includes counselors and psychological support.

References

1. Brown J, Naumann RW, Seckl MJ, Schink J. 15 years of progress in gestational trophoblastic disease: scoring, standardization, and salvage. Gynecol Oncol. 2017;144(1):200–7.
2. Soper JT, Mutch DG, Schink JC, American College of O, Gynecologists. Diagnosis and treatment of gestational trophoblastic disease: ACOG practice bulletin no. 53. Gynecol Oncol 2004;93(3):575–585.
3. http://classics.mit.edu/Hippocrates/airwatpl.7.7.html.
4. Ober WB, Fass RO. The early history of choriocarcinoma. J Hist Med Allied Sci. 1961;16:49–73.
5. Seckl MJ, Sebire NJ, Berkowitz RS. Gestational trophoblastic disease. Lancet. 2010;376(9742):717–29.
6. Soper JT, Creasman WT. Clinical gynecologic oncology. 7th ed. Philadelphia, PA: Elsevier Inc.; 2007.
7. Berkowitz RS, Goldstein DP. Gestational trophoblastic disease. Cancer. 1995;76(10 Suppl):2079–85.
8. Berkowitz RS, Goldstein DP. Chorionic tumors. N Engl J Med. 1996;335(23):1740–8.
9. Berkowitz RS, Goldstein DP. Current advances in the management of gestational trophoblastic disease. Gynecol Oncol. 2013;128(1):3–5.
10. Szulman AE, Surti U. The syndromes of hydatidiform mole. II. Morphologic evolution of the complete and partial mole. Am J Obstet Gynecol. 1978;132(1):20–7.
11. Szulman AE, Surti U. The syndromes of hydatidiform mole. I. Cytogenetic and morphologic correlations. Am J Obstet Gynecol. 1978;131(6):665–71.
12. Szulman AE, Surti U. The clinicopathologic profile of the partial hydatidiform mole. Obstet Gynecol. 1982;59(5):597–602.
13. Vassilakos P, Riotton G, Kajii T. Hydatidiform mole: two entities. A morphologic and cytogenetic study with some clinical consideration. Am J Obstet Gynecol. 1977;127(2):167–70.
14. Bracken MB. Incidence and aetiology of hydatidiform mole: an epidemiological review. Br J Obstet Gynaecol. 1987;94(12):1123–35.
15. Lurain JR. Gestational trophoblastic disease I: epidemiology, pathology, clinical presentation and diagnosis of gestational trophoblastic disease, and management of hydatidiform mole. Am J Obstet Gynecol. 2010;203(6):531–9.
16. Palmer JR. Advances in the epidemiology of gestational trophoblastic disease. J Reprod Med. 1994;39(3):155–62.
17. Smith HO. Gestational trophoblastic disease epidemiology and trends. Clin Obstet Gynecol. 2003;46(3):541–56.
18. Gestational trophoblastic diseases. Report of a WHO Scientific Group. World Health Organ Tech Rep Ser. 1983;692:7–81.
19. Eysbouts YK, Bulten J, Ottevanger PB, Thomas CM, Ten Kate-Booij MJ, van Herwaarden AE, et al. Trends in incidence for gestational trophoblastic disease over the last 20 years in a population-based study. Gynecol Oncol. 2016;140(1):70–5.
20. Semer DA, Macfee MS. Gestational trophoblastic disease: epidemiology. Semin Oncol. 1995;22(2):109–12.
21. Salehi S, Eloranta S, Johansson AL, Bergstrom M, Lambe M. Reporting and incidence trends of

hydatidiform mole in Sweden 1973–2004. Acta Oncol. 2011;50(3):367–72.
22. Wairachpanich V, Limpongsanurak S, Lertkhachonsuk R. Epidemiology of hydatidiform moles in a tertiary hospital in Thailand over two decades: impact of the National Health Policy. Asian Pac J Cancer Prev. 2015;16(18):8321–5.
23. Takeuchi S. Incidence of gestational trophoblastic disease by regional registration in Japan. Hum Reprod. 1987;2(8):729–34.
24. Fatima M, Kasi PM, Baloch SN, Kassi M, Marri SM, Kassi M. Incidence, management, and outcome of molar pregnancies at a tertiary care hospital in Quetta, Pakistan. ISRN Obstet Gynecol. 2011;2011:925316.
25. Igwegbe A, Eleje G. Hydatidiform mole: a review of management outcomes in a tertiary hospital in south-east Nigeria. Ann Med Health Sci Res. 2013;3(2):210–4.
26. Smith HO, Hilgers RD, Bedrick EJ, Qualls CR, Wiggins CL, Rayburn WF, et al. Ethnic differences at risk for gestational trophoblastic disease in New Mexico: a 25-year population-based study. Am J Obstet Gynecol. 2003;188(2):357–66.
27. Martin BH, Kim JH. Changes in gestational trophoblastic tumors over four decades. A Korean experience. J Reprod Med. 1998;43(1):60–8.
28. Parazzini F, Ricci E, Cipriani S, Bulfoni G, Mangili G, Chiaffarino F. Temporal trends in the frequency of hydatidiform mole in Lombardy, northern Italy, 1996–2008. Int J Gynecol Cancer. 2012;22(2):318–22.
29. Matsui H, Iitsuka Y, Yamazawa K, Tanaka N, Seki K, Sekiya S. Changes in the incidence of molar pregnancies. A population-based study in Chiba prefecture and Japan between 1974 and 2000. Hum Reprod. 2003;18(1):172–5.
30. Agrawal N, Sagtani RA, Budhathoki SS, Pokharel HP. Clinico-epidemiological profile of molar pregnancies in a tertiary care centre of Eastern Nepal: a retrospective review of medical records. Gynecol Oncol Res Pract. 2015;2:9.
31. Almasi A, Almassinokiani F, Akbari P. Frequency of molar pregnancies in health care centers of Tehran, Iran. J Reprod Infertil. 2014;15(3):157–60.
32. Jacobs PA, Hunt PA, Matsuura JS, Wilson CC, Szulman AE. Complete and partial hydatidiform mole in Hawaii: cytogenetics, morphology and epidemiology. Br J Obstet Gynaecol. 1982;89(4):258–66.
33. O'Toole BA, Fradkin R, Warkany J, Wilson JG, Mann GV. Vitamin A deficiency and reproduction in rhesus monkeys. J Nutr. 1974;104(11):1513–24.
34. McLaren DS. Present knowledge of the role of vitamin A in health and disease. Trans R Soc Trop Med Hyg. 1966;60(4):436–62.
35. Berkowitz RS, Cramer DW, Bernstein MR, Cassells S, Driscoll SG, Goldstein DP. Risk factors for complete molar pregnancy from a case-control study. Am J Obstet Gynecol. 1985;152(8):1016–20.
36. Parazzini F, La Vecchia C, Mangili G, Caminiti C, Negri E, Cecchetti G, et al. Dietary factors and risk of trophoblastic disease. Am J Obstet Gynecol. 1988;158(1):93–9.
37. Andrijono A, Muhilal M. Prevention of post-mole malignant trophoblastic disease with vitamin A. Asian Pac J Cancer Prev. 2010;11(2):567–70.
38. Coullin P, Diatta AL, Boufettal H, Feingold J, Leguern E, Candelier JJ. The involvement of the trans-generational effect in the high incidence of the hydatidiform mole in Africa. Placenta. 2015;36(1):48–51.
39. Braga A, Growdon WB, Bernstein M, Maesta I, Rudge MV, Goldstein DP, et al. Molar pregnancy in adolescents. J Reprod Med. 2012;57(5–6):225–30.
40. Kashanian M, Baradaran HR, Teimoori N. Risk factors for complete molar pregnancy: a study in Iran. J Reprod Med. 2009;54(10):621–4.
41. Li XL, Du DF, Chen SJ, Zheng SH, Lee AC, Chen Q. Trends in ectopic pregnancy, hydatidiform mole and miscarriage in the largest obstetrics and gynaecology hospital in China from 2003 to 2013. Reprod Health. 2016;13(1):58.
42. Soares RR, Maesta I, Colon J, Braga A, Salazar A, Charry RC, et al. Complete molar pregnancy in adolescents from North and South America: clinical presentation and risk of gestational trophoblastic neoplasia. Gynecol Oncol. 2016;142(3):496–500.
43. Sebire NJ, Foskett M, Fisher RA, Rees H, Seckl M, Newlands E. Risk of partial and complete hydatidiform molar pregnancy in relation to maternal age. BJOG. 2002;109(1):99–102.
44. Parazzini F, La Vecchia C, Pampallona S. Parental age and risk of complete and partial hydatidiform mole. Br J Obstet Gynaecol. 1986;93(6):582–5.
45. Savage PM, Sita-Lumsden A, Dickson S, Iyer R, Everard J, Coleman R, et al. The relationship of maternal age to molar pregnancy incidence, risks for chemotherapy and subsequent pregnancy outcome. J Obstet Gynaecol. 2013;33(4):406–11.
46. Gockley AA, Melamed A, Joseph NT, Clapp M, Sun SY, Goldstein DP, et al. The effect of adolescence and advanced maternal age on the incidence of complete and partial molar pregnancy. Gynecol Oncol. 2016;140(3):470–3.
47. Bagshawe KD, Dent J, Webb J. Hydatidiform mole in England and Wales 1973–83. Lancet. 1986;2(8508):673–7.
48. Rice LW, Lage JM, Berkowitz RS, Goldstein DP, Bernstein MR. Repetitive complete and partial hydatidiform mole. Obstet Gynecol. 1989;74(2):217–9.
49. Berkowitz RS, Im SS, Bernstein MR, Goldstein DP. Gestational trophoblastic disease. Subsequent pregnancy outcome, including repeat molar pregnancy. J Reprod Med. 1998;43(1):81–6.
50. Sand PK, Lurain JR, Brewer JI. Repeat gestational trophoblastic disease. Obstet Gynecol. 1984;63(2):140–4.
51. Garrett LA, Garner EI, Feltmate CM, Goldstein DP, Berkowitz RS. Subsequent pregnancy outcomes in

patients with molar pregnancy and persistent gestational trophoblastic neoplasia. J Reprod Med. 2008;53(7):481–6.
52. Sebire NJ, Fisher RA, Foskett M, Rees H, Seckl MJ, Newlands ES. Risk of recurrent hydatidiform mole and subsequent pregnancy outcome following complete or partial hydatidiform molar pregnancy. BJOG. 2003;110(1):22–6.
53. Berkowitz RS, Bernstein MR, Laborde O, Goldstein DP. Subsequent pregnancy experience in patients with gestational trophoblastic disease. New England Trophoblastic Disease Center, 1965–1992. J Reprod Med. 1994;39(3):228–32.
54. Eagles N, Sebire NJ, Short D, Savage PM, Seckl MJ, Fisher RA. Risk of recurrent molar pregnancies following complete and partial hydatidiform moles. Hum Reprod. 2015;30(9):2055–63.
55. Vargas R, Barroilhet LM, Esselen K, Diver E, Bernstein M, Goldstein DP, et al. Subsequent pregnancy outcomes after complete and partial molar pregnancy, recurrent molar pregnancy, and gestational trophoblastic neoplasia: an update from the New England Trophoblastic Disease Center. J Reprod Med. 2014;59(5-6):188–94.
56. Parazzini F, Mangili G, La Vecchia C, Negri E, Bocciolone L, Fasoli M. Risk factors for gestational trophoblastic disease: a separate analysis of complete and partial hydatidiform moles. Obstet Gynecol. 1991;78(6):1039–45.
57. Acaia B, Parazzini F, La Vecchia C, Ricciardiello O, Fedele L, Battista Candiani G. Increased frequency of complete hydatidiform mole in women with repeated abortion. Gynecol Oncol. 1988;31(2):310–4.
58. Chen CP, Ko TM, Chen CY, Wang TY, Chern SR, Kuo YL, et al. First-trimester molecular diagnosis of complete hydatidiform mole associated with dizygotic twin pregnancy conceived by intrauterine insemination. Taiwan J Obstet Gynecol. 2014;53(4):572–8.
59. Fatima P, Hossain MM, Ishrat S, Rahman D, Hossain HB. Outcome of triplet pregnancy with hydatidiform mole and coexisting twin live fetus following ICSI. Mymensingh Med J. 2014;23(3):590–4.
60. Rao AR, Dafle K, Padmashri G, Rao DR, Sivakumar NC. Pregnancy outcome with coexisting mole after intracytoplasmic sperm injection: a case series. J Hum Reprod Sci. 2015;8(3):178–81.
61. Tariq N, Ghazali U, Uddin Z, Rasheed K, Tariq H. Complete hydatidiform mole coexisting with three viable fetuses in a quadruplet pregnancy. J Coll Physicians Surg Pak. 2016;26(4):326–8.
62. Obeidi N, Tchrakian N, Abu Saadeh F, Mocanu E. Suspected ovarian molar pregnancy after assisted reproductive technology conception: a diagnostic challenge. BMJ Case Rep. 2015;2015
63. Fisher RA, Hodges MD, Newlands ES. Familial recurrent hydatidiform mole: a review. J Reprod Med. 2004;49(8):595–601.
64. Fisher RA, Lavery SA, Carby A, Abu-Hayyeh S, Swingler R, Sebire NJ, et al. What a difference an egg makes. Lancet. 2011;378(9807):1974.
65. Akoury E, Gupta N, Bagga R, Brown S, Dery C, Kabra M, et al. Live births in women with recurrent hydatidiform mole and two NLRP7 mutations. Reprod Biomed Online. 2015;31(1):120–4.
66. Moglabey YB, Kircheisen R, Seoud M, El Mogharbel N, Van den Veyver I, Slim R. Genetic mapping of a maternal locus responsible for familial hydatidiform moles. Hum Mol Genet. 1999;8(4):667–71.
67. Murdoch S, Djuric U, Mazhar B, Seoud M, Khan R, Kuick R, et al. Mutations in NALP7 cause recurrent hydatidiform moles and reproductive wastage in humans. Nat Genet. 2006;38(3):300–2.
68. Wang CM, Dixon PH, Decordova S, Hodges MD, Sebire NJ, Ozalp S, et al. Identification of 13 novel NLRP7 mutations in 20 families with recurrent hydatidiform mole; missense mutations cluster in the leucine-rich region. J Med Genet. 2009;46(8):569–75.
69. Rezaei M, Nguyen NM, Foroughinia L, Dash P, Ahmadpour F, Verma IC, et al. Two novel mutations in the KHDC3L gene in Asian patients with recurrent hydatidiform mole. Hum Genome Var. 2016;3:16027.
70. Altieri A, Franceschi S, Ferlay J, Smith J, La Vecchia C. Epidemiology and aetiology of gestational trophoblastic diseases. Lancet Oncol. 2003;4(11):670–8.
71. Berkowitz RS, Bernstein MR, Harlow BL, Rice LW, Lage JM, Goldstein DP, et al. Case-control study of risk factors for partial molar pregnancy. Am J Obstet Gynecol. 1995;173(3 Pt 1):788–94.
72. Bracken MB, Brinton LA, Hayashi K. Epidemiology of hydatidiform mole and choriocarcinoma. Epidemiol Rev. 1984;6:52–75.
73. Kajii T, Ohama K. Androgenetic origin of hydatidiform mole. Nature. 1977;268(5621):633–4.
74. Ohama K, Kajii T, Okamoto E, Fukuda Y, Imaizumi K, Tsukahara M, et al. Dispermic origin of XY hydatidiform moles. Nature. 1981;292(5823):551–2.
75. Surti U, Szulman AE, O'Brien S. Dispermic origin and clinical outcome of three complete hydatidiform moles with 46,XY karyotype. Am J Obstet Gynecol. 1982;144(1):84–7.
76. Jacobs PA, Wilson CM, Sprenkle JA, Rosenshein NB, Migeon BR. Mechanism of origin of complete hydatidiform moles. Nature. 1980;286(5774):714–6.
77. Candelier JJ. The hydatidiform mole. Cell Adhes Migr. 2016;10(1-2):226–35.
78. Wallace DC, Surti U, Adams CW, Szulman AE. Complete moles have paternal chromosomes but maternal mitochondrial DNA. Hum Genet. 1982;61(2):145–7.
79. Baasanjav B, Usui H, Kihara M, Kaku H, Nakada E, Tate S, et al. The risk of post-molar gestational trophoblastic neoplasia is higher in heterozygous than in homozygous complete hydatidiform moles. Hum Reprod. 2010;25(5):1183–91.

80. Sebire NJ, Fisher RA, Rees HC. Histopathological diagnosis of partial and complete hydatidiform mole in the first trimester of pregnancy. Pediatr Dev Pathol. 2003;6(1):69–77.
81. Joneborg U, Marions L. Current clinical features of complete and partial hydatidiform mole in Sweden. J Reprod Med. 2014;59(1-2):51–5.
82. Sun SY, Melamed A, Goldstein DP, Bernstein MR, Horowitz NS, Moron AF, et al. Changing presentation of complete hydatidiform mole at the New England Trophoblastic Disease Center over the past three decades: does early diagnosis alter risk for gestational trophoblastic neoplasia? Gynecol Oncol. 2015;138(1):46–9.
83. Mosher R, Goldstein DP, Berkowitz R, Bernstein M, Genest DR. Complete hydatidiform mole. Comparison of clinicopathologic features, current and past. J Reprod Med. 1998;43(1):21–7.
84. Castrillon DH, Sun D, Weremowicz S, Fisher RA, Crum CP, Genest DR. Discrimination of complete hydatidiform mole from its mimics by immunohistochemistry of the paternally imprinted gene product p57KIP2. Am J Surg Pathol. 2001;25(10):1225–30.
85. Lipata F, Parkash V, Talmor M, Bell S, Chen S, Maric V, et al. Precise DNA genotyping diagnosis of hydatidiform mole. Obstet Gynecol. 2010;115(4):784–94.
86. Samadder A, Kar R. Utility of p57 immunohistochemistry in differentiating between complete mole, partial mole & non-molar or hydropic abortus. Indian J Med Res. 2017;145(1):133–7.
87. Buza N, Hui P. Partial hydatidiform mole: histologic parameters in correlation with DNA genotyping. Int J Gynecol Pathol. 2013;32(3):307–15.
88. Fisher RA, Tommasi A, Short D, Kaur B, Seckl MJ, Sebire NJ. Clinical utility of selective molecular genotyping for diagnosis of partial hydatidiform mole; a retrospective study from a regional trophoblastic disease unit. J Clin Pathol. 2014;67(11):980–4.
89. Jacobs PA, Szulman AE, Funkhouser J, Matsuura JS, Wilson CC. Human triploidy: relationship between parental origin of the additional haploid complement and development of partial hydatidiform mole. Ann Hum Genet. 1982;46(Pt 3):223–31.
90. Kubelka-Sabit K, Jasar D, Filipovski V, Bozinovski G, Plaseska-Karanfilska D. Molecular and histological characteristics of early triploid and partial molar pregnancies. Pol J Pathol. 2017;68(2):138–43.
91. Wilson Y, Bharat C, Crook ML, Kee AR, Peverall J, Ruba S, et al. Histological comparison of partial hydatidiform mole and trisomy gestation specimens. Pathology. 2016;48(6):550–4.
92. Braga A, Moraes V, Maesta I, Amim Junior J, Rezende-Filho J, Elias K, et al. Changing trends in the clinical presentation and management of complete hydatidiform mole among Brazilian women. Int J Gynecol Cancer. 2016;26(5):984–90.
93. Hou JL, Wan XR, Xiang Y, Qi QW, Yang XY. Changes of clinical features in hydatidiform mole: analysis of 113 cases. J Reprod Med. 2008;53(8):629–33.
94. Sun SY, Melamed A, Joseph NT, Gockley AA, Goldstein DP, Bernstein MR, et al. Clinical presentation of complete hydatidiform mole and partial hydatidiform mole at a regional trophoblastic disease Center in the United States over the past 2 decades. Int J Gynecol Cancer. 2016;26(2):367–70.
95. Soto-Wright V, Bernstein M, Goldstein DP, Berkowitz RS. The changing clinical presentation of complete molar pregnancy. Obstet Gynecol. 1995;86(5):775–9.
96. Ngan HY, Seckl MJ, Berkowitz RS, Xiang Y, Golfier F, Sekharan PK, et al. Update on the diagnosis and management of gestational trophoblastic disease. Int J Gynaecol Obstet. 2015;131(Suppl 2):S123–6.
97. Berkowitz RS, Goldstein DP, Bernstein MR. Natural history of partial molar pregnancy. Obstet Gynecol. 1985;66(5):677–81.
98. Benson CB, Genest DR, Bernstein MR, Soto-Wright V, Goldstein DP, Berkowitz RS. Sonographic appearance of first trimester complete hydatidiform moles. Ultrasound Obstet Gynecol. 2000;16(2):188–91.
99. Fine C, Bundy AL, Berkowitz RS, Boswell SB, Berezin AF, Doubilet PM. Sonographic diagnosis of partial hydatidiform mole. Obstet Gynecol. 1989;73(3 Pt 1):414–8.
100. Santos-Ramos R, Forney JP, Schwarz BE. Sonographic findings and clinical correlations in molar pregnancy. Obstet Gynecol. 1980;56(2):186–92.
101. Fowler DJ, Lindsay I, Seckl MJ, Sebire NJ. Routine pre-evacuation ultrasound diagnosis of hydatidiform mole: experience of more than 1000 cases from a regional referral center. Ultrasound Obstet Gynecol. 2006;27(1):56–60.
102. Naumoff P, Szulman AE, Weinstein B, Mazer J, Surti U. Ultrasonography of partial hydatidiform mole. Radiology. 1981;140(2):467–70.
103. Mundangepfupfu T, Waseem M. Partial hydatidiform mole with false-negative urine human chorionic gonadotropin test in the emergency department. J Emerg Med. 2014;46(3):348–50.
104. Genest DR, Laborde O, Berkowitz RS, Goldstein DP, Bernstein MR, Lage J. A clinicopathologic study of 153 cases of complete hydatidiform mole (1980–1990): histologic grade lacks prognostic significance. Obstet Gynecol. 1991;78(3 Pt 1):402–9.
105. Menczer J, Modan M, Serr DM. Prospective follow-up of patients with hydatidiform mole. Obstet Gynecol. 1980;55(3):346–9.
106. Seckin KD, Baser E, Yeral I, Togrul C, Ozdal B, Gungor T. The impact of ultrasonographic lesion size and initial human chorionic gonadotropin values on treatment success in cases with complete hydatidiform mole. Eur Rev Med Pharmacol Sci. 2013;17(24):3381–4.
107. Romero R, Horgan JG, Kohorn EI, Kadar N, Taylor KJ, Hobbins JC. New criteria for the diagnosis of gestational trophoblastic disease. Obstet Gynecol. 1985;66(4):553–8.

108. Nodler JL, Kim KH, Alvarez RD. Abnormally low hCG in a complete hydatidiform molar pregnancy: the hook effect. Gynecol Oncol Case Rep. 2011;1(1):6–7.
109. Pang YP, Rajesh H, Tan LK. Molar pregnancy with false negative urine hCG: the hook effect. Singap Med J. 2010;51(3):e58–61.
110. Winder AD, Mora AS, Berry E, Lurain JR. The "hook effect" causing a negative pregnancy test in a patient with an advanced molar pregnancy. Gynecol Oncol Rep. 2017;21:34–6.
111. Berkowitz RS, Goldstein DP. Clinical practice. Molar pregnancy. N Engl J Med. 2009;360(16):1639–45.
112. Hancock BW, Tidy JA. Current management of molar pregnancy. J Reprod Med. 2002;47(5):347–54.
113. Tidy JA, Gillespie AM, Bright N, Radstone CR, Coleman RE, Hancock BW. Gestational trophoblastic disease: a study of mode of evacuation and subsequent need for treatment with chemotherapy. Gynecol Oncol. 2000;78(3 Pt 1):309–12.
114. Orr JW Jr, Austin JM, Hatch KD, Shingleton HM, Younger JB, Boots LR. Acute pulmonary edema associated with molar pregnancies: a high-risk factor for development of persistent trophoblastic disease. Am J Obstet Gynecol. 1980;136(3):412–5.
115. Twiggs LB, Morrow CP, Schlaerth JB. Acute pulmonary complications of molar pregnancy. Am J Obstet Gynecol. 1979;135(2):189–94.
116. Montz FJ, Schlaerth JB, Morrow CP. The natural history of theca lutein cysts. Obstet Gynecol. 1988;72(2):247–51.
117. Elias KM, Goldstein DP, Berkowitz RS. Complete hydatidiform mole in women older than age 50. J Reprod Med. 2010;55(5-6):208–12.
118. Hanna RK, Soper JT. The role of surgery and radiation therapy in the management of gestational trophoblastic disease. Oncologist. 2010;15(6):593–600.
119. Giorgione V, Bergamini A, Cioffi R, Pella F, Rabaiotti E, Petrone M, et al. Role of surgery in the management of hydatidiform mole in elderly patients: a single-center clinical experience. Int J Gynecol Cancer. 2017;27(3):550–3.
120. Lang JF, Childers JM, Surwit EA. Laparoscopic hysterectomy for persistent gestational trophoblastic neoplasia. J Am Assoc Gynecol Laparosc. 1995;2(4):475–7.
121. Davis MR, Howitt BE, Quade BJ, Crum CP, Horowitz NS, Goldstein DP, et al. Epithelioid trophoblastic tumor: a single institution case series at the New England Trophoblastic Disease Center. Gynecol Oncol. 2015;137(3):456–61.
122. Namaky D, Basil J, Pavelka J. Placental site trophoblastic tumor presenting as an intramural mass with negative markers: an opportunity for novel diagnosis and treatment with robotic hysterectomy. J Robot Surg. 2010;4(1):57–9.
123. Savelli L, Pollastri P, Mabrouk M, Seracchioli R, Venturoli S. Placental site trophoblastic tumor diagnosed on transvaginal sonography. Ultrasound Obstet Gynecol. 2009;34(2):235–6.
124. Kashimura Y, Kashimura M, Sugimori H, Tsukamoto N, Matsuyama T, Matsukuma K, et al. Prophylactic chemotherapy for hydatidiform mole. Five to 15 years follow-up. Cancer. 1986;58(3):624–9.
125. Limpongsanurak S. Prophylactic actinomycin D for high-risk complete hydatidiform mole. J Reprod Med. 2001;46(2):110–6.
126. Berkowitz RS, Goldstein DP, DuBeshter B, Bernstein MR. Management of complete molar pregnancy. J Reprod Med. 1987;32(9):634–9.
127. Goldstein DP, Berkowitz RS. Prophylactic chemotherapy of complete molar pregnancy. Semin Oncol. 1995;22(2):157–60.
128. Kim DS, Moon H, Kim KT, Moon YJ, Hwang YY. Effects of prophylactic chemotherapy for persistent trophoblastic disease in patients with complete hydatidiform mole. Obstet Gynecol. 1986;67(5):690–4.
129. Uberti EM, Fajardo Mdo C, da Cunha AG, Rosa MW, Ayub AC, Graudenz Mda S, et al. Prevention of postmolar gestational trophoblastic neoplasia using prophylactic single bolus dose of actinomycin D in high-risk hydatidiform mole: a simple, effective, secure and low-cost approach without adverse effects on compliance to general follow-up or subsequent treatment. Gynecol Oncol. 2009;114(2):299–305.
130. Wang Q, Fu J, Hu L, Fang F, Xie L, Chen H, et al. Prophylactic chemotherapy for hydatidiform mole to prevent gestational trophoblastic neoplasia. Cochrane Database Syst Rev. 2017;9:CD007289.
131. Coyle C, Short D, Jackson L, Sebire NJ, Kaur B, Harvey R, et al. What is the optimal duration of human chorionic gonadotrophin surveillance following evacuation of a molar pregnancy? A retrospective analysis on over 20,000 consecutive patients. Gynecol Oncol. 2018;148(2):254–7.
132. Palmieri C, Dhillon T, Fisher RA, Young AM, Short D, Mitchell H, et al. Management and outcome of healthy women with a persistently elevated beta-hCG. Gynecol Oncol. 2007;106(1):35–43.
133. Rotmensch S, Cole LA. False diagnosis and needless therapy of presumed malignant disease in women with false-positive human chorionic gonadotropin concentrations. Lancet. 2000;355(9205):712–5.
134. Cole LA. Phantom hCG and phantom choriocarcinoma. Gynecol Oncol. 1998;71(2):325–9.
135. Fitzmaurice TF, Brown C, Rifai N, Wu AH, Yeo KT. False increase of cardiac troponin I with heterophilic antibodies. Clin Chem. 1998;44(10):2212–4.
136. Cole LA, Shahabi S, Butler SA, Mitchell H, Newlands ES, Behrman HR, et al. Utility of commonly used commercial human chorionic gonadotropin immunoassays in the diagnosis and management of trophoblastic diseases. Clin Chem. 2001;47(2):308–15.
137. Hancock BW. hCG measurement in gestational trophoblastic neoplasia: a critical appraisal. J Reprod Med. 2006;51(11):859–60.
138. Stone M, Dent J, Kardana A, Bagshawe KD. Relationship of oral contraception to development of trophoblastic tumour after evacuation

of a hydatidiform mole. Br J Obstet Gynaecol. 1976;83(12):913–6.
139. Curry SL, Schlaerth JB, Kohorn EI, Boyce JB, Gore H, Twiggs LB, et al. Hormonal contraception and trophoblastic sequelae after hydatidiform mole (a Gynecologic Oncology Group Study). Am J Obstet Gynecol. 1989;160(4):805–9. discussion 9–11.
140. Braga A, Maesta I, Short D, Savage P, Harvey R, Seckl MJ. Hormonal contraceptive use before hCG remission does not increase the risk of gestational trophoblastic neoplasia following complete hydatidiform mole: a historical database review. BJOG. 2016;123(8):1330–5.
141. Dantas PRS, Maesta I, Filho JR, Junior JA, Elias KM, Howoritz N, et al. Does hormonal contraception during molar pregnancy follow-up influence the risk and clinical aggressiveness of gestational trophoblastic neoplasia after controlling for risk factors? Gynecol Oncol. 2017;147(2):364–70.
142. Gaffield ME, Kapp N, Curtis KM. Combined oral contraceptive and intrauterine device use among women with gestational trophoblastic disease. Contraception. 2009;80(4):363–71.
143. Curry SL, Hammond CB, Tyrey L, Creasman WT, Parker RT. Hydatidiform mole: diagnosis, management, and long-term followup of 347 patients. Obstet Gynecol. 1975;45(1):1–8.
144. Hancock BW, Nazir K, Everard JE. Persistent gestational trophoblastic neoplasia after partial hydatidiform mole incidence and outcome. J Reprod Med. 2006;51(10):764–6.
145. Lurain JR, Brewer JI, Torok EE, Halpern B. Natural history of hydatidiform mole after primary evacuation. Am J Obstet Gynecol. 1983;145(5):591–5.
146. Feltmate CM, Growdon WB, Wolfberg AJ, Goldstein DP, Genest DR, Chinchilla ME, et al. Clinical characteristics of persistent gestational trophoblastic neoplasia after partial hydatidiform molar pregnancy. J Reprod Med. 2006;51(11):902–6.
147. Ngan HY, Bender H, Benedet JL, Jones H, Montruccoli GC, Pecorelli S, et al. Gestational trophoblastic neoplasia, FIGO 2000 staging and classification. Int J Gynaecol Obstet. 2003;83(Suppl 1):175–7.
148. Braga A, Torres B, Burla M, Maesta I, Sun SY, Lin L, et al. Is chemotherapy necessary for patients with molar pregnancy and human chorionic gonadotropin serum levels raised but falling at 6months after uterine evacuation? Gynecol Oncol. 2016;143(3):558–64.
149. Berkowitz RS, Goldstein DP. Pathogenesis of gestational trophoblastic neoplasms. Pathobiol Annu. 1981;11:391–411.
150. Morrow CP. Postmolar trophoblastic disease: diagnosis, management, and prognosis. Clin Obstet Gynecol. 1984;27(1):211–20.
151. Elias KM, Shoni M, Bernstein M, Goldstein DP, Berkowitz RS. Complete hydatidiform mole in women aged 40 to 49 years. J Reprod Med. 2012;57(5–6):254–8.
152. Parazzini F, Mangili G, Belloni C, La Vecchia C, Liati P, Marabini R. The problem of identification of prognostic factors for persistent trophoblastic disease. Gynecol Oncol. 1988;30(1):57–62.
153. Rice LW, Berkowitz RS, Lage JM, Goldstein DP, Bernstein MR. Persistent gestational trophoblastic tumor after partial hydatidiform mole. Gynecol Oncol. 1990;36(3):358–62.
154. Gadducci A, Cosio S, Fanucchi A, Tana R, Manacorda S, Pistolesi S, et al. Prognosis of patients with gestational trophoblastic neoplasia and obstetric outcomes of those conceiving after chemotherapy. Anticancer Res. 2016;36(7):3477–82.
155. Gadducci A, Lanfredini N, Cosio S. Reproductive outcomes after hydatiform mole and gestational trophoblastic neoplasia. Gynecol Endocrinol. 2015;31(9):673–8.
156. Joneborg U, Eloranta S, Johansson AL, Marions L, Weibull CE, Lambe M. Hydatidiform mole and subsequent pregnancy outcome: a population-based cohort study. Am J Obstet Gynecol. 2014;211(6):681 e1–7.
157. Bristow RE, Shumway JB, Khouzami AN, Witter FR. Complete hydatidiform mole and surviving coexistent twin. Obstet Gynecol Surv. 1996;51(12):705–9.
158. Matsui H, Sekiya S, Hando T, Wake N, Tomoda Y. Hydatidiform mole coexistent with a twin live fetus: a national collaborative study in Japan. Hum Reprod. 2000;15(3):608–11.
159. Lin LH, Maesta I, Braga A, Sun SY, Fushida K, Francisco RPV, et al. Multiple pregnancies with complete mole and coexisting normal fetus in North and South America: a retrospective multicenter cohort and literature review. Gynecol Oncol. 2017;145(1):88–95.
160. Sebire NJ, Foskett M, Paradinas FJ, Fisher RA, Francis RJ, Short D, et al. Outcome of twin pregnancies with complete hydatidiform mole and healthy co-twin. Lancet. 2002;359(9324):2165–6.
161. Suksai M, Suwanrath C, Kor-Anantakul O, Geater A, Hanprasertpong T, Atjimakul T, et al. Complete hydatidiform mole with co-existing fetus: predictors of live birth. Eur J Obstet Gynecol Reprod Biol. 2017;212:1–8.
162. Di Mattei VE, Carnelli L, Bernardi M, Pagani Bagliacca E, Zucchi P, Lavezzari L, et al. An investigative study into psychological and fertility sequelae of gestational trophoblastic disease: the impact on patients' perceived fertility, anxiety and depression. PLoS One. 2015;10(6):e0128354.
163. Ferreira EG, Maesta I, Michelin OC, de Paula RC, Consonni M, Rudge MV. Assessment of quality of life and psychologic aspects in patients with gestational trophoblastic disease. J Reprod Med. 2009;54(4):239–44.
164. Wenzel L, Berkowitz RS, Habbal R, Newlands E, Hancock B, Goldstein DP, et al. Predictors of quality of life among long-term survivors of gestational trophoblastic disease. J Reprod Med. 2004;49(8):589–94.

165. Quinlivan JA, Ung KA, Petersen RW. The impact of molar pregnancy on the male partner. Psychooncology. 2012;21(9):970–6.
166. Schink JC, Lurain JR. Gestational trophoblastic disease: molar pregnancy and gestational trophoblastic Neoplasia. In: Barakat RR, Berchuck A, Markman M, Randall ME, editors. Principles and practice of gynecologic oncology. 6th ed. Philadelphia, PA: Lippincott Williams & Wilkins; 2013. p. 889.

Transabdominal Cervical Cerclage

28

Sabahattin Anıl Arı, Ali Akdemir, and Fatih Sendag

Definition

Cervical insufficiency is an inadequacy of the uterine cervix to maintain a pregnancy without uterine contractions, preterm premature rupture of membranes, or both, in the second trimester [1]. Wolf et al. reported the incidence of cervical insufficiency as 0.1–1% of all pregnancies.

Pathophysiology

The pathophysiology of cervical insufficiency is unclear. Proposed etiologies for this condition include congenital Müllerian anomalies and deficiencies of cervical collagen and elastin [1].

Obstetric lacerations and surgical trauma caused by conization, loop electrosurgical excision procedures, and mechanical dilatation of the cervix are also acquired reasons. But these are not definitely proven [2].

Diagnosis

Diagnosis of cervical insufficiency is challenging due to lack of definitive criteria. Diagnosis is based on a history of painless cervical dilation in the second trimester without:

- Contractions
- Labor
- Bleeding
- Infection
- Ruptured of membranes

Hysterosalpingography, balloon traction on the cervix, Hegar or Pratt dilatators tests, balloon elastance test, and use of graduated cervical dilatators to calculate a cervical resistance index have been used in the past and have not been validated by scientific studies. Accordingly, these tests should not be used for diagnosis [1].

Treatment Options

Treatment options for cervical insufficiency can be divided into two groups: nonsurgical and surgical treatments. Vaginal pessary is the only nonsurgical approach; however, there was not enough evidence to recommend to high-risk patients. Recently, Saccone et al. published a new meta-analysis about vaginal pessary use in singleton gestations. The only effect according to their

S. A. Arı · A. Akdemir · F. Sendag (✉)
Department of Obstetrics and Gynecology,
Ege University Hospital, Bornova, İzmir, Turkey

C. H. Nezhat (ed.), *Non-Obstetric Surgery During Pregnancy*,
https://doi.org/10.1007/978-3-319-90752-9_28

results is the increase in vaginal discharge [3]. Therefore, the use of vaginal pessary could be limited to selected cases.

Surgical options are transvaginal or transabdominal cervical cerclage. Cervical cerclage provides structural support increasing the resistance of an enfeebled cervix. Modifications of the McDonald and Shirodkar techniques are frequently used in the current approach.

In the McDonald procedure, the cervicovaginal junction is supported by a single nonabsorbable purse-string suture [4]. The dissection of the vesicocervical mucosa and the placement of the nonabsorbable suture at the level of the internal cervical os is the characteristic feature of Shirodkar's technique [5].

Advantages of the suture type or vaginal surgical techniques over the other have not been proven [6], and approximately 13% of pregnancies in women with cervical incompetency treated with transvaginal cerclage will not be accomplished and will deliver previable infants [7].

Transabdominal cervicoisthmic cerclage is usually reserved for patients who have previously unsuccessful transvaginal cerclages or anatomical limitations [8]. Transabdominal cerclage procedures are generally performed in the later part of the first trimester, early second trimester (10–14 weeks of gestation), or prepregnancy and can be left for subsequent pregnancies [9]. The procedure can be performed via open laparotomy or operative laparoscopy.

Indications for Cervical Cerclage in Women with Singleton Pregnancies

The following are the most common indications for cervical cerclage in women with singleton pregnancies:

- History of painless cervical dilation in the second trimester without contractions and labor
- Prior cerclage due to painless cervical dilation in the second trimester
- Painless cervical dilation in the second trimester on physical examination
- Current singleton pregnancy, prior spontaneous preterm birth at less than 34 weeks of gestation and short cervical length (less than 25 mm) before 24 weeks of gestation

Note: In women with twin pregnancies, cerclage is not recommended and can also increase preterm birth [1].

Transabdominal Cerclage

Benson and Durfee first described transabdominal cerclage, also known as transabdominal cervicoisthmic cerclage, 50 years ago. The purpose of this procedure is to increase tissue support at the level of the internal cervical os. The superiorities of abdominal cerclage compared to vaginal cerclage are closer proximity to the internal os, preferable support of the cervical tissue, and lower risk of suture migration [10].

Classic indications for transabdominal cerclage include previously unsuccessful transvaginal cerclage or anatomical limitations like weakness or hypoplasia of the cervix deep cervical laceration or shortening of the cervix by previous procedures.

Studies have found a high rate of pregnancy completion following this procedure. Sneider et al. reported a "take-home baby ratio" of 95% after abdominal cerclage, 73% after vaginal cerclage, and 33% after no cerclage [11]. In spite of this evidence, transabdominal cerclage is underutilized. Surgical risks, caesarean requirement, and low surgical experience are contributing factors to its underutilization. These factors must be addressed in order to increase the future utilization of this procedure.

Procedure

The surgical technique of transabdominal cervical cerclage is simple in theory, but it is redoubtable in practice. Increased paracervical vasculature, blood flow, and softness of the gravid uterus are some of the challenges faced by surgeons. This procedure is less complicated in nonpregnant patients.

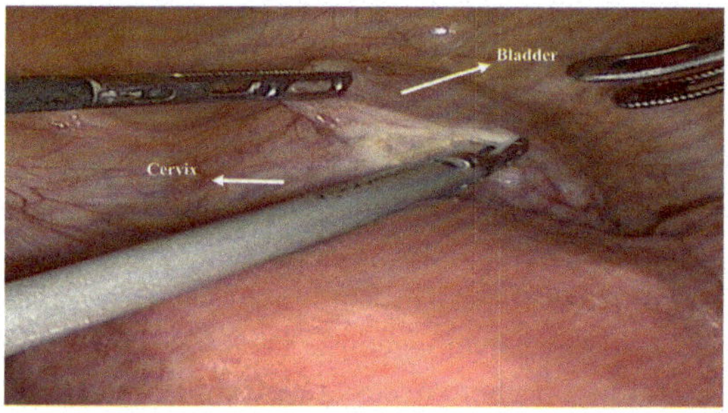

Fig. 28.1 Bladder dissection

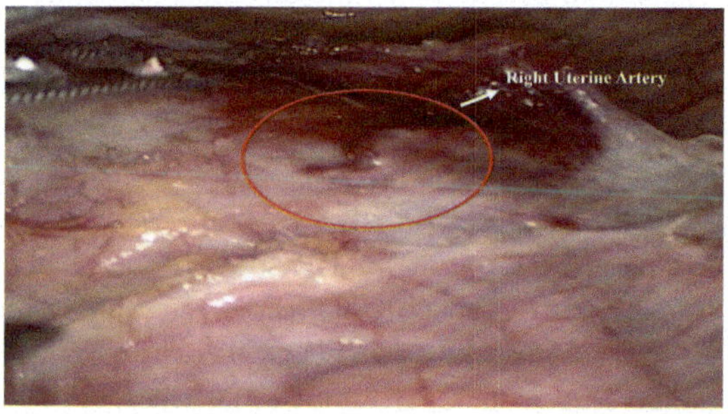

Fig. 28.2 Determining the uterine artery on the right side

In our center, we prefer laparoscopic surgery, when appropriate. Through the general anesthesia and after establishing a pneumoperitoneum, a 10-mm optic port is inserted through the umbilicus for the optic system. Two 5-mm trocars are placed in each lower quadrant laterally at the paramedian line just below the umbilicus, and one 5-mm trocar is placed in the left upper quadrant just above the umbilicus. Subsequently, the bladder is pushed away from the lower uterine segment via sharp and blunt dissection (Fig. 28.1). The uterine arteries are identified, and this is the main step of the procedure (Fig. 28.2). A 5-mm permanent tape with two flat needles is inserted into the abdomen. One suture needle is passed through posterior to anterior medial to the uterine artery at the level of internal cervical os (Figs. 28.3, 28.4, and 28.5). The same steps are then repeated on the other side. Next, the tape is tied anteriorly and the ends are transfixed by a resorbable suture material (Figs. 28.6 and 28.7). Lastly, the visceral peritoneum is covered via a running suture with a resorbable suture material (Fig. 28.8).

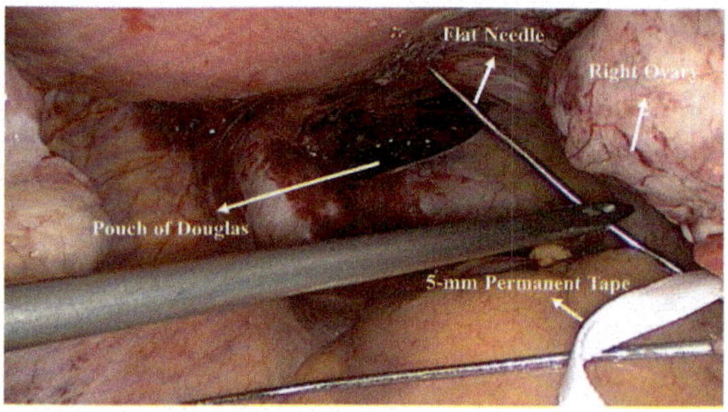

Fig. 28.3 Passing through the needle from posterior to anterior on the right side

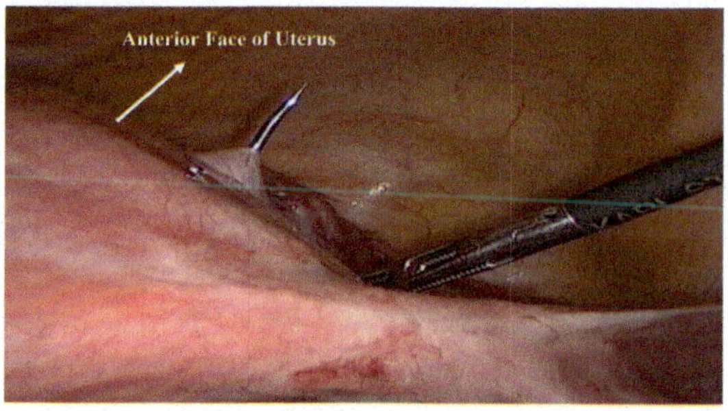

Fig. 28.4 The needle exit from anterior of the uterus

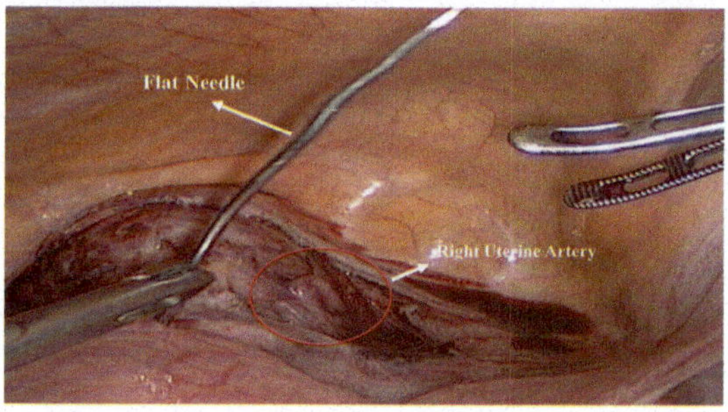

Fig. 28.5 The needle exit from medial to uterine artery on the right side

In other words, a 5-mm permanent tape is placed around the cervix at the level of internal cervical os via fenestrations created on either side of the cervix medial to the uterine artery. The uterine artery is then dissected. Next, a thin grasper is passed through anterior to posterior medial to the uterine artery. After taking one end of the tape, the grasping device is pulled back through, posterior to anterior. The same steps are repeated on the other side. Lastly, the tape is tied anteriorly or posteriorly, according to the

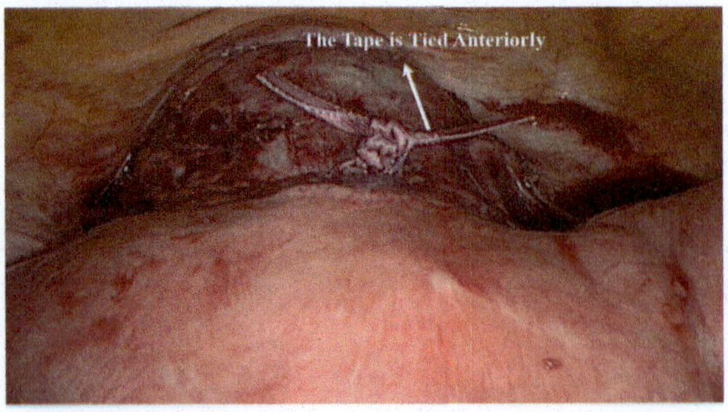

Fig. 28.6 The tape is tied anteriorly

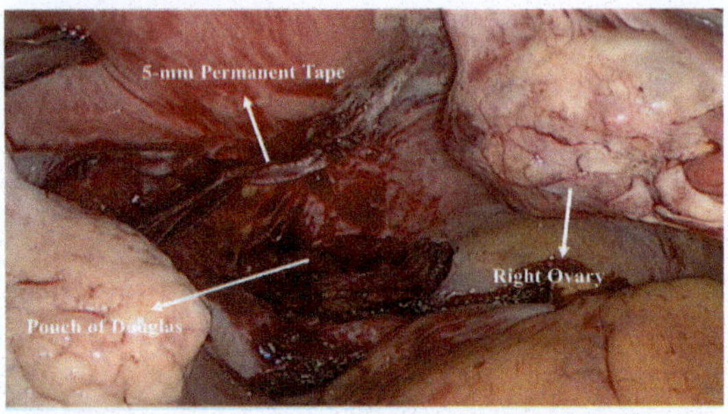

Fig. 28.7 Posterior level of internal cervical os

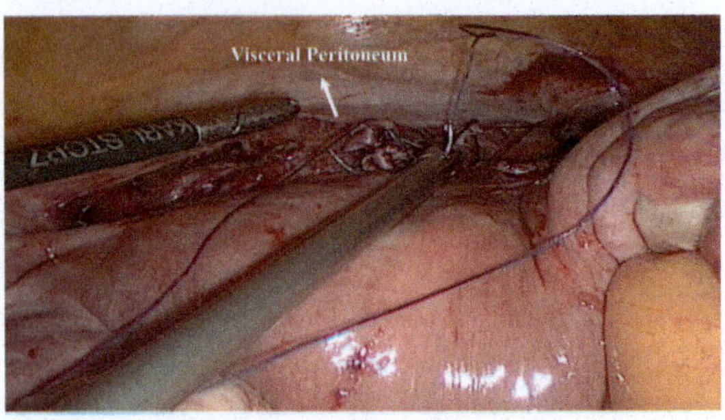

Fig. 28.8 Peritoneum cover

surgeon, and the ends are transfixed by a resorbable suture material.

Hemorrhage is the major risk of the procedure and can be controlled by metal hemostatic clip application. To avoid this complication, the tape can be placed medial to the uterine artery and lateral to the venous plexus. This technique insures the tape compresses the venous plexus [12].

There is no evidence that antibiotics or prophylactic tocolytics increase the effectiveness of cerclage [1].

Advantages of Minimally Invasive Surgery for Transabdominal Cerclage

Conventional and robotic-assisted laparoscopies are the preferred surgical approaches for transabdominal cerclage. These minimal invasive procedures are advantageous because of lower morbidity, higher success rates, shorter hospitalization and recovery time, decreased pain, and also decreased blood loss [13]. Robot-assisted abdominal cerclage has the advantages of three-dimensional visualization and endo-wristed instrumentation when compared to traditional laparoscopy. Such advantages have been previously reported.

Tulandi et al. analyzed 678 pregnancies between 1990 and 2013. The study found no significant difference in deliveries greater than 28 weeks of gestation between the transabdominal cerclages via laparoscopy or laparotomy [14]. In addition, Ades et al. concluded that laparoscopic transabdominal cerclage was associated with a significantly lower rate of complications compared with laparotomy [15].

Finally, a study comparing cervical length after cerclage between vaginal and laparoscopic approaches found that cervical length in the transvaginal group was significantly shorter, while in the laparoscopic group the cervical length remained unchanged [16]. One possible explanation for this finding is that the suture is placed closer to the internal cervical os via laparoscopy compared to the transvaginal approach.

Challenges of transabdominal cervical cerclage include difficulty accessing the lower uterine segment because of the gravid uterus and enhanced vascularization during pregnancy. To overcome these challenges, diversified surgical techniques have been described. One such method is the concomitant use of transvaginal ultrasonography during transabdominal cervical cerclage [17].

The TilePro feature of the da Vinci Surgical System provides simultaneous display of real-time ultrasonography allowing the surgeon to identify the borders of the cervix and the location of the internal cervical ostium. In this way, the surgeon avoids membranes and puts the suture in the right place.

One major risk of this procedure is damage to the vessels and bleeding. Zeybek et al. described the concomitant use of indocyanine green dye with a near-infrared camera system. In their method, 0.1 mg/kg indocyanine green dye was administered intravenous to detect the vascular anatomy before suturing via near-infrared camera system in robotic surgery. In this way, they could see the uterine arteries before passing through the suture. This technique enables identification of vascular anatomy and could prevent complications of hemorrhage [18].

Another challenge is manipulating the gravid uterus. Gibbs et al. reported use of a vaginal fornices delineator with two ring forcep clamps during a robot-assisted abdominal cerclage [19]. In this technique, the Koh Cup, which is clamped along the posterior rim with two ring forceps, is placed on the cervix from vaginal route. Thus, the surgeon could manipulate the uterus, and the Koh Cup is used for a visual landmark during the placement of robot-assisted abdominal cerclage. Jolijn Vissers et al. also described using McCartney tube for the purpose of manipulation during laparoscopy. A McCartney tube is inserted vaginally, and the gravid uterus is manipulated cranially, which provides a fine vision of the vesicouterine fold.

Complications

Risk due to complications varies depending on the timing and reason of cerclage intervention. Uterine rupture and maternal septicemia are mortal and very rarely encountered [20].

Transabdominal cerclage experiences higher complication rates when compared with transvaginal route because it absorbs all risk from open surgery [21].

Surgical complications of transabdominal cerclage are intraoperative hemorrhage, rectovaginal fistula formation, and bladder and bowel injury. Additionally, pregnancy complications may occur when the procedure is performed on a gravid woman. To avoid pregnancy-related complications, preconceptual transabdominal cerclage should be considered [22].

Dawood et al. from the United Kingdom reported preconceptual transabdominal cerclage is more accomplished in preventing repeat spontaneous midtrimester loss and preterm labor and is associated with less surgical and pregnancy-related morbidity compared to first trimester transabdominal cerclage [23].

Fortunately, several studies have reported that cerclage placement before conception does not reduce fertility [23, 24].

Removal of Cerclage

Removal of transvaginal cerclage is recommended at 36–37 weeks of gestation in women without any complications. However, women who undergo transabdominal cerclage will have to deliver via caesarean section. The suture could be removed after delivery via caesarean section or left in place for subsequent pregnancies. Further research into subsequent pregnancies with transabdominal cerclage is necessary.

Management of Preterm Premature Rupture of Membranes with Cerclage

There are no prospective studies or powerful retrospective studies regarding the management of preterm premature rupture of membranes (PPROM) with cerclage. Therefore, there are no evidence-based recommendations. One study has shown a relationship between increased rates of neonatal mortality due to sepsis, neonatal sepsis, respiratory distress syndrome, maternal chorioamnionitis with cerclage retention with PPROM [25]. However, until more evidence is available, clinicians should individualize management based on the clinical circumstances.

Finally, removal of cerclage or consideration of operative delivery is recommended in women experiencing painful regular uterine contractions, with cervical change or heavy vaginal bleeding despite the use of tocolysis.

References

1. American College of Obstetricians and Gynecologists. ACOG Practice Bulletin No.142: Cerclage for the management of cervical insufficiency. Obstet Gynecol 2014;123:372–9.
2. Iams JD, Johnson FF, Sonek J, Sachs L, Gebauer C, Samuels P. Cervical competence as a continuum: a study of ultrasonographic cervical length and obstetric performance. Am J Obstet Gynecol. 1995;172:1097–103.
3. Saccone G, Ciardulli A, Xodo S, Dugoff L, Ludmir J, Pagani G, et al. Cervical pessary for preventing preterm birth in singleton pregnancies with short cervical length: a systematic review and meta-analysis. J Ultrasound Med. 2017;36(8):1535–43. https://doi.org/10.7863/ultra.16.08054. Epub 11 Apr 2017.
4. McDonald IA. Suture of the cervix for inevitable miscarriage. J Obstet Gynaecol Br Emp. 1957;64:346–50.
5. Shirodkar VN. A new method of operative treatment for habitual abortions in the second trimester of pregnancy. Antiseptic. 1955;52:299–300.
6. Berghella V, Szychowski JM, Owen J, Hankins G, Iams JD, Sheffield JS, et al. Suture type and ultrasound-indicated cerclage efficacy. Vaginal Ultrasound Trial Consortium. J Matern Fetal Neonatal Med. 2012;25:2287–90.
7. Harger JH. Cerclage and cervical insufficiency: an evidence based analysis. Obstet Gynecol. 2002;100:1313–27.
8. Davis G, Berghella V, Talucci M, Wapner RJ. Patients with a prior failed transvaginal cerclage: a comparison of obstetric outcomes with either transabdominal or trans-vaginal cerclage. Am J Obstet Gynecol. 2000;183:836–9.
9. Burger NB, Brolmann HA, Einarsson JI, Langebrekke A, Huirne JA. Effectiveness of abdominal cerclage placed via laparotomy or laparoscopy: systematic review. J Minim Invasive Gynecol. 2011;18: 696–704.
10. Romero R, Espinoza J, Erez O, Hassan S. The role of cervical cerclage in obstetric practice: can the patient who could benefit from this procedure be identified? Am J Obstet Gynecol. 2006;194:1–9.
11. Sneider K, Christiansen OB, Sundtoft IB, Langhoff-Roos J. Recurrence rates after abdominal and vaginal cerclages in women with cervical insufficiency: a validated cohort study. Arch Gynecol Obstet. 2017;295(4):859–66. https://doi.org/10.1007/s00404-017-4315-y. Epub 23 Feb 2017.
12. Sumners JE, Kuper SG, Foster TL. Transabdominal cerclage. Clin Obstet Gynaecol. 2016;59(2):295–301.
13. Tusheva OA, Cohen SL, McElrath TF, et al. Laparoscopic placement of cervical cerclage. Rev Obstet Gynecol. 2012;5:e158–65.
14. Tulandi T, Alghanaim N, Hakeem G, et al. Pre- and post-conceptional abdominal cerclage by laparoscopy or laparotomy. J Minim Invasive Gynecol. 2014;21:987–93.
15. Ades A, Dobromilsky KC, Cheung KT, Umstad MP. Transabdominal cervical cerclage: laparoscopy versus laparotomy. J Minim Invasive Gynecol. 2015;22(6):968–73. https://doi.org/10.1016/j.jmig.2015.04.019. Epub 28 Apr 2015.
16. Bolla D, Gasparri ML, Badir S, Bajka M, Mueller MD, Papadia A, et al. Cervical length after cerclage: comparison between laparoscopic and vaginal approach. Arch Gynecol Obstet. 2017;295(4):885–90. https://doi.org/10.1007/s00404-016-4285-5. Epub 3 Mar 2017.
17. Walsh TM, Borahay MA, Fox KA, Kilic GS. Robotic-assisted, ultrasound-guided abdominal cerclage during pregnancy: over- coming minimally invasive surgery limitations? J Minim Invasive Gynecol. 2013;20:398–400.
18. Zeybek B, Borahay MA, Kilic GS. Overcoming the obstacles of visualization in robotically-assisted abdominal cerclage using indocyanine green. J Robot Surg. Published ahead of print 16 Apr 2016. https://doi.org/10.1007/s11701-016-0585-9.
19. Gibbs S, Widelock T, Elkattah R, Depasquale S. Additional uses of a vaginal fornices delineator. Am J Obstet Gynecol. 2015;213:433.e1–3.
20. Althuisius S, Dekker G, Hummel P, Bekedam D, Kuik D, van Geijn H. Cervical incompetence prevention randomized cerclage trial (CIPRACT): effect of therapeutic cerclage with bed rest vs. bed rest only on cervical length. Ultrasound Obstet Gynecol. 2002;20:163–7.
21. Wolfe L, DePasquale S, Adair CD, Torres C, Stallings S, Briery C, et al. Robotic-assisted laparoscopic placement of transabdominal cerclage during pregnancy. Am J Perinatol. 2008;25:653–5.
22. Groom K, Jones BA, Edmonds K, Bennett PR. Preconception transabdominal cervicoisthmic cerclage. Am J Obstet Gynecol. 2004;191(1):230–4.
23. Dawood F, Farquharson RG. Transabdominal cerclage: preconceptual versus first trimester insertion. Eur J Obstet Gynecol Reprod Biol. 2016;199:27–31. https://doi.org/10.1016/j.ejogrb.2016.01.035. Epub 8 Feb 2016.
24. Vousden NJ, Carter J, Seed PT, Shennan AH. What is the impact of preconception abdominal cerclage on fertility: evidence from a randomized controlled trial. Acta Obstet Gynecol Scand. 2017;96:543–6.
25. Laskin MD, Yinon Y, Whittle WL. Preterm premature rupture of membranes in the presence of cerclage: is the risk for intra-uterine infection and adverse neonatal outcome increased? J Matern Fetal Neonatal Med. 2012;25:424–8.

Congenital Uterine Anomalies in Pregnancy

29

Angela L. Du and Joseph S. Sanfilippo

Congenital Uterine Anomalies

Congenital uterine anomalies arise from abnormal formation, incomplete fusion, or incomplete septal resorption of the mullerian ducts during embryologic development of the female reproductive tract. A complete failure of the mullerian ducts to develop results in mullerian agenesis and variable degrees of uterovaginal hypoplasia; this is the most severe mullerian duct anomaly and is incompatible with carrying a pregnancy. Abnormal formation of one mullerian duct results in a unicornuate uterus with a single well-formed uterine cavity that has an asymmetric, ellipsoidal shape, with or without a smaller (rudimentary) horn. If present, this horn can be communicating, non-communicating, or rudimentary, i.e., lacking a uterine cavity. Failure of the two Müllerian ducts to fuse results in uterine didelphys with two separate fundi and cervices (Fig. 29.1). Partial fusion of the mullerian ducts results in a bicornuate uterus with a varying degree of septation of the uterine horns and an indented fundus (≥1 cm). Abnormal resorption of the midline septum after fusion results in a septate or arcuate uterus. A septate uterus is completely or partially divided into two cavities by a muscular or fibrous septum (Fig. 29.2). Unlike a bicornuate uterus, a septate uterus has a fundal indentation usually <1 cm. An arcuate uterus has a slight midline septum and mild fundal indentation; its distinction from the septate uterus is less clearly defined and may be considered a normal variant (Fig. 29.3).

In the general population, the prevalence of congenital uterine anomalies is 4.3–6.7% [1–3]. The most common defects are arcuate and septate uteri, followed by bicornuate uterus. However, the true incidence of congenital uterine anomalies is unknown. Studies are limited by variability in diagnostic techniques and the lack of a universal classification system. Furthermore, many asymptomatic cases remain undiagnosed.

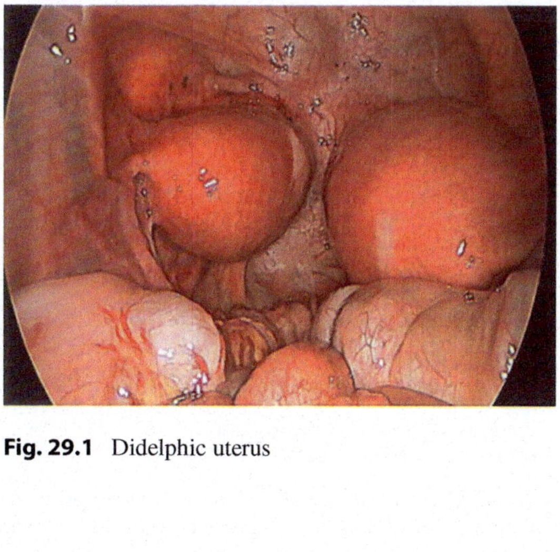

Fig. 29.1 Didelphic uterus

A. L. Du · J. S. Sanfilippo (✉)
Department of Obstetrics, Gynecology and Reproductive Sciences, Magee-Womens Hospital of UPMC, Pittsburgh, PA, USA
e-mail: sanfjs@mail.magee.edu

C. H. Nezhat (ed.), *Non-Obstetric Surgery During Pregnancy*,
https://doi.org/10.1007/978-3-319-90752-9_29

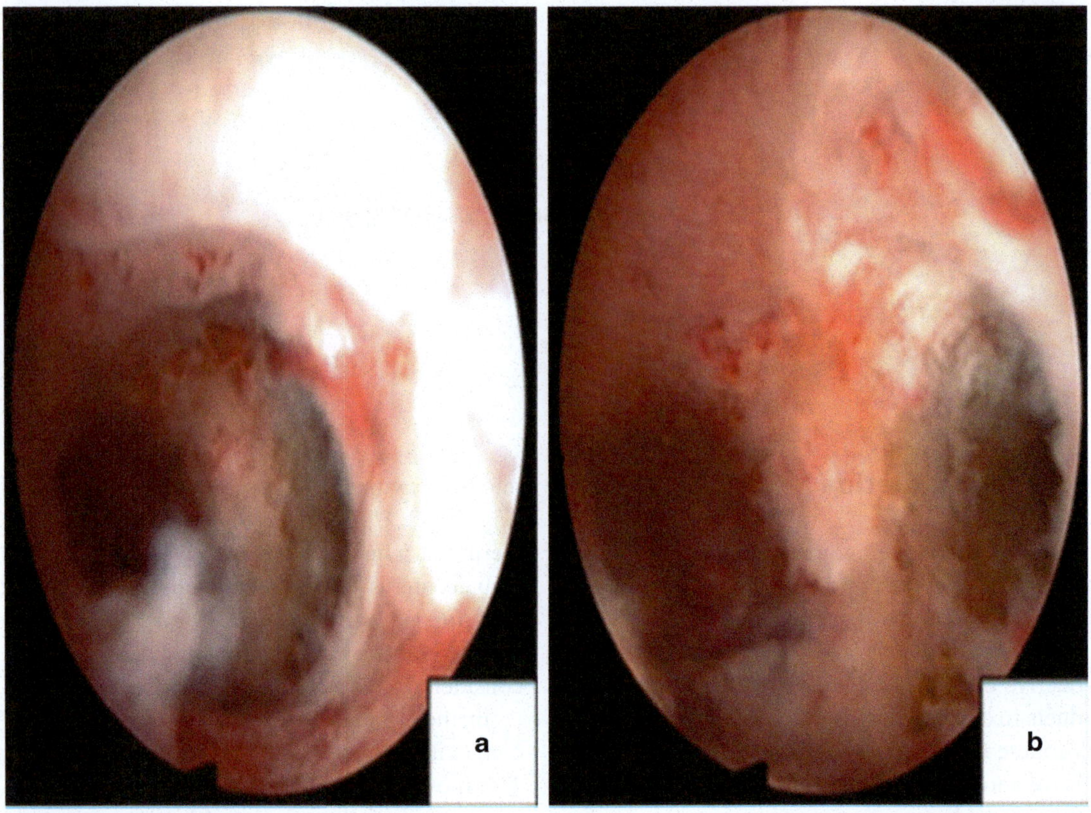

Fig. 29.2 Uterine septum

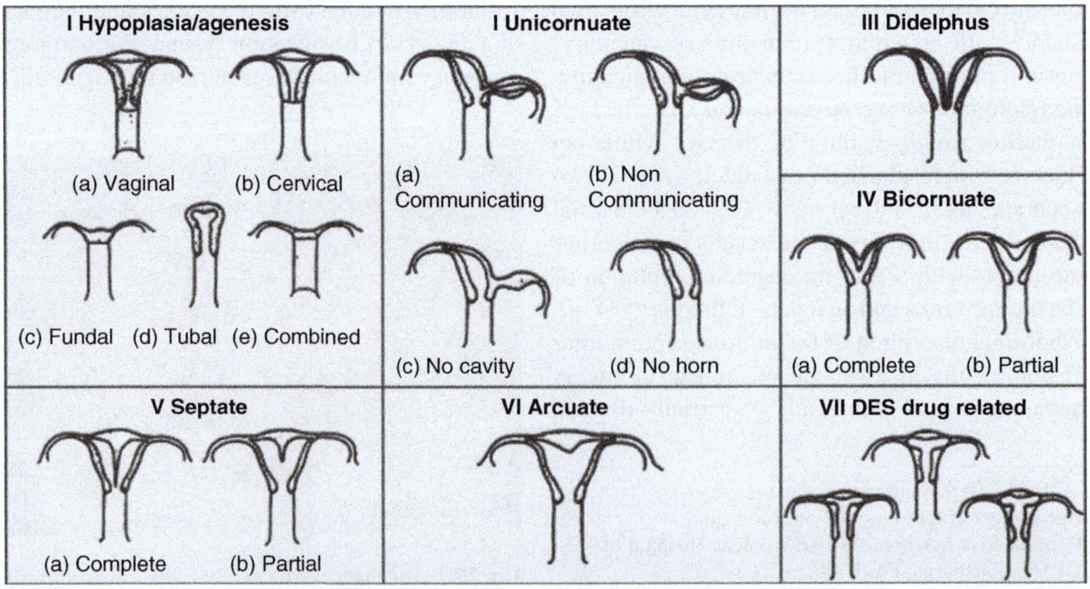

Fig. 29.3 American Fertility Society classification of Müllerian duct anomalies. Reprinted from Fertility and Sterility, 49(6), the American Fertility Society classifications of adnexal adhesions, distal tubal occlusion, tubal occlusion secondary to tubal ligation, tubal pregnancies, Müllerian anomalies, and intrauterine adhesions, 944–55, Copyright 1988 American Society for Reproductive Medicine. Published by Elsevier Inc. All rights reserved [44]

Clinical presentation is variable and includes pelvic pain and dysmenorrhea secondary to obstructed menstrual flow, hypomenorrhea, vaginal discharge, and dyspareunia [4]. However, identification and treatment often occurs in the setting of adverse reproductive outcomes. The uterine anomalies represent a wide spectrum with varying implications on fertility and pregnancy outcomes. Thus, it is important to accurately identify them in order to appropriately manage the associated risks. The following chapter will address these concerns and explore the diagnostic and management options, focusing on surgical management in the setting of optimizing pregnancy outcomes.

Implications for Fertility and Pregnancy

Uterine anomalies have not been decisively shown to be associated with infertility. Studies have found that women with unicornuate, bicornuate, didelphic, and arcuate uteri have similar clinical pregnancy rates compared to women with normal uteri [5–8]. However, the incidence of uterine septa is higher among women with infertility compared to the general population [6, 7, 9, 10], and a meta-analysis on reproductive outcomes in women with congenital uterine anomalies found that women with septate and subseptate uteri had lower clinical pregnancy rates compared to women with normal uteri (RR 0.86, 95% CI 0.77–0.96) [5]. There is evidence that hysteroscopic septum incision is associated with improved clinical pregnancy rates [11, 12], suggesting that the presence of a septum may interfere with implantation.

While most uterine anomalies do not appear to reduce fertility, they are associated with increased rates of first- and second-trimester pregnancy loss [6, 8]. This association is strongest in the septate uterus. The prevalence of uterine anomalies in women with recurrent pregnancy loss is higher than the general population at 12.6–18.2% [1, 3, 13]. Thus, recurrent pregnancy loss is one of the primary indications for treatment of women with uterine malformations.

They are also associated with numerous adverse obstetric outcomes which must be carefully monitored for and managed during pregnancy. This risk does not apply to women with arcuate uteri, as they have been found to have similar reproductive outcomes as women with normal uteri. However, women with unicornuate, bicornuate, and didelphic uteri have a significantly higher probability of giving birth to a low birth weight neonate less than 2500 g and intrauterine growth restriction compared to women with normal uteri [14]. This may be secondary to uteroplacental insufficiency from abnormal vascularization of the uterus [15].

There is a greater risk of fetal malpresentation and preterm birth, often with preterm premature rupture of membranes. As a result, cesarean section is more common among this patient population. Cervical incompetence has also been diagnosed in 30% of patients with uterine malformations [16]. These complications may be secondary to a reduced cavity volume or diminished myometrial function of the abnormal uteri.

Since uterine anomalies are frequently associated with congenital renal anomalies due to the close relationship between the mullerian and mesonephric ducts during development, women with uterine anomalies have increased rates of gestational hypertension and preeclampsia [17]. Renal anomalies, most commonly renal agenesis, are found in 20–30% of women with uterine anomalies, primarily with didelphic and unicornuate uteri [18]. Without renal agenesis, these women have similar rates of preeclampsia compared to the general population [17]. Thus, it is important to evaluate the kidneys for malformations at the time of diagnosis in order to rule out a coexisting renal abnormality and assess risk for secondary complications.

In women with a rudimentary horn, there is a risk of ectopic implantation in the rudimentary horn. This occurs in 1 in 76,000 pregnancies. While there have been cases that have resulted in live birth, 80% of these pregnancies result in uterine rupture at 10–15 weeks gestation due to the poor musculature of the rudimentary horn [19]. This is a life-threatening complication, and early diagnosis and treatment are critical.

Diagnosis

A number of imaging modalities have historically been used to diagnose and categorize uterine anomalies including magnetic resonance imaging (MRI), hysterosalpingography (HSG), saline infusion sonohysterography (SHG), and two- and three-dimensional ultrasonography. MRI is the gold standard for the diagnosis of uterine anomalies as it provides clear delineation of both the internal and external uterine contours. It is a primary imaging modality that can differentiate a bicornuate uterus, which has both fibrous and myometrial components, from a septate uterus with only fibrous tissue. It also has the ability to visualize the extent of the septum in these anomalies.

HSG is excellent for general assessment of the uterine cavity and tubal patency. However, it does not evaluate the external uterine contour, which is often required for definitive diagnosis. It has a diagnostic accuracy of only 55% for differentiating between septate and bicornuate uteri, which requires visualization of the angle between the two horns [20]. Risks of HSG include patient discomfort, radiation exposure, contrast allergy, uterine perforation, and infection. SHG is also useful for evaluating the uterine cavity and has similar diagnostic accuracy as HSG at 95.2% [21]. Thus, it is preferred over HSG in order to avoid the radiation exposure required for HSG when assessing uterine cavity.

Ultrasonography is the more cost-effective and noninvasive method for evaluating both the internal and external uterine contour. However, unlike MRI, ultrasonography cannot as reliably differentiate a septate uterus from a bicornuate uterus or a unicornuate uterus from a normal uterus. However, while two-dimensional ultrasound has historically been used most commonly as the first-line method for evaluating suspected uterine anomalies, the sensitivity of this is only 60% [22]. Three-dimensional ultrasound has emerged as the first-line method because it is more sensitive than two-dimensional ultrasound with similar accuracy as HSG and MRI [23].

Management

Identified uterine anomalies do not require surgical correction unless they are symptomatically bothersome to the patient or have implications for future fertility and pregnancy that can be ameliorated by the surgical procedure. For unicornuate and didelphic uteri, surgery has not been found to improve pregnancy outcomes [13]. Thus, ideally, during pregnancy, these patients are followed closely by, or in consultation with, Maternal-Fetal Medicine physicians and undergo careful monitoring for intrauterine growth restriction and cervical insufficiency. The presence of a hemivagina and associated outflow tract of one horn can lead to partial hematocolpos, hematometra, hematosalpinx, and endometriosis (Figs. 29.4 and 29.5). This is managed with resection of the hemivagina. Other vaginal anomalies are best addressed case by case.

While no surgical intervention is advocated for unicornuate uterus, rudimentary horns with functional endometrium are oftentimes managed with surgical extirpation via minimally invasive approaches. Furthermore, rudimentary horn pregnancies are best excised due to the risk of life-threatening uterine rupture. This has traditionally been accomplished by laparotomy, but laparoscopy is emerging as a minimally invasive technique that allows for horn resection [24].

In women with recurrent pregnancy loss in the setting of a bicornuate uterus, uterine reunification can be effective for increasing rates of fetal

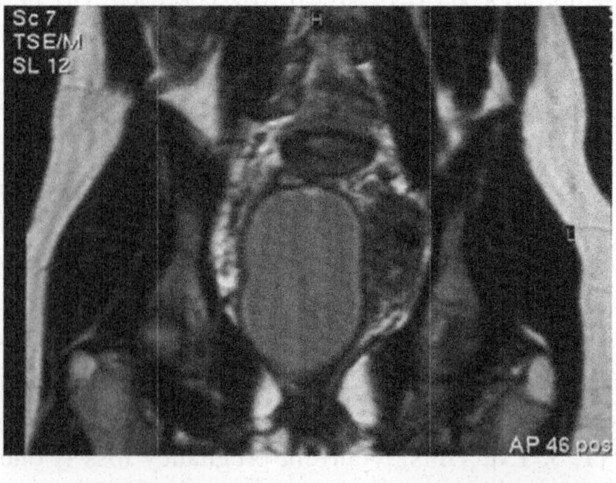

Fig. 29.4 Complete outflow tract obstruction with hematocolpos

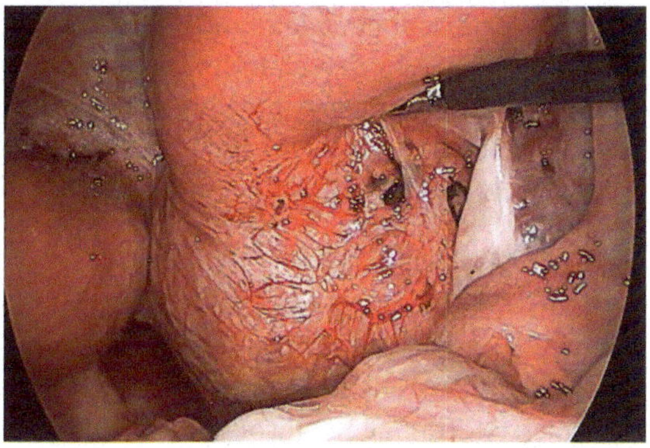

Fig. 29.5 Hematocolpos with endometriosis

survival [25–27]. This typically involves a Strassman metroplasty with wedge resection of septum and subsequent unification of the two cavities, which can be done abdominally or laparoscopically. Following metroplasty, cesarean delivery is indicated due to a high risk for uterine rupture. More often than not, bicornuate uterus is not amenable to surgical correction.

The septate uterus is the most common of the uterine anomalies and is associated with the poorest outcomes. Specifically, it is associated with fetal survival rates of 6–28% and a greater than 60% spontaneous abortion rate [28]. While the finding of a septate uterus per se may not be an indication for surgical intervention, consideration of various etiologies for infertility, implicating the septum, may lead to proceeding with intervention. When the decision is to proceed with surgery, endometrial preparation is important. Some surgeons opt to operate post menses, and others use progestins, gonadotropin-releasing hormone (GnRH) agonists, or danazol to thin the endometrium [28].

Hysteroscopic approaches remain the most popular of options. This is accomplished via hysteroscopic microscissors and electrosurgery (monopolar or bipolar), as well as with laser energy (neodymium-yttrium-aluminum garnet, KTP/532, and argon beam [28]). Either 0- or 12-degree lens provides a normal field of vision.

The two basic techniques of septum resection include [29]:

1. "Shortening" technique – The septum is incised at its apex horizontally across the length of the septum. End points include visualization of vasculature in the operative site, slight bleeding, and/or identification of both cornual ostia when the hysteroscope is held at the internal os.
2. "Thinning" technique – Incisions are made along the sides of the septum with gradual thinning of the septum until a short broad notch remains. This is advocated for wide septa.

Residual septum $\leq$ 1 cm is equated with adequate resection [30].

Some surgeons include intraoperative sonohysterography to determine complete resection. This is in large part physician preference and may be reserved for repeat procedures.

Some clinicians include laparoscopy with hysteroscopic resection and determine the end point by observing completeness of illumination of the hysteroscope when the light source for the laparoscope is temporarily removed. Upon complete resection, a uniform "jack o' lantern" appearance to the uterine fundus is noted [29].

Possible complications of hysteroscopic septum resection include bleeding, uterine perforation, intrauterine adhesions, and uterine rupture in subsequent pregnancies. Postoperative management remains controversial. Use of intrauterine devices, antibiotics, hormonal therapy, and uterine cavity balloon or other types of catheters has not clearly proven beneficial. In a group of 100 patients, there was no statistically significant difference in improved pregnancy outcomes with the use of an intrauterine device, hormone only (estradiol valerate and norgestrel) versus no treatment [31, 32].

Other techniques for uterine septum correction include Jones and Tompkins metroplasties; however, these primarily required laparotomy. The Jones procedure includes wedge resection of the septum. Tompkins approach bisects the uterus (uterine septum or bicornuate) and then incises the medial surface of each horn to result in one unified cavity. More recently robotic approaches have been reported. The uterine septum is surgically excised, and three-layer closure with 2-0 nonreactive suture on an atraumatic needle has been reported [33].

To date, no randomized controlled trials have investigated reproductive outcomes following hysteroscopic septum resection compared to expectant management. However, several observational studies have shown that hysteroscopic septum resection is associated with higher clinical pregnancy rates in women with infertility, decreased rates of spontaneous abortion, and improved live birth rates in women with a history of infertility or recurrent pregnancy loss [12, 34, 35].

Surgical Considerations During Pregnancy

For women with congenital anomalies who require surgery for a non-obstetric indication, the uterine anomaly itself does not pose a unique risk and the patient can be managed similarly to any other pregnant woman. However, in the event of a known uterine anomaly, the surgeon must be aware of associated abnormalities which may have surgical implications.

As mentioned previously, renal anomalies are commonly associated with uterine anomalies, particularly unicornuate and didelphic uteri. These include renal agenesis (most commonly unilateral agenesis), ectopic kidney, renal hypoplasia, horseshoe kidney, malrotation, and duplex kidney. Thorough evaluation of the entire genitourinary tract with renal ultrasound or MRI should be conducted prior to abdominal surgery to identify any associated renal anomalies. Renal anomalies are discussed in more detail in the following section.

Ovarian maldescent, defined as attachment of the upper pole above the common iliac vessels, has been identified in up to 17% of women with congenital uterine anomalies, particularly fusion abnormalities [36, 37]. This would likely be discovered at the time of diagnosis of the uterine anomaly, but surgeons should be aware of this during evaluation of abdominal or pelvic pain and surgical planning.

Outflow tract obstruction is associated with the development of endometriosis due to retrograde menstruation [38, 39]. Endometriosis is a condition in which endometrial glands and stroma are present outside of the uterine cavity, most commonly in pelvic structures including the ovaries, anterior and posterior cul-de-sac, broad ligament, uterosacral ligament, and rectovaginal septum. The rectosigmoid colon and appendix are also commonly involved. Occasionally, endometrial tissue may seed into areas of prior surgical excision such as those following a cesarean delivery. It is hypothesized that retrograde menstrual flow may drive endometrial fragments through the fallopian tubes and into the peritoneal cavity where they can implant, grow, and invade into pelvic structures [40]. Estrogen-dependent inflammation of ectopic endometrial tissue can lead to dysmenorrhea, dyspareunia, and chronic pain. Treatment options for symptomatic endometriosis include medical therapy and surgery. Laparoscopic excision and/or ablation of endometrial implants is the preferred surgical approach that is both diagnostic and therapeutic for women who have failed medical therapy and desire fertility preservation. In the setting of a congenital outflow tract obstruction, endometriosis often resolves spontaneously with correction of the obstruction.

However, surgeons should be aware of the risk of endometriosis in such patients as the majority of women with endometriosis develop extensive intraperitoneal adhesive disease, independent of whether or not they had prior surgery, which may limit the mobility and visualization of internal structures during surgery (Fig. 29.6).

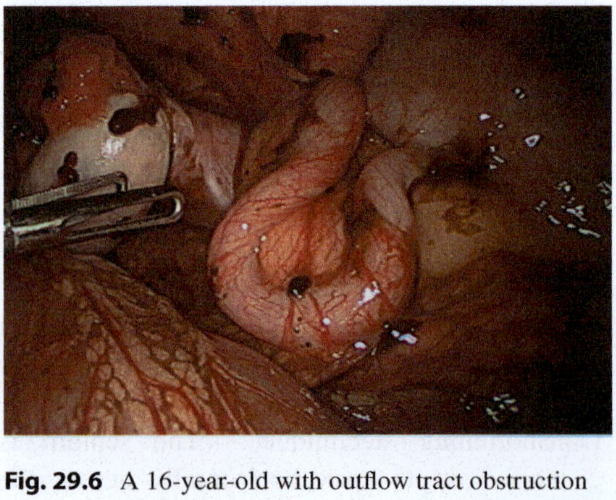

Fig. 29.6 A 16-year-old with outflow tract obstruction

Congenital Renal and Urological Anomalies

Congenital anomalies of the kidney and urinary tract (CAKUT) are a group of multifactorial, heterogeneous disorders that arise from abnormalities in renal parenchymal development, renal migration, or the developing collecting system. It encompasses a spectrum ranging from mild, asymptomatic malformations such as double ureter to severe, life-threatening conditions such as bilateral renal agenesis. These anomalies are often diagnosed during routine antenatal ultrasonography or postnatal ultrasonography.

Abnormal nephron development results in renal parenchymal malformations such as renal dysplasia and renal agenesis. Renal dysplasia is often diagnosed during routine antenatal screening with the presence of oligohydramnios or during postnatal renal ultrasound in a dysmorphic infant. Bilateral dysplasia may present as impaired renal function at birth with subsequent progressive renal failure, but patients with unilateral renal agenesis have excellent long-term outcomes in the setting of a normal contralateral kidney. Renal agenesis, on the other hand, is the complete absence of renal parenchymal tissue. While bilateral renal agenesis is incompatible with life, unilateral renal agenesis is often asymptomatic and detected incidentally. Patients are at increased risk for long-term chronic renal disease. In both unilateral renal dysplasia and renal agenesis, the contralateral normal kidney should be monitored with serial ultrasonography for compensatory hypertrophy.

Abnormal renal embryonic migration can result in an ectopic kidney or fusion abnormalities. An ectopic kidney is abnormally located below, above, or contralateral to the normal anatomic kidney location. Fusion abnormalities include horseshoe kidney and crossed fused renal ectopy. Horseshoe kidney is more common and is characterized by the fusion of one pole of each kidney. The separate excretory renal units and ureters are usually preserved as the vast majority of cases involve fusion at the lower poles. Crossed fused renal ectopy is a condition in which an ectopic kidney and ureter cross the midline and fuse with the contralateral kidney. Patients with these abnormalities are often asymptomatic and may have normal renal function. However, they are at risk for other genitourinary abnormalities, most commonly vesicoureteral reflux, which may lead to frequent urinary tract infections, renal calculi, hydronephrosis, and renal injury. No treatment is necessary in the absence of obstruction or kidney damage.

Anomalies of the collecting system may involve abnormalities at the level of the renal pelvis, ureter, and bladder. At the renal pelvis, ureteropelvic junction obstruction can lead to partial or total intermittent blockage of the flow of urine. In asymptomatic patients, observation and monitoring with serial ultrasounds and diuretic renography is sufficient. However, in patients who develop symptoms secondary to hydronephrosis, surgical pyeloplasty is recommended to relieve the obstruction.

An ectopic ureter is one in which the ureteral orifice opens caudal to the normal insertion on the bladder trigone. Females present with incontinence during childhood, and surgical reconstruction via ureteroureterostomy in the setting of a duplex kidney or nephroureterectomy in the setting of a single kidney has good long-term outcomes.

Duplex kidney, the most common congenital anomaly of the urinary tract, is characterized by complete or partial duplication of the renal collecting system. In complete duplication, there are two separate pelvicaliceal systems with separate ureters. The ureter associated with the lower collecting system usually enters the bladder at its normal insertion site in the trigone, while the ureter from the upper collecting system may insert in the trigone or an ectopic site which may result in obstruction or vesicoureteral reflux. In partial duplication, the two separate pelvicaliceal systems have either a single ureter or separate ureters which unite prior to insertion into the bladder. Surgical repair is indicated in the setting of complications such as recurrent urinary tract infections or hydronephrosis secondary to obstruction.

Bladder exstrophy is defined as exposure of the bladder on the outer surface of the abdomen. This occurs secondary to in utero rupture of the cloacal membrane during development, which leads to herniation of the lower abdominal contents through the abdominal wall. It is associated with numerous other malformations including diastasis of the symphysis pubis, low-set umbilicus, shortened urethra and vagina, and epispadias with a bifid clitoris and small, laterally displaced labia minora. Optimal management involves early closure of the bladder during infancy, but periodic assessment is required due to the risk of long-term complications including pelvic organ prolapse and malignancy. During pregnancy, bladder exstrophy is associated with a higher risk of antepartum pyelonephritis, urinary retention, ureteral obstruction, pelvic organ prolapse, and breech presentation.

Surgical Considerations During Pregnancy

Prior to surgery, renal function must be evaluated and anatomy be assessed for surgical planning. During pregnancy, numerous adaptations to renal physiology occur to support a healthy pregnancy. These changes include dilatation of the urinary collecting system, an increase in renal plasma flow and glomerular filtration rate, and net vasodilation via alterations in hormones including mediators of the renin-angiotensin-aldosterone system. Glomerular hyperfiltration results in a physiologically lower serum creatinine levels and proteinuria. These changes must be taken into account when interpreting the results of renal function tests. Furthermore, for women with advanced chronic renal disease, there is a risk of progression of kidney injury during pregnancy [41].

CAKUT, if clinically significant, is typically identified and corrected at an early age. However, extensive adhesions following prior repair may alter the internal anatomy and complicate future surgery. Furthermore, any anatomical anomalies should be taken into account during surgical planning. In the setting of an ectopic or fused kidney, abnormal rotation of the developing kidney results in a renal pelvis that is directed anteriorly rather than medially. In a fusion abnormality, the ureters lie over the isthmus of the horseshoe kidney or the anterior surface of the fused kidney. The blood supply is variable and may originate from the iliac arteries, aorta, hypogastric arteries, or middle sacral arteries.

It is important to note that infection or obstruction of abnormal genitourinary organs can mimic appendicitis [42]. Pregnancy itself poses a diagnostic challenge in appendicitis due to variable anatomic positioning and nonspecific symptoms throughout pregnancy. During pregnancy, appendicitis may present as right upper or lower quadrant pain, nausea, vomiting, diarrhea, uterine contractions, dysuria, rectal pain, and vaginal tenderness. MRI is recommended as the first-line imaging study for pregnant women with such symptoms [43].

Conclusion

Congenital anomalies pose a unique diagnostic and therapeutic challenge in the setting of pregnancy. Congenital uterine anomalies are associated with adverse reproductive outcomes including recurrent pregnancy loss, IUGR, preterm delivery, fetal malpresentation, and rudimentary horn pregnancy with subsequent uterine rupture. MRI, SHG, and three-dimensional ultrasound all have acceptable diagnostic accuracy. Surgery is not recommended for unicornuate and didelphic uteri nor for the most part with bicornuate as it has not been shown to significantly improve pregnancy outcomes. However, there are a number of minimally invasive therapeutic options that have been shown to improve rates of fetal survival in women with septate uteri. Thus, in women with infertility, prior pregnancy loss, or poor obstetrical outcomes, surgical correction of such anomalies merits appropriate consideration on a case-by-case basis depending on the anomaly. Non-obstetric surgery during pregnancy is not contraindicated but may be complicated by associated renal anomalies, ovarian maldescent, or endometriosis.

Congenital anomalies of the renal system and urinary tract encompass a spectrum of abnormalities in renal parenchymal development, renal migration, and the developing collecting system. Most of these anomalies are diagnosed in the antenatal or postnatal period, and if clinically significant, they are often corrected during infancy. Even so, pregnant women with a history of CAKUT may have reduced renal function and altered anatomy secondary to anatomic abnormalities or adhesions from prior surgery. These factors must be taken into account prior to non-obstetric surgery in these patients.

References

1. Chan YY, Jayaprakasan K, Zamora J, Thornton JG, Raine-Fenning N, Coomarasamy A. The prevalence of congenital uterine anomalies in unselected and high-risk populations: a systematic review. Hum Reprod Update. 2011;17(6):761–71.
2. Grimbizis GF, Camus M, Tarlatzis BC, Bontis JN, Devroey P. Clinical implications of uterine malformations and hysteroscopic treatment results. Hum Reprod Update. 2001;7(1):161–74.
3. Saravelos SH, Cocksedge KA, Li TC. Prevalence and diagnosis of congenital uterine anomalies in women with reproductive failure: a critical appraisal. Hum Reprod Update. 2008;14(5):415–29.
4. Golan A, Langer R, Bukovsky I, Caspi E. Congenital anomalies of the mullerian system. Fertil Steril. 1989;51(5):747–55.
5. Chan YY, Jayaprakasan K, Tan A, Thornton JG, Coomarasamy A, Raine-Fenning NJ. Reproductive outcomes in women with congenital uterine anomalies: a systematic review. Ultrasound Obstet Gynecol. 2011;38(4):371–82.
6. Acien P. Reproductive performance of women with uterine malformations. Hum Reprod. 1993;8(1):122–6.
7. Shuiqing M, Xuming B, Jinghe L. Pregnancy and its outcome in women with malformed uterus. Chin Med Sci J. 2002;17(4):242–5.
8. Woelfer B, Salim R, Banerjee S, Elson J, Regan L, Jurkovic D. Reproductive outcomes in women with congenital uterine anomalies detected by three-dimensional ultrasound screening. Obstet Gynecol. 2001;98(6):1099–103.
9. Raga F, Bauset C, Remohi J, Bonilla-Musoles F, Simon C, Pellicer A. Reproductive impact of congenital anomalies. Hum Reprod. 1997;12(10):2277–81.
10. Tomazevic T, Ban-Frangez H, Virant-Klun I, Verdenik I, Pozlep B, Vrtacnik-Bokal E. Septate, subseptate and arcuate uterus decrease pregnancy and live birth rates in IVF/ICSI. Reprod Biomed Online. 2010;21(5):700–5.
11. Mollo A, De Franciscis P, Colacurci N, Cobellis L, Perino A, Venezia R, et al. Hysteroscopic resection of the septum improves the pregnancy rate of women with unexplained infertility: a prospective controlled trial. Fertil Steril. 2009;91(6):2628–31.
12. Shokeir T, Abdelshaheed M, El-Shafie M, Sherif L, Badawy A. Determinants of fertility and reproductive success after hysteroscopic septoplasty for women with unexplained primary infertility: a prospective analysis of 88 cases. Eur J Obstet Gynecol Reprod Biol. 2011;155(1):54–7.
13. Grimbizis GF. Clinical implications of uterine malformations and hysteroscopic treatment results. Hum Reprod Update. 2001;7(2):161–74.
14. Venetis CA, Papadopoulos SP, Campo R, Gordts S, Tarlatzis BC, Grimbizis GF. Clinical implications of congenital uterine anomalies: a meta-analysis of comparative studies. Reprod Biomed Online. 2014;29(6):665–83.
15. Burchell RC, Creed F, Rasoulpour M, Whitcomb M. Vascular anatomy of the human uterus and pregnancy wastage. Br J Obstet Gynaecol. 1978;85(9):698–706.
16. Golan A, Langer R, Neuman M, Wexler S, Segev E, David MP. Obstetric outcome in women with congenital uterine malformations. J Reprod Med. 1992;37(3):233–6.
17. Heinonen PK. Gestational hypertension and preeclampsia associated with unilateral renal agenesis in women with uterine malformations. Eur J Obstet Gynecol Reprod Biol. 2004;114(1):39–43.
18. Oppelt P, von Have M, Paulsen M, Strissel PL, Strick R, Brucker S, et al. Female genital malformations and their associated abnormalities. Fertil Steril. 2007;87(2):335–42.
19. Nahum GG. Rudimentary uterine horn pregnancy. The 20th-century worldwide experience of 588 cases. J Reprod Med. 2002;47(2):151–63.
20. Reuter KL, Daly DC, Cohen SM. Septate versus bicornuate uteri: errors in imaging diagnosis. Radiology. 1989;172(3):749–52.
21. Ludwin A, Ludwin I, Banas T, Knafel A, Miedzyblocki M, Basta A. Diagnostic accuracy of sonohysterography, hysterosalpingography and diagnostic hysteroscopy in diagnosis of arcuate, septate and bicornuate uterus. J Obstet Gynaecol Res. 2011;37(3):178–86.
22. Saravelos SH, Cocksedge KA, Li TC. The pattern of pregnancy loss in women with congenital uterine anomalies and recurrent miscarriage. Reprod Biomed Online. 2010;20(3):416–22.
23. Deutch TD, Abuhamad AZ. The role of 3-dimensional ultrasonography and magnetic resonance imaging in the diagnosis of mullerian duct anomalies: a review of the literature. J Ultrasound Med. 2008;27(3):413–23.
24. Dulemba JF, Midgett WA, Freeman MVR. Laparoscopic management of a rudimentary horn pregnancy. J Am Assoc Gynecol Laparosc. 1996;3(4, Suppl):S10–1.
25. Ayhan A, Yucel I, Tuncer ZS, Kisnisci HA. Reproductive performance after conventional metroplasty: an evaluation of 102 cases. Fertil Steril. 1992;57(6):1194–6.

26. Lolis DE, Paschopoulos M, Makrydimas G, Zikopoulos K, Sotiriadis A, Paraskevaidis E. Reproductive outcome after Strassman metroplasty in women with a bicornuate uterus. J Reprod Med. 2005;50(5):297–301.
27. Rechberger T, Monist M, Bartuzi A. Clinical effectiveness of Strassman operation in the treatment of bicornuate uterus. Ginekol Pol. 2009;80(2):88–92.
28. Homer HA, Li TC, Cooke ID. The septate uterus: a review of management and reproductive outcome. Fertil Steril. 2000;73(1):1–14.
29. March CM, Israel R. Hysteroscopic management of recurrent abortion caused by septate uterus. Am J Obstet Gynecol. 1987;156(4):834–42.
30. Fedele L, Bianchi S, Marchini M, Mezzopane R, Di Nola G, Tozzi L. Residual uterine septum of less than 1 cm after hysteroscopic metroplasty does not impair reproductive outcome. Hum Reprod. 1996;11(4):727–9.
31. Tonguc EA, Var T, Yilmaz N, Batioglu S. Intrauterine device or estrogen treatment after hysteroscopic uterine septum resection. Int J Gynaecol Obstet. 2010;109(3):226–9.
32. Practice Committee of the American Society for Reproductive Medicine. Electronic address Aao, Practice Committee of the American Society for Reproductive M. Uterine septum: a guideline. Fertil Steril. 2016;106(3):530–40.
33. Chen YJ, Twu NF, Horng HC, Yen MS, Chao KC. Robotic modified Jones metroplasty for uterine unification. J Minim Invasive Gynecol. 2010;17(6):S11–S2.
34. Saygili-Yilmaz E, Yildiz S, Erman-Akar M, Akyuz G, Yilmaz Z. Reproductive outcome of septate uterus after hysteroscopic metroplasty. Arch Gynecol Obstet. 2003;268(4):289–92.
35. Tonguc EA, Var T, Batioglu S. Hysteroscopic metroplasty in patients with a uterine septum and otherwise unexplained infertility. Int J Gynaecol Obstet. 2011;113(2):128–30.
36. Allen JW, Cardall S, Kittijarukhajorn M, Siegel CL. Incidence of ovarian maldescent in women with mullerian duct anomalies: evaluation by MRI. Am J Roentgenol. 2012;198(4):W381–5.
37. Dabirashrafi H, HMohammad K, Moghadami-Tabrizi N. Ovarian malposition in women with uterine anomalies. Obstet Gynecol. 1994;83(2):293–4.
38. Gell JS. Mullerian anomalies. Semin Reprod Med. 2003;21(4):375–88.
39. Sanfilippo JS, Wakim NG, Schikler KN, Yussman MA. Endometriosis in association with uterine anomaly. Am J Obstet Gynecol. 1986;154(1):39–43.
40. Vercellini P, Vigano P, Somigliana E, Fedele L. Endometriosis: pathogenesis and treatment. Nat Rev Endocrinol. 2014;10(5):261–75.
41. Hladunewich MA. Chronic kidney disease and pregnancy. Semin Nephrol. 2017;37(4):337–46.
42. Dalpiaz A, Gandhi J, Smith NL, Dagur G, Schwamb R, Weissbart SJ, et al. Mimicry of appendicitis symptomatology in congenital anomalies and diseases of the genitourinary system and pregnancy. Curr Urol. 2017;9(4):169–78.
43. Karul M, Berliner C, Keller S, Tsui TY, Yamamura J. Imaging of appendicitis in adults. Rofo. 2014;186(6):551–8.
44. The American Fertility Society classifications of adnexal adhesions, Distal tubal occlusion, tubal occlusion secondary to tubal ligation, tubal pregnancies, Müllerian anomalies and intrauterine adhesions. Fertil Steril. 1988;49(6):944–55.

Uterine Incarceration During Pregnancy

30

Tracey H. DeYoung, Laura Marie Fluke, and Joy A. Greer

Epidemiology

Uterine incarceration during pregnancy is a rare but potentially serious diagnosis [1]. This complication is reported to affect 1 in 3000–10,000 pregnancies [2–4] and has been reported in the literature for the past three centuries [5–10].

Pathophysiology

In a majority of women, the uterus is anteverted and is positioned ventral to the sacral promontory [11, 12]. During pregnancy, the uterus enlarges and transitions from a pelvic to an abdominal organ at the end of the first trimester of pregnancy. As an abdominal organ, the uterus continues to grow through the third trimester until delivery at around 40 weeks gestation [3, 13].

In 11–19% of pregnancies, the uterus can be retroflexed or retroverted; this is considered a normal variant and is not associated with poor pregnancy outcomes [11, 14, 15]. By 12 weeks gestation, most retroflexed or retroverted uteri will become ventral to the sacral promontory as pregnancy processes. However, in rare cases, a retroverted or retroflexed uterus may become wedged between the sacral promontory and the pubic symphysis, preventing the enlarging uterus from transitioning to an abdominal organ [1, 3]. As the uterus becomes entrapped, the cervix, bladder neck, and urethra are displaced anteriorly, and the rectum is pushed more posteriorly by the uterine fundus [16]. Additionally, the uterus enlarges anteriorly, distorting normal anatomy and causing thinning of the anterior uterine wall and lower uterine segment around the gestational sac in a process known as "classic" sacculation (Fig. 30.1) [6, 17–19].

While a retroverted uterus in the first trimester is the most common risk factor for incarceration of the gravid uterus, many other risk factors have also been described in the literature. Other anatomic variations that can predispose women to uterine incarceration during pregnancy include a deep sacral concavity with an overlying sacral promontory or Müllerian anomalies such as a bicornuate or didelphic uterus [1, 20, 21]. Pelvic masses such as ovarian cysts or leiomyomas have been linked to incarceration as well as pelvic adhesive disease from endometriosis or previous abdominal or pelvic surgery [1, 22, 23]. The only reported potentially pregnancy-related risk factor

T. H. DeYoung · J. A. Greer (✉)
Department of Women's Health, Naval Medical Center Portsmouth, Norfolk, VA, USA
e-mail: joy.a.greer.mil@mail.mil

L. M. Fluke
Department of General Surgery, Naval Medical Center Portsmouth, Portsmouth, VA, USA

C. H. Nezhat (ed.), *Non-Obstetric Surgery During Pregnancy*,
https://doi.org/10.1007/978-3-319-90752-9_30

is a multifetal gestation [1]. History of a uterine incarceration in a prior pregnancy can additionally increase the risk of recurrence [17].

Diagnosis

Initially, many women with this complication will present with non-specific symptoms between 14 and 16 weeks gestation. Patients may present earlier if there is a multifetal gestation or pelvic mass contributing to the incarceration [1, 24]. Presenting symptoms are usually secondary to mechanical compression and can involve pregnancy-specific complaints or nonpregnancy-related complaints involving the genitourinary, gastrointestinal, or musculoskeletal system (Table 30.1) [1, 2, 21, 25–29]. The differential diagnosis includes ovarian cyst, leiomyoma, extrauterine pregnancy, pelvic hematocele, simple uterine sacculation, and classic sacculation [14].

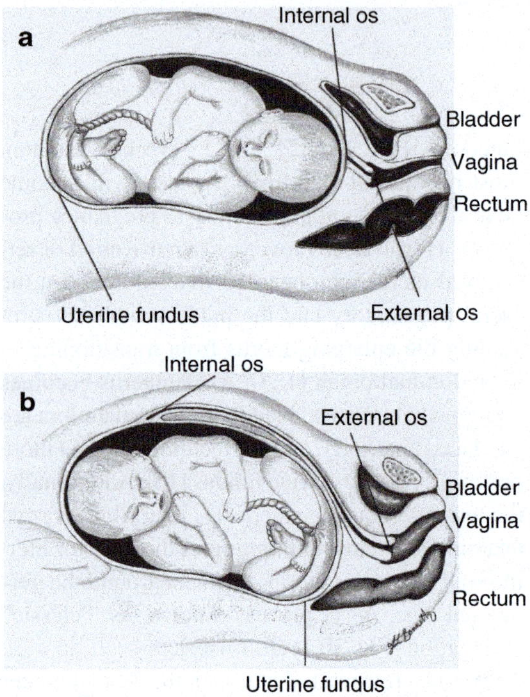

Fig. 30.1 (**a**) Artistic rendering of a gravid uterus at term. (**b**) Artistic rendering of an incarcerated gravid uterus at term. Note the fundal location, elongated cervix, and potential injuries if a cesarean delivery would be accomplished in the traditional fashion

Clinical examination should include an assessment of the abdomen and pelvic exam for patients presenting with any of the symptoms listed in Table 30.1 in addition to other more targeted assessments [1]. Fetal heart tones should be assessed by Doppler or ultrasound. The abdominal exam should evaluate for the presence of extrauterine masses and a measurement of fundal height. The pelvic exam should include a speculum exam, bimanual exam, and recto-vaginal exam. Pertinent findings on the abdominal and pelvic examinations that are suggestive of a retroverted uterus and potential uterine incarceration include fundal height less than expected for gestational age, an anteriorly displaced cervix that is difficult to visualize on speculum exam or difficult to palpate on bimanual exam, and a palpable mass in the posterior cul-de-sac [21, 23].

Imaging adjuncts can be used to confirm the diagnosis or make the diagnosis in women who are asymptomatic or present with vague symptoms of abdominal pain. Ultrasound findings suggestive of an incarcerated uterus in pregnancy include a retroverted uterus with posterior or fundal fibroids that appear trapped in the pelvis or a

Table 30.1 Potential symptoms of uterine incarceration in pregnancy

Timing	Gastrointestinal	Genitourinary	Musculoskeletal	Obstetric
Early	Abdominal pain Constipation Tenesmus Rectal pressure	Urinary retention	Back pain	Spontaneous abortion
Delayed	Same as above	Overflow incontinence Hydronephrosis Bladder atony Bladder ischemia Bladder rupture	Lower extremity swelling Thromboembolus	Fundal height less than expected for gestation age Intrauterine growth restriction Uterine rupture

cervix that is anteriorly and superiorly displaced and elongated. However, in the second and third trimesters, the cervix may be poorly visualized [30]. The most consistent clinical and sonographic finding is the anterior location of the cervix. The lower uterine segment is located where the fundus is usually found, in the anterior curve of the pelvis [31]. Abnormal positioning of the products of conception deep within the pelvis may also be noted. The bladder can be seen anterior, rather than inferior, to the products of conception [32]. With the uterine fundus located deep within the pelvis, a fundal placenta will appear to be overlying the vagina, giving a misleading appearance of a placenta previa on ultrasound [33–35].

Magnetic resonance imaging (MRI) is considered superior to pelvic ultrasound to confirm sacculation, placental location, and anatomic relationships. It can be especially useful to confirm the diagnosis and assist with preoperative planning [1, 12]. MRI can also clarify abnormal placentation which has been observed concomitantly and helps to avoid misdiagnoses of intraperitoneal pregnancy, fetal malpresentation, or placenta previa [31, 35–37]. On T2-weighted scans, the cervix is a hypointense linear structure. When the gravid uterus is incarcerated, the cervix will frequently be thin and elongated and is located parallel to the vagina [38].

Misdiagnosis or delayed diagnosis is unfortunately common with an unsuspected uterine incarceration. Reported misdiagnoses include acute appendicitis resulting in an unnecessary appendectomy, ectopic pregnancy, or abdominal pregnancy [6, 16, 28, 39, 40]. Uterine rupture and/or vaginal delivery of an intrauterine fetal demise have also been described in cases where the diagnosis has been significantly delayed [10, 41].

A high level of clinical suspicion, a thorough pelvic examination, and imaging adjuncts with pelvic ultrasound and MRI aid prompt diagnosis [1]. Early diagnosis permits optimal management with fewer complications and thus improved outcomes for the mother and fetus [3].

Treatment

Treatment of uterine incarceration complicating pregnancy depends greatly on the gestational age when the diagnosis is made as the risks and benefits of treatment vary [1]. Early diagnosis is essential for successful treatment. *Manual reduction of the uterus* is recommended if the gestational age is earlier than 20 weeks gestation [1, 40]. After 20 weeks gestation, manual reduction has been described [42] but is less likely to be successful and carries an increased risk of morbidity to include preterm labor, preterm premature rupture of membranes, and intrauterine fetal demise [1, 43, 44]. Lettieri and colleagues suggest that an attempted reduction after 20 weeks should be limited to patients who are significantly symptomatic [28].

Figure 30.2 lists sequential steps contributing to a successful manual reduction of an incarcerated pregnancy. Anesthesia can range from sedation to regional or general and should be used as needed for patient tolerance [24, 42, 45]. If initial manual reduction is unsuccessful, Lettieri and colleagues suggest repeating an attempt at manual reduction 1 week later if patient remains asymptomatic [28]. Once successful reduction has occurred, a pessary (Fig. 30.3) can be placed to help maintain the uterine position until the uterus is large enough to avoid a recurrent incarceration during the pregnancy, typically in the mid-second trimester. Gynecologic consultation is recommended to assist with successful pessary placement if it has not already been obtained. Alternatively, if a pessary cannot be successfully fitted, other authors suggest sleeping in a prone position and knee-chest exercises along with frequent bladder emptying, reduced liquid at night, and avoidance of Valsalva voiding [3, 26, 46, 47]. RhoGAM treatment should be provided for those women who are Rh negative regardless of whether the manual reduction is successful [4].

If the manual reduction is unsuccessful and the patient remains symptomatic, other mechanisms to achieve reduction have been reported and are described below. Due to the rarity of the condition, superiority of any one treatment

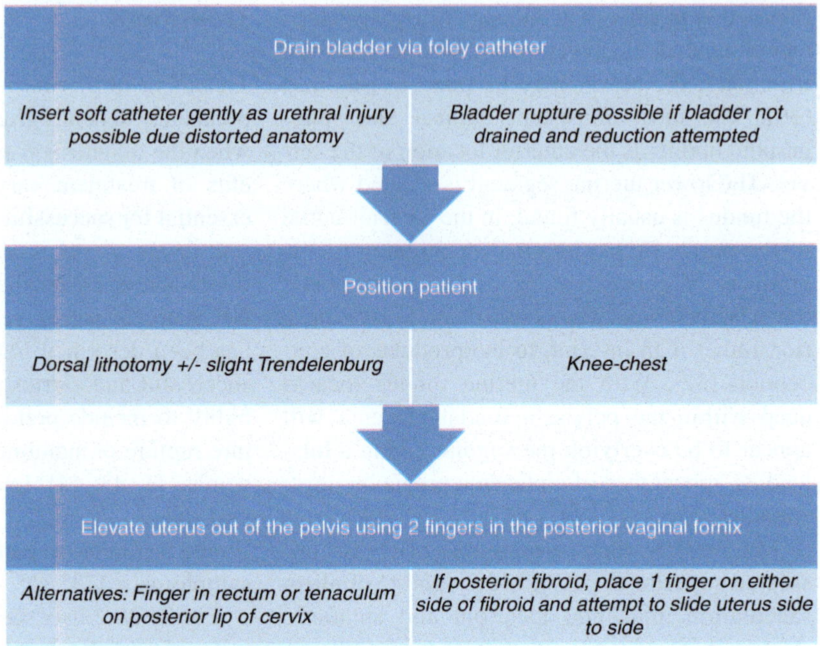

Fig. 30.2 Manual reduction of uterine incarceration in pregnancy

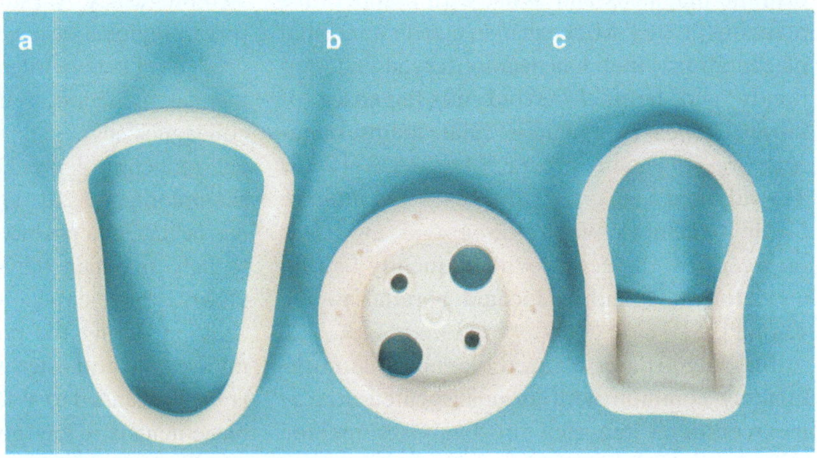

Fig. 30.3 Common pessaries used to maintain uterine position after manual reduction of uterine incarceration. (**a**) #3 Smith pessary. (**b**) #3 Ring pessary. (**c**) #1 Hodge pessary

method has not been established. Ultimately, the choice of treatment should take into consideration the suspected etiology for the incarceration, the gestational age of the fetus, and the anticipated risks and benefits.

Colonoscopy-Assisted Reduction of Uterine Incarceration

Colonoscopy-assisted uterine reduction has been described as follows: (1) enemas are given prior to the procedure to clear the rectal vault; (2) the endoscope is passed through the rectum and sigmoid colon and into the distal descending colon, allowing formation of a loop within the sigmoid colon; and (3) this loop of sigmoid colon then provides enough pressure to reduce the fundus of the uterus anteriorly, allowing it to ascend into the abdominal cavity [25, 48]. While this has been described successfully and without resulting morbidity in gestations up to 22 weeks [25], Newell and colleagues describe a case where rectal insufflation with an endoscope was attempted unsuccessfully in a patient at 22 + 6 weeks gestational age [44].

Beyond the likelihood of success at correcting the incarceration, there are several risks that must be considered prior to undertaking this procedure. There is no reported higher risk of perforation than a normal diagnostic colonoscopy or flexible sigmoidoscopy, which carries a 0.16–5% [49, 50] and 0.027–0.088% risk, respectively [51, 52]. However, given the small number of case reports in which it is performed, the true incidence of complications is difficult to discern, and the patient should be counseled accordingly. Pressure safety thresholds required to prevent perforating the bowel yet reduce the incarceration have not been reported. Furthermore, the forceful insertion of an endoscope with sigmoid loop formation is the leading cause of antimesenteric, longitudinal bowel perforation [52, 53], and a hallmark principle of endoscopy includes the prevention of loop formation [54]. An additional known risk factor for colon perforation during endoscopy is adhesions from prior abdominal or pelvic surgery. Adhesions cause tethering of the colon, which can lead to tearing within the fixed loop [55]. Tethering of the colon due to adhesions could be translated to fixation within the boney pelvis due to uterine incarceration. Thus, this method should be used judiciously and be performed only by an experienced endoscopist.

Laparoscopy or laparotomy should be considered only when the patient is in extremis and all other interventions have failed. These techniques are associated with a high risk of fetal loss or hysterectomy [17]. When the laparoscopic approach is chosen, an additional attempt at manual reduction should be made after the pneumoperitoneum has been obtained. The pneumoperitoneum has been hypothesized to help break the seal between the uterine serosa and the pelvic peritoneum [28]. If the pneumoperitoneum alone is insufficient to reduce the incarceration, Fernandes and colleagues describe laparoscopic assistance to grasp the round ligaments and exert steady traction to augment the vaginal hand to reduce the incarceration [31]. *Adhesiolysis* has also been described and is recommended if the adhesions are thought to be contributing to the incarceration [56]. Pabuccu and colleagues describe a case of recurrent uterine incarceration in the same pregnancy which was successfully managed using *ventrofixation* of the uterus which was performed through a laparotomy in the second trimester. The pregnancy progressed to full term, resulting in a vaginal delivery [57].

Abdominal myomectomy to relieve uterine incarceration has been reported in a few cases. Kim and colleagues removed a pedunculated subserosal leiomyoma resolving the uterine incarceration and resulting in a successful vaginal delivery at 39 weeks gestation [58]. In contrast, Chauleur and Vulliez reported two cases of myomectomy during the second trimester of pregnancy [26]. One case resulted in ongoing pregnancy; however, the second resulted in a spontaneous miscarriage. Suggested criteria for considering a myomectomy include rapid growth of a complex fibroid, failure to relieve fibroid-related symptoms after a 72-hour trial of conservative treatment, and a greater than 5-mm distance between the myoma and the endometrial cavity [2, 26].

While uncommon, there have also been two reports of spontaneous resolution of uterine incarceration. Hill describes a spontaneous resolution in one pregnancy between 24 and 26 weeks gestation [34]. Katopodis also reports the spontaneous necrosis of a fibroid leading to resolution [59].

Delivery

If manual reduction is unsuccessful prior to 20 weeks gestation, it is recommended that the pregnancy is followed with serial ultrasounds to assess fetal growth and amniotic fluid to help optimize timing of delivery [1, 21]. In reported cases of vaginal delivery, the infants did not survive [10, 60]. Therefore, the recommended route of delivery is via cesarean section when the uterine incarceration cannot be corrected; however, the optimal timing of delivery is unknown, and the risks and benefits need to be weighed [1].

Once the determination is made to proceed with delivery, a preoperative MRI is recommended to evaluate maternal anatomy and specifically identify the lower uterine segment.

Several authors have reported that the lower uterine segment was located above the umbilicus rather than suprapubically [6, 17, 35, 61].

At term gestation, a midline vertical skin incision extended above the umbilicus is recommended to extend the field of view [14, 17, 20, 41, 61]. If normal maternal anatomy cannot be restored with gentle manipulation, a vertical hysterotomy should be performed on the anterior wall of the uterus and extended cephalad with bandage scissors to avoid injury to the bladder, cervix, and vagina [28, 35, 43]. Once the fetus is delivered, the hysterotomy should be repaired. There are conflicting reports on the benefit of uterine suspension or anterior fixation of the uterus to prevent recurrent uterine incarceration [1, 28, 57]. Uterine suspension does not reliably prevent recurrence, and there is the potential increased risk and morbidity of subsequent surgery due to the development of adhesive disease.

Obstetric Complications

There are multiple obstetric complications that may arise secondary to uterine incarceration. Compression of the pelvic vasculature leads to impaired uterine blood flow, which can result in decidual hemorrhage and subsequent spontaneous abortion or intrauterine fetal demise [3]. Additionally, by similar mechanism, fetal growth restriction can occur; therefore serial growth scans are recommended [1]. Preterm labor and preterm premature rupture of membranes are commonly described [33, 35, 62]. There are multiple reports of abnormal placentation associated with uterine incarceration. This is hypothesized to result due to the thinning of the anterior uterine wall, especially in cases of prior cesarean delivery. Thus, in any patient with a prior cesarean delivery and uterine incarceration, placenta accreta should be considered [37, 63].

With the onset of labor and delivery, additional complications arise, especially in a patient with uterine incarceration not previously diagnosed. The abnormal polarity of the uterus inhibits the ability of contractions to cause cervical change; therefore, if inadvertently allowed to labor, labor dystocia ensues [6, 20]. The stress of labor may also lead to intrapartum fetal demise and uterine rupture [2, 21, 64]. Following delivery, there is an increased risk of postpartum hemorrhage and retained placenta [6, 60].

At the time of cesarean delivery, the distorted maternal anatomy leads to increased surgical risk. The maternal vagina, cervix, and bladder are pulled anteriorly and superiorly into the location where a low transverse uterine incision is typically made. Failure to recognize this distorted anatomy may lead to inadvertent transection of the vagina, cervix, or bladder with delivery through a hysterotomy on the posterior wall of the uterus [11, 36, 65]. Case reports describe necessity for cesarean hysterectomy after complete transection through the anterior and posterior walls of the vagina resulting in detachment of the uterus from the vagina [66, 67]. This supports the importance of clear documentation and preoperative planning for delivery, with the aid of diagnostic imaging adjuncts, to decrease the risk of intraoperative complications.

Non-obstetric Complications

Due to the compression and displacement of adjacent pelvic structures, there are a number of non-obstetric complications that arise secondary to uterine incarceration. Compression on the pelvic vasculature causes impaired venous return and venous stasis resulting in hypertension and lower extremity edema with an increased risk of venous thromboembolism and pulmonary embolism, especially in the hypercoagulable postpartum state [25, 44, 60, 66].

Gastrointestinal complications include the sensation of rectal pressure, constipation, and tenesmus due to added pressure on the rectum at the pelvic inlet due to compression between the sacral promontory and the uterus [25]. While rectal gangrene has been quoted in the literature, the original reference given by Gibbons in 1969 quotes chapters written by Huffman and Jeffcoate in 1962, neither of which describe rectal gangrene as a complication [3, 68]. Furthermore, the rectum has a robust blood supply, and even in the setting of primary pathogenesis of the rectum or compression from large pelvic masses, this is not seen. Uterine rupture or gangrene, especially in the setting of posterior sacculation [68], may be a cause of peritonitis; however, this would be a late finding. Additionally, appendicitis is a possible misdiagnosis, and further imaging with ultrasound or MRI should help delineate between these diagnoses.

The urologic system is at significant risk of complications resulting from uterine incarceration. Prolonged compression of the bladder or urethra results in urinary retention. Chronic urinary retention can lead to persistent bladder atony, infections, and lower and upper urinary tract injury. Overdistention of the bladder can cause persistent bladder atony via chronic neuromuscular dysfunction resulting in bladder ischemia, necrosis, and rupture if untreated [21, 69]. Treatment of urinary retention can be managed with prolonged indwelling urethral catheter, intermittent self-catheterization, or suprapubic catheter placement [26, 70]. Infectious complications include urinary tract infection and pyelonephritis [28, 32]. Pyelonephritis in pregnancy can cause significant morbidity including sepsis and acute respiratory distress syndrome [71]. Hydronephrosis results from either chronic bladder outlet obstruction or ureteral compression due to the incarcerated uterus [44, 67]. In severe cases, renal failure can develop [66]. Cystoscopically placed ureteral stents followed by nephrostomy tubes, if needed, can be placed to prevent calyceal rupture [64]. Due to the multifactorial and complex nature of these possible complications, urologic consultation should be performed. After relief of the obstruction by repositioning, catheterization, or nephrostomy tube placement, monitoring of urine output and serum electrolytes is recommended due to risk of post-obstructive diuresis with resultant electrolyte derangements [72].

Subsequent Pregnancy

Recurrent uterine incarceration has been described by several authors [3, 38, 64]. Recurrence is more common in patients with uterine anomalies, leiomyomas, and pelvic adhesive disease that are not addressed medically or surgically between the pregnancies. It is recommended that all patients with a history of uterine incarceration in previous pregnancies undergo serial bimanual exams in the first and second trimesters to ensure the proper assent of the uterus. Early use of a pessary and knee-chest exercises has also been described to assist in enabling a successful outcome with future pregnancies complicated by either a retroverted uterus or recurrent incarceration [3, 64]. A trial of labor after cesarean delivery can be determined based on the usual criteria [73], but it is strongly recommended that medical records and operative reports be reviewed in detail to determine the location of prior hysterotomy to aid in counseling regarding mode of delivery.

Conclusion

Though rare, uterine incarceration is a serious complication of pregnancy. It occurs when the growing, retroverted, gravid uterus becomes wedged between the pubic symphysis and sacral promontory. Evaluation for uterine incarceration should be performed in any patient presenting with new onset urinary retention in pregnancy. Physical exam findings of an anteriorly displaced cervix, posterior mass within the cul-de-sac, and size measuring less than dates should prompt further imaging with pelvic US and/or pelvic MRI. If less than 20 weeks gestation or symptomatic, manual reduction should be attempted. Alternative methods of reduction are described and can be attempted in a patient who has failed conservative management. Choice of procedure should be based on the suspected etiology of incarceration. If in labor or diagnosed at a later gestational age, delivery by cesarean section is recommended. Preoperative MRI is recommended to assist with surgical planning. Early recognition and intervention are critical for optimizing maternal and fetal outcomes.

Acknowledgments We thank Ms. Jean Bonnette from Visual Information Department, Naval Medical Center, Portsmouth, Virginia, for her artistic assistance.

References

1. Shnaekel KL, Wendel MP, Rabie NZ, Magann EF. Incarceration of the gravid uterus. Obstet Gynecol Surv. 2016;71(10):613–9.
2. Barton-Smith P, Kent A. Asymptomatic incarcerated retroverted uterus with anterior sacculation at term. Int J Gynaecol Obstet. 2007;96(2):128.
3. Gibbons JM Jr, Paley WB. The incarcerated gravid uterus. Obstet Gynecol. 1969;33(6):842–5.
4. Hess LW, Nolan TE, Martin RW, Martin JN Jr, Wiser WL, Morrison JC. Incarceration of the retroverted gravid uterus: report of four patients managed with uterine reduction. South Med J. 1989;82(3):310–2.
5. Freeth D, Dring AP. Incarceration and sacculation of the uterus with rupture of the cervix. Br Med J. 1953;1(4803):202.
6. Gottschalk EM, Siedentopf JP, Schoenborn I, Gartenschlaeger S, Dudenhausen JW, Henrich W. Prenatal sonographic and MRI findings in a pregnancy complicated by uterine sacculation: case report and review of the literature. Ultrasound Obstet Gynecol. 2008;32(4):582–6.
7. Hammond H Jr. Incarceration of the retrodisplaced gravid uterus. Stanford Med Bull. 1949;7(3):127–9.
8. Mendoza JT. Incarceration of 6 month gravid uterus; report of a case. Philipp J Surg. 1948;3(2):60–3.
9. Hunter RW. Medical observations and inquiries. 2nd ed. London, UK; 1771.
10. Merriman S. Retroversion of the womb. Med Physical J. 1806;XVI(98):386–93.
11. Feusner AH, Mueller PD. Incarceration of a gravid fibroid uterus. Ann Emerg Med. 1997;30(6):821–4.
12. van Beekhuizen H, Bodewes HW, Tepe EM, Oosterbaan HP, Kruitwagen R, Nijland R. Role of magnetic resonance imaging in the diagnosis of incarceration of the gravid uterus. Obstet Gynecol. 2003;102(5):1134–7.
13. Jacobsson B, Wide-Swensson D. Recurrent incarceration of the retroverted gravid uterus—a case report. Acta Obstet Gynecol Scand. 1999;78(8):737.
14. Fadel HE, Misenhimer HR. Incarceration of the retroverted gravid uterus with sacculation. Obstet Gynecol. 1974;43(1):46–9.
15. Weekes AR, Atlay RD, Brown VA, Jordan EC, Murray SM. The retroverted gravid uterus and its effect on the outcome of pregnancy. Br Med J. 1976;1(6010):622–4.
16. Gerscovich EO, Maslen L. The retroverted incarcerated uterus in pregnancy: imagers beware. J Ultrasound Med. 2009;28(10):1425–7.
17. Dierickx I, Mesens T, Van Holsbeke C, Meylaerts L, Voets W, Gyselaers W. Recurrent incarceration and/or sacculation of the gravid uterus: a review. J Matern Fetal Neonatal Med. 2010;23(8):776–80.
18. Frei KA, Duwe DG, Bonel HM, Durig P, Schneider H. Posterior sacculation of the uterus in a patient presenting with flank pain at 29 weeks of gestation. Obstet Gynecol. 2005;105(3):639–41.
19. McGann KP, Griffin WT. Recurrent classical sacculation of the pregnant uterus. J Fam Pract. 1988;26(3):339–41.
20. Evans AJ, Anthony J, Masson GM. Incarceration of the retroverted gravid uterus at term. Case report. Br J Obstet Gynaecol. 1986;93(8):883–5.
21. Van Winter JT, Ogburn PL Jr, Ney JA, Hetzel DJ. Uterine incarceration during the third trimester: a rare complication of pregnancy. Mayo Clinic Proc. 1991;66(6):608–13.
22. Hirsch E. Anterior uterine incarceration. Int J Gynaecol Obstet. 1997;57(2):195–7.
23. Matsushita H, Kurabayashi T, Higashino M, Kojima Y, Takakuwa K, Tanaka K. Incarceration of the retroverted uterus at term gestation. Am J Perinatol. 2004;21(7):387–9.
24. Childs AJ, Goldkrand JW. Uterine incarceration in a 9-week multifetal pregnancy resulting from in vitro fertilization. A case report. J Reprod Med. 2003;48(12):992–4.
25. Dierickx I, Van Holsbeke C, Mesens T, Gevers A, Meylaerts L, Voets W, et al. Colonoscopy-assisted reposition of the incarcerated uterus in mid-pregnancy: a report of four cases and a literature review. Eur J Obstet Gynecol Reprod Biol. 2011;158(2):153–8.
26. Chauleur C, Vulliez L, Seffert P. Acute urine retention in early pregnancy resulting from fibroid incarceration: proposition for management. Fertil Steril. 2008;90(4):1198.e7–10.
27. Yohannes P, Schaefer J. Urinary retention during the second trimester of pregnancy: a rare cause. Urology. 2002;59(6):946.
28. Lettieri L, Rodis JF, McLean DA, Campbell WA, Vintzileos AM. Incarceration of the gravid uterus. Obstet Gynecol Surv. 1994;49(9):642–6.
29. Edminster SC, Raabe RD, Kates RB. The incarcerated gravid uterus. Ann Emerg Med. 1987;16(8):910–2.
30. Gunn AP. Incarcerated gravid uterus mimicking placenta praevia. Australas Radiol. 1993;37(1):93–4.
31. Fernandes DD, Sadow CA, Economy KE, Benson CB. Sonographic and magnetic resonance imaging findings in uterine incarceration. J Ultrasound Med. 2012;31(4):645–50.
32. Laing FC. Sonography of a persistently retroverted gravid uterus. Am J Roentgenol. 1981;136(2):413–4.

33. Jackson D, Elliott JP, Pearson M. Asymptomatic uterine retroversion at 36 weeks' gestation. Obstet Gynecol. 1988;71(3 Pt 2):466–8.
34. Hill LM, Chenevey P, DiNofrio D. Sonographic documentation of uterine retroversion mimicking uterine sacculation. Am J Perinatol. 1993;10(5):398–400.
35. Hachisuga N, Hidaka N, Fujita Y, Fukushima K, Wake N. Significance of pelvic magnetic resonance imaging in preoperative diagnosis of incarcerated retroverted gravid uterus with a large anterior leiomyoma: a case report. J Reprod Med. 2012;57(1–2):77–80.
36. Charova J, Yunus D, Sarkar PK. Incarcerated retroverted gravid uterus presenting as placenta praevia. J Obstet Gynaecol. 2008;28(5):537–9.
37. DeFriend DE, Dubbins PA, Hughes PM. Sacculation of the uterus and placenta accreta: MRI appearances. Br J Radiol. 2000;73(876):1323–5.
38. Gardner CS, Jaffe TA, Hertzberg BS, Javan R, Ho LM. The incarcerated uterus: a review of MRI and ultrasound imaging appearances. Am J Roentgenol. 2013;201(1):223–9.
39. Emery D, Nolan R. Ultrasonography of an incarcerated uterus during pregnancy. Can Assoc Radiol J. 1994;45(5):397–8.
40. van der Tuuk K, Krenning RA, Krenning G, Monincx WM. Recurrent incarceration of the retroverted gravid uterus at term—two times transvaginal caesarean section: a case report. J Med Case Rep. 2009;3:103.
41. Renaud MC, Bazin S, Blanchet P. Asymptomatic uterine incarceration at term. Obstet Gynecol. 1996;88(4):721.
42. Grossenburg NJ, Delaney AA, Berg TG. Treatment of a late second-trimester incarcerated uterus using ultrasound-guided manual reduction. Obstet Gynecol. 2011;118(2 Pt 2):436–9.
43. Al Wadi K, Helewa M, Sabeski L. Asymptomatic uterine incarceration at term: a rare complication of pregnancy. J Obstet Gynaecol Can. 2011;33(7):729–32.
44. Newell SD, Crofts JF, Grant SR. The incarcerated gravid uterus: complications and lessons learned. Obstet Gynecol. 2014;123(2 Pt 2 Suppl 2):423–7.
45. Algra LJ, Fogel ST, Norris MC. Anesthesia for reduction of uterine incarceration: report of two cases. Intl J Obstet Anesth. 1999;8(2):142–3.
46. Sweigart AN, Matteucci MJ. Fever, sacral pain, and pregnancy: an incarcerated uterus. West J Emerg Med. 2008;9(4):232–4.
47. Yang JM, Huang WC. Sonographic findings of acute urinary retention secondary to an impacted pelvic mass. J Ultrasound Med. 2002;21(10):1165–9.
48. Seubert DE, Puder KS, Goldmeier P, Gonik B. Colonoscopic release of the incarcerated gravid uterus. Obstet Gynecol. 1999;94(5 Pt 1):792–4.
49. Repici A, Pellicano R, Strangio G, Danese S, Fagoonee S, Malesci A. Endoscopic mucosal resection for early colorectal neoplasia: pathologic basis, procedures, and outcomes. Dis Colon Rectum. 2009;52(8):1502–15.
50. Rathgaber SW, Wick TM. Colonoscopy completion and complication rates in a community gastroenterology practice. Gastrointest Endosc. 2006;64(4):556–62.
51. Gatto NM, Frucht H, Sundararajan V, Jacobson JS, Grann VR, Neugut AI. Risk of perforation after colonoscopy and sigmoidoscopy: a population-based study. J Natl Cancer Inst. 2003;95(3):230–6.
52. Lohsiriwat V, Sujarittanakarn S, Akaraviputh T, Lertakyamanee N, Lohsiriwat D, Kachinthorn U. Colonoscopic perforation: a report from world gastroenterology organization endoscopy training center in Thailand. World J Gastroenterol. 2008;14(43):6722–5.
53. Gedebou TM, Wong RA, Rappaport WD, Jaffe P, Kahsai D, Hunter GC. Clinical presentation and management of iatrogenic colon perforations. Am J Surg. 1996;172(5):454–7. discussion 7–8.
54. Hawari R, Pasricha PJ. Going for the loop: a unique overtube for the difficult colonoscopy. J Clin Gastroenterol. 2007;41(2):138–40.
55. Hansen AJ, Tessier DJ, Anderson ML, Schlinkert RT. Laparoscopic repair of colonoscopic perforations: indications and guidelines. J Gastrointest Surg. 2007;11(5):655–9.
56. Inaba F, Kawatu T, Masaoka K, Fukasawa I, Watanabe H, Inaba N. Incarceration of the retroverted gravid uterus: the key to successful treatment. Arch Gynecol Obstet. 2005;273(1):55–7.
57. Pabuccu EG, Kiseli M, Gursoy AY, Bostanci A, Caglar GS, Cengiz SD. Successful vaginal delivery at term following ventro-fixation procedure for uterine incarceration. J Obstet Gynaecol. 2016;36(7):869–72.
58. Kim SC, Lee YJ, Jeong JE, Joo JK, Lee KS. Incarceration of gravid uterus by growing subserosal myoma: case report. Clin Exp Obstet Gynecol. 2016;43(1):131–3.
59. Katopodis C, Menticoglou S, Logan A. Incarcerated fibroid uterus: the role of conservative management. J Obstet Gynaecol Can. 2013;35(6):536–8.
60. Singh MN, Payappagoudar J, Lo J, Prashar S. Incarcerated retroverted uterus in the third trimester complicated by postpartum pulmonary embolism. Obstet Gynecol. 2007;109(2 Pt2):498–501.
61. Dietz HP, Teare AJ, Wilson PD. Sacculation and retroversion of the gravid uterus in the third trimester. Aust N Z J Obstet Gynaecol. 1998;38(3):343–5.
62. Lee SW, Kim MY, Yang JH, Moon MH, Cho JY. Sonographic findings of uterine sacculation during pregnancy. Ultrasound Obstet Gynecol. 2008;32(4):595–7.
63. Ozyurek ES, Kahraman AA, Yildirim D, Karacaoglu UM. Clinical presentation of placenta percreta with uterine incarceration in the second trimester. J Obstet Gynaecol. 2015;35(6):641–3.
64. Hooker AB, Bolte AC, Exalto N, Van Geijn HP. Recurrent incarceration of the gravid uterus. J Matern Fetal Neonatal Med. 2009;22(5):462–4.

65. Hankins GD, Cedars MI. Uterine incarceration associated with uterine leiomyomata: clinical and sonographic presentation. J Clin Ultrasound. 1989;17(5):385–8.
66. Uma R, Olah KS. Transvaginal caesarean hysterectomy: an unusual complication of a fibroid gravid uterus. BJOG. 2002;109(10):1192–4.
67. Keating PJ, Walton SM, Maouris P. Incarceration of a bicornuate retroverted gravid uterus presenting with bilateral ureteric obstruction. Br J Obstet Gynaecol. 1992;99(4):345–7.
68. Huffman J. Uterine displacements. In: Gynecology and obstetrics. Philadelphia, PA: Saunders; 1962. p. 821–30.
69. Jeffcoate TN. Principles of gynaecology. 2nd ed. London: Butterworth; 1962.
70. Silva PD, Berberich W. Retroverted impacted gravid uterus with acute urinary retention: report of two cases and a review of the literature. Obstet Gynecol. 1986;68(1):121–3.
71. Cunningham FG, Leveno KJ, Bloom SL, Spong CY, Dashe JS, Hoffman BL, et al. Renal and urinary tract disorders. In: Williams obstetrics. 24th ed. New York: McGraw-Hill Education; 2013.
72. Swartz EM, Komins JI. Postobstructive diuresis after reduction of an incarcerated gravid uterus. J Reprod Med. 1977;19(5):262–4.
73. American College of Obstetricians and Gynecologists. ACOG practice bulletin no. 115: vaginal birth after previous cesarean delivery. Obstet Gynecol. 2010;116(2 Pt 1):450–63.

31 Spontaneous Uterine Rupture During Pregnancy

Andrea Tinelli, Ospan A. Mynbaev, Michael Stark, Radmila Sparic, Sasa Kadija, Sandro Gerli, and Antonio Malvasi

Introduction

Uterine rupture is a life-threatening obstetric complication, an obstetric catastrophe associated with high maternal and perinatal morbidity and mortality [1].

Spontaneous rupture of the uterus, as well as a very rare event, is an unpredictable event, requiring a high index of suspicion for diagnosis [2].

In developed countries, uterine rupture is rare and is most commonly a complication of previous cesarean section (CS); in low-resource poor countries, it is commonly associated with prolonged obstructed labor due to fetopelvic disproportion, fetal malpresentation or malposition (such as neglected transverse lie), and injudicious or inappropriate use of uterine stimulants [3].

Hofmeyr et al. [4], in a research published over a decade ago, showed that uterine rupture was reported to be lower in a community-based study (median 0.053%, range 0.016–0.030%) compared to facility-based study (0.031, 0.012–2.9%). This prevalence was also higher in less developed countries (sub-Saharan Africa particularly) than in the developed countries [4].

Uterine rupture may be incomplete when uterine serosa remains intact or complete in cases of

A. Tinelli (✉)
Division of Experimental Endoscopic Surgery, Imaging, Technology and Minimally Invasive Therapy, Department of Obstetrics and Gynecology, Vito Fazzi Hospital, Lecce, Italy

Laboratory of Human Physiology, Phystech BioMed School, Faculty of Biological and Medical Physics, Moscow Institute of Physics and Technology (State University), Moscow Region, Russia

O. A. Mynbaev
Laboratory of Human Physiology, Phystech BioMed School, Faculty of Biological and Medical Physics, Moscow Institute of Physics and Technology (State University), Moscow Region, Russia

Division of Molecular Technologies, Research Institute of Translational Medicine, N.I. Pirogov Russian National Research Medical University, Moscow, Russia

Institute of Numerical Mathematics, RAS, Moscow, Russia

M. Stark
New European Surgical Academy, Berlin, Germany

R. Sparic
Clinic for Gynecology and Obstetrics, Clinical Centre of Serbia, Belgrade, Serbia

Medical Faculty, University of Belgrade, Belgrade, Serbia

S. Kadija · S. Gerli
Clinic for Gynecology and Obstetrics, Clinical Centre of Serbia, Belgrade, Serbia

A. Malvasi
Laboratory of Human Physiology, Phystech BioMed School, Faculty of Biological and Medical Physics, Moscow Institute of Physics and Technology (State University), Moscow Region, Russia

Department of Obstetrics and Gynecology, Santa Maria Hospital GVM Care and Research, Bari, Italy

C. H. Nezhat (ed.), *Non-Obstetric Surgery During Pregnancy*,
https://doi.org/10.1007/978-3-319-90752-9_31

disruption of the full thickness of uterine wall including uterine serosa, thus resulting in a direct connection between the peritoneal space and the uterine cavity with or without protrusion or expulsion of the fetus and/or placenta into the peritoneal cavity (Fig. 31.1).

Incomplete uterine rupture is almost always the result of a dehiscence of a previous cesarean delivery scar and is often asymptomatic, only discovered at the time of repeated cesarean delivery or during manual exploration of the uterus after a successful vaginal delivery after previous cesarean delivery [5].

It is a rare peripartum complication that occurs in around 7/10,000 women, but this rate increases to 20–80/10,000 in those with uterine scars, mostly as a result of previous cesarean section [6].

Rupture of the unscarred pregnant uterus is a rare event, estimated to occur in one in 5700 to one in 20,000 pregnancies [7].

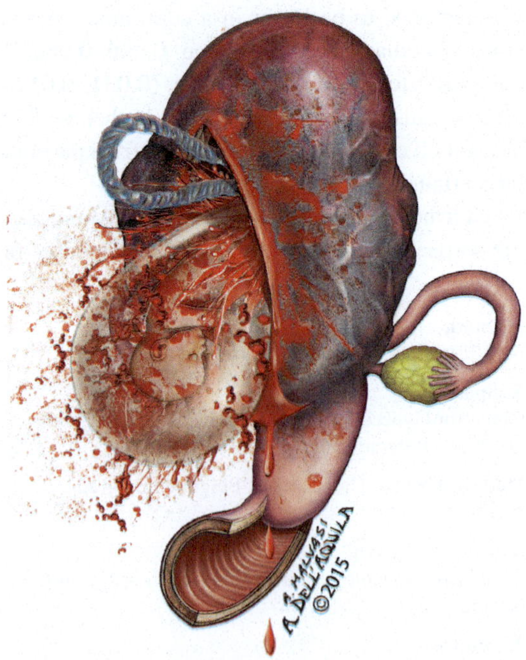

Fig. 31.1 A description of a complete uterine rupture, with the sudden pregnancy extrusion outside uterine cavity (Reprinted from Management and therapy of early pregnancy complications: first and second trimesters, edited by Malvasi A, Tinelli A, Di Renzo GC, Spontaneous uterine rupture prior to twenty weeks of gestation, 2016, Guseh SH, Carusi DA, Tinelli A, Gargiulo AR. With permission of Springer)

Definition of Uterine Rupture

Uterine rupture is divided into two main categories: rupture in a scarred uterus and rupture in an intact uterus. The term "scarred uterus" is referred to the uterus of a woman that has previously undergone gynecological operations, predominantly CS, which constitutes the principal cause of overall uterine ruptures.

Ruptures of the gravid uterus are generally described as "spontaneous" or "traumatic." Most authors who use the term "spontaneous rupture" mean that the uterus has ruptured during labor without other precipitating traumas [8].

Generally, labor involves vigorous, sustained myometrial contractions occurring for a prolonged period; thus, to call intrapartum uterine rupture "spontaneous" is misleading. An additional factor(s) is almost always present when a uterus ruptures. Very rare cases of uterine rupture in nonlaboring, nulliparous (or primigravid) women with unscarred uterus have been reported [9].

Trends of Uterine Rupture

Uterine rupture prevalence is estimated at 1% in patients with uterine scar [1]. Uterine rupture in a previously unscarred uterus is a rare event, estimated at 1:17,000–20,000 [10].

A study of Al-Zirqi et al. [6] evaluated women giving birth in 21 maternity units in Norway during the period 1967–2008. They identified 359 uterine ruptures among a total on 1,441,712 maternities, with an incidence of 2.5/10,000. Cited authors documented a sharply growing trend of uterine rupture. The increase was largely a result of the increasing percentages of scarred uteri (mainly from previous cesarean section) and augmentation of labor with oxytocin. Although the increase was observed among both intact and scarred uteri, scarred uteri showed a considerably higher incidence, with an increase from 14.2 to 66.8 in 10,000 maternities from the second to the fourth decade, respectively. Among scarred uteri, induction of labor with prostaglandins and combined prostaglandins and oxytocin played an important role. The authors concluded that uterine rupture is rare in Norway, but there has been a sharp increase in recent years. This increase was partly linked to increases in scarred uteri (as a result of increasing rates of cesarean section), induced labor with prostaglandins or combined prostaglandins and oxytocin, and augmented labor with oxytocin.

Another study of Berhe and Wall [3] reviewed the clinical experience with uterine rupture in resource-poor countries. By their analysis, authors detected that in industrialized, high-resource countries, uterine rupture occurs most often in women who have had a previous cesarean delivery, whereas in resource-poor nations, uterine rupture is more commonly associated with obstructed labor, injudicious obstetric interventions/manipulations (often performed by untrained birth attendants), lack of antenatal care, grand multiparity, and poor access to emergency obstetric care. In resource-poor settings, uterine rupture is a reflection of ill-equipped, badly managed, and under-resourced healthcare systems that seem largely indifferent to the reproductive health needs of women [3].

The ultimate success (or failure) of these countries depends in large part upon their commitment to maintaining a healthy and productive female population.

With the advent of misoprostol, a prostaglandin E1 analog is cheap and accessible to most health facilities in Cameroon and most other countries in sub-Saharan Africa; the rates of uterine rupture have increased noticeably. Although much attention is paid to scar rupture associated with uterotonic agents, 13% of ruptures occurred in unscarred uteri, and 72% occurred during spontaneous labor [11].

Moreover, the low rates of partogram use in most countries in sub-Saharan Africa could have obstetric consequences, especially given the high likelihood that, under such circumstances, parturients are administered oxytocin or prostaglandins and are not properly followed up by hourly or 2-hourly examinations [12].

Reports from the study in Mali show that uterine rupture occurred in 87.4% (415/475) of cases in unscarred uterus vs. 12.6% (60/475) in a scarred uterus. Observed risk factors for primary uterine rupture included contracted pelvis, 12.0% (57/475); fetal macrosomia, 9.7% (46/475); and contracted pelvis associated with macrosomia, 3.4% (16/475). Malpresentation was recorded in 12.4% (59/475). Dystocia associated with oxytocin and/or traditional medicines labor augmentation has been observed in 12.6% of cases (60/475). Grand multiparity (≥7 deliveries in obstetric history) accounted for 12.4% (59/475) of all uterine ruptures, while short inter-pregnancy interval has been observed in 12.0% of all uterine ruptures (57/475) [13].

Risk Factors of Spontaneous Uterine Rupture

Risk factors for third-trimester uterine rupture in labor are well known; nevertheless, data on spontaneous second- and early third-trimester uterine rupture before labor remain very limited [11].

Unscarred uterine rupture is a rare event that usually occurs in late pregnancy or during labor. Risk factors for this condition include high parity, placental abnormalities (Fig. 31.2), and uterine anomaly [14]. Women with a classical incision that run vertically on the corpus uteri run a higher risk of uterine rupture than those with a low uterine segment transverse incision [15].

Nevertheless, there is still no consensus on the best gestational age in which to perform an iterative cesarean section, to prevent uterine rupture [16].

Surico et al. [17] evaluated the main risk factors for uterine rupture in a case series. It was previous cesarean section (5/10, 50%), but three of the ten cases of uterine rupture had no demonstrable risk factors. Thus, uterine rupture also occurred in the absence of risk factors in three cases (30%).

The major common predisposing factors of uterine rupture are poverty, ignorance, illiteracy, traditional practices, high parity, poor infrastructure, cephalopelvic disproportion, previous uterine scars, and poor obstetric care. Obviously such etiological factors are more present in low-resource countries. For example, in Nigeria, uterine rupture is a frequent obstetric complication, and reported incidence rates vary from 1 in 81 to 1 in 426 deliveries; these rates are largely similar to rates from sub-Saharan African countries [18].

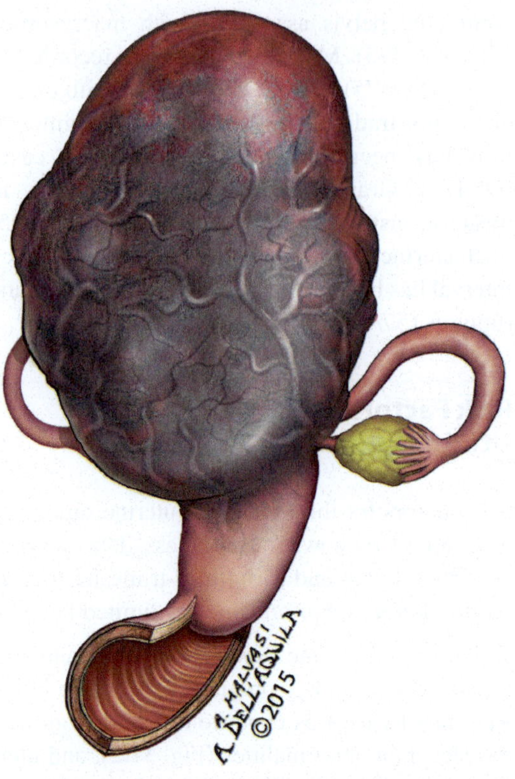

Fig. 31.2 A description of a placenta accreta at the site of prior cesarean sections could be a possible risk factor for uterine rupture (Reprinted from Management and therapy of early pregnancy complications: first and second trimesters, edited by Malvasi A, Tinelli A, Di Renzo GC, Spontaneous uterine rupture prior to twenty weeks of gestation, 2016, Guseh SH, Carusi DA, Tinelli A, Gargiulo AR. With permission of Springer)

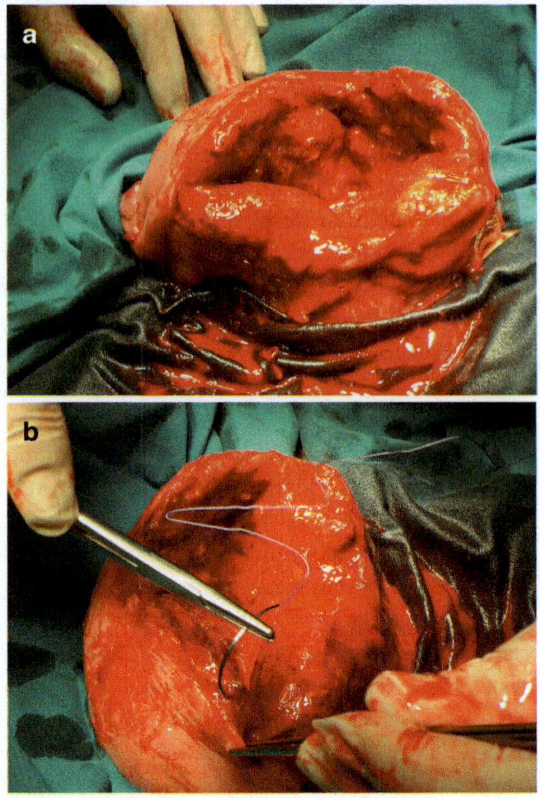

Fig. 31.3 A uterine rupture during pregnancy, in primigravida at 34 weeks, following Bret-Palmer metroplasty. Patient was urgently operated in laparotomy, showing a complete fundal uterine rupture (**a**), treated by a conservative hysterorrhaphy (**b**)

Ehlers-Danlos syndrome is an inherited collagen disorder connected with the risk of uterine rupture [19].

Ruptures may also occur, spontaneously, in a congenital abnormal uterus, after uterine repair of congenital anomalies (Fig. 31.3) and in patients with history of invasive mole [1, 14].

Incidence rate of pregnancy in a rudimentary horn with a bicornuate uterus was estimated as 1 case per 100.000 up to 140.000 pregnancies. Studies indicated to a vast variation in rupture period congenital abnormal uterus, ranging from 5 to 35 weeks and that was attributed to the ability of the horn musculature to hypertrophy and dilate, but it has been identified that around 70–90% occur before 20 weeks and these lead to catastrophic results [20].

Several studies have shown that the shorter the time between a cesarean delivery and a subsequent delivery, the higher the rate of uterine rupture. Commonly, thresholds of 18 and 24 months have been examined. Adjusted odds ratios range from 2.5 to 3.0 for an increased rate of uterine rupture in the women with less time between deliveries. The biologic plausibility of this effect is related to the amount of time required for the uterine scar to heal completely and to nutritional factors [21–23].

Uccella et al. [24] published a review of pre-labor uterine rupture in primiparous women and found that 52.2% of the identified cases had history of infertility. In almost half of them, partial uterine wall defect was the principal recognizable risk factor for pre-labor uterine rupture. The patient they presented had a uterine hysteroscopic

5 mm perforation. At the same time, she had premature ovarian failure, so the authors speculated that wasting of myometrial tissue due to aging and gonadal hormone depletion played a role in uterine dehiscence on the site of previous perforation.

Rarely, rupture can occur following unrecognized injury to the uterus at a previous difficult delivery or dilatation and curettage, iatrogenic uterine perforation, salpingectomy with cornual resection, and deep cornual resection [25, 26].

A Canadian research group reported a single-layer closure of the previous lower segment incision is the most influential factor and is associated with a fourfold increase in the risk of uterine rupture compared with a double-layer closure [27]. This data was defeated by Malvasi et al. [28], in a study on uterine scar evaluated by light microscopy and scanning electron microscopy. The problem of scar resistance depends on biological factors such as whether or not the visceral peritoneum is closed. If the visceral peritoneum is closed, the uterine scar becomes worse in its biological quality. It is therefore advisable to always open the visceral peritoneum, after LUS suture, during cesarean section. Moreover, Malvasi et al. [29] successively confirmed these data in another experimental study, so as Cochrane review [27].

Moreover, Malvasi et al. [30] demonstrated by light microscopy and by immunohistochemistry, for the morphometric quantification of neurotransmitter fibers in the lower uterine segment (LUS) after CS. The substance P (SP) levels are higher in repeat CS, whereas vasoactive intestinal polypeptide (VIP) levels are reduced in the LUS. The increase of SP is probably linked to the attempt to achieve cervical ripening in post-CS LUS, with the possible consequences of dystocia during vaginal birth after CS. However, the decrease of VIP probably affects the relaxation of the internal uterine orifice, compromising the LUS formation and cervical ripening.

A study of Di Tommaso et al. [31] mapped the concentration of neurotransmitters in the non-pregnant uterus; the cervix is the uterine part highly rich in neurotransmitters.

Anything that compromises the distribution of neurotransmitters and neurofibers during labor and/or cesarean delivery may ultimately compromise LUS during gestation or during delivery. It is therefore the case of dystocia or obstructed labor, which causes hypoxia, hysterectomy, and necrosis in the LUS for a relatively long period of time, with subsequent denervation of the uterus area and risk of uterine rupture. Or, it is also the case of the LUS suture type after hysterotomy, in which the visceral peritoneum must not be closed [32].

Researchers, in another investigation on neurotransmitters and neurofibers during pregnancy, concluded that it is not advisable to wait a long time in the case of dystocia or obstructed labor before deciding for cesarean section, because the damage to tissue denervation will be definitive and the LUS will subsequently be at risk of rupture during the subsequent pregnancy [33].

Previous rupture of the scar makes the risk of subsequent rupture even more high. Factors that may influence the incidence of the rupture in cases of scarred uterus are related to individual healing characteristic related to the production of growth factors and collagen deposition. These factors have not been much investigated. Any kind of myometrial injury leads to a growth factor production, thus causing proliferation of the connective tissue forming scar. After each surgical procedure on the uterus, those individual wound healing characteristics may predispose to a uterine rupture. Uterine scars cannot remodel during pregnancy as normal myometrial tissue. Thus, there is a concern about the ability of scarred uterus to withstand pregnancy and labor, and the myometrial tensile strength in the scar is decreased [1].

Spontaneous rupture of the uterus is, in rare cases, also associated with previously performed salpingectomy. Authors [34] reviewed literature on such topic, reporting 33% of cases of uterine rupture following salpingectomy occurred during intrauterine pregnancy, whereas the rest was associated with interstitial ectopic pregnancy. Laparoscopic salpingectomy more often resulted in rupture of the uterus during non-ectopic pregnancy as compared to laparotomy (4 vs. 2 cases, respectively).

Another potential complication of salpingectomy that could lead to uterine rupture is the inter-

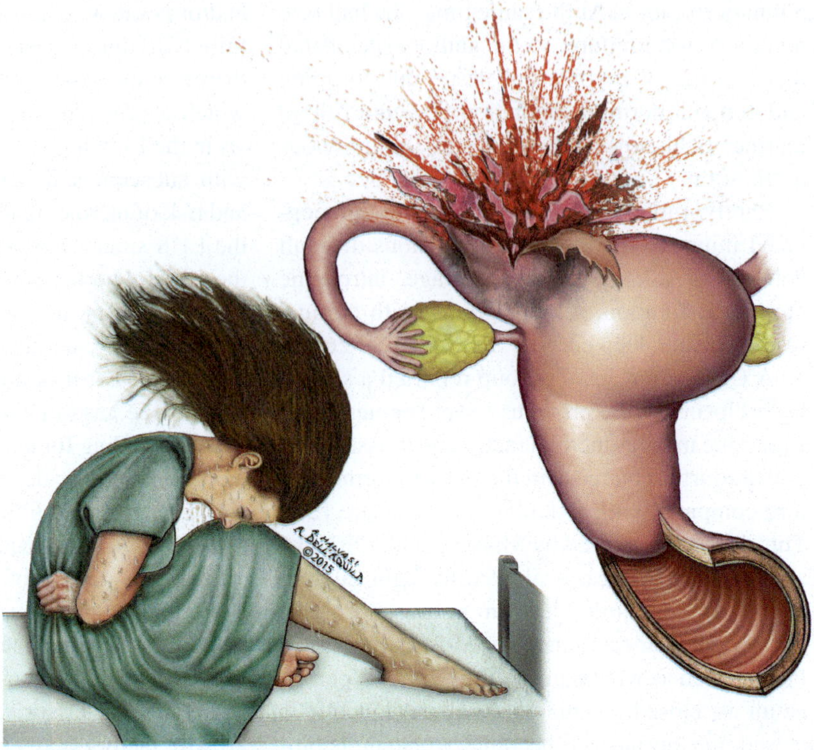

Fig. 31.4 The picture shows an interstitial pregnancy with sudden rupture and painful and hemorrhagic shock of the woman

stitial pregnancy (Fig. 31.4), a rare type of ectopic pregnancy that is responsible for approximately 2.4% of all extrauterine gestations. When interstitial pregnancies were excluded, uterine rupture was a cause of fetal death in 67% of reported gestations. There were no cases of maternal mortality. Conservative treatment was the preferred management option, and total hysterectomy was performed in only two women [34].

Uterine fundal pressure (UFP) is widely used to speed up the time of the second stage of delivery. UFP involves the application of manual pressure on the uppermost part of the uterus, directed toward the birth canal [35].

A survey in the USA found that in 80% of institutions, UFP was applied—there is scarce data about its association with uterine rupture [36]. Thereby, the intrauterine pressure in the second stage of labor transiently increases by up to 86% [37], which might pose a relevant factor in the pathophysiology of uterine rupture. Generally, the use of UFP is only indicated in case of complications such as prolonged second stage of labor, which represents another risk factor for uterine rupture itself, although there is scarce data about its safety. Also the adenomyosis can be a risk factor for uterine rupture due to the weakening of the uterine muscle fibers. In a case report with review of literature, Nikolaou et al. [38] reported a rare case of spontaneous uterine rupture of an unscarred uterus caused by adenomyosis in the early third trimester.

Nagao et al. [39] observed a case of spontaneous uterine rupture in a patient during the 35th week of gestation, after a laparoscopic adenomyomectomy. At a scheduled date in the 35th week of gestation, after combined spinal epidural anesthesia and frequent uterine contractions, a weak pain suddenly ensued. After 13 min of uterine contractions, vaginal bleeding was evident. A CS was performed, and the uterine rupture was found in the scar.

A review published by Morimatsu et al. showed that the rate of uterine rupture after adenomyomectomy during pregnancy is 6.0% [40].

Nagao et al. [39] speculated on some reasons why uterine rupture frequently occurs in pregnant women with prior laparoscopic adenomyo-

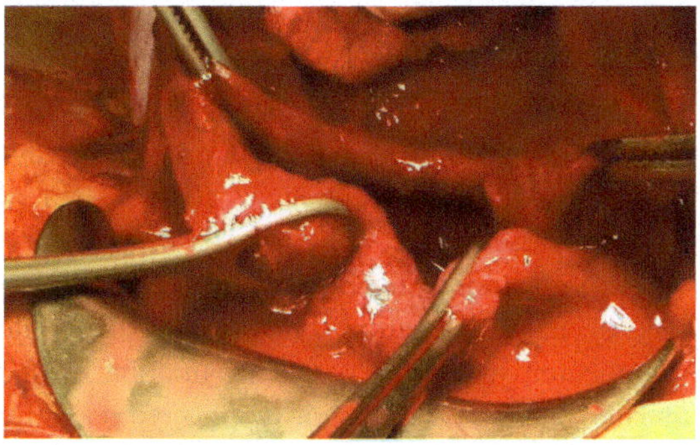

Fig. 31.5 An intraoperatory image of uterine diverticulum, highlighted with ring forceps

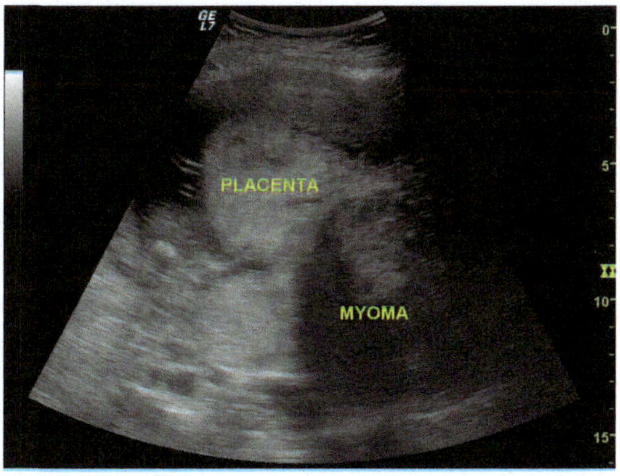

Fig. 31.6 An ultrasonographic image showing a large myoma in pregnancy

mectomies. The boundary between the normal uterine muscle layer and the lesion is unclear. A lesion of adenomyosis tends to remain around the edges of excisions and the area to be sutured, which might lead to weak connections between sutured edges. If a lesion of adenomyosis is enucleated widely to eliminate the lesion, the uterus will be small and irregular in shape, which leads to a diminished capacity to expand. With a laparoscopic adenomyomectomy, it is particularly difficult to delineate the border of the lesion because of a lacking sense of touch and deep sensation.

Agarwal et al. [41] reported a case of intrapartum unscarred uterine fundal rupture in a case of drug abuse. A careful history of drug abuse must be elicited when the common causes of uterine rupture have been excluded or the rupture site is unusual. There are other described cases of uterine rupture associated with cocaine abuse, as well [42].

Also, the cause of uterine rupture could be uterine diverticulum, frequently misunderstood and reported as uterine sacculation [43]. Uterine diverticulum (Fig. 31.5) has a narrow connection with the uterine cavity and a thicker wall than in sacculation. While uterine sacculation is usually observed during pregnancy, diverticulum is usually detected in nonpregnant women. Uterine diverticula as a complication during pregnancy are rare.

Finally, also uterine torsion could be assumed among risk factors of uterine rupture [44]. Uterine torsion is defined as the rotation of the uterus on its long axis by more than 45° [45]. The round ligaments, broad ligaments, and uterosacral ligaments normally stabilize the position of the uterus. Excessive traction on the uterus can cause rotation of the uterus on its long axis [46]. Most reported cases of uterine torsion occur during pregnancy. The most common cause of nongravid uterine torsion is a myomatous uterus but also during pregnancy (Fig. 31.6) [47]. Other causes of nongravid uterine torsion include a bicornuate uterus, pelvic adhesions, adnexal masses, and bowel peristalsis [45]. A review of the literature revealed only three published cases of uterine torsion secondary to an ovarian cyst [44].

Uterine Rupture After Myomectomy

Myomectomy, both in minimally invasive and in traditional open method, is one of the most important gynecological surgeries performed in the woman.

The problem of the appropriateness of myomectomy is to optimize postsurgical reproductive outcomes, including subsequent fertility and ultimately the safe delivery of a healthy neonate.

In the light of advanced age of obstetric population, there is a substantial risk of uterine rupture on the site of previous myomectomy scar (Fig. 31.7). Both myomectomy and cesarean delivery can either directly, or indirectly predisposing formation of abnormally invasive placenta, influence the occurrence of uterine rupture.

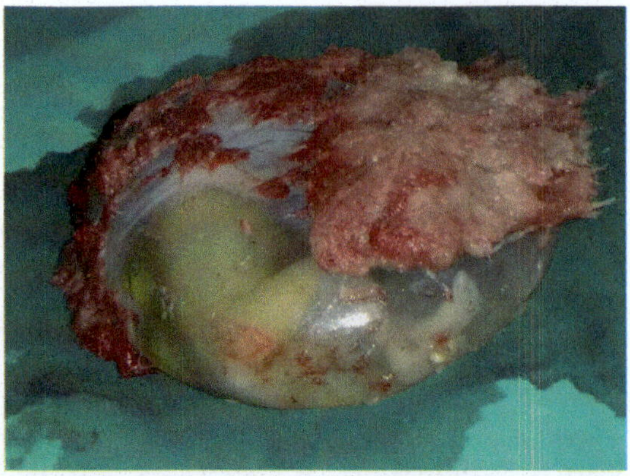

Fig. 31.7 Uterine rupture in a 15-week pregnant woman. The fetus was totally evacuated, with amniotic sac and placenta, in the abdominal cavity. The uterus was unscarred, and the uterine rupture was sutured during laparotomy

In 1964, Garnet [48] identified 3 (4%) uterine ruptures among 83 women who had scars from a previous abdominal myomectomy.

Koo et al. [49] performed a large retrospective review of obstetrical outcomes in women who underwent laparoscopic myomectomy. A total of 523 women with completed pregnancy data after laparoscopic myomectomy were studied. The rate of uterine rupture was 0.6% (3 of 523 deliveries). Although in two cases of uterine rupture the overall maternal-fetal outcomes were favorable, one case occurring at 21 weeks was associated with placenta accreta, hemorrhage, hysterectomy, and fetal demise. The study examined characteristics of the myomas removed, including number size and location. Uterine rupture did not appear to correlate with any of these factors. Literature data published later suggest that the uterine rupture rate following myomectomy is 0.7–1%. Trial of labor after myomectomy is associated with a 0.47% risk of uterine rupture [50].

Today, the use of minimally invasive techniques and laparoscopic and robotic-assisted myomectomies is being performed in greater numbers today than ever before, since minimally invasive surgery has been associated with improvements in perioperative surgical variables [51].

There are, however, many concerns about the minimally invasive surgical benefits of reproduction and birth labor, such as, for example, the risk of uterine rupture.

Sizzi et al. [52] in a multicenter study on laparoscopic myomectomy complications reported 1 rupture among 386 pregnancies (0.26%) out of 2050 operations.

Several studies have demonstrated a 0–1% risk of uterine rupture following laparoscopic myomectomy, even if a true evaluation of the uterine rupture rate after endoscopic myomectomy is difficult as information about this comes primarily from case reports [53, 54].

Many surgeons have proposed various suture techniques to improve the quality of the scar, but no one has ever scientifically demonstrated the benefits of a technique on the other (Fig. 31.8). For example, some surgeons affirm that a multi-

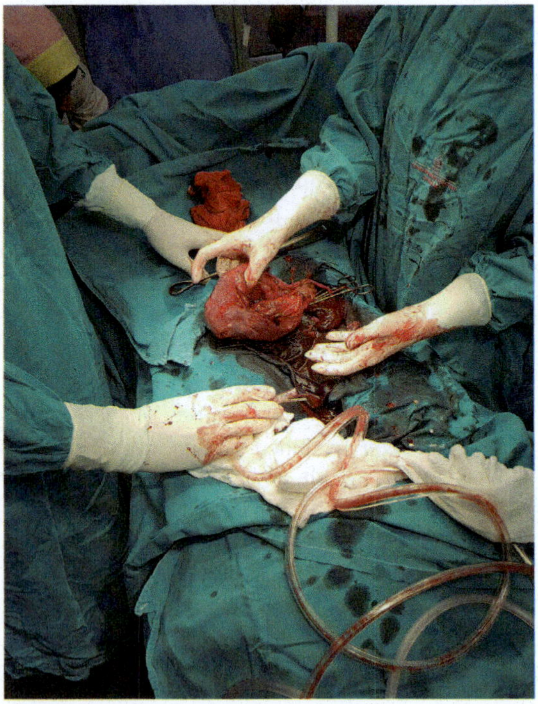

Fig. 31.8 Post-laparoscopic myomectomy uterine rupture in pregnancy. Patient arrived at the hospital in emergency for a uterine rupture at 36.4 weeks in the fundal region. The fetus was mostly in the abdomen, with head, one arm, and placenta in the uterus. Prior to the cesarean section in emergency, the fetal heart rate was 40 bpm. The uterus was sutured, and the mother had an uneventful recovery (Image courtesy of Dr. Radmila Ćirić, Clinic for Gynecology and Obstetrics, Clinical Center of Serbia, Belgrade)

layer repair can improve the strength of the wound and decrease the risk of postoperative hematoma formation, which can also interfere with optimal tissue healing. Anyway, the use of barbed suture (Fig. 31.9) in a continuous suture is a newer adaptation that may increase the tensile strength of the defect. Moreover, the use of electrosurgery should be limited owing to a theoretical risk of devascularization. When possible, alternative energy sources (such as ultrasonic energy) may be preferred. Thus, many surgeons say that it is best to avoid entering the uterine cavity during myomectomy to avoid healing problems.

The influence of myomectomy technique on the incidence of the rupture is still a matter of debate [55]. The rate of uterine rupture after abdominal myomectomy has been estimated as <1% in most, but not all, studies [54].

It is not clear whether the laparoscopic procedure is associated with higher risk of subsequent rupture or whether these cases are being more systematically reported [56].

The myometrial healing following either laparoscopically or at laparotomy performed myomectomy is influenced by the used technique during myomectomy: (1) method and/or instrumentation used for uterine incision, (2) achievement of hemostasis during surgery, (3) myorrhaphy, (4) the potential hematoma formation within the myometrium, and (5) patients' individual characteristics that influence the healing process [57].

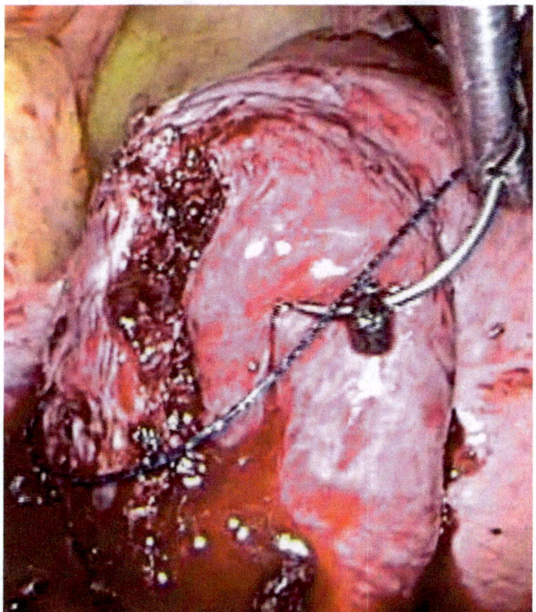

Fig. 31.9 A barbed suture used for myorraphy in continuous suturing

For example, non-expert laparoscopists hardly suture adequately by laparoscopy than by laparotomy. During laparotomy, closure of the myometrial defect is usually accomplished by a multilayered suture. During laparoscopy, failure to suture adequately myometrial defects and lack of hemostasis with subsequent hematoma formation may interfere with wound healing and increase the successive risk of uterine rupture [57].

Moreover, inappropriate use of electrocautery may induce in-depth necrosis of the myometrium with an adverse effect on healing. Excessive use of diathermocoagulation (with inflammation, hypoxia, necrosis, fibrosis, and neuropeptides damaging) can lead to delay in the correct uterine healing and generate a weaker uterine scar.

In Dubuisson et al. [54] study, one rupture occurred on the site of later myomectomy in another institute, due to placenta percreta over the second scar. Although the authors did not calculate this case in their count, second myomectomy was the most probable causative mechanism of forming an abnormally invasive placenta. The other rupture case had a rupture on the site of myomectomy scar which was re-sutured during second-look laparoscopy 7 weeks after the surgery.

Pistofidis and coworkers [56] investigated all seven cases of uterine rupture after laparoscopic myomectomy reported to the Greek Board of Endoscopic Gynecologic Surgery from 1998 to 2011. Only one of those patients had intramural myoma, and the endometrial cavity was not opened in any of the patients. Bipolar diathermy was the sole method of hemostasis in 28.6% of cases and could be characterized as excessive in 87.5% of patients. Most of the ruptures occurred at 34 weeks of gestation or later, with one case at 24 weeks of gestation in twin pregnancy. Those authors concluded that it seems reasonable that women who have undergone laparoscopic myomectomy would best avoid multiple pregnancies because of potentially increased risk of rupture.

Parker et al. [58] investigated 19 cases of uterine rupture following laparoscopic myomectomy and concluded that it's reasonable to use in laparoscopy to techniques similar to those adopted for open myomectomy, as bipolar diathermy during laparoscopic procedures has potentially detrimental effect on the healing process.

Robotic-assisted laparoscopic surgery is relatively new innovation in the field of gynecologic surgery. An advantage of robotic-assisted laparoscopic myomectomy is the ability to perform an identical multilayer closure to the abdominal approach that controls hemostasis without the need for significant use of electrosurgical instruments [59]. The incidence of uterine rupture in pregnancy after robotic-assisted myomectomy reported by Pitter et al. [60] was 1.1%. The uterine rupture in this study occurred in 33 weeks of gestation in a patient who conceived 18 weeks after the robotic multiple myomectomy without entering the endometrial cavity.

Recurrent uterine rupture rate in patients with prior repair is 4–19% [61]. In the Pistofidis study [56], out of seven cases of uterine rupture after laparoscopic myomectomy, there were two cases of recurrent rupture (28.6%).

The integrity of the hysterotomy scar and the risk of uterine rupture following laparoscopic myomectomy remain topics of debate.

Tinelli et al. [62] evaluated the problem of myometrial healing after myomectomy, analyzing the data of their research on neurotransmission in the nonpregnant uterus and on the uterine myomas. Myometrial healing is an interactive, dynamic process involving neuropeptides, angiogenetic factors, neuromodulators, blood cells, the extracellular matrix, and parenchymal cells. It follows three complex and overlapping phases: inflammation, tissue formation, and tissue remodeling.

Growth factors present in leiomyoma pseudocapsule vessels (Fig. 31.10) promote angiogenesis, a process probably enhanced by leiomyoma, who excites the formation of surrounding vascular structure, ensuring autonomic blood supply for its growth. Biochemical data showed many growth factors and related receptors to be deregulated in leiomyoma tissue. Investigations on leiomyoma pseudocapsule gene expression outlined an angiogenic profile in the pseudocapsule. Scientific evidences suggest to preserve myoma pseudocapsule during myomectomy (Fig. 31.11), since pseudocapsule contains such important peptides and other biologically active molecules [62].

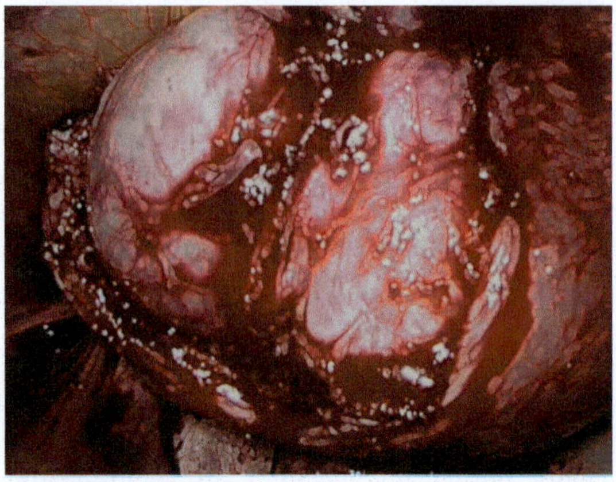

Fig. 31.10 A multi-lobulated myoma surrounded by pseudocapsule vessels

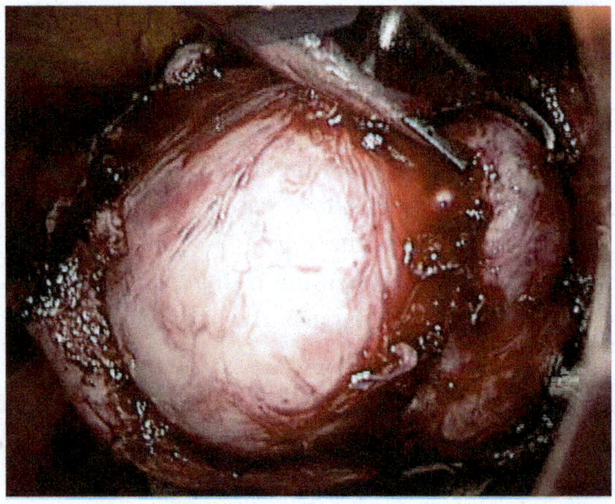

Fig. 31.11 Myoma enucleation during an intracapsular myomectomy pseudocapsule sparing

Even if papers assert the indisputable benefits of myomectomy on fertility in woman affected by leiomyoma-related infertility, so far, literature lacks data regarding surgical technique rationale, explaining all the steps of surgical techniques.

Tinelli et al. [63] explained the rationale for reproductive surgery procedures aiming at leiomyoma enucleation with the preservation of its pseudocapsule, promoter and enhancer of a correct myometrial healing, with positive impact on successive pregnancy and delivery.

Uterine Rupture During Labor

There are no precise diagnostic criteria of uterine rupture during pregnancy and labor.

According to a systematic review of maternal morbidity and mortality by the World Health Organization in 2005, the median incidence of uterine rupture is 5.3 per 10,000 deliveries [4].

The most common sign in women with a uterine rupture without a scar is shock, followed by uterine bleeding, severe abdominal pain, and easily palpable fetal parts. Traditionally, primigravidae and unscarred uteri are considered immune to rupture.

Most reported cases of uterine rupture are associated with previous scarring of the uterus, multiparity, a short length of time (less than 18 months) since the last cesarean section, the number of previous cesarean sections, single-layer closure instead of two-layer closure, placenta previa, and the use of prostaglandins or oxytocin for labor induction or augmentation [23, 64, 65].

Rupture after a prolonged labor is commonly due to obstructed labor, with formation of a retraction or Bandl's ring. First described by Ludwig Bandl in 1875, it represents marked thinning of the lower segment and increased retraction of the upper uterine segment. The tear begins in the lower uterine segment, may extend up to the fundus or down into the vagina, or proceed laterally into the broad ligament. If the tear is posterior, it may go through the posterior vaginal fornix into the pouch of Douglas [66].

A multiparous patient in the obstructed labor will continue to have tetanic contractions until the uterus ruptures, while primiparas will usually go out of labor. The contractions usually stop when the fetus is expelled into the peritoneal cavity (Fig. 31.12).

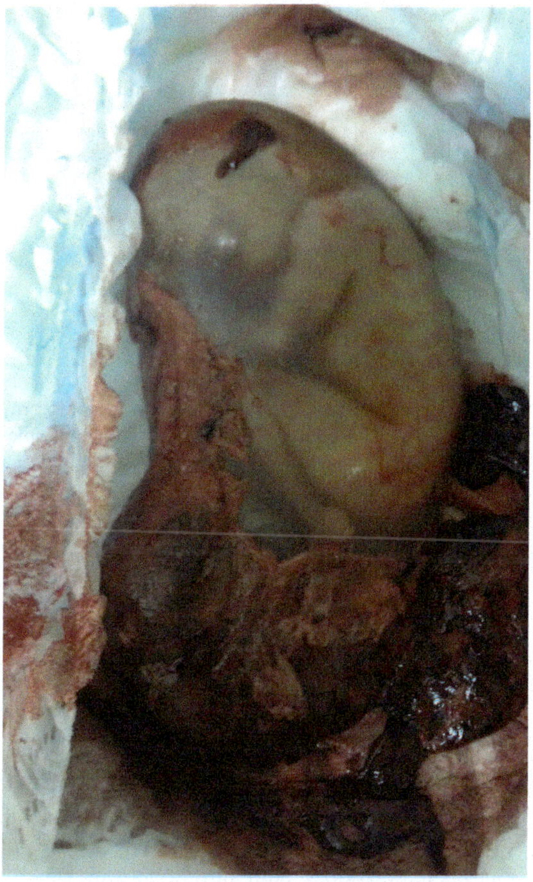

Fig. 31.12 A complete fetal expulsion after uterine rupture in abdominal cavity, with amniotic sac and placenta, at 18 weeks of pregnancy

Fetal heart rate abnormality, most commonly bradycardia, is the most common presentation of uterine rupture. Uterine rupture can also present as abdominal pain, vaginal bleeding, and altered uterine contractions. More rarely, it can present as hypotension, shock, hematuria, and shoulder tip pain and scar tenderness. The most common combination of these symptoms is an abnormal fetal heart rate with abdominal pain [65].

Rupture of the unscarred uterus is generally sudden accompanied by severe abdominal pain with the fetal bradycardia or absence of fetal heart sounds and cessation of uterine contractions in conjunction with vaginal bleeding and followed by vascular collapse.

It causes significant morbidity and mortality rate in both the fetus and the mother.

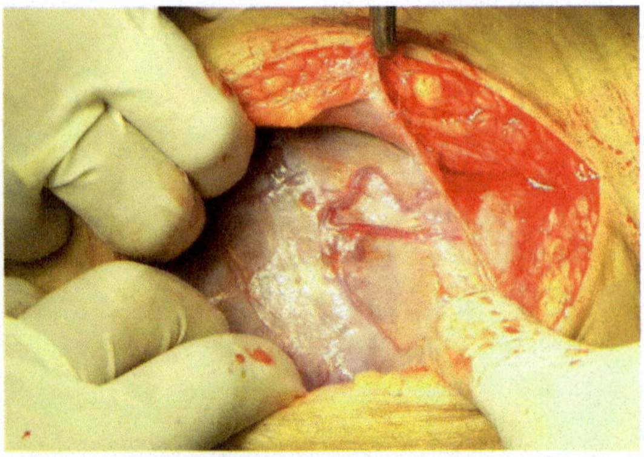

Fig. 31.13 An urgent suprapubic transversal laparotomy for uterine rupture; after the abdomen opening, the placenta attachments appear directly in the pelvis

In less developed countries, it is a significant cause of maternal mortality, contributing for 9.3–14.6% of maternal deaths [3].

Maternal tachycardia is an alarming sign that can, along with another medical signs, alert the physician to the possibility of uterine rupture [67].

From the time of diagnosis to delivery, generally only 10–31 min are available before clinically significant fetal morbidity becomes inevitable (Fig. 31.13). Fetal morbidity occurs as a result of massive hemorrhage, fetal anoxia, or both [68].

Clinical Presentation of Uterine Rupture

Although rare, primary uterine rupture is particularly morbid [69, 70]. An unscarred gravid uterus has the potential for catastrophic hemorrhage, in comparison with rupture or dehiscence of a previous cesarean scar, which can be bloodless [71].

Uterine rupture can occur at any time during gestation and may be difficult to predict [72]. Uterine anomalies are a reported cause of rupture of the unscarred uterus in the first trimester in patients with uterine anomalies [73].

In the differential diagnosis of uterine rupture, placental abruption, placenta previa, uterine inversion, cervical tear, vaginal tear, coagulopathy, uterine atony, and uterine artery rupture may be considered [74, 75].

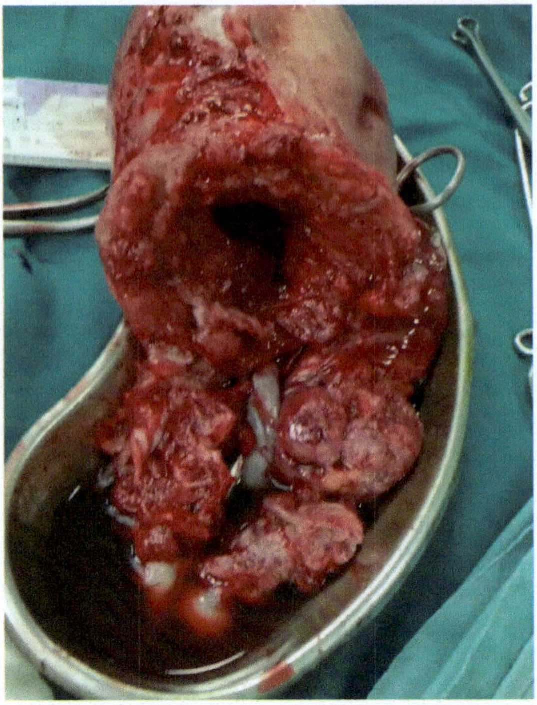

Fig. 31.14 An hysterectomized uterus after a uterine rupture, with a placenta accreta inside the uterus

Endometriosis can cause erosion of the utero-ovarian vessels, resulting in severe hemorrhage [76].

Generally, the most frequent site of uterine rupture is the LUS, the site of the previous CS, but no assumptions can be made concerning the site of rupture or the involvement of other structures. Intra-abdominal bleeding is rare during the first trimester of pregnancy. In the first trimester of pregnancy, most cases of intraabdominal bleeding are related to extrauterine pregnancy [77].

Hemoperitoneum in the second trimester can be attributed to both obstetric and non-obstetric causes. The site of rupture may be posterior, fundal, lateral (sometimes involving one or both uterine arteries), as well as anterior or may extend from the lower segment up to the fundus or down into the cervix and/or the vagina [78].

The causes of these cases can be divided into placental (Fig. 31.14), uterine, and vascular. Placenta percreta is a rare placental abnormality that can cause severe complications, such as hemoperitoneum [78, 79].

Placental abruption is not a cause of hemoperitoneum in the absence of uterine rupture.

However, during pregnancy, the clinical features of hemoperitoneum can trigger a suspicion of placental abruption because these conditions share similar clinical features, and these similarities can cause diagnostic difficulties [80].

Patients with uterine rupture are usually moribund, in severe hypovolemic shock with air hunger. They present with a grossly distended and tender pregnant abdomen with signs of peritonitis. Often very little can be palpated abdominally because of the distention and guarding. However, sometimes fetal limbs are abnormally easy to feel, or the uterus can be separated from the fetus [81].

Typical presenting features include abdominal pain, tachycardia, hypotension, shock, coma, vaginal bleeding, fetal parts palpable through the abdominal wall, and sepsis, depending on the length of time that has elapsed between rupture and arrival at the hospital [82].

Another issue is silent uterine rupture; this has potential risk for complete uterine rupture, which leads to acute life-threatening complications for both the mother and baby. It is difficult to determine whether to manage complete uterine rupture expectantly or surgically, including repair of the uterine wall or termination of the pregnancy, especially in the early second trimester [73].

Instrumental Diagnosis of Uterine Rupture

Possible sites of rupture include the posterior uterine wall, the anterior wall, the lateral uterine side, the fundus, and the lower uterine segment.

Ultrasonography can be a useful tool for the timely detection of uterine rupture in stable patients who have atypical presentations suspicious of uterine rupture. The typical ultrasound manifestations of uterine rupture are the empty uterus and the gestational sac above the uterus.

Ultrasonography can allow for a rapid preliminary survey of uterine wall integrity, which could aid decision-making on the need for immediate surgical intervention.

Other sonographic findings are intrauterine blood and large uterine mass with gas bubbles [83].

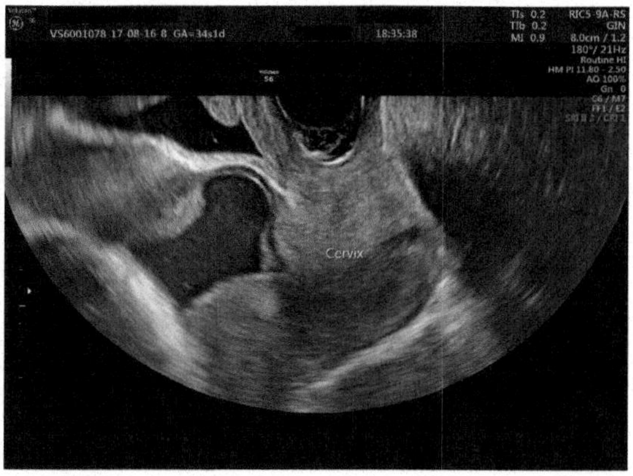

Fig. 31.15 A 34-weeks pregnant patient with a lower uterine thickness of <2.3 mm. The patient had a pre-cesarean section and was hospitalized for high risk of uterine rupture, with urgent cesarean iterative surgery

A secondary assessment of fetal well-being could also be done by cardiotocography.

Ultrasonography has been studied to predict uterine rupture.

Bujold et al. [84] performed an investigation on 125 women with previous CS, undergoing trial of labor. Their analysis determined that optimal cutoff is a LUS thickness of <2.3 mm (Fig. 31.15), with the rate of uterine rupture being 9.1% for this group. The limitation of this study includes the fact that most women with a lower uterine thickness < 2.0 mm did not undergo trial of labor. This might suggest an established practice pattern which might limit future studies using ultrasound to predict uterine rupture.

Kok et al. [85] evaluated the accuracy of antenatal sonographic measurement of LUS thickness in the prediction of risk of uterine rupture during a trial of labor (TOL) in women with a previous CS. Their meta-analysis included 21 studies with a total of 2776 analyzed patients. The estimated sROC curves showed that measurement of LUS thickness seemed promising in the prediction of occurrence of uterine defects (dehiscence and rupture) in the uterine wall. The pooled sensitivity and specificity of myometrial LUS thickness for cutoffs between 0.6 and 2.0 mm were 0.76 (95% CI, 0.60–0.87) and 0.92 (95% CI, 0.82–0.97); cutoffs between 2.1 and 4.0 mm reached a sensitivity and specificity of 0.94 (95% CI, 0.81–0.98) and 0.64 (95% CI,

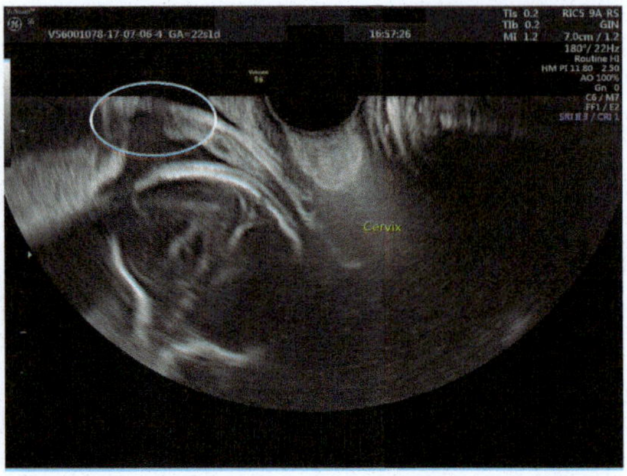

Fig. 31.16 A transvaginal scan evaluating LUS thickness throughout pregnancy in a patient without a previous cesarean section at 22 weeks

0.26–0.90). The pooled sensitivity and specificity of full LUS thickness for cutoffs between 2.0 and 3.0 mm were 0.61 (95% CI, 0.42–0.77) and 0.91 (95% CI, 0.80–0.96); cutoffs between 3.1 and 5.1 mm reached a sensitivity and specificity of 0.96 (95% CI, 0.89–0.98) and 0.63 (95% CI, 0.30–0.87).

Recently, Fukuda et al. [86] evaluated the normal ranges of LUS thickness throughout pregnancy in women without a previous CS (Fig. 31.16) and evaluated the relationship between ultrasound and intraoperative LUS thickness. They performed 20,307 LUS thickness measurements in between 119 and 944 women at each week of gestation, in 944 women during labor, and in 936 women after delivery. They observed a strong relationship between transabdominal and transperineal ultrasound ($p < 0.001$) and an inverse correlation between LUS thickness and gestational age ($p < 0.001$), with a mean thickness of 5.1 ± 1.4 mm at 20 weeks, 3.6 ± 1.3 mm at 30 weeks, and 2.3 ± 0.6 mm at 40 weeks of gestation.

In women undergoing elective CS, we observed a strong relationship between antepartum and intraoperative LUS thickness ($p < 0.001$), with mean thicknesses of 2.2 ± 0.7 mm in 28 women without thinning of LUS, 0.8 ± 0.1 mm in 4 women with grade II uterine scar dehiscence, and 0.4 ± 0.1 mm in 3 women with grade III dehiscence. Authors concluded that a LUS myometrial thickness less than 1.2 mm could have predicted all grade II and grade III uterine scar dehiscence, without false-positive cases.

Barzilay et al. [87] investigated the thickness of the LUS during active labor phase in women with or without a history of a previous CS, by transabdominal sonography in the midsagittal position with a full urinary bladder. They compared a total of 28 women with a previous cesarean delivery, to 29 women without a history of uterine surgery. The median LUS was significantly thinner in women with a uterine scar both during (4 vs. 5 mm, $p = 0.001$) and between contractions (5 vs. 7 mm, $p = 0.011$). Paired comparison of LUS thickness between and during contractions within each group showed that thinning of LUS during contraction was significant for both the previous CS group ($p < 0.001$) and the control group ($p < 0.001$). Authors found that LUS was significantly thinner in women after a previous CS and that the LUS was significantly thinner during contraction, and they showed no correlation between LUS thickness and chances of successful trial of labor after cesarean (TOLAC).

Useful as it is, computerized tomography (CT) is not the first choice for imaging examination of pregnant women with abdominal pain because of the radiation problem.

But in some recent surveys, CT is performed to evaluate pregnant women with abdominal pain, for the benefits are thought to outweigh the risks [88]. Hruska et al. [89] reported the importance of the MRI examination for assessment of pregnant patients in case of uterine rupture.

Authors evaluated tocogram characteristics associated with uterine rupture during trial of labor after CS by a systematic review. Three tocogram characteristics were associated with uterine rupture: (1) hyper-stimulation was more frequently observed compared with controls during the delivery (38% vs. 21% and 58% vs. 53%) and in the last 2 h prior to birth (19% vs. 4%), results of meta-analysis: OR 1.68 (95% CI, 0.97–2.89) and $p = 0.06$; (2) decrease of uterine activity was observed in 14–40%; and (3) an increasing baseline in 10–20%. Five studies documented no changes in uterine activity or Montevideo units. A direct comparison between external tocodynamometer and intrauterine pressure catheters was not feasible. Authors concluded that uterine rupture can be preceded or accompanied by several types of changes in uterine contractility, including hyperstimulation, reduced number of contractions, and increased or reduced baseline tonus [90].

Management of Uterine Rupture

Early diagnosis and immediate preoperative resuscitation are of great importance in ruptured uterus. Sudden fetal heart abnormalities in laboring patients should be taken as a potential sign of danger. With awareness, prompt diagnosis, rapid replacement of blood loss, and improved techniques in surgical management and neonatal care, maternal and fetal morbidity and mortality can be lowered remarkably. It is possible to reduce fetal and maternal mortality with a prompt intervention, less than 18 min from onset of prolonged deceleration to delivery [23].

The managing clinician should also be aware of the physiologic pregnancy adaptations, where blood and erythrocyte volume increase by 50% and 30%, respectively. A pregnant woman is physiologically prepared to lose blood up to 2 L without any detectable hemodynamic changes. When blood loss approaches 2.5 L, she can deteriorate dramatically [91].

Reports have been published regarding repair of uterine rupture in the second trimester by suturing and/or patching. There have been reported cases of diagnosis of uterine defect in second and third trimester of pregnancy, diagnosed on ultrasound, which were repaired and the pregnancy continued till fetal maturity [92–94].

The management of complete uterine rupture is surgical, and a delay in treatment is often fatal (Fig. 31.17). An emergency laparoscopy or laparotomy is needed for correct diagnosis and to allow the appropriate treatment to take place. Early surgical intervention is usually the key to successful treatment of uterine rupture (Fig. 31.18). Generally, the best chance for

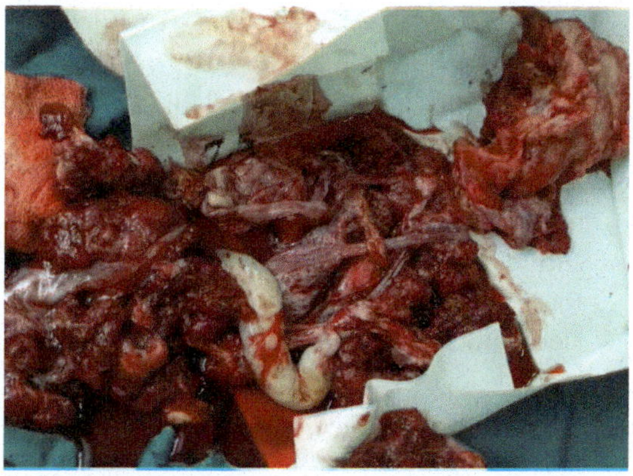

Fig. 31.17 The postoperative image shows a complete uterine rupture with a sort of explosion of pregnant uterus during pregnancy

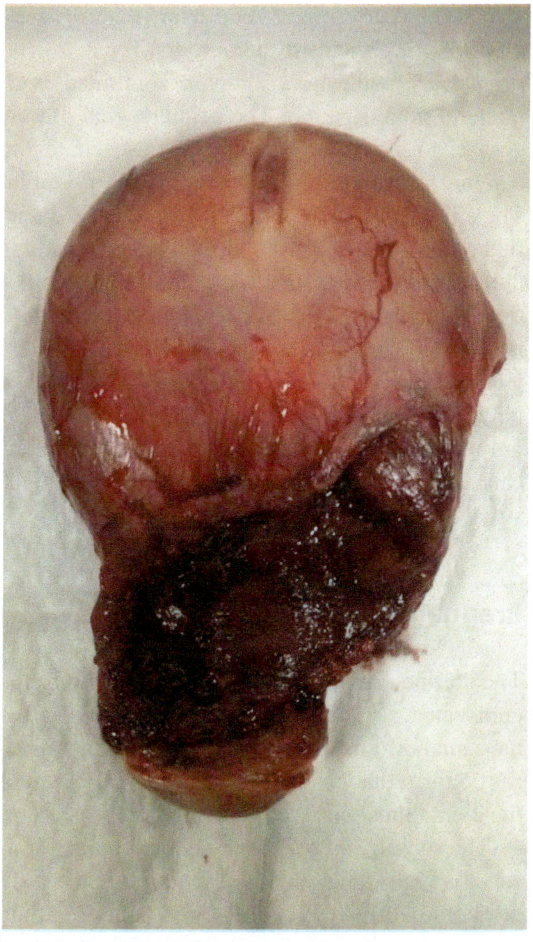

Fig. 31.18 A removed uterus with a complete rupture in a patient with two previous cesarean sections at 24 weeks of pregnancy. The uterus is completely open at the old scars

maternal survival is prompt laparotomy in non-expert laparoscopists.

Although resuscitation of the patient with fluids and blood transfusion is desirable, it is mandatory to explore immediately the pelvis. Once the abdomen is open, the specific clinical circumstance can be assessed. The fetus and the placenta must be removed immediately in case of complete uterine rupture and fetus expulsion in the abdomen. In the vast majority of cases, the fetus will be dead or dying. The rate of perinatal death in cases of uterine rupture is extremely high. Treatment will primarily depend on the extent of the lesion, parity, age and condition of the patient, and expertise of the surgeon [78].

The surgical choices usually come down to one of the four options: total hysterectomy, subtotal (supracervical) hysterectomy, repair of the rupture by suturing, or repair combined with bilateral tubal ligation. The primary goal of surgery is to stop the hemorrhage, resuscitate the patient, and stabilize her as rapidly as possible. The circumstances in which the operation is carried out may be desperate. Often, the operation is undertaken by a surgeon without extensive experience, using inadequate equipment, and who lacks adequate anesthesia and nursing support. Under these circumstances, the best operation may be simple suture repair of the rupture. Not only does this meet the patient's immediate clinical needs, but it preserves the uterus and menstrual function along with it [3].

Pregnancy After Uterine Rupture

The uterine rupture is a very rare and serious circumstance, so there are not many studies that have analyzed this incident. Few literature analyses confirm that postpartum delivery after cuts of the uterus must be faced by CS.

The subsequent pregnancy outcome after conservative management of uterine rupture has only been studied in small case series, among which the prevalence of recurrence ranged from approximately 0 to 33% [95]. Ritchie et al. [96] estimated the rate of involuntary infertility after uterine rupture to be approximately 33%, probably because of the formation of abdominal adhesions and tubal occlusion.

In scientific literature, there are some case reports that describe pregnancies after uterine rupture. Surico et al. [17] published a second trimester uterine rupture repair, on 40-year-old women at 15 weeks and 5 days. Her first pregnancy had resulted in preterm cesarean delivery at 27 weeks of gestation for placental abruption, leading to stillbirth. The initial diagnosis was appendicitis or ovarian torsion, so exploratory laparoscopy was performed. Before the medical procedure, the patient was advised about the potential risks and benefits of the intervention, and she gave her informed consent. Hemoperitoneum (1000 g of blood loss) was found with a myometrial defect on the anterior uterine wall. Uterine rupture with complete opening of the uterine wall at the site of the previous transverse scar was found, with protrusion of the placenta. Conversion to open surgery was necessary. The ruptured uterus was repaired using two layered separate stitch sutures of 1-0 polyglactin 910 (Coated Vicryl, Ethicon, Inc., Somerville, NJ, USA). The patient's postoperative recovery was uneventful, and she was discharged on the fifth postoperative day. She was informed of the potential risks of this conservative management and was discharged home. A healthy baby (weight 2640 g, normal Apgar scores) was delivered by elective traditional cesarean section because of placenta previa at 36 weeks of gestation.

Conclusion

Uterine rupture is a clinical diagnosis, and there must be a high index of suspicion by the healthcare provider. Uterine rupture, whether in a previously scarred uterus or in an unscarred uterus, is potentially life-threatening for both the mother and fetus, and it is associated with significant mortality and morbidity.

Risk factors for such ruptures may include previous uterine scar, short birth spacing, and use of uterotonic (oxytocin/prostaglandin) medications. It can occur during pregnancy, early in labor or following the prolonged labor, most frequently near or at term. Rarely, the uterus can rupture during early to midpregnancy. A scarred uterus is not a necessary precondition for uterine rupture. The survival of patients after uterine rupture depends on the time interval between rupture and intervention and the availability of blood products for transfusion.

It is very important in clinical trials to have a large number of clinical cases so that one can have safe and reliable clinical indications, avoiding drawing conclusions from studies with few numbers, believed by Tversky and Kahneman [97], who won the Nobel Prize discussing "the error of small numbers."

References

1. Tinelli A. Uterine rupture: up to date. JDReAM. 2017;1(1):61–74.
2. Dane B, Dane C. Maternal death after uterine rupture in an unscarred uterus: a case report. J Emerg Med. 2009;37(4):393–5.
3. Berhe Y, Wall LL. Uterine rupture in resource-poor countries. Obstet Gynecol Surv. 2014;69(11): 695–707.
4. Hofmeyr GJ, Say L, Gülmezoglu AM. Systematic review: WHO systematic review of maternal mortality and morbidity: the prevalence of uterine rupture. BJOG. 2005;112(9):1221–8.
5. Turner MJ. Uterine rupture. Best Pract Res Clin Obstet Gynaecol. 2002;16(1):69–79.
6. Al-Zirqi I, Stray-Pedersen B, Forsen L, Daltveit A, Vangen S. Uterine rupture: trends over 40 years. BJOG. 2016;123(5):780–7.
7. Gibbins KJ, Weber T, Holmgren CM, Porter TF, Varner MW, Manuck TA. Maternal and fetal morbidity associated with uterine rupture of the unscarred uterus. Am J Obstet Gynecol. 2015;213(3):382.e1–6.
8. Sun HD, Su WH, Chang WH, Wen L, Huang BS, Wang PH. Rupture of a pregnant unscarred uterus in an early secondary trimester: a case report and brief review. J Obstet Gynaecol Res. 2012;38(2):442–5.
9. Walsh CA, O'Sullivan RJ, Foley ME. Unexplained prelabor uterine rupture in a term primigravida. Obstet Gynecol. 2006;108(3 Pt 2):725–7.
10. Ofir K, Sheiner E, Levy A, Katz M, Mazor M. Uterine rupture: differences between a scarred and an unscarred uterus. Am J Obstet Gynecol. 2004;191(2):425–9.
11. Zwart JJ, Richters JM, Öry F, de Vrics JI, Bloemenkamp KW, van Roosmalen J. Uterine rupture in the Netherlands: a nationwide population-based cohort study. BJOG. 2009;116(8):1069–78. discussion 1078–80.
12. Egbe TO, Halle-Ekane GE, Tchente CN, Nyemb JE, Belley-Priso E. Management of uterine rupture: a case report and review of the literature. BMC Res Notes. 2016;9(1):492.
13. Teguete I, Dolo A, Sissoko A, Thera A, Traore M, Djire MY, et al. Determining factors of cesarean delivery trends in developing countries: lessons from point G National Hospital (Bamako-Mali). Croatia: INTECH Open Access; 2012. p. 161–202.
14. Sparić R, Kadija S, Tadić J, Dokić M, Milenković V. Intrapartal resection of the bicornuete uterus for placenta membranacea percreta. Srp Arh Celok Lek. 2007;135(1–2):85–7.
15. Halperin ME, Moore DC, Hannah WJ. Classical versus low-segment transverse incision for preterm caesarean section: maternal complications and outcome of subsequent pregnancies. Br J Obstet Gynaecol. 1988;95(10):990–6.
16. Landon MB, Lynch CD. Optimal timing and mode of delivery after cesarean with previous classical incision or myomectomy: a review of the data. Semin Perinatol. 2011;35(5):257–61.
17. Surico D, Amadori R, Vigone A, D'Agostino C, Dessole M, Surico N. Successful delivery after surgical repair of uterine rupture at 15 weeks of gestation: case report and brief review. Eur J Obstet Gynecol Reprod Biol. 2016;204:5–8.
18. Eze JN, Anozie OB, Lawani OL, Ndukwe EO, Agwu UM, Obuna JA. Evaluation of obstetricians' surgical decision making in the management of uterine rupture. BMC Pregnancy Childbirth. 2017;17(1):179.
19. McCarthy F, Germain S. Connective tissue disorders and dermatological disordres in pregnancy. Obstet Gynaecol Reprod Med. 2013;23(3):71–80.
20. Al Qarni AA, Al-Braikan N, Al-Hanbali MM, Alharmaly AH. Rupture rudimentary horn pregnancy at 31 week. Saudi Med J. 2017;38(2):201–3.
21. Bujold E, Mehta SH, Bujold C, Gauthier RJ. Interdelivery interval and uterine rupture. Am J Obstet Gynecol. 2002;187(5):1199–202.
22. Stamilio DM, DeFranco E, Paré E, Odibo AO, Peipert JF, Allsworth JE, et al. Short interpregnancy interval: risk of uterine rupture and complications of vaginal birth after cesarean delivery. Obstet Gynecol. 2007;110(5):1075–82.
23. Bujold E, Gauthier RJ. Risk of uterine rupture associated with an interdelivery interval between 18 and 24 months. Obstet Gynecol. 2010;115(5):1003–6.
24. Uccella S, Cromi A, Bogani G, Zaffaroni E, Ghezzi F. Spontaneous prelabor uterine rupture in a primigravida: a case report and review of the literature. Am J Obstet Gynecol. 2011;205(5):e6–8.
25. Mittal S, Misra SL. Uterine perforation following medical termination of pregnancy by vacuum aspiration. Int J Gynaecol Obstet. 1985;23(1):45–50.
26. Grindler NM, Ng J, Tocce K, Alvero R. Considerations for management of interstitial ectopic pregnancies: two case reports. J Med Case Rep. 2016;10(1):106.
27. Bamigboye AA, Hofmeyr GJ. Closure versus non-closure of the peritoneum at caesarean section: short- and long-term outcomes. Cochrane Database Syst Rev. 2014;(8):CD000163.
28. Malvasi A, Tinelli A, Farine D, Rahimi S, Cavallotti C, Vergara D, et al. Effects of visceral peritoneal

closure on scar formation at cesarean delivery. Int J Gynaecol Obstet. 2009;105(2):131–5.
29. Malvasi A, Tinelli A, Guido M, Cavallotti C, Dell'Edera D, Zizza A, et al. Effect of avoiding bladder flap formation in caesarean section on repeat caesarean delivery. Eur J Obstet Gynecol Reprod Biol. 2011;159(2):300–4.
30. Malvasi A, Tinelli A, Cavallotti C, Bettocchi S, Di Renzo GC, Stark M. Substance P (SP) and vasoactive intestinal polypeptide (VIP) in the lower uterine segment in first and repeated cesarean sections. Peptides. 2010;31(11):2052–9.
31. Di Tommaso S, Cavallotti C, Malvasi A, Vergara D, Rizzello A, De Nuccio F, et al. A qualitative and quantitative study of the innervation of the human non pregnant uterus. Curr Protein Pept Sci. 2016;18(2):140–8.
32. Malvasi A, Cavallotti C, Gustapane S, Giacci F, Di Tommaso S, Vergara D, et al. Neurotransmitters and neuropeptides expression in the uterine scar after cesarean section. Curr Protein Pept Sci. 2016;18(2):175–80.
33. Malvasi A, Cavallotti C, Resta L, Mynbaev OA, Di Tommaso S, Vergara D, et al. Laminin and collagen IV: two polypeptides as marker of dystocic labor. Curr Protein Pept Sci. 2016;18(2):149–54.
34. Stanirowski PJ, Trojanowski S, Słomka A, Cendrowski K, Sawicki W. Spontaneous rupture of the pregnant uterus following salpingectomy: a literature review. Gynecol Obstet Investig. 2015;80(2):73–7.
35. Api O, Balcin ME, Ugurel V, Api M, Turan C, Unal O. The effect of uterine fundal pressure on the duration of the second stage of labor: a randomized controlled trial. Acta Obstet Gynecol Scand. 2009;88(3):320–4.
36. Verheijen EC, Raven JH, Hofmeyr GJ. Fundal pressure during the second stage of labour. Cochrane Database Syst Rev. 2009(4):CD006067.
37. Buhimschi CS, Buhimschi IA, Malinow AM, Kopelman JN, Weiner CP. The effect of fundal pressure manoeuvre on intrauterine pressure in the second stage of labour. BJOG. 2002;109(5):520–6.
38. Nikolaou M, Kourea HP, Antonopoulos K, Geronatsio K, Adonakis G, Decavalas G. Spontaneous uterine rupture in a primigravid woman in the early third trimester attributed to adenomyosis: a case report and review of the literature. J Obstet Gynaecol Res. 2013;39(3):727–32.
39. Nagao Y, Osato K, Kubo M, Kawamura T, Ikeda T, Yamawaki T. Spontaneous uterine rupture in the 35th week of gestation after laparoscopic adenomyomectomy. Int Med Case Rep J. 2015;9:1–4.
40. Morimatsu Y, Matsubara S, Okuchi A, et al. Pregnancy after adenomyomectomy—literature review of uterine rupture and obstetrical management. Japan J Obstet Gynaecol. 2007;74(9):1047–53.
41. Agarwal R, Gupta B, Radhakrishnan G. Rupture of intrapartum unscarred uterus at the fundus: a complication of passive cocaine abuse? Arch Gynecol Obstet. 2011;283(Suppl 1):53–4.
42. Palmer JM, Indermaur MD, Tebes CC, Spellacy WN. Placenta increta and cocaine abuse in a grand multipara leading to a second trimester rupture of an unscarred uterus: a case report. South Med J. 2008;101(8):834–5.
43. Rajiah P, Eastwood KL, Gunn ML, Dighe M. Uterine diverticulum. Obstet Gynecol. 2009;113(2 Pt 2):525–7.
44. Yap FY, Radin R, Tchelepi H. Torsion, infarction, and rupture of a nongravid uterus: a complication of a large ovarian cyst. Abdom Radiol (NY). 2016;41(12):2359–63.
45. Sparić R, Pervulov M, Stefanović A, Tadić J, Gojnić M, Milićević S, Berisavac M. Uterine torsion in term pregnancy. Srp Arh Celok Lek. 2007;135(9–10):572–5.
46. Jeong YY, Kang HK, Park JG, Choi HS. CT features of uterine torsion. Eur Radiol. 2003;13(Suppl 6):L249–50.
47. Luk SY, Leung JL, Cheung ML, So S, Fung SH, Cheng SC. Torsion of a nongravid myomatous uterus: radiological features and literature review. Hong Kong Med J. 2010;16(4):304–6.
48. Garnet JD. Rupture of the uterus in pregnancy. Postgrad Med. 1964;36:28–33.
49. Koo YJ, Lee JK, Lee YK, Kwak DW, Lee IH, Lim KT, Lee KH, Kim TJ. Pregnancy outcomes and risk factors for uterine rupture after laparoscopic myomectomy: a single-center experience and literature review. J Minim Invasive Gynecol. 2015;22(6):1022–8.
50. Gambacorti-Passerini Z, Gimovsky AC, Locatelli A, Berghella V. Trial of labor after myomectomy and uterine rupture: a systematic review. Acta Obstet Gynecol Scand. 2016;95(7):724–34.
51. Barakat EE, Bedaiwy MA, Zimberg S, Nutter B, Nosseir M, Falcone T. Robotic-assisted, laparoscopic, and abdominal myomectomy: a comparison of surgical outcomes. Obstet Gynecol. 2011;117(2 Pt 1):256–65.
52. Sizzi O, Rossetti A, Malzoni M, Minelli L, La Grotta F, Soranna L, Panuzi S, Spagnolo R, Imperato F, Landi S, Fiaccamento A, Stola A. Italian multicenter study on complications of laparoscopic myomectomy. J Minim Invasive Gynecol. 2007;14(4):453–62.
53. Seracchioli R, Manuzzi L, Vianello F, Gualerzi B, Paradisi R, Venturoli S. Obstetric and delivery outcome of pregnancies achieved after laparoscopic myomectomy. Fertil Steril. 2006;86(1):159–65.
54. Dubuisson JB, Fauconnier A, Deffarges JV, Norgaard C, Kreiker G, Chapron C. Pregnancy outcome and deliveries following laparoscopic myomectomy. Hum Reprod. 2000;15(4):869–73.
55. Sparić R, Malvasi A, Kadija S, Babović I, Nejković L, Tinelli A. Cesarean myomectomy trends and controversies: an appraisal. J Matern Fetal Neonatal Med. 2017;30(9):1114–23.
56. Pistofidis G, Makrakis E, Balinakos P, Dimitriou E, Bardis N, Anaf V. Report of 7 uterine rupture cases after laparoscopic myomectomy: update of the literature. J Minim Invasive Gynecol. 2012;19(6):762–7.
57. Tinelli A. Concepts and thoughts about modern uterine intramural and subserosal myomectomy. Int J Gynecol Obstet Neonat Care. 2017;4:11–9.

58. Parker WH, Einarsson J, Istre O, Dubuisson JB. Risk factors for uterine rupture after laparoscopic myomectomy. J Minim Invasive Gynecol. 2010;17(5):551–4.
59. Tinelli A, Malvasi A, Gustapane S, Buscarini M, Gill IS, Stark M, Nezhat FR, Mettler L. Robotic assisted surgery in gynecology: current insights and future perspectives. Recent Pat Biotechnol. 2011;5(1):12–24.
60. Pitter MC, Gargiulo AR, Bonaventura LM, Lehman JS, Srouji SS. Pregnancy outcomes following robot-assisted myomectomy. Hum Reprod. 2013;28(1):99–108.
61. Abbas AM, Sheha AM, Ali MK, Ali SS, Salem NZ, Talaat E, Hassan A. Second-trimester spontaneous uterine rupture after laparoscopic electromyolysis in nulligravida: a case report. Middle East Fertil Soc J. 2017;22:73–6.
62. Tinelli A, Mynbaev OA, Sparić R, Vergara D, Di Tommaso S, Salzet M, Maffia M, Malvasi A. Angiogenesis and vascularization of uterine leiomyoma: clinical value of pseudocapsule containing peptides and neurotransmitters. Curr Protein Pept Sci. 2016;18(2):129–39.
63. Tinelli A, Malvasi A. Uterine fibroid pseudocapsule. In: Tinelli A, Malvasi A, editors. Uterine myoma, myomectomy and minimally invasive treatments. Cham, Switzerland: Springer Publisher; 2015. p. 73–93.
64. Hagneré P, Denoual I, Souissi A, Deswarte S. Spontaneous uterine rupture after myomectomy. Case report and review of the literature. J Gynecol Obstet Biol Reprod (Paris). 2011;40(2):162–5.
65. Abdalla N, Reinholz-Jaskolska M, Bachanek M, Cendrowski K, Stanczak R, Sawicki W. Hemoperitoneum in a patient with spontaneous rupture of the posterior wall of an unscarred uterus in the second trimester of pregnancy. BMC Res Notes. 2015;8:603.
66. Tinelli A, Di Renzo GC, Malvasi A. The intrapartum ultrasonographic detection of the Bandl ring as a marker of dystocia. Int J Gynaecol Obstet. 2015;131(3):310–1.
67. Sweeten KM, Graves WK, Athanassiou A. Spontaneous rupture of the unscarred uterus. Am J Obstet Gynecol. 1995;172(6):1851–5.
68. Carlin A, Alfirevic Z. Intrapartum fetal emergencies. Semin Fetal Neonatal Med. 2006;11(3):150–7.
69. Endres LK, Barnhart K. Spontaneous second trimester uterine rupture after classical cesarean. Obstet Gynecol. 2000;6(5 Pt 2):806–8.
70. Ijaz S, Mahendru A, Sanderson D. Spontaneous uterine rupture during the 1st trimester: a rare but life-threatening emergency. J Obstet Gynaecol. 2011;31(8):772.
71. Sun CH, Liao CI, Kan YY. "Silent" rupture of unscarred gravid uterus with subsequent pelvic abscess: successful laparoscopic management. J Minim Invasive Gynecol. 2005;12(6):519–21.
72. Iemura A, Kondoh E, Kawasaki K, Fujita K, Ueda A, Mogami H, Baba T, Konishi I. Expectant management of a herniated amniotic sac presenting as silent uterine rupture: a case report and literature review. J Matern Fetal Neonatal Med. 2015;28(1):106–12.
73. Tola EN. First trimester spontaneous uterine rupture in a young woman with uterine anomaly. Case Rep Obstet Gynecol. 2014;2014:967386.
74. Mazzone ME, Woolever J. Uterine rupture in a patient with an unscarred uterus: a case study. WMJ. 2006;105(2):64–6.
75. Berisavac M, Sparić R, Pervulov M, Arsenijević L, Spremović Radjenović S, Vrzić Petronijević S, Marković N, Milićević S. Spontaneous intraabdominal bleeding in twin pregnancy-case report. Srp Arh Celok Lek. 2008;136(5–6):299–301.
76. Williamson H, Indusekhar R, Clark A, Hassan IM. Spontaneous severe haemoperitoneum in the third trimester leading to intrauterine death: case report. Case Rep Obstet Gynecol. 2011;2011:173097.
77. Agdi M, Tulandi T. Surgical treatment of ectopic pregnancy. Best Pract Res Clin Obstet Gynaecol. 2009;23(4):519–27.
78. Guseh S, Carusi D, Tinelli A, Gargiulo A. Spontaneous uterine rupture prior to twenty weeks of gestation. In: Malvasi A, Tinelli A, Di Renzo GC, editors. Management and therapy of early pregnancy complications. Cham, Switzerland: Springer Publisher; 2016. p. 255–67.
79. Sparić R, Mirković L, Ravilić U, Janjić T. Obstetric complications of placenta praevia percreta. Vojnosanit Pregl. 2014;71(12):1163–6.
80. Vyjayanthi S, Rajesh U, Bloomfield TH. Haemoperitoneum due to placenta percreta in the third trimester mimicking placental abruption. J Obstet Gynaecol. 2002;22(6):690–1.
81. Groen GP. Uterine rupture in rural Nigeria: review of 144 cases. Obstet Gynecol. 1974;44(5):682–7.
82. Gessessew A, Melese MM. Ruptured uterus: eight year retrospective analysis of causes and management outcome in Adigrat Hospital, Tigray Region, Ethiopia. Ethiop J Health Dev. 2002;16(3):241–5.
83. Bedi DG, Salmon A, Winsett MZ, Fagan CJ, Kumar R. Ruptured uterus: sonographic findings. J Clin Ultrasound. 1986;14(7):529–33.
84. Bujold E, Jastrow N, Simoneau J, Brunet S, Gauthier RJ. Prediction of complete uterine rupture by sonographic evaluation of the lower uterine segment. Am J Obstet Gynecol. 2009;201(3):320.e1–6.
85. Kok N, Wiersma IC, Opmeer BC, de Graaf IM, Mol BW, Pajkrt E. Sonographic measurement of lower uterine segment thickness to predict uterine rupture during a trial of labor in women with previous cesarean section: a meta-analysis. Ultrasound Obstet Gynecol. 2013;42(2):132–9.
86. Fukuda M, Fukuda K, Shimizu T, Bujold E. Ultrasound assessment of lower uterine segment thickness during pregnancy, labour, and the postpartum period. J Obstet Gynaecol Can. 2016;38(2):134–40.
87. Barzilay E, Shay A, Lahav-Ezra H, Shina A, Perlman S, Achiron R, Gilboa Y. Sonographic assessment of the

lower uterine segment during active labor in women with or without a uterine scar—a prospective study. J Matern Fetal Neonatal Med. 2017:1–4. https://doi.org/10.1080/14767058.2017. [Epub ahead of print].
88. Lazarus E, Mayo-Smith WW, Mainiero MB, Spencer PK. CT in the evaluation of nontraumatic abdominal pain in pregnant women. Radiology. 2007;244(3):784–90.
89. Hruska KM, Coughlin BF, Coggins AA, Wiczyk HP. MRI diagnosis of spontaneous uterine rupture of an unscarred uterus. Emerg Radiol. 2006;12(4):186–8.
90. Vlemminx MW, de Lau H, Oei SG. Tocogram characteristics of uterine rupture: a systematic review. Arch Gynecol Obstet. 2017;295(1):17–26.
91. Hill CC, Pickinpaugh J. Trauma and surgical emergencies in the obstetric patient. Surg Clin North Am. 2008;88(2):421–40.
92. Vaknin Z, Maymon R, Mendlovic S, Barel O, Herman A, Sherman D. Clinical, sonographic, and epidemiologic features of second- and early third-trimester spontaneous antepartum uterine rupture: a cohort study. Prenat Diagn. 2008;28(6):478–84.
93. Dow M, Wax JR, Pinette MG, Blackstone J, Cartin A. Third-trimester uterine rupture without previous cesarean: a case series and review of the literature. Am J Perinatol. 2009;26(10):739–44.
94. Damiani GR, Gaetani M, Landi S, Lacerenza L, Barnaba M, Spellecchia D, Pellegrino A. Uterine rupture in a nulliparous woman with septate uterus of the second trimester pregnancy and review in literature. Int J Surg Case Rep. 2013;4(3):259–61.
95. Ofir K, Sheiner E, Levy A, Katz M, Mazor M. Uterine rupture: risk factors and pregnancy outcome. Am J Obstet Gynecol. 2003;189(4):1042–6.
96. Ritchie EH. Pregnancy after rupture of the pregnant uterus. A report of 36 pregnancies and a study of cases reported since 1932. J Obstet Gynaecol Br Commonw. 1971;78(7):642–8.
97. Tversky A, Kahneman D. Belief in the law of small numbers. Psychol Bull. 1971;76(2):105–10.

In Utero Surgery for Spina Bifida Aperta

32

Jan Deprest, Roland Devlieger, Frank Van Calenbergh, Sarah Devroe, Hannes Van der Merwe, Liesbeth Lewi, Luc De Catte, and Luc Joyeux

Introduction

Congenital malformations occur in 2–4% of all births. Despite their low prevalence, they are responsible for approximately 30% of perinatal deaths and considerable infant morbidity. Congenital anomalies were previously typically diagnosed in the second trimester; current first trimester screening programs, improved imaging hardware, and skills should allow for an early diagnosis. One of the conditions that may be picked up are neural tube defects (NTD). NTD are the most common anomaly of the central nervous system, with a prevalence in Europe of around 9 per 10,000 births [1]. Spina bifida (SB) aperta (including myelomeningocele [MMC] and myeloschisis, Fig. 32.1) refers to the subtype caused by the failed closure of the distal neural tube during the embryonic period (referred to as "first hit"). It is characterized by the extrusion of the meninges and the spinal cord through a bony and soft tissue defect that appears cystic (MMC) or not (myeloschisis). The exposure of the developing spinal cord and nerves to the amniotic fluid as well as direct trauma causes progressive damage (the "second" hit). The functional impact is highly dependent on the level and extension of the lesion [2, 3]. Clinically this means, upper extremity sensori-motor disruption of function, along with orthopedic disabilities, as well as in lower lesions; in sacral lesions we have bowel, bladder and sexual dysfunction [2, 4, 5]. Leakage of the cerebrospinal fluid leads to the downward displacement of the cerebellum and brain (Chiari malformation type II—CM II) and potentially also ventriculomegaly [2]. That caudal displacement is already visible at 11–13 weeks [6], yet clinically most cases are still diagnosed in the second trimester [7]. The prenatal diagnosis of SB today has become relevant because the most common form, spina bifida aperta (SBA), is amenable for fetal surgery, as an additional option next to expectant management or termination of pregnancy. SBA has a prevalence of 4.9 per 10,000 live births in

Electronic Supplementary Material The online version of this chapter (https://doi.org/10.1007/978-3-319-90752-9_32) contains supplementary material, which is available to authorized users.

J. Deprest (✉) · L. De Catte · L. Lewi · R. Devlieger
Department of Obstetrics and Gynaecology, University Hospitals Leuven, Campus Gasthuisberg, Leuven, Belgium
e-mail: jan.deprest@uzleuven.be

F. Van Calenbergh
Department of Neurosurgery, University Hospitals Leuven, Campus Gasthuisberg, Leuven, Belgium

S. Devroe
Department of Anesthesiology, University Hospitals Leuven, Campus Gasthuisberg, Leuven, Belgium

H. Van der Merwe · L. Joyeux
Department of Development and Regeneration, Cluster Woman and Child, Katholieke Universiteit Leuven, Leuven, Belgium

C. H. Nezhat (ed.), *Non-Obstetric Surgery During Pregnancy*,
https://doi.org/10.1007/978-3-319-90752-9_32

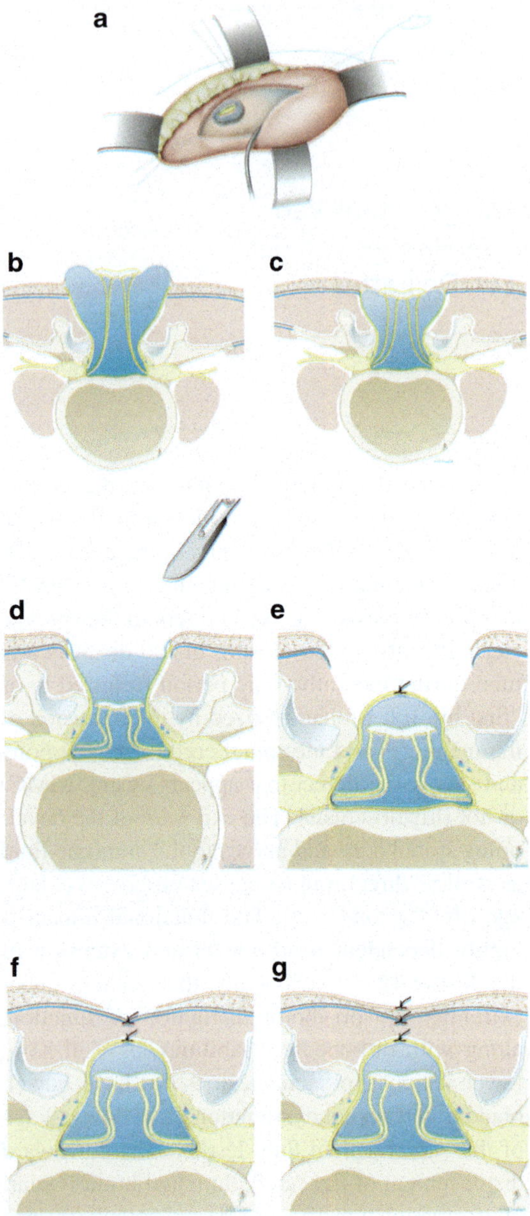

Fig. 32.1 Schematic drawings of the steps of open fetal surgical repair. (**a**) Laparotomy and exposition of the uterus; stapled hysterotomy and exposition of a myelomeningocele (MMC); (**b**) schematic drawing of a myelomeningocele, with the placode being part of the bulging cystic lesion; (**c**) schematic drawing of a case of myeloschisis, with the placode surfacing on a collapsed arachnoidal space; (**d**) dissection and untethering of the neural placode. This is followed by anatomical closure in three layers: closure of the dural sac (**e**), the myofascial flaps (**f**), and the skin (**g**). There are other techniques being used, i.e., using patches or at times closing the lesion in less or even more layers. Drawings by Myrthe Boymans. Copyright UZ Leuven, Leuven, Belgium

Europe and 3.17 in the USA [1, 8–10]. Despite improved prevention, early diagnosis, and specialized postnatal management, SBA remains a major source of morbidity and mortality throughout the world [2]. Over 80% of children require lifelong ventriculoperitoneal shunting or an alternative, of whom up to 50% will have shunt complications in the first year of life [11].

The in utero progressive nature of the condition led to the concept of fetal intervention, which arrests or reverses the process. Successful layered anatomical repair of SBA with improved functional outcome was first experimentally described in the late 1990s [12]. This was translated clinically with encouraging early results in several case series [13, 14]. Because there was no objective evidence of the benefit of fetal repair, the National Institutes of Health sponsored a randomized controlled trial, entitled Management of Myelomeningocele Study (MOMS), while at the same time embargoing this procedure in the USA to be offered outside this trial. The MOMS trial demonstrated that mid-gestational layered repair reduces the need for ventriculoperitoneal shunting, improves the degree of hindbrain herniation, and better preserves motor function when compared to postnatal surgery. Fetal repair is however not without significant risks, such as premature delivery and maternal complications. Additionaly, the corporeal scar compromises uterine integrity.

Indications and Operative Technique

The selection criteria for this operation are summarized in Table 32.1. The procedure requires maternal general inhalational anesthesia, which provides uterine relaxation and fetal anesthesia. The fetus is manually positioned such that the myelomeningocele sac is in the center of the future hysterotomy (Figs. 32.1a and 32.2a). That location is also dependent on the placental location, which is to be avoided at all price. In most centers, this incision is made with specifically designed resorbable uterine staplers. The fetus is given an additional intramuscular injection of fentanyl and a muscle relaxant. Then a catheter is connected to an

Table 32.1 Inclusion and exclusion criteria of the randomized MOMS trial

Inclusion criteria
• Maternal age ≥18 years
• Gestational age at randomization 19 weeks, 0 day–25 weeks, 6 days
• Normal karyotype
• S1-level lesion or higher
• Confirmed CM II type II malformation on prenatal ultrasound and magnetic resonance imaging
Exclusion criteria
• Multiple gestation pregnancy
• Insulin-dependent pregestational diabetes (meanwhile well-controlled diabetes is accepted)
• Additional fetal anomalies unrelated to myelomeningocele
• Fetal kyphosis ≥30 degrees
• History of incompetent cervix and/or short cervix <20 mm by ultrasound scan
• Placenta previa
• Other serious maternal medical conditions
• Obesity defined by body mass index of ≥35 (this has meanwhile been raised to 40)
• Previous spontaneous singleton delivery <37 weeks gestation
• Maternal-fetal Rh isoimmunization
• Positive maternal human immunodeficiency virus or hepatitis B or known hepatitis C positivity
• No support person to stay with the pregnant women at the center
• Uterine anomaly
• Psychosocial limitations
• Inability to comply with travel and follow-up protocols

irrigator which can maintain sufficient amniotic fluid levels during the surgery (not all centers do this). The actual MMC repair is not different from what is typically done after birth. The neurosurgery starts with the dissection of the placode, so that the spinal cord can sink into the spinal canal (Figs. 32.1b–d, 32.2b and 32.3a; Video 32.1). The dura is either closed primarily, or in case of a large defect, a patch can be used (Figs. 32.1e and 32.3b) [15]. Lumbodorsal fascial flaps are mainly freed and used to cover the dural repair (Figs. 32.1f and 32.3c). Finally the skin is closed (Figs. 32.1g and 32.3d). This technique is usually referred to as "anatomical repair," hence the same as is done postnatally [15, 16]. For larger defects skin substitutes can be used as well while others have been using relaxing incisions (Fig. 32.4).

The uterus is closed in two layers with prior restoration of amniotic fluid and antibiotic administration and covered with an omental patch. Prophylactic tocolytics are started (in the USA this is typically magnesium sulfate (24 h); in Europe this will be atosiban, which reduces maternal side effects). The other perioperative drug used for 48 h is indomethacin though that, together with maternal hyperoxygenation and deep inhalation anesthesia, may affect fetal cardiac contractility. Oral nifedipine is continued until 37 weeks. Typical hospital stay is 4 days. Elective cesarean delivery by lower uterine incision is at 37 weeks.

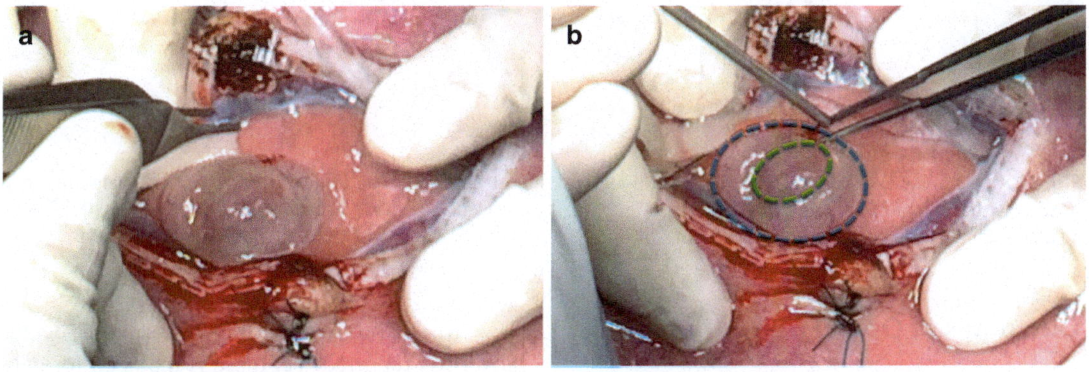

Fig. 32.2 Exposition and dissection of a myelomeningocele during open fetal surgery. These are pictures from a surgery in a 25-week fetus exposed via laparotomy and hysterotomy (**a**). First, the junction line between the skin (blue circle) and sac (green circle) is circumferentially sharply dissected, with preservation of all neural components as much as possible (**b**). Any pathological elements that are attached to the placode, i.e., the sac, zona epitheliosa, and junction line, are resected. Copyright UZ Leuven, Leuven, Belgium

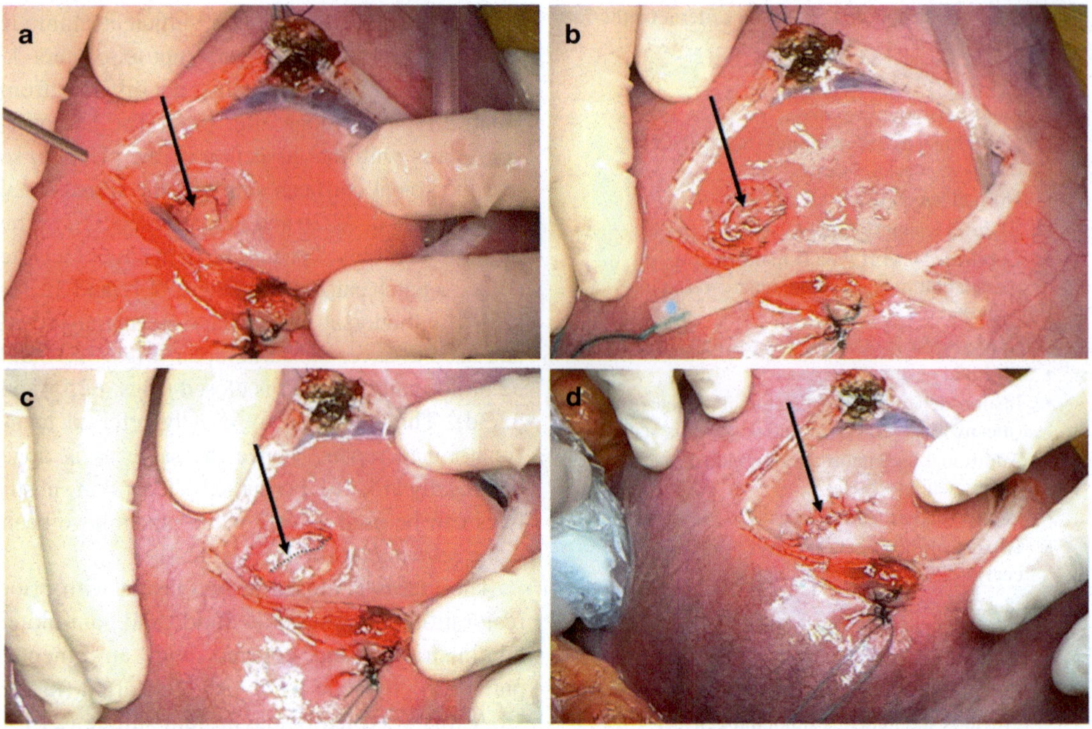

Fig. 32.3 Technique of primary anatomical layered repair of a myelomeningocele. Once dissection is completed, the neural placode is untethered and spontaneously drops into the spinal canal (**a**). Then anatomical closure in three layers is attempted. First, the dural sac (**b**) is closed with a 6/0 running suture. Then the skin is undermined, and paraspinal myofascial flaps are raised and closed over the closed dura (**c**). Finally the skin is closed (**d**) using a 4/0 running monofilament suture. Copyright UZ Leuven, Leuven, Belgium

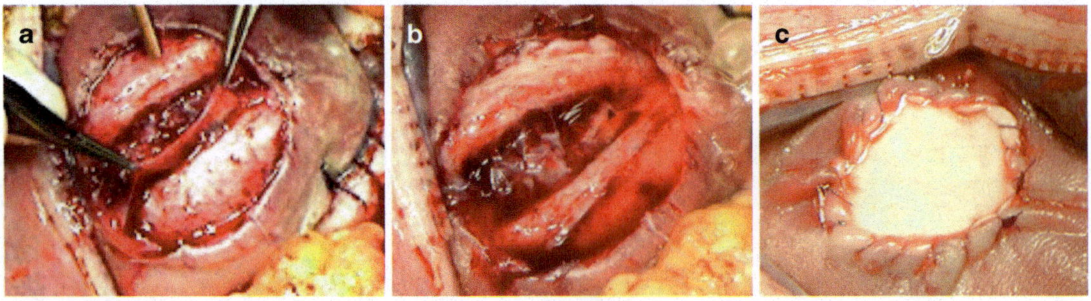

Fig. 32.4 Technique of patch repair of a large myelomeningocele. In 20% of cases, the lesion may be so large that a skin patch (**c**) may be required after closure of dura (**a**) and fascia (**b**) underneath. Alternatively, relaxing incisions may be made lateral to the defect over the flanks (not shown). Copyright UZ Leuven, Leuven, Belgium

Outcomes of Open Fetal Surgery

Immediate Maternal and Fetal Outcomes

Open SBA repair via hysterotomy has a number of inherent risks and postoperative complications [17, 18]. To our knowledge, no maternal deaths have been reported. Yet there is the need for general anesthesia and the administration of drugs with potential side effects, such as pulmonary edema. There is also the impact of laparotomy (Table 32.2) [17, 19]. Following corporeal hysterotomy to expose the lesion, uterine dehiscence

Table 32.2 Maternal outcomes comparing open fetal surgery to postnatal surgery for SBA as in the MOMS randomized clinical trial [19]

	Open fetal repair	Postnatal repair	Statistical analysis	
Number of pregnancies/fetuses	78 (MOMS trial) 91 (complete trial cohort)	80 (MOMS trial) 92 (complete trial cohort)	Relative risk (95% CI)	*P* value
Fetal profile				
Gestational age at randomization	23.7 ± 1.4	23.9 ± 1.3	NS	≥0.5
Operative outcomes				
Intraoperative incomplete closure (abandoned procedure)	0% (0/91)	0% (0/92)	NA	NA
Bradycardia during repair	10.3% (8/78)	0% (0/80)	NA	**0.003**
Mean operation time (skin-to-skin in min)	105.2 ± 21.8*	NA	NA	NA
Maternal outcomes				
Placental abruption	6.6 (6/91)	0% (0/92)	NA	**0.01**
Pulmonary edema	5.5% (5/91)	0% (0/92)	NA	**0.03**
Chorioamnionitis	2.2% (2/91)	0% (0/92)	NA	0.25
Oligohydramnios	20% (19/91)	3.3% (3/92)	6.40 (1.96–20.89)	**<0.001**
Chorioamniotic membrane separation	30% (33.0)	0% (0/92)	NA	**<0.001**
Preterm premature rupture of membranes (PPROM)	44% (40/91)	7.6% (7/92)	5.78 (2.73–12.22)	**<0.001**
Hemorrhage requiring transfusion at delivery	8.8% (8/91)	1.1% (1/92)	8.09 (1.03–63.37)	**0.02**
Hysterotomy scar thinning or dehiscence at delivery	35.3% (31/88)	NA	NA	NA

NA not applicable, *NS* not stated
p values in bold indicate significance
*Plus–minus values are means ±SD

may develop. In analogy to any other corporeal incision, mothers are not allowed to labor and deliver vaginally in the index and future pregnancies. On the fetal side, there is the intraoperative occurrence of reduced heart contractility and/or bradycardia, seldom leading to cardiac arrest [19]. Also the risk for peripartal hemorrhage is higher.

Elective, or in case of preterm labor or any other complication, delivery is by lower uterine cesarean section. Mothers are advised not to become pregnant within the next 2 years [17, 19, 20]. Results from other similar fetal surgeries suggest that the reproductive outcome is not compromised [20].

The reduced heart contractility and/or bradycardia seldom leading to cardiac arrest which are believed to be caused by the effects of inhalational anesthesia, yet traction on the skin and intra-abdominal compression may also contribute. In the MOMS trial, the perinatal mortality of fetal surgery was comparable to that of postnatal surgery (1–2%), yet the causes are different [18, 19]. In essence, in prenatally managed cases, deaths are due to fetal distress at the time of surgery or preterm birth. In postnatally managed cases, mortality is due to the consequences of symptomatic CM II. Preterm birth may cause respiratory distress syndrome (20.8%) and other prematurity-related problems (Table 32.3).

From a neurosurgical viewpoint, postnatal surgery is rarely needed. Reintervention for postnatal wound healing problems such as persisting cerebrospinal fluid leak or dehiscence is rare (2.6%). In about one fifth of cases, a patch may be required, and depending on the exact material used, a wound revision may be needed.

1- and 2.5-Year Neurologic Outcomes

In the MOMS trial, the need for ventriculoperitoneal shunting at 12 months was reduced (see Table 32.3). The exact rate of shunting was depen-

Table 32.3 Fetal and pediatric outcomes comparing open fetal surgery to postnatal surgery for SBA as in the MOMS randomized clinical trial [19]

Results of the MOMS trial	Open fetal repair	Postnatal repair	Statistical analysis	
Number of pregnancies/fetuses	78 (MOMS trial) 91 (complete trial cohort)	80 (MOMS trial) 92 (complete trial cohort)	Relative risk (95% CI)	*P* value
Fetal profile				
Lesion level on ultrasonography				
– Thoracic	5.1% (4/78)	3.7% (3/80)	NS	≥0.5
– L1–L2	27% (21/78)	12.5% (10/80)	NS	≥0.5
– L3–L4	38.5% (30/78)	56.2% (45/80)	NS	≥0.5
– L5–S1	29.5% (23/78)	27.5% (22/80)	NS	≥0.5
Fetal and neonatal outcomes[a]				
Perinatal mortality[a]	2.2% (2/91)	2.2% (2/92)	1.01 (0.1–9.34)	1.00
Mean gestational age at birth (weeks)	34.0 ± 3.0	37.3 ± 1.1	NA	**<0.001**
Preterm birth <30 weeks	11% (10/91)	0% (0/92)	NA	**0.001**
Mean birth weight (g)	2383 ± 688	3039 ± 469	NA	**<0.001**
Partial dehiscence at repair site not requiring reoperation	13% (10/77)	6.3% (5/80)	2.05 (0.73–5.73)	0.16
Postnatal additional SBA surgical repair[b]	2.6% (2/77)[c]	NS	NA	NA
Respiratory distress syndrome	20.8% (16/77)	6.3% (5/80)	3.32 (1.28–8.63)	**0.008**
Periventricular leukomalacia	5.2% (4/77)	2.5% (2/80)	2.08 (0.39–11.02)	0.44
Necrotizing enterocolitis	1.3% (1/77)	0% (0/80)	NA	0.49
Pediatric outcomes				
At 1 year	*Improvement of structures of central nervous system*			
Primary outcome (fetal/neonatal death or the need for CSF shunt)	72.5% (66/91)[d]	97.8% (90/92)[d]	0.74 (0.65–0.85)[d]	**<0.001**[d]
Placement of CSF shunt	44.0% (40/91)[d]	83.7% (77/92)[d]	0.53 (0.41–0.67)[d]	**<0.0001**[d]
Shunt revision	15.4% (14/91)	40.2% (37/92)	0.38 (0.22–0.66)	**<0.001**[d]
Any hindbrain herniation	64.3% (45/70)	95.6% (66/69)	0.67 (0.56–0.81)	**<0.001**
Complete reversal of Chiari malformation	35.7% (25/70)	4.3% (3/69)	NS	**<0.001**
Chiari malformation decompression surgery	1.3% (1/77)	5% (4/80)	0.26 (0.03–2.24)	0.37
Surgery for tethered cord	7.8% (6/77)	1.2% (1/80)	6.15 (0.76–50.00)	0.06
At 2.5 years	*Improvement of function of peripheral nervous system*			
Primary outcome[e]	199.4 ± 80.5	166.6 ± 76.7	NA	**0.004**
Bayley Mental Development Index[f]	89.5 ± 15.0	86.2 ± 18.1	NA	0.22
Difference between motor function and anatomical levels[g]	−0.80 ± 5.5	−1.56 ± 4.7	NA	**0.002**
≥2 levels better	26.4% (23/87)	11.4% (10/88)		
1 level better	11.5% (10/87)	8.0% (7/88)		
No difference	26.4% (23/87)	21.6% (19/88)		

Results of the MOMS trial	Open fetal repair	Postnatal repair	Statistical analysis	
1 level worse	19.5% (17/87)	27.3% (24/88)		
≥2 levels worse	16.1% (14/87)	31.8% (28/88)		
Independent walking (ability to walk without orthotics or devices)	44.8% (39/87)	23.9% (21/88)	1.88 (1.21–2.92)	**0.004**
Bayley Psychomotor Development Index[f] (mean)	63.9 ± 17.3	58.9 ± 15.1	NA	**0.03**
Peabody developmental motor scales (locomotion)	3.0 ± 1.8	2.1 ± 1.5	NA	**0.001**
WeeFIM score (degree of disability)[h]				
– Mobility – Self-care – Cognitive	19.6 ± 6.5 20.8 ± 4.4 25.0 ± 5.7	16.2 ± 6.2 19.0 ± 4.3 24.9 ± 6.3	NA NA NA	**<0.001** **0.006** 0.74
At 2.5 years	*Urologic outcomes*			
Number of children	56	59	RR (95% CI)	*P* value
Primary outcome (death or need for CIC by 30 months)	52% (29/56)	66% (39/59)	0.78 (0.57–1.07)	0.133
Death at 2.5 years	0% (0/56)	0% (0/59)	NA	1.00
Patients on CIC use	38% (21/56)	51% (30/59)	0.74 (0.48–1.12)	0.189
Bladder trabeculations on urodynamics and ultrasound	8% (4/51)	33% (17/52)	0.39 (0.19–0.79)	**0.003**
Open bladder neck on urodynamics	26% (13/51)	44% (23/52)	0.71 (0.46–1.09)	0.063
At 2.5 years	*Impact on family and parental stress*			
Number of women	87	88	RR (95% CI)	*P* value
Total parental stress (PSI-SF)	61.3 ± 21.3	60.3 ± 15.4	NA	0.89
Familial-social impact (IFS)	14.0 ± 3.8	15.3 ± 3.7	NA	**0.004**
IFS score	24.6 ± 6.5	26.8 ± 6.6	NA	**0.02**

p values in bold indicate significance

When data are available from the complete trial cohort, only the latter ones are displayed [17, 18, 21]. Further there is data from two substudies evaluating urological outcomes [22] and the impact on family and parental stress [23]. *P* value indicates statistically significant values

SBA spina bifida aperta, *MOMS* Management Of Myelomeningocele Study, *CM* Chiari II malformation, *NS* nonspecified, *NA* non-applicable, *GA* gestational age, *CSF* cerebrospinal fluid, *CIC* clean intermittent catheterization, *RR* relative risk, *CI* confidence interval, *PSI-SF* 36-item Parenting Stress Index-Short Form, *IFS* 15-item Impact on Family Scale

[a]Based on the number of live-born infants. Like in the MOMS trial, perinatal mortality was defined by the number of fetal and neonatal (within 28 days of life) deaths

[b]Postnatal reoperation in case of dehiscence of all layers

[c]Data from our previous systematic review [24]

[d]One-year outcomes for the complete MOMS trial: only ventricular size is associated with the need for shunting, and prenatal surgery does not improve shunt outcome when ventricular size is ≥15 mm; lesion level and degree of CM had no effect on the eventual need for shunting [21]

[e]Primary outcome at 2.5 years: score derived from the Bayley Mental Development Index and the difference between functional and anatomical levels of the lesion

[f]On the Bayley Scales of Infant Development II, the Mental Development Index and the Psychomotor Development Index are both scaled to have a population mean (±SD) of 100 ± 15, with a minimum score of 50 and a maximum score 150. Higher scores indicate better performance

[g]For the difference between the motor function level and the anatomical level, positive values indicate function that is better than expected on the basis of the anatomical level

[h]The WeeFIM score (functional independence measure for children) measures the degree of disability in children. On the WeeFIM evaluation, the score on the self-care measurement ranges from 8 to 56, and scores on the mobility and cognitive measurements range from 5 to 35, with higher scores indicating greater independence

dent on prenatal ventricular dimensions. When the ventricles were ≥15 mm (normal range <10 mm), the shunting rate was as high as in postnatally operated cases [21]. The reduction in shunting was maximal in those fetuses with normal ventricles. Fetal surgery also improved motor outcomes at 30 months (see Table 32.3) [18, 19, 21]. Children were more likely to have a level of function that was on average two levels better than expected based on the anatomical level. Postnatal motor function showed no correlation with either prenatal ventricular size or postnatal shunt placement [18]. The effects on the bladder were mixed [22]. There was a reduction in bladder trabeculation, a marker of bladder outlet obstruction, and less frequently an open bladder neck on video-urodynamic examination, a marker of bladder dysfunction, yet the rate of clean intermittent catheterization at 30 months was not different (see Table 32.3) [22].

One of the major postoperative neurosurgical complications of spina bifida repair in general is tethered cord syndrome. This is the secondary attachment of the spinal cord to the scar, in some cass leading to dysfunction and pain. There are no good numbers yet that can determine whether tethered cord is more likely after fetal surgery or not. Data from patients operated in the pre-MOMS era show that the incidence is identical to what was earlier reported in postnatally repaired cohorts. However, tethered cord in prenatally operated patients occurred more often in association with the development of cutaneously derived intradural inclusion cysts [15, 25].

Prenatal rather than postnatal repair had a positive impact on the family, yet parental stress remained comparable [26]. The main determinants of such outcomes were the ability of the child to walk independently and greater family resources.

5-Year Outcomes

The long-term outcomes of the MOMS cohort are not yet known at the time of this writing. Therefore one has to rely on data from operations done before that study. The Philadelphia team reported on a prospective cohort of 58 children who met the majority of the MOMS criteria operated in utero. They all had a ventricular size <17 mm and conserved motor function in the lower limbs at the time of fetal surgery [27]. Children operated in utero had brain stem function and lower extremity neuromotor function better than expected yet not in the normal range [27]. Preschool neurodevelopmental outcomes, especially intelligence quotient, were within the normal range [28]. Though better than expected, preschool functional independence did not fall within the normal range. Total, neurocognitive and mobility independence were higher in non-shunted than shunted patients and in children with average neurodevelopmental scores. Self-care independence tended to be higher [28]. There was no increase in behavioral problems, impaired social interactions, and restricted behavior patterns [29]. Quality of life outcome data of families and their children has not yet been reported in this population.

10-Year Outcomes

Open fetal surgery (OFS) for SBA improved long-term neurodevelopmental and neurofunctional outcomes as well as long-term ambulatory status compared to historical controls [30]. Concerning the social outcomes, there are no data so far; however one can speculate that also this would be better after OFS. Whereas this surgery certainly does not cure the disease, much of it will depend on whether there is an improved self-care capacity, which can increase the opportunity for peer relationships, decrease prolonged caregiver dependency, and increase community acceptance. On the other hand, OFS increases independent mobility, which would justify to expect a long-term benefit. In a cross-sectional study on 122 children with SBA operated postnatally, good mental ability, muscle strength, and being independent in mobility were the best predictors of daily life function and quality of life [31].

Alternative Techniques

The downside of OFS is the increased maternal morbidity and the risk of prematurity—mainly due to membrane rupture—and the large uterine incision, which may lead to dehiscence in 10% of cases. Uterine scarring may have an effect on the index and future pregnancies, which is a limitation [20]. Therefore, teams have been exploring what is possible by fetoscopy, which would obviate most likely the latter problem, as demonstrated in mothers undergoing fetoscopic laser ablation for transfusion syndrome or balloon occlusion for congenital diaphragmatic hernia [32, 33]. Currently fetoscopic SBA repair is still technically challenging. The operation times are very long, and the initial surgical failure rate is high. Moreover, the fetal loss rate is higher, and there is an ongoing vivid debate about the potential side effects of carbon dioxide insufflation [34–38]. Surgeons also have to resort to alternative neurosurgical repair techniques, either covering the dissected defect in two layers by a combination of patch and skin closure or a single layer (patch or skin) (Fig. 32.5). Most of these techniques seem to evolve as experience grows. However, one should realize that the experimental basis for these is often lacking [42]. Ideally, these alternative surgical techniques need to be formally weighed against the gold standard, which is the open layered repair, ideally in a head-to-head comparison.

Reducing invasiveness should however be investigated for two reasons: first, from a maternal perspective, to avoid the abdominal incision but, more importantly, to reduce the uterine scar

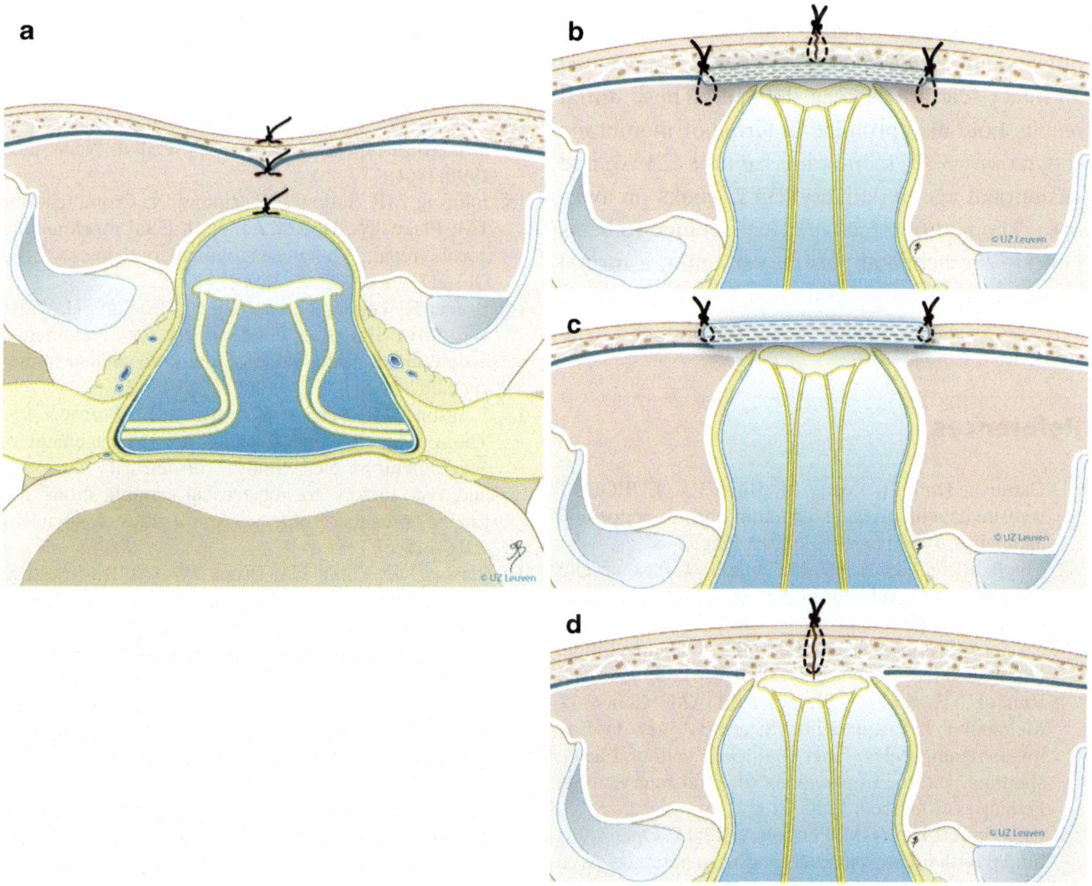

Fig. 32.5 Comparison of closure techniques. Schematic representation of neurosurgical closure following dissection and untethering, either (**a**) through multilayered repair involving the dura, musculofascial structures, and skin, as in the previous figures, or (**b**) using a dural substitute, consisting of a biocellulose patch, as described in [39, 40] or (**c**) a skin substitute. In some reports, two grafts are used to assist myofascial and skin closure. More recently a technique with only skin closure (**d**) was reported [26, 41]. Drawings by Myrthe Boymans. Copyright UZ Leuven, Leuven, Belgium

with its persistent consequences. The second reason is that it may reduce membrane rupture rates hence preterm delivery. Counterintuitively, this seems not to be the case when systematically reviewing the initial fetoscopy experience [24]. However, in the most recent experience by the Houston group exteriorizing the uterus through laparotomy, the placement of two ports, and surgical closure of puncture sites; early results suggest a lower membrane rupture rate [41, 43]. There is, however, one other approach which may reconciliate the best of both worlds. These Brazilian surgeons perform a multilayer anatomical repair under the operation microscope through a 3-cm mini-hysterotomy [44]. In other words, they do not compromise on the operative technique formally tested in a randomized trial, while on the other hand, the uterine access is much smaller. Of 45 patients operated, 95% had an intact scar at cesarean delivery. These initial results hold also promise in terms of membrane separation (3%), membrane rupture (23%), and gestational age at delivery (35.2 weeks on average). The neuroprotective effect seemed to be as good in the neonatal period, yet again, a formal comparison is not possible given other selection criteria.

References

1. Garne E, Dolk H, Loane M, Boyd PA. EUROCAT website data on prenatal detection rates of congenital anomalies. J Med Screen. 2010;17(2):97–8.
2. Mitchell LE, Adzick NS, Melchionne J, Pasquariello PS, Sutton LN, Whitehead AS. Spina bifida. Lancet. 2004;364(9448):1885–95.
3. Bruner JP, Tulipan N. Tell the truth about spina bifida. Ultrasound Obstet Gynecol. 2004;24(6):595–6.
4. Rintoul NE, Sutton LN, Hubbard AM, Cohen B, Melchionni J, Pasquariello PS, et al. A new look at myelomeningoceles: functional level, vertebral level, shunting, and the implications for fetal intervention. Pediatrics. 2002;109(3):409–13.
5. Oakeshott P, Hunt GM, Poulton A, Reid F. Open spina bifida: birth findings predict long-term outcome. Arch Dis Child. 2012;97(5):474–6.
6. Engels AC, Joyeux L, Brantner C, De Keersmaecker B, De Catte L, Baud D, et al. Sonographic detection of central nervous system defects in the first trimester of pregnancy. Prenat Diagn. 2016;36(3):266–73.
7. Ovaere C, Eggink A, Richter J, Cohen-Overbeek TE, Van Calenbergh F, Jansen K, et al. Prenatal diagnosis and patient preferences in patients with neural tube defects around the advent of fetal surgery in Belgium and Holland. Fetal Diagn Ther. 2015;37(3):226–34.
8. Khoshnood B, Loane M, de Walle H, Arriola L, Addor MC, Barisic I, et al. Long term trends in prevalence of neural tube defects in Europe: population based study. BMJ. 2015;351:h5949.
9. European Surveillance of Congenital Anomalies [Internet]. www.eurocat-network.eu.
10. Canfield MA, Mai CT, Wang Y, O'Halloran A, Marengo LK, Olney RS, et al. The association between race/ethnicity and major birth defects in the United States, 1999–2007. Am J Pub Health. 2014;104(9):e14–23.
11. Caldarelli M, Di Rocco C, La Marca F. Shunt complications in the first postoperative year in children with meningomyelocele. Childs Nerv Syst. 1996;12(12):748–54.
12. Meuli M, Meuli-Simmen C, Hutchins GM, Yingling CD, Hoffman KM, Harrison MR, et al. In utero surgery rescues neurological function at birth in sheep with spina bifida. Nat Med. 1995;1(4):342–7.
13. Adzick NS, Sutton LN, Crombleholme TM, Flake AW. Successful fetal surgery for spina bifida. Lancet. 1998;352(9141):1675–6.
14. Tulipan N, Bruner JP. Myelomeningocele repair in utero: a report of three cases. Pediatr Neurosurg. 1998;28(4):177–80.
15. Johnson MP, Sutton LN, Rintoul N, Crombleholme TM, Flake AW, Howell LJ, et al. Fetal myelomeningocele repair: short-term clinical outcomes. Am J Obstet Gynecol. 2003;189(2):482–7.
16. Bruner JP, Tulipan N, Paschall RL, Boehm FH, Walsh WF, Silva SR, et al. Fetal surgery for myelomeningocele and the incidence of shunt-dependent hydrocephalus. JAMA. 1999;282(19):1819–25.
17. Johnson MP, Bennett KA, Rand L, Burrows PK, Thom EA, Howell LJ, et al. The Management of Myelomeningocele Study: obstetrical outcomes and risk factors for obstetrical complications following prenatal surgery. Am J Obstet Gynecol. 2016;215(6):778.e1–9.
18. Farmer DL, Thom EA, Brock JW 3rd, Burrows PK, Johnson MP, Howell LJ, et al. The Management of Myelomeningocele Study: full cohort 30 month pediatric outcomes. Am J Obstet Gynecol. 2018;218(2):256.e1–256.e13.
19. Adzick NS, Thom EA, Spong CY, Brock JW 3rd, Burrows PK, Johnson MP, et al. A randomized trial of prenatal versus postnatal repair of myelomeningocele. N Engl J Med. 2011;364(11):993–1004.
20. Wilson RD, Lemerand K, Johnson MP, Flake AW, Bebbington M, Hedrick HL, et al. Reproductive outcomes in subsequent pregnancies after a pregnancy complicated by open maternal-fetal surgery (1996–2007). Am J Obstet Gynecol. 2010;203(3):209.e1–6.
21. Tulipan N, Wellons JC 3rd, Thom EA, Gupta N, Sutton LN, Burrows PK, et al. Prenatal surgery for myelomeningocele and the need for cerebrospinal fluid shunt placement. J Neurosurg Pediatr. 2015;16:1–8.

22. Brock JW 3rd, Carr MC, Adzick NS, Burrows PK, Thomas JC, Thom EA, et al. Bladder function after fetal surgery for Myelomeningocele. Pediatrics. 2015;136(4):e906–13.
23. Antiel RM, Adzick NS, Thom EA, Burrows PK, Farmer DL, Brock JW 3rd, et al. Impact on family and parental stress of prenatal vs postnatal repair of myelomeningocele. Am J Obstet Gynecol. 2016;215(4):522.e1–6.
24. Joyeux L, Engels AC, Russo FM, Jimenez J, Van Mieghem T, De Coppi P, et al. Fetoscopic versus open repair for spina bifida aperta: a systematic review of outcomes. Fetal Diagn Ther. 2016;39(3):161–71.
25. Danzer E, Adzick NS, Rintoul NE, Zarnow DM, Schwartz ES, Melchionni J, et al. Intradural inclusion cysts following in utero closure of myelomeningocele: clinical implications and follow-up findings. J Neurosurg Pediatr. 2008;2(6):406–13.
26. Belfort M, Deprest J, Hecher K. Current controversies in prenatal diagnosis 1: in utero therapy for spina bifida is ready for endoscopic repair. Prenat Diagn. 2016;36(13):1161–6.
27. Danzer E, Gerdes M, Bebbington MW, Zarnow DM, Adzick NS, Johnson MP. Preschool neurodevelopmental outcome of children following fetal myelomeningocele closure. Am J Obstet Gynecol. 2010;202(5):450.e1–9.
28. Danzer E, Gerdes M, Bebbington MW, Koh J, Adzick SN, Johnson MP. Fetal myelomeningocele surgery: preschool functional status using the functional independence measure for children (WeeFIM). Childs Nerv Syst. 2011;27(7):1083–8.
29. Danzer E, Gerdes M, Bebbington MW, Koh J, Adzick NS, Johnson MP. Preschool neurobehavioral outcome following fetal myelomeningocele surgery. Fetal Diagn Ther. 2011;30(3):174–9.
30. Danzer E, Thomas NH, Thomas A, Friedman KB, Gerdes M, Koh J, et al. Long-term neurofunctional outcome, executive functioning, and behavioral adaptive skills following fetal myelomeningocele surgery. Am J Obstet Gynecol. 2016;214(2):269.e1–8.
31. Schoenmakers MA, Uiterwaal CS, Gulmans VA, Gooskens RH, Helders PJ. Determinants of functional independence and quality of life in children with spina bifida. Clin Rehabil. 2005;19(6):677–85.
32. Gregoir C, Engels AC, Gomez O, DeKoninck P, Lewi L, Gratacos E, et al. Fertility, pregnancy and gynecological outcomes after fetoscopic surgery for congenital diaphragmatic hernia. Hum Reprod. 2016;31(9):2024–30.
33. Vergote S, Lewi L, Gheysen W, de Catte L, Devlieger R, Deprest J. Subsequent fertility, pregnancy and gynecologic outcomes after fetoscopic laser therapy for twin-twin transfusion syndrome compared to normal monochorionic twin gestations. Am J Obstet Gynecol. 2018;218(4):447.e1–7. https://doi.org/10.1016/j.ajog.2018.01.013.
34. Flake A. Percutaneous minimal-access fetoscopic surgery for myelomeningocele—not so minimal! Ultrasound Obstet Gynecol. 2014;44(5):499–500.
35. Mazzone L, Meuli M. Re: Fetoscopic repair of spina bifida: safer and better? Ultrasound Obstet Gynecol. 2016;48(6):802.
36. Moise KJ Jr, Flake A. Fetoscopic open neural tube defect repair: development and refinement of a two-port, carbon dioxide insufflation technique. Obstet Gynecol. 2017;130(3):648.
37. Shanmuganathan M, Sival DA, Eastwood KA, Morris K, Cartmill J, Heep A, et al. Prenatal surgery for spina bifida: a therapeutic dilemma. Proceedings of the SHINE conference, Belfast. Ir J Med Sci. 2017. https://doi.org/10.1007/s11845-017-1709-6.
38. Belfort MA. In reply. Obstet Gynecol. 2017;130(3):648.
39. Pedreira DA, Zanon N, de Sa RA, Acacio GL, Ogeda E, Belem TM, et al. Fetoscopic single-layer repair of open spina bifida using a cellulose patch: preliminary clinical experience. J Matern Fetal Neonatal Med. 2014;27(16):1613–9.
40. Pedreira DA, Zanon N, Nishikuni K, De Sa RA, Acacio GL, Chmait RH, et al. Endoscopic surgery for the antenatal treatment of myelomeningocele: the CECAM trial. Am J Obstet Gynecol. 2016;214(1):111.e1–111.e11.
41. Belfort MA, Whitehead WE, Shamshirsaz AA, Bateni ZH, Olutoye OO, Olutoye OA, et al. Fetoscopic open neural tube defect repair: development and refinement of a two-port, carbon dioxide insufflation technique. Obstet Gynecol. 2017;129(4):734–43.
42. Joyeux L, De Bie F, Danzer E, Van Mieghem T, Flake AW, Deprest J. Safety and efficacy of fetal surgery techniques to close a spina bifida defect in the fetal lamb model: a systematic review. Prenat Diagn. 2018;38(4):231–42. https://doi.org/10.1002/pd.5222.
43. Kabagambe SK, Jensen GW, Chen YJ, Vanover MA, Farmer DL. Fetal surgery for myelomeningocele: a systematic review and meta-analysis of outcomes in fetoscopic versus open repair. Fetal Diagn Ther. 2018;43(3):161–74. https://doi.org/10.1159/000479505. [Epub ahead of print].
44. Botelho RD, Imada V, Rodrigues da Costa KJ, Watanabe LC, Rossi Junior R, De Salles AAF, et al. Fetal Myelomeningocele repair through a mini-hysterotomy. Fetal Diagn Ther. 2017;42(1):28–34.

Laser Treatment of Twin-Twin Transfusion Syndrome

33

Rubén A. Quintero, Eftichia V. Kontopoulos, and Ramen H. Chmait

Introduction

The treatment of twin-twin transfusion syndrome (TTTS) has evolved through the years and has included expectant medical management [1], *sectio parva* [2], serial amniocenteses [3–5], and the current treatment using laser photocoagulation of the placental vascular anastomoses [6–11]. The rationale for the use of laser photocoagulation in TTTS stems from the fact that:

1. TTTS occurs via placental vascular anastomoses, which are responsible for the net imbalance sharing of blood volume between two (or more) fetuses.
2. As a corollary, TTTS does not occur in the absence of placental vascular anastomoses (e.g., dichorionic twins).
3. TTTS should resolve if all the placental vascular anastomoses are successfully ablated.

R. A. Quintero (✉) · E. V. Kontopoulos
The Fetal Institute, Miami, FL, USA

The USFetus Research Consortium, Miami, FL, USA
e-mail: quintero@usfetus.org

R. H. Chmait
The USFetus Research Consortium, Miami, FL, USA

Department of Obstetrics and Gynecology, Keck School of Medicine, University of Southern California, Los Angeles, CA, USA

Therefore, the goal of the laser surgery is to correctly identify and ablate all of the placental vascular anastomoses responsible for the syndrome. This raises two fundamental issues:

1. Can all of the placental vascular anastomoses be indeed identified?
2. Can all of the placental vascular anastomoses actually be ablated?

Step One: Identification of the Placental Vascular Anastomoses

Classic placental pathology studies have shown the presence of three different types of placental vascular anastomoses: arteriovenous (AV) (so-called deep anastomoses), arterio-arterial (A-A), and veno-venous (V-V) anastomoses (A-A and V-V are also called "superficial" anastomoses) [12]. All of the anastomoses can be seen on the surface of the placenta, even if the actual anastomotic exchange occurs deep within the substance of the placenta. While some authors have suggested that in fact there are anastomoses deep within the placental parenchyma that cannot be seen on the surface of the placenta [13], such arguments have proven untenable because in fact, based on clinical experience and placental pathological evaluation, all anastomoses can be seen on the placental surface. While in principle

C. H. Nezhat (ed.), *Non-Obstetric Surgery During Pregnancy*,
https://doi.org/10.1007/978-3-319-90752-9_33

all the placental vascular anastomoses are visible on the surface of the placenta, their endoscopic identification may be hindered by a variety of factors, including the fetuses themselves, the location or the angle of the endoscope relative to the anastomosis, and/or the amniotic fluid discoloration.

How can all the anastomoses be identified? In the early days of laser surgery, this was an issue of contention. The original reports suggested that the anastomoses could be identified based on their appearance, i.e., based on specific patterns and angles, with drawings intended to aid in this process (identification based on pattern recognition) [14]. Soon it became clear that a gestalt approach to the identification of the placental vascular anastomoses was both inaccurate and impractical, given the myriad of vascular patterns that the anastomoses can actually have. Furthermore, non-anastomotic vessels could be mistaken for an anastomosis using a pattern recognition approach. The lack of a practical and accurate way to identify placental vascular anastomoses was one of the most important hindrances in establishing laser surgery as a valid approach for the treatment of TTTS. This limitation led to the development of what we called "the nonselective technique."

The Nonselective Technique

The nonselective technique was based on lasering all of the vessels that would cross the dividing membrane. By definition, this technique did not attempt to differentiate anastomotic from non-anastomotic vessels but rather to catch as many anastomoses as possible based on three assumptions:

1. The dividing membrane should lie parallel to the vascular equator.
2. All vessels crossing the dividing membrane are vascular anastomoses.
3. The vascular anastomoses (vascular equator) are all within the sac of the recipient twin (where the endoscope is inserted).

Although these three assumptions could be true in many cases, they do not guarantee that only anastomotic vessels will be targeted. First, the location of the dividing membrane may or may not be parallel to the so-called vascular equator, the area of the placenta where the anastomoses are located. Indeed, the location of the dividing membrane relative to the fetal placental surface may be:

- At an angle to the vascular equator (such that some of the anastomoses may be in the sac of the donor twin and some in the sac of the recipient twin)
- Completely within the sac of the donor twin, such that all of the anastomoses are inside the sac of the donor twin

Second, and as a corollary, not all of the vessels crossing the dividing membrane are anastomotic vessels. Therefore, by lasering all of the vessels that would cross the dividing membrane, the risk of ablating normal vessels (i.e., non-anastomotic) could be high. Third, in the rare cases where all of the anastomoses are within the sac of the donor twin, lasering of all the vessels crossing the dividing membrane from within the sac of the recipient twin would aim only at recipient vessels (with or without anastomoses), with a high risk of demise for this fetus. The increased risk for harm to either twin from the use of a nonselective technique can be appreciated in the report by Ville et al. in 1995, where the use of the nonselective technique was associated with a dual fetal survival of only 35% and a rate of single intrauterine fetal demises of 35% as well [9]. Subsequent clinical studies showed that the use of a nonselective technique, which unnecessarily targeted non-anastomotic vessels, was associated with an increased risk for demise of one or both twins [9]. Clearly, using the dividing membrane as a surrogate for the identification of the placental vascular anastomoses was suboptimal, albeit an improvement over the previously nondescriptive reports. Thus, a better way of identifying the actual anastomoses was needed.

The Selective Technique

In 1998, Quintero et al. described the selective laser photocoagulation of communicating vessels technique (coined as "SLPCV") [10]. This was the first description of a precise anatomical method of identifying the placental vascular anastomoses endoscopically and differentiating them from non-anastomotic vessels. The technique required a systematic assessment of the vascular equator from one end of the placenta to the other. Basically, this meant following each vessel on the surface of the placenta to its terminal end. If the terminal end of the artery of one twin had a returning vein to the same fetus, this was labeled as a non-anastomotic pair. On the other hand, if the terminal end of an artery was followed by a vein returning to the other twin, this was identified labeled as an AV anastomosis. Arterio-arterial (A-A) anastomoses were apparent, since the artery of one twin would continue as an artery to the other twin as well. Similarly, veno-venous (V-V) anastomoses could be identified by following an uninterrupted vein from one twin to the other. The identification of the anastomoses using the SLPCV technique did not rely on the location of the dividing membrane relative to the vascular equator. This avoided missing anastomoses located in the sac of the donor twin, regardless of whether this involved a few or even all of the placental vascular anastomoses. Identification of the anastomoses within the sac of the donor by looking through the dividing membrane was also shown to be possible. This was in contrast to previous reports which had stated that anastomoses within the sac of the donor would not be visible due to the presence of two layers of amnion [14]. In fact, the two layers of amnion do not preclude visualization of anastomoses located within the sac of the donor twin, particularly if severe oligohydramnios or anhydramnios is present in the sac of that fetus. The selective technique provided a reproducible way of identifying all of the vascular anastomoses, independent of their location, a first step in the proper performance of the laser surgical technique. Quintero et al. also commented on how to document the identified vascular anastomoses. This included mentioning the type (AV, A-A, V-V), size (e.g., "hair," small, medium, large, extra-large), as well as their direction (AVDR, an AV anastomosis from donor to recipient, or AVRD, an AV anastomosis from recipient to donor) [15]. The direction of flow in A-A or V-V anastomoses could be determined in some cases, provided there was significant color differences in these vessels resulting from differences in fetal SpO_2 [16]. This led to the concept of the "hemodynamic equator" or HE, which represents the collision front between the two fetal circulations within an A-A or a V-V anastomosis [17]. The HE allowed for the first time a better understanding of the actual functional behavior of A-A or V-V anastomoses, which until then were thought to be bidirectional in all cases. Indeed, if the HE moves back and forth between draining vessels of either twin, the behavior of the A-A or V-V anastomosis is truly bidirectional. On the other hand, if the HE only reaches a draining vessel of one twin, the function of such superficial vessel is essentially no different than an AV anastomosis (and as such, labeled as fAVDR if from donor to recipient, or fAVRD if from recipient to donor). Lastly, if the HE does not reach any draining vessel, the net exchange of blood between the fetuses through that vessel is zero.

The selective technique also assumed that once the vascular equator was entirely mapped, the anastomoses could all be photocoagulated (a two-step process).

The acronym used for the selective technique, i.e., SLPCV, defined the systematic approach that needs to take place to identify and photocoagulate all of the vascular anastomoses. Other acronyms used to describe the performance of the laser surgery may or may not be similar to the Quintero SLPCV technique. For example, while performing SLPCV, the dividing membrane is always respected. Purposeful injury to the dividing membrane, or the so-called septostomy, is not part of the SLPCV technique [18]. Though not implicit, the performance of a laparotomy to access the amniotic cavity is also not part of the SLPCV technique. While general anesthesia was originally used in our cases [19], surgery can be best performed under local anesthesia [20]. Therefore, the acronym SLPCV should apply only to those surgeries in which access to the amniotic cavity is performed under local anesthesia, percutaneously and following a systematic and thorough identification and obliteration only of placental vascular anastomoses [10, 21, 22].

Lasering Healthy Interanastomotic Placental Tissue: The "Solomon" Technique

As centers began to adopt the selective technique, it became apparent that the rate of residual patent placental vascular anastomoses after laser surgery (as shown on surgical pathology of the placenta) varied significantly between centers (Table 33.1). Similarly, the incidence of failed surgery, defined as persistent or reverse TTTS, which is the clinical manifestation of residual patent placental vascular anastomoses after laser surgery, also varied significantly (Table 33.2). In a study by Robyr et al., the rate of failed surgery was 22% [28]. Anemia of a surviving twin after demise of the co-twin, which is reflective of incomplete occlusion of all placental vascular anastomoses, was also noted as a common complication. Lopriore et al. reported an incidence of 33% of residual patent placental vascular anastomoses in 52 TTTS patients treated with laser at their institution [29]. In comparison, the rate of residual patent placental vascular anastomoses after SLPCV by our groups, using a similar technique and similar technology, has consistently been less than 5%, with no anemia after demise of the co-twin, and an incidence of reverse or persistent TTTS of only 1–1.5% (USFetus Consortium) [33] (see Tables 33.1 and 33.2).

In view of the relatively high incidence of residual patent placental vascular anastomoses seen by some groups, some authors proposed "connecting the dots" between photocoagulated areas on the surface of the placenta [34]. The premise behind this idea was that, by lasering areas between laser-ablated placental vascular anastomoses, such "blind lasering" would capture "anastomoses" that would have been presumably missed ("not visible") [13]. The argument was based on the assumption by such authors that not all of the placental vascular anastomoses can be identified endoscopically [13] and that, therefore, ablating only the visible ones using the selective technique could miss vascular

Table 33.2 Reported incidence of clinical outcomes after laser therapy reflecting residual patent placental vascular anastomoses

Author	Reverse or persistent TTTS	*p*
Chmait [24]	1/100 (1%)	–
Kontopoulos [27]	5/417 (1.5%)	1.0
Robyr [28]	14/101 (13.8%)	0.0006
Lopriore [29]	2/52 (3.8%)	0.27
Slaghekke [30]		
"Standard"	9/135 (6.7%)	0.046
Solomon	2/137 (1.5%)	1.0
Baschat [31]		
"Selective"	6/71 (8.5%)	0.02
Solomon	3/76 (3.9%)	0.31
Ruano [32]		
"Selective"	4/76 (5.3%)	0.17
Solomon	0/26 (0%)	1

Comparisons made relative to the lowest reported rate

Table 33.1 Reported incidence of residual patent placental vascular anastomoses after laser surgery on surgical pathology analysis of the placentas

Author	Residual patent placental vascular anastomoses	P1	P2
Quintero (SLPCV) [23]	5/143 (3.5%)	–	
Chmait (SLPCV) [24]	5/100 (5%)	0.74	
Lopriore ("fetoscopic laser surgery") [25]	17/52 (33%)	<0.001	
Slaghekke [26]			
"Standard"	26/77 (34%)	<0.001	>0.05
Solomon	14/74 (19%)	<0.001	

Comparisons made relative to the lowest reported rate (P1) or between the "standard" and the Solomon techniques (P2)

anastomoses. This would explain their high rate of residual patent placental vascular anastomoses. The resulting surgical technique of lasering healthy interanastomotic areas of the placenta was dubbed "the Solomon technique" [30] in reference to the biblical passage where, in order to resolve a dispute between two alleging mothers of a child, King Solomon proposed to cut the baby in half (1 Kings 3:16–28, NIV). The analogy, therefore, is that by lasering the areas of the placenta between endoscopically identified and laser-ablated vascular anastomoses, the placenta would be "cut in half." Recent studies suggest that indeed, relative to the surgical groups' prior experience with the selective technique, the use of the Solomon technique was associated with improved perinatal outcomes [31, 32].

To test whether the Solomon technique could indeed reduce the rate of residual patent placental vascular anastomoses, an open-label randomized clinical trial was conducted in Europe (the Solomon trial) comparing the Solomon technique versus the "standard" technique [30]. The latter, although not directly mentioned, was intended to refer to the selective technique (SLPCV). The primary outcome was a composite of the rate of twin anemia polycythemia sequence (TAPS), recurrence of TTTS, perinatal mortality, or severe neonatal morbidity. No statistical differences were detected in the composite outcome between the two groups. However, the study did show a decreased rate of persistent or reverse TTTS (2/137, 1% vs. 9/135, 7%, Solomon vs. "standard," respectively, $p = 0.03$) and of TAPS (4/137, 2.9% vs. 21/135, 15.5%, Solomon vs. "standard," respectively, $p \leq 0.001$). Interestingly, the actual rate of persistent residual patent placental vascular anastomoses was no different between the two techniques (14/74, 19% vs. 23/77, 29.8%, Solomon vs. "standard," respectively, $p = 0.12$). Although the primary outcome of the study was no different between the groups, the authors concluded that the Solomon technique was superior to the "standard" technique. Two additional observational studies comparing the Solomon technique with the selective technique also appeared to show favorable results with the former technique [31, 32].

Table 33.1 shows the rate of residual patent placental vascular anastomoses reported by the different groups using either the Quintero selective (SLPCV) technique (i.e., the "standard" approach) or the Solomon technique. As can be seen, the rate of residual patent placental vascular anastomoses is lowest using the Quintero SLPCV. Table 33.2 shows that the Quintero SLPCV technique is also associated with a lower rate of persistent or reverse TTTS than that of the "standard" technique in the Solomon trial and the "selective technique" of other authors and that the Solomon technique in all studies achieves the same rate of persistent or reverse TTTS than that reported with the Quintero SLPCV technique. Given that the Solomon technique is still associated with approximately 20% of residual patent placental vascular anastomoses, the initial rationale for the technique, i.e., to reduce the high rate of residual patent placental vascular anastomoses, does not appear to hold. Furthermore, given that the proponents of the Solomon technique have also shown that most missed anastomoses are located in the margins of the placenta [29], lasering inexistent placental vascular anastomoses in otherwise healthy placental tissue between vascular anastomoses within the main body of the placenta is incongruent with the rationale (Table 33.3) (Fig. 33.1a, b). Altogether, the Solomon technique would seem to represent a backward step in the ability to correctly identify all of the placental vascular anastomoses, by accepting the unproven theory of the presence of non-visible placental vascular anastomoses on otherwise healthy-appearing fetal surface of the placenta. Alternatively, we have shown that *all* of the placental vascular anastomoses can be clearly identified without having to ablate inexistent anastomoses in healthy placental areas. Stated differently, the use of the "Solomon technique" may simply represent an attempt to achieve similar results as those that can be obtained with the performance of the Quintero SLPCV technique, rather than a true advantage over the SLPCV technique, at the expense of lasering healthy placental tissue.

Table 33.3 Principles and results of the use of the Solomon technique to identify and ablate all placental vascular anastomoses in twin-twin transfusion syndrome

Purpose of the surgery	Purported location of the residual patent placental vascular anastomoses	Actual location of the additional laser ablations	Rate of residual patent placental vascular anastomoses [30]	Rate of residual patent placental vascular anastomoses (USFetus group) [23, 24]
To decrease the rate of residual patent placental vascular anastomoses after laser therapy	Mostly on the margins of the placenta	Within the body of the placenta, between endoscopically identified vascular anastomoses	30% ("standard") vs. 19% (Solomon) $p > 0.05$	5% $p < 0.05$ relative to Solomon technique

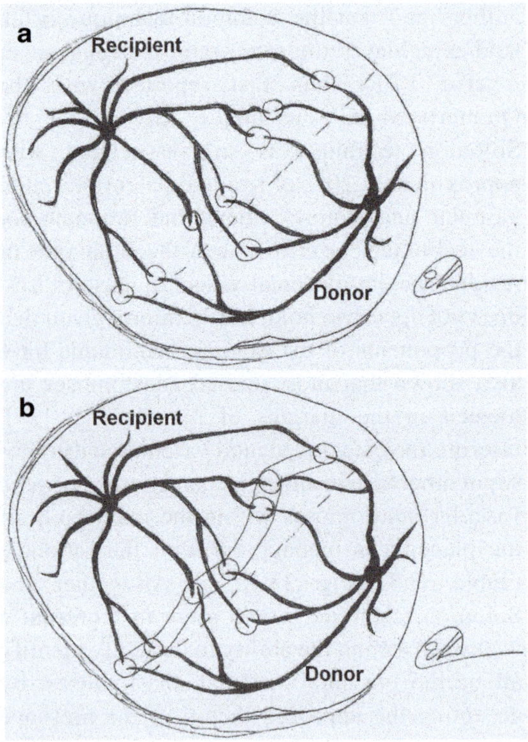

Fig. 33.1 (**a**) Selective photocoagulation of communicating vessels (SLPCV). All of the anastomoses are photocoagulated, regardless of their location relative to the dividing membrane while sparing non-anastomotic vessels. Rate of residual patent placental vascular anastomoses, 3.5–5% [24, 27]. (**b**) Solomon modification of the SLPCV technique. The fetal surface of the placenta between endoscopically identified anastomoses is also lasered, to occlude "anastomoses" not visible by the endoscope. Rate of residual patent vascular anastomoses, 20% [30]

Step Two: Ablation of the Placental Vascular Anastomoses

Assuming that there is a conceptual agreement on how to identify the anastomoses, the next step consists of being able to ablate them. Successful ablation of the placental vascular anastomoses assumes that the surgeon can adapt to the different clinical scenarios and overcome the various challenges that may be present in each case. Particular known surgical challenges include:

- The location of the placenta (anterior, posterior)
- Interference with the visualization of the anastomoses by the donor twin that is "stuck" along the vascular equator from severe oligohydramnios (unmovable donor)
- The presence of discolored fluid within the sac of the recipient twin from prior procedures (amniocenteses) or from prior intra-amniotic bleeding
- Triplet (or higher order multiple) gestations, whether monochorionic or not
- Close proximity of the umbilical cord placental insertions
- Large anastomotic vessels
- Tangential access to the placenta (whether the placenta is anterior or posterior)
- Anastomoses located behind the site of trocar entry
- High maternal BMI

The management of each of these challenges requires the use of special techniques or technology, including the use of fluid management systems, blunt probes, trocar assistance [23], and special laser photocoagulation techniques, which are beyond the scope of this article [35]. A recent Delphi study outlined the multitude of steps needed to perform the surgery. Most authors agreed on the basic surgical goal (the purpose of the Delphi survey), including the ablation of all of the placental vascular anastomoses along the vascular equator, without injuring healthy placenta or non-anastomotic vessels [36]. The question is: how often can these goals be accomplished while overcoming the various challenges mentioned above? One way to address this question is by noting both how often the placenta can be adequately assessed as well as how often can the vessels be selectively ablated.

Adequate Placental Assessment

Adequate placental assessment refers to the ability of the surgeon to survey the entire vascular equator. For example, in a sub-analysis of the Solomon trial, the authors reported that they were able to adequately assess the placenta in only 65 out of 74 patients in the Solomon group (87%) and in only 69 out of 77 (89%) in the "standard" group [37]. The reasons behind the inability of the surgeons to adequately assess the placenta in more than 10% of the cases in each group were not stated. Obviously, if the placenta cannot be adequately assessed, this is likely to result in missed anastomoses and thus an increased likelihood for adverse clinical outcomes, including persistent or reverse TTTS. In contrast, our group has shown consistently the ability to assess the placenta adequately in over 99% of the patients [38].

Selective Ablation of the Anastomoses

Another surgical competency benchmark refers to the ability of the surgeon to selectively ablate the vascular anastomoses without including non-anastomotic vessels. A "selectivity index" (SI) was proposed by Stirnemann et al., as SI = log (SC + 1)/(NSC + 1), where SC are the selectively coagulated vessels and NSC are the non-anastomotic vessels. NSC were also vessels that were considered presumed anastomoses but that could not be followed to their terminal end and were nonetheless lasered. In their experience, most surgeries involved lasering both anastomotic and non-anastomotic vessels [34, 39]. A "high" SI defined as −0.25 was reported by the authors to correlate with improved postnatal survival at 28 days of at least one twin and both twins. Crisan et al. have shown that the selectivity index proposed by Stirnemann et al. is mathematically inaccurate and should not be used to assess the adequacy of the laser surgery [38]. Instead, a simpler index consisting of a ratio between how often the surgery can be done using the Quintero selective technique vs. nonselectively is more representative and easier to understand: $\left(\mathrm{QSI} = 100 * \frac{\mathrm{SLPCV} - \mathrm{NSLPCV}}{\mathrm{SLPCV}}\right)$, where QSI is the Quintero selectivity index, SLPCV is a surgery performed selectively, and NSLPCV is a surgery where at least one vessel was not clearly identified as an anastomosis but was lasered. For example, in that same article, the authors showed that they were able to perform a selective surgery in only 34% of cases [39]. In another report of 123 patients, surgery could not be completed in five cases for a stuck twin obscuring the equator (2), poor visualization (2), and a large anastomotic vessel (1) [29]. Obviously, the goal is to try to perform the surgery selectively as close to 100% of the time as possible [22, 27, 38].

Accuracy of Laser Therapy

Theoretically, one could combine the rate of adequate placental assessment and of selective laser surgery with the rate of either residual patent placental vascular anastomoses (when available) and the rate of persistent or reverse TTTS to determine how accurate the laser surgery is being performed at a given center or by a given

Table 33.4 Accuracy of laser surgery for twin-twin transfusion syndrome (TTTS)

Author	Rate of selectively performed surgeries (%)	1—Rate of residual patent placental vascular anastomoses	1—Rate of persistent/reverse TTTS	Accuracy of SLPCV (%)
USFetus group [27, 38]	98.7	0.95	0.99	92
Solomon [30]	87	0.81	0.99	69.7
Solomon [30] "standard"	89	0.66	0.93	54

surgeon. Accuracy of SLPCV could thus be defined as:

$$\text{AccSLPCV} = \text{QSI} * (1 - \text{RPPVA}) * (1 - \text{PRTTTS})$$

where AccSLPCV is the accuracy in performing SLPCV, QSI is the rate of Quintero selectively performed surgeries, RPPVA is the rate of residual patent placental vascular anastomoses (when available), and PRTTTS is the rate of persistent or reverse TTTS. Table 33.4 shows such a theoretical calculation and its use to compare different reports.

Should the Rate of Twin-Anemia-Polycythemia Sequence (TAPS) Be Included as a Benchmark for the Performance of Laser Therapy in TTTS?

The rate of twin-anemia-polycythemia sequence (TAPS) has been included as a measure of failed laser therapy for TTTS, in addition to the rate of residual patent placental vascular anastomoses and persistent/reverse TTTS [24, 30–32, 37]. The decision stems from the purported etiology of TAPS, which presumably results from the transfer of blood between two monochorionic twins through small placental vascular anastomoses in such a way that one fetus develops anemia and the other twin develops polycythemia, but without the net blood volume inequalities typical of TTTS [25]. Presumably, the syndrome occurs through small caliber AV anastomoses, in contrast to larger size vessels typically seen in TTTS. In actuality, such a theory is even less plausible than the contested theory of TTTS (in which all indirect and circumstantial evidence does point to placental vascular anastomoses as being the etiological factor for TTTS and indirectly confirmed by resolution of the syndrome with occlusion of all placental vascular anastomoses). The proposed theory of TAPS is thus suspect for many reasons:

Table 33.5 Role of placental vascular anastomoses in the etiology of twin-twin transfusion syndrome (TTTS) and twin-anemia-polycythemia sequence (TAPS)

	TTTS	TAPS
Can exist in the presence of placental vascular anastomoses	Yes	Yes
Can exist in the absence of placental vascular anastomoses	No	Yes [27, 40]
Is eliminated by ablating the placental vascular anastomoses	Yes	Yes? [26]

- The original theory was based on the presence of residual patent placental vascular anastomoses. Given the high incidence of residual patent placental vascular anastomoses reported from such groups (20–33%), it is not possible to discern what role, if any, these anastomoses play in the etiology of TAPS.
- While TAPS has been described in the presence of residual patent placental vascular anastomoses, they are not indispensable. We and others have recently reported on the presence of TAPS without apparent placental vascular anastomoses [27, 40].
- Contrary to TTTS, ablation of residual patent placental anastomoses in cases of TAPS may not necessarily eliminate the condition in all cases. Table 33.5 compares TTTS with TAPS

relative to the role of placental vascular anastomoses.

- Depending on the order the vascular communications are ablated, there may be preferential intraoperative transfusion from one twin to another twin. Thus, the findings of anemia in one twin and polycythemia of the other in the postoperative period may be a reflection of the surgical procedure itself. See the sequential technique section below for further details of this phenomenon.

Therefore, the assumption that TAPS is only the result of unsuccessful laser therapy may not be entirely accurate. Thus, in our opinion, the inclusion of TAPS as a benchmark of failed laser therapy should be used with caution.

Functional Ablation of the Placental Vascular Anastomoses: The Sequential Technique

The development of the selective technique represented an important historical step in the surgical treatment of twin-twin transfusion syndrome. SLPCV is indeed an anatomical surgical technique, which involves the identification and selective laser obliteration of the placental vascular anastomoses, while preserving non-anastomotic vessels and healthy placental tissue. However, despite precise identification and ablation of placental vascular anastomoses, intrauterine fetal demise of one of the fetuses after SLPCV would still occur in approximately 9–29% of cases with this technique [10, 41]. A potential explanation for this complication could lie in the sequence with which the anastomoses were obliterated during surgery. Indeed, since TTTS occurs from an excessive transfer of blood from the donor twin to the recipient twin, ablation of the anastomoses from the donor to the recipient first would stop immediately the transfer of blood from this twin to the recipient twin. Furthermore, during this interval, however brief, the recipient twin would be transfusing the donor twin back through placental vascular anastomoses from recipient to donor. As a result, the donor twin, which is presumed hypotensive, would stop losing blood as soon as the laser process started while at the same time receive an intraoperative transfusion from the recipient twin. The photocoagulation of the vascular anastomoses from donor to recipient first followed by from recipient to donor second was called the "sequential technique" or SQLPCV. Using the sequential technique, our group showed a reduction in the rate of intrauterine fetal demise of the donor twin from 21% to 7% and an increase in the double survival rate from 56% to 75% [42]. Our group is currently assessing the merits of performing the sequential technique through a randomized clinical trial of the USFetus group [43]. While a sequential technique may not necessarily be required in all cases, it could have an indication in patients where the condition of the donor twin would be most compromised.

Is There a Role for Umbilical Cord Occlusion in TTTS?

Interruption of the blood exchange between the fetuses can also be accomplished by occluding one of the two umbilical cords. This procedure should be contemplated only as a last resort to treat the syndrome. Unfortunately, the availability of bipolar photocoagulation and radiofrequency ablation has resulted in an unwarranted high number of selective feticide in many centers on patients that otherwise could have perhaps been treated best with laser surgery [34, 44]. Umbilical cord occlusion should not be offered as an alternative to laser because of limitations of the surgeon or the center, unless the patient cannot be referred to another center capable of offering laser. Umbilical cord occlusion should be offered to patients with twin-twin transfusion syndrome in which additional complicating circumstances may exist. This may be the case of patients with a severe congenital anomaly of one of the twins or a moribund hydropic fetus. Since such cases are rare, the performance of selective feticide via umbilical cord occlusion in twin-twin transfusion syndrome should be an exception, rather than the rule. Indeed, the counseling of our patients involves mentioning a survival rate of approximately 90% with a 5% risk of neurological damage if laser therapy is chosen, compared to 90% survival and a 5% risk of neurological damage to the surviving co-twin if umbilical cord occlusion is chosen. Therefore, since both survival and morbidity statistics are similar between the two procedures, but with umbilical cord occlusion one of the fetuses is denied the chance to survive, the justification is not there to offer feticide to an otherwise anatomically normal fetus.

Conclusion

It's been more than 20 years since laser therapy was first proposed for the treatment of twin-twin transfusion syndrome. Significant strides have been made both in establishing the scientific merit of using laser to ablate the placental vascular anastomoses to treat the condition [45] as well as in the various steps, techniques, and other technical aspects that allow for such therapy. Selectively interrupting the placental vascular anastomoses without injuring healthy portions of the placenta using the Quintero selective technique, while obvious as a concept and as a surgical goal, has been associated with markedly different outcome results between centers. The Solomon technique has been proposed as a way to mitigate such differences, but has not shown to lower the high rate of residual patent placental vascular anastomoses that prompted its development. A properly performed Quintero SLPCV technique is associated with the highest rate of clinical success and with the lowest rate of failed therapy either by surgical pathology or clinical criteria. Further improvements in clinical outcomes with the use of the sequential technique, particularly for specific situations in which the donor may be at a unique disadvantage, could be expected and is being addressed in the ongoing randomized clinical trial conducted by our groups comparing SLPCV with SQLPCV. Selective feticide via umbilical cord occlusion should be the exception rather than the rule for severe cases of TTTS, and should not be performed to compensate for physician or surgical center limitations. Improvements in the surgical equipment and other ancillary technology, while difficult to pursue, should continue to remain among the objectives of caregivers in this field. The education of next-generation surgeons using the wealth of information thus far gathered by the different centers should also be a main focus of all programs.

References

1. Jones J, Sbarra A, Dilillo L, Cetrulo CL, D'Alton ME. Indomethacin in severe twin-to-twin transfusion syndrome. Am J Perinatol. 1993;10:24.
2. Urig MA, Simpson GF, Elliott JP, Clewell WH. Twin-twin transfusion syndrome: the surgical removal of one twin as a treatment option. Fetal Ther. 1988;3(4):185–8.
3. Wax JR, Blakemore KJ, Blohm P, Callan NA. Stuck twin with cotwin nonimmune hydrops: successful treatment by amniocentesis. Fetal Diagn Ther. 1991;6(3–4):126–31.
4. Saunders NJ, Snijders RJ, Nicolaides KH. Therapeutic amniocentesis in twin-twin transfusion syndrome appearing in the second trimester of pregnancy. Am J Obstet Gynecol. 1992;166(3):820–4.
5. Dennis LG, Winkler CL. Twin-to-twin transfusion syndrome: aggressive therapeutic amniocentesis. Am J Obstet Gynecol. 1997;177(2):342–7. discussion 7–9.
6. De Lia JE, Cruikshank DP, Keye WR Jr. Fetoscopic neodymium:YAG laser occlusion of placental vessels in severe twin-twin transfusion syndrome. Obstet Gynecol. 1990;75(6):1046–53.
7. Ville Y, Hecher K, Ogg D, Warren R, Nicolaides K. Successful outcome after Nd:YAG laser separation of chorioangiopagus-twins under sonoendoscopic control. Ultrasound Obstet Gynecol. 1992;2(6):429–31.
8. De Lia JE, Kuhlmann RS, Harstad TW, Cruikshank DP. Fetoscopic laser ablation of placental vessels in severe previable twin-twin transfusion syndrome. Am J Obstet Gynecol. 1995;172(4 Pt 1):1202–8. discussion 8–11.
9. Ville Y, Hyett J, Hecher K, Nicolaides K. Preliminary experience with endoscopic laser surgery for severe twin-twin transfusion syndrome. N Engl J Med. 1995;332:224–7.
10. Quintero R, Morales W, Mendoza G, Allen M, Kalter C, Giannina G, et al. Selective photocoagulation of placental vessels in twin-twin transfusion syndrome: evolution of a surgical technique. Obstet Gynecol Surv. 1998;53(12):s97–s103.
11. Hecher K, Diehl W, Zikulnig L, Vetter M, Hackeloer BJ. Endoscopic laser coagulation of placental

anastomoses in 200 pregnancies with severe mid-trimester twin-to-twin transfusion syndrome. Eur J Obstet Gynecol Reprod Biol. 2000;92(1):135–9.
12. Benirschke K, Kaufmann P. Pathology of human placenta. New York: Springer-Verlag; 1995. p. 719–827.
13. Lewi L, Jani J, Cannie M, Robyr R, Ville Y, Hecher K, et al. Intertwin anastomoses in monochorionic placentas after fetoscopic laser coagulation for twin-to-twin transfusion syndrome: is there more than meets the eye? Am J Obstet Gynecol. 2006;194(3):790–5.
14. De Lia J, Kuhlmann R, Cruikshank D, O'Bee LR. Current topic: placental surgery: a new frontier. Placenta. 1993;14:477.
15. Quintero R, Quintero L, Pivatelli A, Bornick P, Allen M, Johnson P. The donor-recipient (D-R) score: *in vivo* endoscopic evidence to support the hypothesis of a net transfer of blood from donor to recipient in twin-twin transfusion syndrome. Prenat Neonat Med. 2000;5:84–91.
16. Quintero RA, Chmait RH, Carver J, Bornick PW, Allen MH, Kontopoulos EV. In utero fetal oximetry via visible light spectroscopy in twin-twin transfusion syndrome. Am J Obstet Gynecol. 2008;199(6):639.e1–4.
17. Chang YL, Chmait RH, Bornick PW, Allen MH, Quintero RA. The role of laser surgery in dissecting the etiology of absent or reverse end-diastolic velocity in the umbilical artery of the donor twin in twin-twin transfusion syndrome. Am J Obstet Gynecol. 2006;195(2):478–83.
18. Harkness UF, Crombleholme TM. Twin-twin transfusion syndrome: where do we go from here? Semin Perinatol. 2005;29(5):296–304.
19. Rossi AC, Kaufman MA, Bornick PW, Quintero RA. General vs local anesthesia for the percutaneous laser treatment of twin-twin transfusion syndrome. Am J Obstet Gynecol. 2008;199(2):137.e1–7.
20. Ville Y, Hecher K, Gagnon A, Sebire N, Hyett J, Nicolaides K. Endoscopic laser coagulation in the management of severe twin-to-twin transfusion syndrome. Br J Obstet Gynaecol. 1998;105(4):446–53.
21. Quintero R. Selective laser photocoagulation of communicating vessels in twin-twin transfusion syndrome. In: Quintero R, editor. Diagnostic and operative fetoscopy. New York: The Parthenon Publishing Group; 2002. p. 43–54.
22. Chmait RH, Kontopoulos EV, Korst LM, Llanes A, Petisco I, Quintero RA. Stage-based outcomes of 682 consecutive cases of twin-twin transfusion syndrome treated with laser surgery: the USFetus experience. Am J Obstet Gynecol. 2011;204(5):393.e1–6.
23. Quintero RA, Chmait RH, Bornick PW, Kontopoulos EV. Trocar-assisted selective laser photocoagulation of communicating vessels: a technique for the laser treatment of patients with twin-twin transfusion syndrome with inaccessible anterior placentas. J Matern Fetal Neonatal Med. 2010;23(4):330–4.
24. Chmait RH, Assaf SA, Benirschke K. Residual vascular communications in twin-twin transfusion syndrome treated with sequential laser surgery: frequency and clinical implications. Placenta. 2010;31(7):611–4.
25. Lopriore E, Middeldorp JM, Oepkes D, Kanhai HH, Walther FJ, Vandenbussche FP. Twin anemia-polycythemia sequence in two monochorionic twin pairs without oligo-polyhydramnios sequence. Placenta. 2007;28(1):47–51.
26. Slaghekke F, Favre R, Peeters SH, Middeldorp JM, Weingertner AS, van Zwet EW, et al. Laser surgery as a management option for twin anemia-polycythemia sequence. Ultrasound Obstet Gynecol. 2014;44(3):304–10.
27. Kontopoulos E, Chmait R, Baker B, Llanes A, Quintero R. USFetus surgical benchmarks of selective laser therapy for twin-twin transfusion syndrome. Am J Obstet Gynecol. 2015;212(1):S91–2.
28. Robyr R, Lewi L, Salomon LJ, Yamamoto M, Bernard JP, Deprest J, et al. Prevalence and management of late fetal complications following successful selective laser coagulation of chorionic plate anastomoses in twin-to-twin transfusion syndrome. Am J Obstet Gynecol. 2006;194(3):796–803.
29. Lopriore E, Middeldorp JM, Oepkes D, Klumper FJ, Walther FJ, Vandenbussche FP. Residual anastomoses after fetoscopic laser surgery in twin-to-twin transfusion syndrome: frequency, associated risks and outcome. Placenta. 2007;28(2–3):204–8.
30. Slaghekke F, Lopriore E, Lewi L, Middeldorp JM, van Zwet EW, Weingertner AS, et al. Fetoscopic laser coagulation of the vascular equator versus selective coagulation for twin-to-twin transfusion syndrome: an open-label randomised controlled trial. Lancet. 2014;383(9935):2144–51.
31. Baschat AA, Barber J, Pedersen N, Turan OM, Harman CR. Outcome after fetoscopic selective laser ablation of placental anastomoses vs equatorial laser dichorionization for the treatment of twin-to-twin transfusion syndrome. Am J Obstet Gynecol. 2013;209(3):234.e1–8.
32. Ruano R, Rodo C, Peiro JL, Shamshirsaz A, Haeri S, Nomura ML, et al. Fetoscopic laser ablation of the placental anastomoses in twin-twin transfusion syndrome using the "Solomon technique". Ultrasound Obstet Gynecol. 2013;42(4):434–9.
33. Quintero RA. Twin-twin transfusion syndrome. London: InformaHealth; 2007.
34. Chalouhi GE, Essaoui M, Stirnemann J, Quibel T, Deloison B, Salomon L, et al. Laser therapy for twin-to-twin transfusion syndrome (TTTS). Prenat Diagn. 2011;31(7):637–46.
35. Quintero R. Laser treatment for twin-twin transfusion syndrome. In: Quintero R, editor. Twin-twin transfusion syndrome. London: InformaHealth; 2007.
36. Peeters SH, Akkermans J, Westra M, Lopriore E, Middeldorp JM, Klumper FJ, et al. Identification of essential steps in laser procedure for twin-twin transfusion syndrome using the Delphi methodology: SILICONE study. Ultrasound Obstet Gynecol. 2015;45(4):439–46.

37. Slaghekke F, Lewi L, Middeldorp JM, Weingertner AS, Klumper FJ, Dekoninck P, et al. Residual anastomoses in twin-twin transfusion syndrome after laser: the Solomon randomized trial. Am J Obstet Gynecol. 2014 Sep;211(3):285.e1–7.
38. Crisan LS, Kontopoulos EV, Quintero RA. Appraisal of the selectivity index in a cohort of patients treated with laser surgery for twin-twin transfusion syndrome. Am J Obstet Gynecol. 2010;202(2):157.e1–5.
39. Stirnemann JJ, Nasr B, Quarello E, Ortqvist L, Nassar M, Bernard JP, et al. A definition of selectivity in laser coagulation of chorionic plate anastomoses in twin-to-twin transfusion syndrome and its relationship to perinatal outcome. Am J Obstet Gynecol. 2008;198(1):62.e1–6.
40. Taniguchi K, Sumie M, Sugibayashi R, Wada S, Matsuoka K, Sago H. Twin anemia-polycythemia sequence after laser surgery for twin-twin transfusion syndrome and maternal morbidity. Fetal Diagn Ther. 2015;37(2):148–53.
41. Quintero RA, Comas C, Bornick PW, Allen MH, Kruger M. Selective versus non-selective laser photocoagulation of placental vessels in twin-twin transfusion syndrome. Ultrasound Obstet Gynecol. 2000;16(3):230–6.
42. Quintero RA, Ishii K, Chmait RH, Bornick PW, Allen MH, Kontopoulos EV. Sequential selective laser photocoagulation of communicating vessels in twin-twin transfusion syndrome. J Matern Fetal Neonatal Med. 2007;20(10):763–8.
43. Chmait RH, Kontopoulos EV, Quintero RA. Sequential laser surgery for twin-twin transfusion syndrome. Am J Perinatol. 2014;31(Suppl 1):S13–8.
44. Chalouhi GE, Stirnemann JJ, Salomon LJ, Essaoui M, Quibel T, Ville Y. Specific complications of monochorionic twin pregnancies: twin-twin transfusion syndrome and twin reversed arterial perfusion sequence. Semin Fetal Neonatal Med. 2010;15(6):349–56.
45. Senat MV, Deprest J, Boulvain M, Paupe A, Winer N, Ville Y. Endoscopic laser surgery versus serial amnioreduction for severe twin-to-twin transfusion syndrome. N Engl J Med. 2004;351(2):136–44.

Index

C. H. Nezhat (ed.), *Non-Obstetric Surgery During Pregnancy*,
https://doi.org/10.1007/978-3-319-90752-9

D

M

P

V

The manufacturer's authorised representative in the EU is Springer Nature Customer Service Centre GmbH, Europaplatz 3, 69115 Heidelberg, Germany. If you have any concerns regarding our products, please contact ProductSafety@springernature.com

Printed and bound by CPI Group (UK) Ltd, Croydon, CR0 4YY
02/10/2026
02227391-0001